PAIN

clinical and experimental perspectives

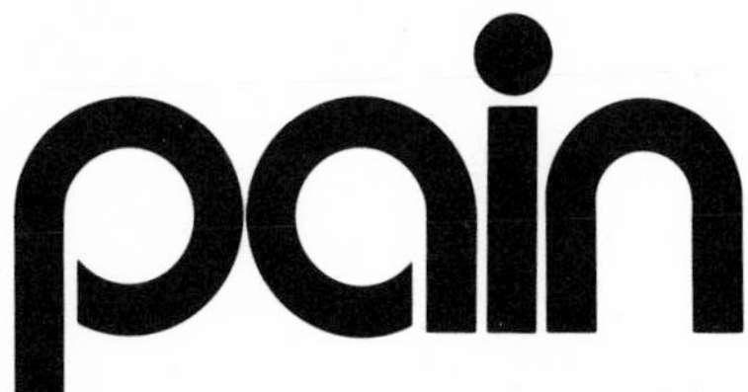

clinical and experimental perspectives

EDITED BY

Matisyohu Weisenberg, Ph.D.

Assistant Professor, Department of Behavioral Sciences
and Community Health, The University of Connecticut Health Center,
Farmington, Connecticut

WITH 86 ILLUSTRATIONS

The C. V. Mosby Company

SAINT LOUIS **1975**

Printed in the United States of America

Distributed in Great Britain by Henry Kimpton, London

Library of Congress Cataloging in Publication Data

Weisenberg, Matisyohu, 1936-
Pain.

Bibliography: p.
Includes index.
1. Pain. 2. Analgesics. I. Title. [DNLM:
1. Pain. WL700 W427p]
RB127.W44 616.07'2 74-28276
ISBN 0-8016-5387-8

C/M/M 9 8 7 6 5 4 3 2 1

Preface

Pain is one of the most dramatic, complex, and universal phenomena. Adequate definitions of it are hard to state. To the person experiencing pain it signifies a hurt, physical damage, impending danger, fear, anxiety, punishment, and love or loss of it. It can also be a means for communicating to others, a reason for obtaining or avoiding treatment, a means of judging how good the treatment is, or any combination of the above. To the professional it is an important area of research in psychology, sociology, anthropology, psychiatry, physiology, neurology, pharmacology, and anesthesiology. It is also a major reason for the dispensing of clinical treatment by health practitioners over a wide range of specialties.

Researchers and clinicians alike are aware of the complexity of factors that influence the pain reaction. They are aware of the differences between laboratory and clinical pathological pain. Whereas in the laboratory it is possible to achieve more accurate measurement of stimulus and response parameters, the circumstances may be considered artificial, lacking the intensity, fear, and anxiety concerning impending death or disfigurement that is found in clinical pathological pain. In the clinic there is less control of both the stimulus and the response. Objective measurement becomes difficult and clinical acumen must be relied on. If there is one point of agreement, it is that no single discipline has the answer. Each field can contribute to the developing pool of information. There has thus become an increasing interest in teaching comprehensive, multidisciplinary courses on pain in schools of dentistry, medicine, and nursing. However, teaching and research material is scattered throughout the many journals in a dozen different fields. Hence, the purpose of this book is to assemble, in one place, selected samples from the voluminous literature dealing with pain.

In most cases the articles selected present data based on research. In a few cases articles without data beyond the single case history were included when they illustrated an important point.

The book contains eight major groups of readings and an annotated bibliography on pain. Preceding each major section there are comments by me regarding some of the basic concepts and issues covered in the selected readings.

In almost every section selections were made of both experimental and clinical studies in the area. Readings were chosen to present both a general and a detailed view of pain from the perspective of different research and clinical disciplines. Illustrations of pain reactions and their correlates were also selected from several different types of diseases commonly associated with pain.

From an experimental view the emphasis has been on the measurement of pain, its correlates, and the variables that have been used to manipulate the pain reaction. From a clinical view the emphasis has been on measurement, surgery, and clinical techniques independent of drugs for the relief of pain.

It is hoped that this collection of readings can provide researchers with new insights, stimulate clinicians to new treatment approaches, and perhaps thereby lessen human suffering somewhat.

I would like to thank Nancy A. Stilwell for her assistance in preparing this book. Appreciation is also expressed to my secretaries, Sharon Siton and Marilyn Glenn, for their typing and assembling of the manuscript.

MATISYOHU WEISENBERG

Contents

SECTION EIGHT

Pain control associated with selected diseases

PAIN

clinical and experimental perspectives

Introduction

Sensory psychologists and physiologists have mostly viewed pain as a separate sensation along with temperature and other cutaneous senses (Geldard, 1972; Kenshalo, 1971; Mountcastle, 1974; Hardy, Wolff, and Goodell, 1952). Each author mentions that emotional factors are very important in affecting the reaction to pain. However, they then proceed to an almost purely sensory discussion of pain. They describe the qualities of pain (pricking, burning, and aching), compare laboratory methods for arousing pain, and discuss the specific nervous pathways.

Pain is defined as a reaction related to actual or impending tissue damage on the basis of the stimuli that arouse it and on the basis of the responses measured to indicate evidence of its presence. Stimuli that arouse pain are mechanical (pressure), electrical (shock), thermal (radiant heat), and chemical (bradykinin) (see Section two). Responses measured are verbal (expressions of hurt), behavioral (withdrawal), and physiological (changes in blood pressure).

These sensory approaches have made a major contribution to the scientific analysis of pain. Laboratory study has led to the development of a finely controlled methodology for the exploration of pain phenomena. This methodology includes the mapping of the surface of the body for sensitivity, an analysis of neural pathways from the periphery to central areas, and the development of finely controlled methods of stimulation that can be used in some clinical situations.

However, as clinical experience has demonstrated, these studies have great limitations because the so-called emotional component of pain has been excluded from them. For example, the definition of pain as a reaction to actual or impending tissue damage would imply that the greater the tissue damage, the greater the reaction. Aside from the problem of spatial summation, the classical study of Beecher (1956) has demonstrated how the setting can affect the reaction more than the actual tissue destruction. Of 215 men seriously wounded in battle, only 25% wanted a narcotic for pain relief. In comparison, over 80% of civilian patients studied wanted relief from the pain of a surgical wound made with the patient under anesthesia. Beecher attributes the difference in reaction to the significance assigned to the wound rather than to the extent of physical tissue damage. In battle the wound meant a ticket to safety, but in civilian life the surgery meant disaster.

A simplistic view of pain as merely a sensation has also implied a simplistic clinical view, and the outcomes of such a view have been unfavorable. A simplistic view regarding pain in the same manner as any other sensation suggests that there are straightforward pain pathways. To stop pain, all that would be needed, therefore, would be to interrupt the pain pathway. Surgical results, however, indicate a rather disappointing record of success (see Section seven).

Defining pain in stimulus and response terms is inadequate clinically; pain for which no apparent stimuli can be demonstrated exists. Psychiatric illness, especially depression, has been associated with complaints of pain (see Reading 41). In instances of central pain observed pathology outside of the nerves, spinal cord, or brain is not present in sufficient degree to account for the pain (Loeser, 1975). Peripheral input does not seem to account for central pain, nor is there a favorable result with peripheral surgical procedures (except for tic douloureux).

The paradoxical aspect of some pain, such as causalgia (a burning pain associated with deformation of nerves by bullets and other high-velocity missiles), is that it persists months after the tissue damage has healed.

The problems involved in the experimental study of pain do not mean that this study should be abandoned. Even something as difficult to explain as phantom limbs has been experimentally studied (Melzack and Bromage, 1973). The sensation of a phantom limb occurs in most amputees almost immediately following an amputation. As described by Melzack (1973), in about 8% to 10% of patients, a pain develops that is often very severe. It endures after the stump tissues have healed and can be triggered in certain zones of the body by gentle pressure or even a pinprick on another limb of the body. It develops mostly in patients who have had pain in the limb for some time prior to the amputation. The pain is sometimes permanently abolished by the injection of a local anesthetic into the stump tissue even though the anesthesia wears off in a couple of hours.

These mysterious aspects of pain demonstrate the complexity of defining and examining the pain response. Experimental study of pain must include a great deal more than the examination of simple sensory processes. Over the past 10 years there has been an increase in experimental studies that have viewed pain as a complex psychological phenomenon that includes cognitive, emotional, and affective components. Central processes have been given a much stronger role (Melzack, 1973). The reaction to pain has been shown to be manipulatable and affected by cultural and other background factors. The principles of learning and social influence have been used effectively to modify pain reactions. Unfortunately, many clinicians are still not aware of the many possible ways, other than surgical or pharmacological, of influencing the pain reaction.

On the other hand, it is only very recently that distress and suffering have come into the laboratory as important variables (see Reading 24). It is through the clinical examination of pain that many of these forgotten and important variables have been brought to the attention of the experimentalist. Importantly, pain reactions often convey a great deal more than a signal that tissue damage is occurring. As Szasz (1957), Plainfield and Adler (1962), Zborowski (1969), and others have pointed out in discussing human reactions to pain, communication aspects are frequently overlooked. Pain reactions can mean "Don't hurt me"; "Help me"; "It's legitimate for me to get out of my daily responsibilities"; "Look, I'm being punished"; "Hey, look, I'm a real man"; or "I'm still alive."

It is hoped that the following sections will convey to the experimentalists some of the many variables that should be examined under controlled conditions. In turn, it is hoped that clinicians will become aware of the variety of methods for influencing the reactions to pain. We are still at a stage in our knowledge where multidisciplinary contributions would enhance our understanding and ability to control one of the human race's most demanding problems—pain and suffering.

REFERENCES

Beecher, H. K. 1956. Relationship of significance of wound to the pain experienced, Journal of the American Medical Association **161:**1609-1613.

Geldard, F. A. 1972. The human senses, John Wiley & Sons, Inc., New York.

Hardy, J. D., Wolff, H. G., and Goodell, H. 1952. Pain sensations and reactions, Hafner Publishing Co., New York.

Kenshalo, D. R. 1971. The cutaneous senses. In Kling, J. W., and Riggs, L. A., editors: Woodworth and Schlossberg's experimental psychology, Holt, Rinehart and Winston, Inc., New York.

Loeser, J. D. 1975. Mechanisms of central pain. In Weisenberg, M., editor: The control of pain, Psychological Dimensions, Inc., New York.

Melzack, R. 1973. The puzzle of pain, Basic Books, Inc., Publishers, New York.

Melzack, R., and Bromage, P. R. 1973. Experimental phantom limbs, Experimental Neurology **39:**261-269.

Mountcastle, V. B. 1974. Pain and temperature sensibilities. In Mountcastle, V. B., editor: Medical physiology, The C. V. Mosby Co, St. Louis.

Plainfield, S., and Adler, N. 1962. The meaning of pain, The Dental Clinics of North America, 659-668.

Szasz, T. A. 1957. Pain and pleasure, Basic Books, Inc., Publishers, New York.

Zborowski, M. 1969. People in pain, Jossey-Bass, Inc., Publishers, San Francisco.

SECTION ONE

General and theoretical concepts of pain reactions

There have been many theories of pain. Some have looked at pain as an emotion; others have looked at pain as a unique sensation with all the characteristics of any other sensory modality. Hardy, Wolff, and Goodell (1952) have reviewed the earlier views of pain. Melzack and Wall (1965) have critically examined current concepts of pain processes and presented their famous gate control theory of pain. Reading 1 is an updated version of Melzack and Wall's earlier paper.

Melzack and Wall review the specifity and pattern theories of pain perception and reject them. There may be specialization such as that found with A-delta and C fibers at receptor sites that respond to particular types and ranges of physical energy. However, specialization is not specificity. Specificity implies responding to one, and only one, given kind of stimulus. Melzack and Wall reject specificity and accept specialization. Many things happen at various levels of energy stimulation; aside from the activation of specific fibers, changes occur in the total number of neurons responding, as well as in their temporal and spatial relationships. However, a pattern theory of pain by itself appears to contradict physiological evidence.

Pain has a sensory component similar to other sensory processes. It is discriminable in time, space, and intensity. However, pain also has an essential aversive cognitive-motivational and emotional component that leads to behavior designed to escape or avoid the stimulus. Different neurophysiological mechanisms have been described for each system.

Pain perception can be modulated by the peripheral gating mechanism that can prevent pain stimulation from entering the system. It can also be controlled by a central control process that can modify stimulation once it has entered the system. Exact neurophysiological connections involved in each mechanism are still not firmly established. Strong criticism of the gate control model has thus been made because specific neurophysiological mechanisms do not support it. "I think therefore that one ought at this stage to strongly support Schmidt in his attempt to prevent the Gate hypothesis from taking root in the field of neurology" (Iggo, 1972, p. 127).

However, regardless of the accuracy of the specific wiring diagrams involved, the gate control theory of pain has been the most influential and important current theory of pain perception. It ties together many of the puzzling aspects of pain perception and control; it has had profound influence on pain research and the clinical control of pain; and it has generated new interest in pain perception, stimulating a multidisciplinary view of pain for research and treatment. There is little doubt that research will produce changes in the original gate control conceptions. There is also little doubt that the theory has had a great impact on the field.

Pain is a psychological experience. Behavioral and emotional variables can affect the manner in which it is perceived. Emotional and psychological factors can also cause pain. Merskey (Reading 2) reviews evidence of these factors exhibited in medical and psychiatric practice. Thirty-eight percent of patients with pain and 40% of patients without pain at a medical clinic were found to be there because of psychological illness (Devine and Merskey, 1965).

Merskey views pain as an unpleasant experience primarily associated with tissue damage, described in terms of tissue damage even when none is apparent, or by a combination of the two. Psychogenic pain is caused mainly or wholly by psychological factors, and organic pain is caused mainly or wholly by physical factors. From the patient's viewpoint, the subjective experience may not be different.

Psychogenic pain occurs under three main circumstances: (1) as hallucinations (schizophrenia), (2) with muscle tension caused by psychological factors (tension headaches), and (3) by conversion hysteria.

Pain due to stress has become the focus of new treatment approaches. One of the most exciting of these new approaches is the use of biofeedback, a procedure whereby a biological function is continuously measured and played back to the person being measured. Through these means the person is able to learn to control many difficult body processes. Muscle tension feedback, for example, is now being used in the treatment of tension headache (Budzynski, Stoyva, and Alder, 1970).

Whether pain is mainly psychogenic or organic is not always easy to determine. Multidisciplinary clinics can be most helpful in this regard. It is often very easy to place the cause of pain on a physical lesion, yet it is not always easy to prove that the lesion is the cause since there may be many people who have a similar lesion without any complaints of pain. In turn, it is possible to have a patient with a history of conversion symptoms whose pain this time is really being caused by a lesion. A multidisciplinary approach would more likely consider both of these issues.

There are many psychological variables that affect the reactions to pain. Murray (Reading 3) has reviewed some of the cognitive and affective variables that affect the pain reaction. Of these, anticipation and anxiety have been found to be extremely important. Many implications can be derived from studies that have been made in the clinic and in the laboratory, both for the clinical treatment of pain and for a theory of pain. Distraction, for example, is one way of reducing the reaction to pain. It seems that the human body cannot simultaneously accept two competing stimuli—that of distraction and that of pain.

Keele (Reading 4) looks at the importance of pain sensitivity for the evaluation of symptoms presented to a physician. Using myocardial infarction as an illustration, Keele points to the great variation in patient behavior. There are some patients who, even when having a severe myocardial infarction, do not react much. Other patients react a great deal even to mild physical damage. Having an independent estimate of pain sensitivity would allow the physician to know what the proper treatment should be. Tursky (1975) has argued that an individual's unique way of reacting to pain should become a routine part of a medical record, along with blood pressure and other vital signs. Knowing this information would provide for pain control efforts best suited to the condition. For some patients morphine might be indicated, but for others reassurance concerning their prognosis would be adequate.

This section includes readings to give the reader an appreciation of some of the major experimental and clinical approaches to pain control. In subsequent sections many of these topics are expanded or applied. The reading by White (Reading 38, Section eight) for example, shows how a counterirritant can produce relief from pain. The reading does not mention it directly, but this approach is a direct application of the gate control theory of pain.

REFERENCES

Budzynski, T., Stoyva, J., and Adler, C. 1970. Feedback—induced muscle relaxation: application to tension headache, Journal of Behavior Therapy and Experimental Psychiatry **1**:205-211.

Devine, R., and Merskey, H. 1965. The description of pain in psychiatric and general medical patients, Journal of Psychosomatic Research **9**:311-316.

Iggo, A. 1972. Critical remarks on the gate control

theory. In Janzen, R., and others, editors: Pain: basic principles, pharmacology, therapy, Georg Thieme Verlag KG, Stuttgart, Germany.

Hardy, J. D., Wolff, H. G., and Goodell, H. 1952. Pain sensations and reactions, Hafner Publishing Co., New York.

Melzack, R., and Wall, P. D. 1965. Pain mechanisms: a new theory, Science **150:**971-979.

Tursky, B. 1975. The measurement of pain reactions: laboratory studies. In Weisenberg, M., editor: The control of pain, Psychological Dimensions, Inc., New York.

1

Psychophysiology of pain*

Ronald Melzack and Patrick D. Wall

EVOLUTION OF PAIN THEORIES

Theories of pain mechanisms, since the beginning of the century, have undergone evolutionary changes based partly on the accumulation of new experimental evidence and partly on imaginative assumptions derived from clinical and psychological observations. New biological-medical theories, like theories in the physical sciences [4], are accepted reluctantly; old theories are dogmatically maintained in the face of contrary evidence until a new theory supersedes them that can account for both the older and newer facts. In this process of evolution there is usually a characteristic swing of the pendulum between two major theoretical concepts (such as the phlogiston versus oxygen theories of combustion), until one of them eventually dominates. Another feature of this evolution in science [4] is that a theory may be conceptually correct although the particular explanatory *mechanism* that is postulated may well be wrong in one or more details. The theoretical concept thus often awaits widespread acceptance until a satisfactory mechanistic explanation is proposed.

Overriding all these features of the scientific process is the bitter controversy generated between opposing schools of thought. The problems of cutaneous mechanisms in general, and pain in particular, have given rise to vituperation that, according to Dallenbach [5], is unparalleled in the biological sciences. The early three-cornered fight involving von Frey, Goldscheider, and Marshall (whose emotion—or quale—theory of pain was soon pushed out of the ring, despite Sherrington's [42] sympathy with Marshall's view) marks the beginning of a controversy that has continued throughout this century.

Part of the reason for the bitterness engendered by the battle may be the obvious clinical implications that derive from any theoretical advance. The practice of medicine, because it deals with human lives, is generally conservative so that old ideas that have worked (even imperfectly) are cherished and newer ideas are viewed with suspicion and often antipathy. It is in the light of this understanding of scientific processes that we shall here review two major theoretical concepts of pain—the specificity and pattern theories—that are the basis of much of the bitter controversy on pain mechanisms in this century, and describe a third theory—gate control theory—that we have proposed as an alternative to both.

Specificity theory

Specificity theory proposes that a mosaic of specific pain receptors in body tissue projects to a pain center in the brain. It maintains [44] that free nerve endings are pain receptors and generate pain impulses that are carried by A-delta and C fibers in peripheral nerves and by the lateral spinothalamic tract in the spinal cord to a pain center in the thalamus. Despite its apparent simplicity, the theory contains an

Reprinted with permission of Little, Brown and Co. from The International Anesthesiology Clinics **8**:3-34. Copyright 1970.
*Supported by contract SD-193 (to R. M.) from the Advanced Research Projects Agency of the U. S. Department of Defense, and by grants (to P. D. Wall) from the British Medical Research Council, Foundations Fund for Research in Psychiatry, and Merck Sharp & Dohme.

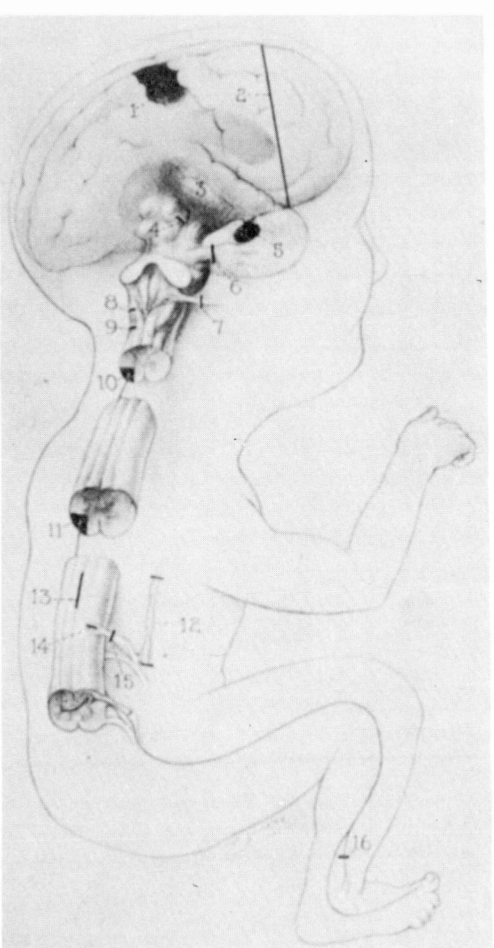

Fig. 1. MacCarty and Drake's [23] schematic diagram of the pain pathway, illustrating various surgical procedures designed to alleviate pain. 1: Gyrectomy. 2: Prefrontal lobotomy. 3: Thalamotomy. 4: Mesencephalic tractotomy. 5: Hypophysectomy. 6: Fifth-nerve rhizotomy. 7: Ninth-nerve neurectomy. 8: Medullary tractotomy. 9: Trigeminal tractotomy. 10: Cervical chordotomy. 11: Thoracic chordotomy. 12: Sympathectomy. 13: Myelotomy. 14: Lissauer tractotomy. 15: Posterior rhizotomy. 16: Neurectomy.

explicit statement of physiological specialization and an implicit psychological assumption [20, 31, 32]. Consider the proposition that the skin contains pain receptors. To say that a receptor responds only to intense, noxious stimulation of the skin is a physiological statement of fact; it says that the receptor is specialized to respond to a particular kind of stimulus. To call a receptor a *pain* receptor, however, is a psychological assumption: it implies a direct connection from the receptor to a brain center where pain is felt (Figs. 1, 2A, and 5A), so that stimulation of the receptor must always elicit pain and only the sensation of pain. The facts of physiological specialization provide the power of specificity theory; its psychological assumption is its weakness [31, 32].

There can no longer by any doubt that the receptors and fibers of the skin sensory system exhibit a high degree of specialization of function. There is no convincing evidence, however, to substantiate the view that there is a special class of receptor-fiber units that comprise an exclusive pain modality. In the search for peripheral fibers that respond exclusively to high intensity stimulation, Burgess and Perl [3] have recently discovered a specialized class of A-delta small-diameter myelinated fibers with slow conduction velocity. They are attached to true nociceptors since they transmit impulses only when the skin is actually damaged. It is reasonable to assume that these fibers carry impulses which contribute to pain processes, but they cannot be considered as modality-specific "pain fibers" because: (1) pain may be triggered by stimuli (particularly in neuralgic patients) that are inadequate to fire these fibers, (2) noxious heat, cold, and bradykinin (a noxious chemical) do not fire them, (3) they adapt fairly rapidly, and (4) there is no after-discharge. We see, then, that while these fibers may, on occasion, contribute to the afferent barrage which triggers pain, they do not have the required properties of explaining all cutaneous pains or the variable relationship between stimulus and response.

These data suggest that a small number of specialized fibers may exist that respond only to intense stimulation, but this does not mean that they are "pain fibers"—that they must always produce pain, and only pain, when they are stimulated. It is more likely that they represent the extreme of a continuous distribution of receptor-fiber thresholds rather than a special category. The transduction properties of receptor-fiber units are a function of many physiological variables: (1) threshold to mechanical distortion, (2) threshold to negative and positive temperature change, (3) peak sensitivity to temperature change, (4) threshold to chemical change, (5) stimulus strength-response curve, (6) rate of adaptation, and (7) after-discharge. Each receptor-fiber unit must be specified accurately in terms of its coordinates with respect to these variables instead of being forced into a preconceived, oversimplified, psychological modality class. Similarly, experiments that appear to correlate loss of pain sensation with selective block of C fibers by pharmacological agents are usually interpreted to mean that C fibers are pain fibers. However, there is an alternative interpretation: that pain results when the total integral of the afferent barrage in all fibers exceeds a critical preset level and that the only way to exceed the level is by activation of C fibers. Indeed, all experiments that attempt to correlate sensory modalities with particular groups of nerve fibers on the basis of selective block by cocaine, ischemia, and the like, can be interpreted in terms of interaction among fiber groups rather than specific modalities.

This distinction between physiological specialization and psychological assumption also applies to central projection systems [31]. There is, without question, evidence that central nervous system pathways have specialized functions that play a role in pain mechanisms. Surgical lesions of the lateral spinothalamic tract [44] or portions of the thalamus [25] may on occasion abolish pain of pathological origin. But the fact that these areas carry signals related to pain does not mean that they comprise a specific pain system. The lesions have multiple effects: They reduce the total number of responding neurons; they change the temporal and spatial relationships among all ascending systems; and they affect the descending feedback that controls transmission from peripheral fibers to dorsal horn cells. Moreover, pain frequently recurs after apparently successful cordotomy [37]. Physiological specialization is a fact that can be recognized without acceptance of the psychological assumption that pain is determined entirely by impulses in a straight-through transmission system from the skin to a pain center in the brain.

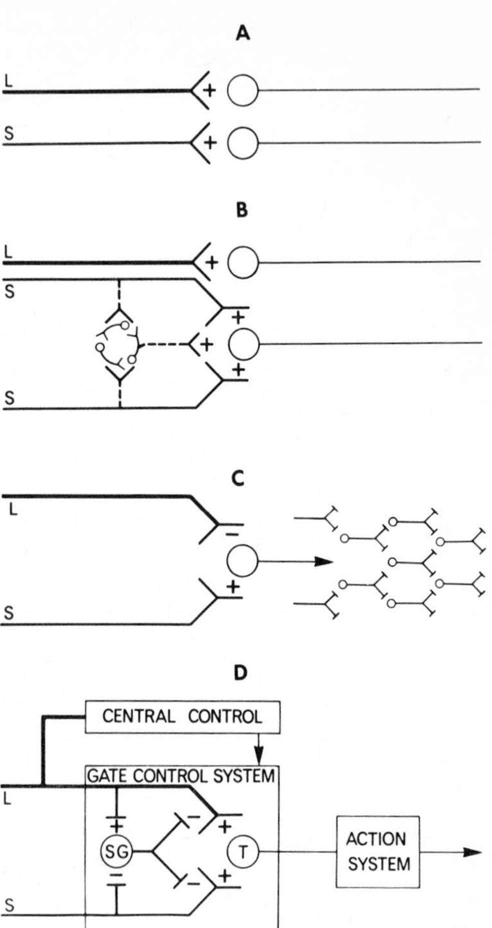

Fig. 2. Schematic representation of conceptual models of pain mechanisms. (A) Specificity theory. Large (L) and small (S) fibers are assumed to transmit touch and pain impulses respectively, in separate, specific, straight-through pathways to touch and pain centers in the brain. (B) Summation theory, showing convergence of small fibers onto a dorsal horn cell. The central network projecting to the central cell represents Livingston's [20] conceptual model of reverberatory circuits underlying pathological pain states. Touch is assumed to be carried by large fibers. (C) Sensory interaction theory, in which large (L) fibers inhibit (−) and small (S) fibers excite (+) central transmission neurons. The output projects to spinal cord neurons which are conceived by Noordenbos [38] to comprise a multisynaptic afferent system. (D) Gate control theory. The large (L) and small (S) fibers project to the substantia gelatinosa (SG) and first central transmission (T) cells. The central control trigger is represented by a line running from the large fiber system to central control mechanisms, which in turn project back to the gate control system. The T cells project to the entry cells of the action system. + = excitation; − = inhibition. (From Melzack and Wall [32].)

Pattern theory

As a reaction against the psychological assumption in specificity theory, new theories have been proposed which can be grouped under the general heading of *pattern theory*. Goldscheider [10] was the first to propose that stimulus intensity and central summation are the critical determinants of pain. Goldscheider (Fig. 2B) proposed that the large cutaneous fibers comprise a specific touch system, while the smaller fibers converge on dorsal horn cells which summate their input and transmit the pattern to the brain where it is perceived as pain. Other theories have been proposed, within the framework of Goldscheider's concept, which stress central summation mechanisms. Livingston [20] was the first to suggest specific neural mechanisms to account for the remarkable summation phenomena in clinical pain syndromes. He proposed that intense, pathological stimulation of the body sets up reverberating circuits (central circuit incorporated into Fig. 2B) in spinal internuncial pools that can then be triggered by normally nonnoxious inputs and generate abnormal volleys that are interpreted centrally as pain.

Related to theories of central summation is the theory that a specialized input-controlling system normally prevents summation from occurring, and that destruction of this system leads to pathological pain states. Basically, this theory proposes the existence of a rapidly conducting fiber system which inhibits synaptic transmission in a more slowly conducting system that carries the signal for pain [51]. These two systems are identified as the epicritic and protopathic [13], fast and slow [18], phylogenetically new and old [2], and myelinated and unmyelinated [38] fiber systems. Under pathological conditions, the slow system establishes dominance over the fast, and the result is protopathic sensation [13], slow pain [18], diffuse burning pain [2], or hyperalgesia [38]. It is important to note the transition from specificity theory to the pattern concept: Noordenbos [38] does not associate psychological quality with each system but attributes to the rapidly conducting system the ability to modify the input pattern transmitted through the slowly conducting, multisynaptic system in the spinal cord (Fig. 2C).

The concepts of central summation and input control have shown remarkable power in their ability to explain many of the clinical phenomena of pain. The various specific theoretical mechanisms that have been proposed, however, fail to comprise a satisfactory general theory of pain. They lack unity, and no single theory so far proposed is capable of integrating the diverse theoretical mechanisms.

A recent variant of pattern theory has been proposed by Weddell [50] and Sinclair [43] based on the earlier suggestion by Nafe [36] that all cutaneous qualities are produced by spatiotemporal patterns of nerve impulses rather than by separate modality-specific transmission routes. The theory proposes that all fiber endings (apart from those that innervate hair cells) are alike, so that the pattern for pain is produced by intense stimulation of nonspecific receptors. The physiological evidence, however, reveals [31] high degree of receptor-fiber specialization. The pattern theory proposed by Weddell and Sinclair, then, fails as a satisfactory theory of pain because it ignores the facts of physiological specialization. It is more reasonable to assume that the specialized physiological properties of each receptorfiber unit, such as response ranges, adaptation rates, and thresholds to different stimulus intensities, play an important role in determining the characteristics of the temporal patterns that are generated when a stimulus is applied to the skin.

Summary

In summary, we believe that the specific modality and pattern theories of pain, although they appear to be mutually exclusive, both contain valuable concepts that supplement one another. Recognition of receptor specialization for the transduction of particular kinds and ranges of cutaneous stimulation does not preclude acceptance of the concept that the information generated by skin receptors is coded in the form of patterns of nerve impulses. The law of the adequate stimulus can be retained without also accepting a narrow, fixed relationship between receptor specialization and perceptual and behavioral response. Similarly, the original hopes for a monopolization of a particular modality by a specific fiber-diameter group have not materialized. The evidence permits only a loose association of function with fiber diameter. Moreover, the evidence suggests that central projection pathways are specialized for the transmission of particular kinds of information, but there is no evidence that allows us, even at this central level, to assume a one-to-one relationship between physiological specialization and psychological events.

There can no longer be any doubt that temporal and spatial patterns of nerve impulses provide the basis of our sensory perceptions. The coding of information in the form of nerve impulse patterns is a fundamental concept in contemporary neurophysiology and psychology. Yet pattern theory, because of its vagueness, fails to provide an adequate account of somesthesis. The inadequacies of specificity and pattern theories of pain have therefore necessitated the formulation of alternative conceptions. Indeed, the fact that so many forms of pain still resist pharmacological or surgical control demands exploration of new approaches and new concepts.

Gate control theory

We have recently proposed a new theory of pain in which a gate control system modulates sensory input from the skin before it evokes pain perception and response [32]. Stimulation of skin evokes nerve impulses that are transmitted to three spinal cord systems (Fig. 2D): the cells of the substantia gelatinosa in the dorsal horn, the dorsal column fibers that project toward the brain, and the central transmission (T) cells in the dorsal horn. We proposed that (1) the substantia gelatinosa functions as a gate control mechanism that modulates the afferent patterns before they influence the T cells; (2) the afferent patterns in the dorsal column system act, in part at least, as a central control trigger which activates selective brain processes that then influence, by way of descending fibers, the modulating properties of the gate control system; and (3) the T cells activate neural mechanisms which comprise the action system responsible for perception and response. The theory suggests that pain phenomena are determined by interactions among these three systems.

Figure 2D shows the factors involved in the transmission of impulses from peripheral nerve to T cells in the cord. We proposed that the control over transmission is affected by two factors: by the afferent impulses acting on a gating mechanism and by impulses descending from the brain. Impulses in large-diameter fibers were assumed to decrease the effectiveness of afferent volleys, while small afferents increased it. The substantia gelatinosa was suggested as the actual control mechanism and the presynaptic terminals of afferent fibers as the site of action. Thus, in the model (Fig. 2D), volleys in large fibers are effective initially in firing the T cells, but their later effect is reduced by the presynaptic inhibitory gating mechanism. In contrast, volleys in fine fibers reduce the presynaptic inhibition and thereby exaggerate the effect of arriving impulses. Figure 2D shows only presynaptic control, but postsynaptic control mechanisms are also presumed to contribute to the observed input-output function. Furthermore, descending impulses from the brain control the presynaptic mechanism so that the ease with which impulses penetrate the cord cells is determined both by the afferent activity and by central control processes originating in the brain. The output of the T cells, then, is determined by the number of active fibers and their rate of firing, by the balance of large- and small-fiber activity in the afferent barrage, and by the activity of central structures.

We proposed [32] that the signal which triggers the action system responsible for pain perception and response occurs when the output of the T cells reaches or exceeds a critical level. That is, there is a temporal summation or integration of the arriving barrage by central cells which finally results in pain perception and response when the integral exceeds a preset level. The clinical and pharmacological implications of the theory will be discussed after it is first evaluated in the light of recent evidence.

GATE CONTROL THEORY: RECENT EVIDENCE

Recent physiological evidence necessitates a revision of gate control theory. The laminar organization of the dorsal horns is now better understood and, moreover, in-

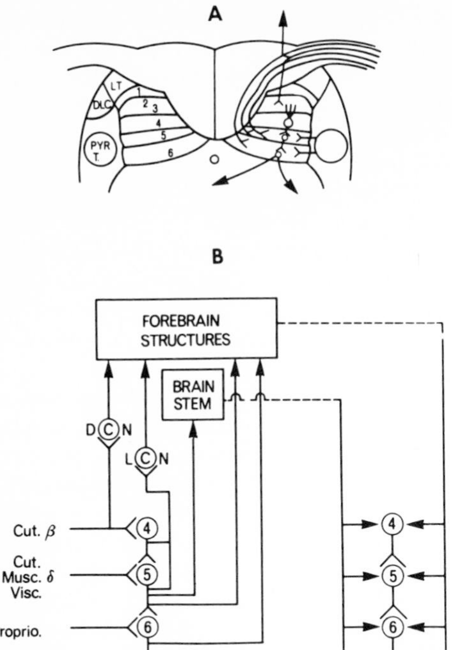

Fig. 3. (A) Representation of the laminar organization and some of the connections and projections in the dorsal spinal cord. (B) Schematic representation of major connections and projections of the somatic sensory system. 4, 5, 6 represent the dorsal horn laminae (shown in [A]). DLC = dorsolateral column; PYR T. = pyramidal tract; LT = Lissauer's tract; DCN = dorsal column nuclei; LCN = lateral cervical nucleus. Cutaneous, muscular, visceral, and proprioceptive inputs are indicated.

dicates a convergence of visceral afferent impulses onto the T cells. In addition, new questions are raised on the actual mechanisms underlying gate control; although the concept of the balance of large-fiber versus small-fiber activity appears to be valid, the actual explanatory *mechanism* still needs to be determined unequivocally.

Spinal cord mechanisms and control of entering impulses

Since the gate control theory of pain was proposed in 1965, further research has been done on the dorsal horns, and a much more specific but still highly speculative picture of the process of reception and transmission can be presented. The reason for the necessity for speculation is that it is not yet possible to collect the crucial evidence. The anatomical gaps are produced by the difficulty in staining substantia gelatinosa cells, the extreme complexity of the interconnections, uncertainty about the morphology of functional synapses, and ignorance of the ultimate destination of projecting axons. The physiological ignorance comes from the fact that recordings can be made only from outside a minority of cells and from inside an even smaller number. It is not even certain that the small cells of substantia gelatinosa generate nerve impulses. Under these circumstances, it is not surprising that important details are unknown about the passage of impulses from afferent fibers to central transmitting cells. A final serious problem is the assessment of the significance of the powerful descending influences from the brain on the dorsal horn. We know from physiological experiments that these pathways exist but we cannot know under what circumstances they actually work until they have been studied during behavior. In spite of these difficulties a lot of important results have been generated in the last few years and we can again attempt a summary in the form of an extension of our earlier gate control theory.

Anatomy. Cutaneous afferent fibers terminate in the dorsal two-thirds of the dorsal horn (Fig. 3). These fibers end on cells which are arranged in a series of laminae. The most dorsal of these is the thin scattered layer of marginal cells whose significance remains unknown. Next is the substantia gelatinosa, lamina 2, which contains three components: the terminals of afferent fibers, the dendrites of deeper cells, and the small cells and their interconnections. The fibers which terminate in this lamina must be of a special variety since their terminals degenerate within 48 hours of root section [14]. Golgi staining suggests that these are fine afferents which project directly into the dorsal gray from the dorsal roots by way of the medial part of the Lissauer tract [8, 45]. The dendrites rise up from the large deeper cells. These dendrites form broad fans which run rostrocaudally and subdivide the lamina into compartments [39]. The small cells interconnect with each other by short axons and by longer axons running in the lateral part of the Lissauer tract. The region contains large numbers of axo-axonic contacts and many of the receiving axons are presumed to be peripheral afferents [45]. The small cells receive contacts from each other, probably from afferents, and probably from a special type of small cell in the third lamina.

The third lamina contains the same three component types as the second, but the afferents ending here are known to be in part the large myelinated cutaneous afferents which follow a curved course bending back on themselves to project dense fans of terminal arbors intermeshed with the fan-shaped dendrites of the deeper cells. The small cells, some of which are pyramidal in shape, receive primary afferents and project their axons into lamina 2. Below this layer, there is a layer of cells (lamina 4) with large cell bodies; their dendrites project into laminae 2 and 3 and some of their axons travel in the ipsilateral dorsolateral tract, at least in the lower mammals. In the cat these axons project to the lateral cervical nucleus and from there to thalamus and cortex. It is debatable if an analogous nucleus exists in the primates.

Finally, in the narrowest part of the dorsal horn there is lamina 5, which receives afferent fibers and projects in a number of directions. A small number of these cells send their axons in the dorsolateral white matter on the same side. Some may project by way of the dorsal columns to unknown end-stations in the brain and some may project to thalamus by way of the ventral crossed spinothalamic tract [7]. All five laminae receive axons descending from the brain, including some by way of the pyramidal tract.

Physiology of changes in terminals. The original gate control theory was based on the fact that changes are produced in the membrane potential of terminal axons following the arrival of impulses from the periphery. Impulses arriving in large-diameter cutaneous afferents produce a large, prolonged depolarization of the terminals of the active fibers and their passive neighbors. Schmidt, Senges, and Zimmermann [40] have suggested that this depolarizing interaction is particularly strongly produced by certain specific types of afferents. Mendell and Wall [34] believed that the smaller afferents (A-delta and C fibers), in contrast to the large fibers, produce a hyperpolarization of terminals so that the actual membrane potential is determined by the balance of large versus small fibers active in the afferent volley. The reported effect of C fibers, however, has recently been challenged.

Whatever the outcome may be, it is clear that the membrane potential of the terminals is controlled by some central mechanism which is in turn controlled by the rival effects of certain large versus certain small afferents. The mechanism is still believed to involve cells in laminae 2 and 3. The membrane potential of the terminal arborization was thought to determine the postsynaptic effectiveness of the arriving impulses, either by a block of impulses in the fine terminal filaments or by controlling the amount of transmitter released. Now, however, it is not at all certain that these purely presynaptic mechanisms exist in isolation. The presynaptic membrane potential control exists but it may be coupled with a simultaneous change in the postsynaptic membrane.

Physiology of the transmitting cells

While poor progress has been made in unravelling the details of synaptic transmission from cutaneous afferents to transmitting cells, a great deal more is now known about the input and output functions of these cells. The cells in lamina 4 are poor candidates as the transmitters of impulses likely to trigger pain reactions, because they fail to respond to intense cutaneous pressure stimuli or to electrical stimuli of peripheral nerves involving A-delta and C afferents. In contrast, the lamina 5 cells are the best candidates so far discovered as the first central transmission cells in a pain-signalling pathway because their properties fulfill a number of requirements needed to explain actual phenomena. While summarizing present knowledge and suggesting a pain mechanism, it is essential to remember that the data are based on a partial survey of cell types because present techniques do not permit recording from smaller cells.

There are five laminae in the dorsal horn containing cells which receive cutaneous afferents (Fig. 3). We believe that the cells of lamina 5 are the most likely transmitter cells concerned with triggering pain reactions. The cells of lamina 1 are very few in number, have large receptive fields with a multiple convergence from skin and muscle, and are not known to be concerned with projection in the crucial contralateral ventral white matter. The cells of laminae 2 and 3 have an unknown physiology but their anatomy suggests that they modulate the flow of impulses from the afferents to the larger cells. The cells of lamina 4 have small cutaneous receptive fields and project to the ipsilateral white matter and probably to lamina 5 cells. They respond to light pressure stimuli and to A-beta afferent volleys, but they fail to increase their response to A-delta or C volleys. In contrast, the cells of lamina 5 have somewhat larger cutaneous receptive fields, respond to all types of cutaneous stimuli, and are also involved in the reception of impulses from deep and visceral structures.

The cutaneous receptive fields of lamina 5 cells have three components. In the center, there is a region where low pressure stimuli and hair movements excite the cell. Very low level electrical stimuli sufficient to excite A-beta afferents excite the cell, probably by way of the lamina 4 cells. This region is superimposed on top of a wider area of skin from which the cell is excited by intense electrical or mechanical stimuli. The excitation produced by small fibers is followed by a very prolonged period of after-discharge. Finally, these two regions are superimposed on top of an even larger region from which low threshold fibers produce inhibition. This combination of convergences produces a three-zoned receptive field: In the center the cell is excited by the full range of mechanical stimuli, but inhibition follows after light stimuli and facilitation follows heavy stimuli; the firing rate increases with increasing intensity of stimulation, and intense stimulation produces very prolonged repetitive discharges. Around this zone is a region where light stimuli or large-fiber stimulation produces inhibition while heavy stimuli or small-fiber stimulation produces excitation and some facilitation. The two excitatory fields are surrounded by an even larger zone in which no natural stimuli excite but, instead, produce inhibition. The mechanism of the inhibition produced by the large fibers and the facilitation produced by the small fibers is unknown, but it may involve both postsynaptic and presynaptic changes and the small cells of laminae 2 and 3. Certain components of the facilitatory mechanism must be sensitive to barbiturate, since Hillman and Wall [15] never observed prolonged facilitation in the presence of barbiturate anesthesia, confirming Mendell and Wall [35].

In the decerebrate or barbiturate anesthetized cat, powerful tonic descending impulses from the brainstem arrive in the cord and excite the local inhibitory mechanism (Fig. 3B). This means that the number of impulses leaving a lamina 5 cell after stimulation is controlled by brain structures.

The organization of convergence with associated inhibitory and facilitatory mechanisms allows the cells to operate in several modes. For light stimuli or large-diameter afferents there is a small receptive field with inhibitory surround. For heavy mechanical stimuli, there is a larger receptive field and a facilitatory mechanism which competes with the inhibition. The intensity of inhibition is controlled by the brainstem. For a particular cell, the small-fiber influence may come from one of three sources: the cutaneous delta afferents, the small muscle afferents, or the small visceral afferents. All cells are excited by small afferents, whatever their origin, and inhibited by large-diameter afferents of cutaneous origin. We propose that if the frequency of nerve impulses leaving any of these cells ever rises above some critical level, then pain reactions will be triggered. The presence of convergence, interaction, and control at the entry point help to explain many pain phenomena, particularly those associated with diseases of peripheral nerves.

Beyond the gate

We assume that the gating of the input at the dorsal horn level of the spinal cord marks the beginning of repeated modulation, filtering, and abstraction of the input as it ascends toward and into the brain. It is obvious that barbiturates and other analgesics act on the action system as well as gate mechanisms in the spinal cord. Melzack and Casey [26] have noted (Figs. 4, 5B) that the output of the dorsal horn T

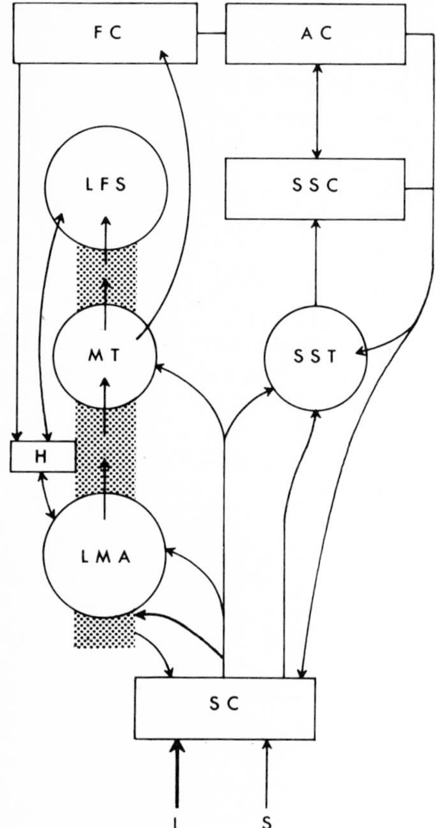

Fig. 4. Schematic diagram of the anatomical foundation of proposed pain model in Figure 5B. (Right) Thalamic and neocortical structures subserving discriminative capacity. (Left) Reticular and limbic systems subserving motivational-affective functions. Ascending pathways from the spinal cord (SC) are: (1) dorsal column-lemniscal and dorsolateral tracts (right ascending arrow) projecting to the somatosensory thalamus (SST) and cortex (SSC), and (2) anterolateral pathway (left ascending arrow) to somatosensory thalamus via neospinothalamic tract, and to reticular formation (stippled area), limbic midbrain area (LMA) and medial thalamus (MT) via paramedial ascending system. Descending pathways to spinal cord originate in somatosensory and associated cortical areas (AC) and in the reticular formation. Polysynaptic and reciprocal relationships in limbic and reticular systems are indicated. Other abbreviations: FC = frontal cortex; LFS = limbic forebrain structures (hippocampus, septum, amygdala, and associated cortex); H = hypothalamus. (From Melzack and Casey [26].)

cells is transmitted toward the brain by fibers in the anterolateral spinal cord and is projected into two major brain systems: via neospinothalamic fibers into the ventrobasal and posterolateral thalamus and the somatosensory cortex, and via medially coursing fibers, that comprise a paramedial ascending system, into the reticular formation and medial intralaminar thalamus and the limbic system (Fig. 4). Electrical stimulation of the tooth at noxious intensities evokes activity in both projection systems, and discrete lesions in each may strikingly diminish pain perception and response [16, 30]. Moreover, analgesic doses of nitrous oxide produce a striking reduction of the amplitude of potentials evoked by tooth stimulation in both systems [12]. Barbiturates and ether are also known to reduce potentials in the reticular formation [9]. The connections and functional properties of the spinal cord and brain projection and relay systems are complex and still controversial. Since this literature is reviewed in detail elsewhere in this issue, we will here only sketch the major central pathways and their interactions.

Recent behavioral and physiological studies have led Melzack and Casey [26] to propose (Fig. 5B) that (1) the selection and modulation of the sensory input through the neospinothalamic projection system provides, in part at least, the neurological basis of the sensory-discriminative dimension of pain [41]; (2) activation of reticular and limbic structures through the paramedial ascending system underlies the powerful motivational drive and unpleasant affect that trigger the organism into action; and (3) neocortical or higher central nervous system processes, such as evaluation of the input in terms of past experience, exert control over activity in both the discriminative and motivational systems. It is assumed that these three categories of activity interact with one another to provide perceptual information regarding the location, magnitude, and spatiotemporal properties of the noxious stimulus, motivational tendency toward escape or attack, and cognitive information based on analysis of multimodal information, past experience, and probability of outcome of different response strategies. All

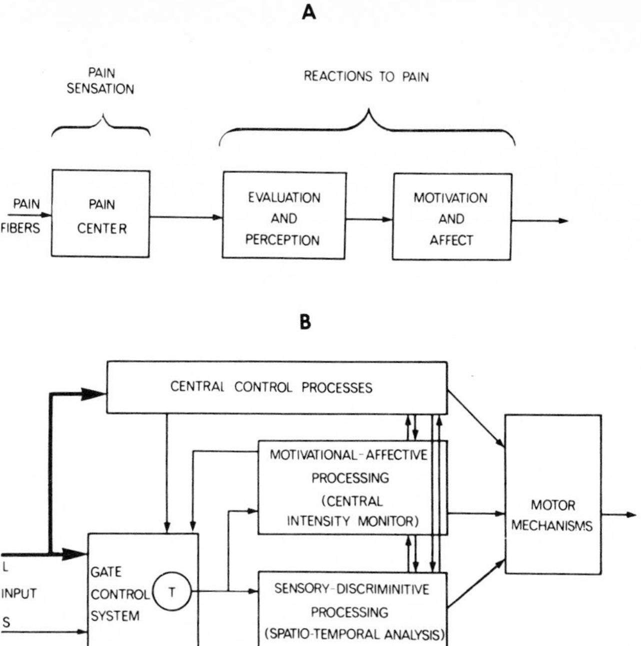

Fig. 5. (A) Conceptual model of the basis of pain experience according to specificity theory. (B) Conceptual model of the sensory, motivational, and central control determinants of pain. The output of T cells of the gate control system projects to the sensory-discriminative system (via neospinothalamic fibers) and the motivational-affective system (via the paramedial ascending system). The central control trigger (comprising the dorsal column and dorsolateral projection systems) is represented by a line running from the large-fiber system to central control processes; these, in turn, project back to the gate control system, and to the sensory-discriminative and motivational-affective systems. All three systems interact with one another and project to the motor system. (From Melzack and Casey [26].)

three forms of activity could then influence motor mechanisms responsible for the complex pattern of overt responses that characterize pain.

There is now a convincing body of evidence that stimulation of reticular and limbic system structures produces strong aversive drive and behavior typical of responses to naturally occurring painful stimuli. These data together with related evidence (reviewed by Melzack and Casey [26]) on the effects of ablation indicate that limbic structures, although they play a role in many other functions, provide a neural basis for the aversive drive and affect that comprise the motivational dimension of pain. Melzack and Casey propose that the reticular and limbic systems function as a central intensity monitor: that their activities are determined, in part at least, by the intensity of the T cell output (the total number of active fibers and their rate of firing) after it has undergone modulation by the gate control system in the dorsal horns. They suggest that the output of the T cells, beyond a critical intensity level, activates those areas underlying negative affect and aversive drive. Signals from these structures to motor mechanisms set the stage for response patterns that are aimed at dealing with the input on the basis of both sensory information and cognitive processes.

It is now firmly established that stimulation of the brain activates descending efferent fibers [22] which can influence afferent conduction at the earliest synaptic levels of the somesthetic system. Thus it is possible for central nervous system activities subserving attention, emotion, and memories of prior experience to exert control over the sensory input. There is evidence [11, 47] to suggest that these central influences are mediated through the gate control system. While some central activities, such as anxiety or excitement, may open or close the gate for all inputs at any site of the body, others obviously involve selective, localized gate activity. For example, men wounded in battle may feel little or no pain from the wound (because it signifies that they survived the battle) but may complain bitterly about an inept vein puncture [1]. The signals, then, must be identified, evaluated in terms of prior experience, localized, and inhibited before the action system responsible for pain perception and response is activated. We propose, therefore, that there exists in the nervous system a mechanism, which we call the *central control trigger,* that activates the particular, selective brain processes that exert control over the sensory input (Fig. 2D).

We have already noted [32] that the dorsal column-medial lemniscal and dorsolateral systems could fulfill the functions of the central control trigger. They carry precise information about the nature and location of the stimulus, and they conduct so rapidly that they may not only set the receptivity of cortical neurons for subsequent afferent volleys but may, by way of central control efferent fibers, also act on the gate control system. At least part of their function, then, could be to activate selective brain processes that influence information which is still arriving over slowly conducting fibers or is being transmitted up more slowly conducting pathways.

IMPLICATIONS OF THE MODEL FOR PAIN CONTROL

We have already noted [32] that gate control theory is able to account for many pain phenomena. If, for example, there is a selective destruction of large peripheral nerve fibers (leaving the small fibers relatively intact), as in diabetic or alcoholic neuropathy, the normal presynaptic and postsynaptic inhibition of the input by the gate control system does not occur. Thus the input arriving over the remaining smaller fibers is transmitted through the unchecked, open gate produced by the C fiber input and provides the basis for intense, pathological pain. Moreover, since the total number of peripheral fibers is reduced, it may take a considerable time before the T cells can be wound up to the discharge level necessary to trigger pain, which would account for the delays often observed in pathological pain states [38].

Similar mechanisms may account for neuralgic pains: Kerr and Miller [17] have recently demonstrated that the trigeminal ganglia and adjacent posterior rootlets in patients with trigeminal neuralgia show marked proliferative-degenerative changes in the myelin sheaths of the large fibers. Comparable experimental demyelination [24] produces a striking reduction of conduction velocities in formerly rapidly conducting fibers. This relative decrease in the large-fiber input provides a possible mechanism for the pain of anesthesia dolorosa and the "spontaneous" pains which develop in these syndromes. Spatial summation would also occur easily under such conditions. The phenomena of referred pain, spread of pain, and trigger points at some distance from the original site of body damage point toward summation mechanisms which can be understood in terms of the model, since the substantia gelatinosa at any level receives inputs from both sides of the body and (by way of Lissauer's tract) from the substantia gelatinosa in neighboring body segments.

In addition to the sensory influences on the gate control system, there is a tonic input to the system from the brain which exerts an inhibitory affect on the sensory input [47]. Thus, any lesion that impairs the normal downflow of impulses to the gate control system would open the gate. Central nervous system lesions associated with hyperalgesia and spontaneous pain could have this effect. On the other hand, any central nervous system condition that increases the flow of descending impulses would tend to close the gate. The model also suggests that psychological factors such as past experience, attention, and emotion influence pain response and perception by acting on the gate control system. The balance between sensory facilitation and central inhibition of the input after peripheral-nerve lesion could account for the variability of pain even in cases of severe nerve injury.

The recent discovery that the small visceral afferents project directly or indirectly into lamina 5 cells provides gate control theory with still further power in explaining referred pain. It is evident that the phenomenon of referred pain is not simply a mislocation of the origin of a visceral afferent barrage. Somewhere in the nervous system there must be a convergence and summation of nerve impulses from the diseased viscera and from the area of skin to which the pain is referred. The pain is exaggerated if skin is touched in the area where the pain is located. Local anesthesia of skin to which pain is referred abolishes or diminishes the pain. Many theories have suggested possible locations for the convergence between cutaneous and visceral afferents. Lamina 5 cells exhibit this convergence and are monosynaptically connected to visceral afferents. They are therefore good candidates for explaining the phenomenon of referred pain as well as pain of direct cutaneous origin. Both inhibitory and excitatory interactions exist between the converging visceral and cutaneous inputs, which would account for both inhibitory and excitatory interactions at the clinical perceptual level, although the particular conditions necessary for each is not yet clear.

The role of the autonomic nervous system in pain is also comprehensible in terms of gate control theory. There are obvious signs in a number of severe pain syndromes such as causalgia and Raynaud's disease that the sympathetic system plays a role in pain and, indeed, sympathectomy may abolish the pain [20].

There are three possible mechanisms of autonomic action. (1) Neurohumoral substances released by autonomic efferent activity may change the sensitivity of afferent nerve endings. In the frog there is good evidence that this is the case. In mammalian skin we have indirect evidence that the effect, if present, must be small because sensitivities of particular endings have been shown to be stable over long periods of time and in the presence of various anesthetics which would be expected to vary the sympathetic outflow. (2) The removal of normal pain-producing metabolites such as bradykinin, which are associated with tissue breakdown, are controlled by local circulation which in turn is affected by the autonomic nervous system. Thus, part of the analgesic effect of sympathectomy in such conditions as intermittent claudication and Raynaud's disease may be the consequence of the vasodilation produced by the abolition of sympathetic activity. (3) Somatic afferents pass through the sympathetic ganglia. When sympathetic ganglia are surgically removed or blocked by local anesthesia, an important group of small myelinated and unmyelinated afferent fibers are destroyed in addition to the efferent fibers. Chemical sympathectomy affects only the efferents. Where pains are not relieved by chemical sympathectomy but are relieved by surgical sympathectomy, it seems reasonable to conclude that the pain was produced by the afferents passing through the ganglia and not by any efferent control of peripheral sensitivity. All three of these possibilities imply changes in the *number* of impulses per unit time that impinge on lamina 5 cells. Thus, the autonomic nervous system may act directly or indirectly on receptor-fiber sensitivity and central cell activity levels. In either case the tendency to summation and facilitation are increased, with an attendant increased probability that the critical level necessary to trigger pain will be exceeded.

Gate control theory has important implications for pain control. Neurosurgery represents only one method of pain control, and not necessarily the best one. Noordenbos [38] has noted that neurosurgical section of so-called pain pathways in the spinal cord produces a high proportion of failures, particularly in attempts to control the neuralgias, causalgia, and phantom limb pain. He has specifically labeled the phenomenon *the leak* and has proposed that the diffuse multisynaptic connections of the anterolateral pathways (Fig. 2C) are such that "the leak" is almost inevitable. To be sure, surgical section of the anterolateral pathway cuts down the number of centrally conducting fibers, which would decrease the summation of inputs at brainstem or higher levels. Control of pain from cancer, however, while often effective, frequently fails. Nathan [37] notes that bilateral or unilateral cordotomy (astonishingly, the former is not more effective than the latter) produces good relief of pain in about 50 percent of patients and only fair relief in 25 percent. A full 25 percent of patients are not significantly helped. Even more important, however, is the frequency of undesired side effects, such as loss of urinary control, dysesthesias, and so on. Nathan notes that these are sufficiently frequent and unpleasant that they should induce the neurosurgeon to try all other possibilities before proceeding with surgical intervention. There is, therefore, a need for other approaches, and gate control theory has implications for pharmacological, sensory, and psychological control of pain.

Pharmacological control of pain

Pharmacological agents may act at a variety of levels in the nervous system. They may act at the receptor level, at the level of the dorsal horn, or at higher levels such as the brainstem. A given drug may possibly act at all three sites.

Analgesics that act at peripheral receptors would presumably have the effect of decreasing the amount of their output. Inflammation is associated with tissue breakdown, swelling, vasodilation, and pain. Neither the swelling nor the vasodilation seems to be sufficient to cause the pain. Active research is now in progress to detect and analyze tissue and serum breakdown products which cause pain [19]. Aspirin and phenylbutazone appear to antagonize the action of one of these compounds—bradykinin (which produces pain when injected into the body)—at the receptors [19]. It is not known how this interaction occurs but it may be that the accumulation of the substance is prevented rather than that there is a direct interaction at receptor sites. Similarly the analgesic effect of cortisone occurs presumably because it prevents the appearance or the accumulation of the compounds. Knowledge of the actual nature of the compounds will become particularly important because it will offer the possibility of preventing their synthesis by the body or of flooding the region with a competitive blocking agent which would occupy the receptor sites without producing nerve impulses. Such compounds would be true peripheral analgesics, as would be drugs which speeded the destruction of pain-producing substances.

Drugs may also affect the transmission of input at the spinal cord level. The gate control model suggests that a better understanding of the substantia gelatinosa may lead to new ways of controlling pain. The resistance of the substantia gelatinosa to nerve cell stains suggests that its chemistry differs from that of other neural tissue. Drugs affecting excitation or inhibition of substantia gelatinosa activity may be of particular importance in future attempts to control pain. There is already some evidence on the effects of pharmacological agents on gate control mechanisms. There are three ways in which anesthetics might be acting at the level of the dorsal horns: (1) by decreasing the excitatory effect of individual impulses, (2) by increasing the inhibitory effect of individual impulses, or (3) by disorganizing the spatial and temporal pattern of bombardment. These are not alternative modes of action; all three may be found to occur simultaneously. Recently, Mendell and Wall [34] have demonstrated that the purely positive dorsal root potential evoked by C fibers is completely abolished by light anesthetic doses of barbiturate. Thus, the positive effect exerted by the C fibers via the substantia gelatinosa, which normally facilitates the transmission of input from peripheral fibers to T cells, is abolished, permitting maximal presynaptic and postsynaptic inhibition and a reduction of the afferent barrage below the critical level necessary for pain. De Jong and Wagman [6] have also reported that halothane produces a marked suppression of activity in cells in the dorsal horns.

The effects of anesthetics and analgesics on transmission in the reticular formation is well documented. Nitrous oxide, at analgesic levels, strikingly diminishes the amplitude of potentials evoked in the midbrain reticular formation by supramaximal stimulation of the toothpulp [12]. The powerful effects of barbiturates and other anesthetics at this level have been described and evaluated by French et al. [9]. At least part of the effects on pain may be the prevention of summation of sensory inputs so that the critical level necessary to trigger pain reactions is not exceeded.

Sensory control of pain

Interactions between sensory inputs have long been used as a method to control pain. Scratching to relieve itch, application of mustard plasters to decrease chest pain, and acupuncture fall into this category. The gate control model suggests that control of pain may be achieved by selectively enhancing the large-fiber input. Thus, Livingston [21] found that causalgia could be effectively cured by therapy such as bathing the limb in gently moving water, followed by massage, which would increase the input in the large-fiber system. Similarly, Trent [46] reports a case of pain of central nervous system origin which could be brought under control when the patient tapped his fingers on a hard surface.

The control of itch by scratching or vibration provides further evidence of these effects. Vibration, like scratching, decreases the perceived intensity of mild or moderate itch, but may turn severe itch into frank pain [29, 48]. Melzack, Wall, and Weisz [33] also examined the interaction between a single brief pressure stimulus and a single brief electric shock. It was found that the pressure pulse raised the threshold for the detection of the occurrence of the electric shock and for the level at which the shock produced a sharp pricking sensation. However, if the strength of the electric shock was further raised so that it produced severe pain, then the pressure stimulus increased the severity of the pain. It is therefore apparent that there is a complex interaction between pressure stimuli and painful electrical stimuli. The inhibitory effect of the pressure stimulus was the same if it preceded or if it followed the electrical stimulus by 50 milliseconds. This phenomenon, which is called *metacontrast,* shows that the decision to trigger pain reactions is not made by an instantaneous reading of the arriving information but must involve a prolonged analysis of the incoming signals. The extent to which spatial summation mechanisms are involved is indicated by the fact that vibration of the wrist of one hand decreases itch intensity experienced at the wrist of the other hand [29].

These interactions between sensory inputs also help make sense of the puzzling phenomena produced by stimulation of the skin with very small-diameter tactile or thermal probes. Touching the skin, particularly the lip, with a von Frey hair frequently sets off a tingling or afterflow sensation that may persist for several minutes [27]. The afterflow sometimes spreads beyond the site of stimulation, and occasionally the mirror-area on the other side of the lip may begin to tingle. There is characteristically a delay in the onset of the afterglow. These effects are even more pronounced when a small-diameter warm probe stimulates the skin. The afterglow appears after a delay, wells up into a sharp stinging pain, and persists long after stimulation. Stimulation of a larger area of skin with a probe of the same temperature produces only reports of warmth sensation. These effects are not found uniformly across the skin, but only in particular regions, which may vary in location from one testing period to the next [28]. The tendency for these effects to occur is diminished if the skin is vibrated immediately before stimulation with the probes.

These effects of delay, spread, aftersensations, and unusual, unpleasant sensory qualities are reminiscent of the properties of the neuralgias, and it is interesting to speculate that the underlying mechanisms may be essentially alike. Lamina 5 cells receive, directly or indirectly, inputs from the A-delta as well as the A-beta fibers (Fig. 3B). These connections provide the large triple receptive field previously described. It is possible, then, that from time to time a small-diameter stimulus would activate the predominantly excitatory center of the three superimposed fields with minimal stimulation of the inhibitory peripheral region. As we have already noted in the foregoing discussion of neuralgia, the decreased inhibitory influence would tend to open the dorsal horn "gate," which would be the basis for delayed, long-lasting, hyperesthetic sensations.

One of the most exciting applications of the principle of sensory interaction is Wall and Sweet's [49] investigation of the effect of electrical stimulation of large diameter nerve fibers originating from a painful region. The stimulation, which is just above threshold and causes a mild tingling sensation, interferes with the perception of pain.

In patients with peripheral nerve lesions, the effect of 10 minutes of stimulation may last for a half-hour or more. In patients with carcinoma, the pain was blocked but returned shortly after stimulation. This method, we believe, holds great promise as an effective tool for the control of pain.

Psychological control of pain

Finally, it is important to recognize the role of cognitive or "higher central nervous system" activities such as anxiety, attention, and suggestion in pain processes. The model suggests that psychological factors such as past experience, attention, and emotion influence pain response and perception by acting on the gate control system. The degree of central control, however, would be determined, in part at least, by the temporal-spatial properties of the input patterns. Some of the most unbearable pains, such as cardiac pain, rise so rapidly in intensity that the patient is unable to achieve any control over them. On the other hand, more slowly rising temporal patterns are susceptible to central control and may allow the patient to "think about something else" or use other stratagems to keep the pain under control.

It is clear that the surgical and pharmacological attack on pain might well profit by redirecting thinking toward the neglected and almost forgotten contributions of motivational and cognitive processes. Pain can be treated not only by trying to cut down the sensory input by anesthetic block, surgical intervention, and the like, but also by influencing the motivational-affective and cognitive factors as well. Relaxants, tranquillizers, sedatives, suggestion, placebos, and hypnosis are known to exert a profound influence on pain [1], but the historical emphasis on sensory mechanisms and the relative neglect of the motivational and cognitive contributions to pain has made these forms of therapy suspect, seemingly fraudulent, almost a sideshow in the mainstream of pain treatment. Yet, if we can recover from historical accident, these methods deserve more attention than they have received.

REFERENCES

1. Beecher, H. K. *Measurement of Subjective Responses.* New York: Oxford University Press, 1959.
2. Bishop, G. H. The relation between nerve fiber size and sensory modality: Phylogenetic implications of the afferent innervation of cortex. *J. Nerv. Ment. Dis.* 128:89, 1959.
3. Burgess, P. R., and Perl, E. R. Myelinated afferent fibres responding specifically to noxious stimulation of the skin. *J. Physiol.* (London) 190:541, 1967.
4. Conant, J. B. *On Understanding Science,* New York: Mentor Books, 1951.
5. Dallenbach, K. M. Pain: History and present status. *Amer. J. Psychol.* 52:331, 1939.
6. de Jong, R. H., and Wagman, I. H. Block of afferent impulses in the dorsal horn of monkey: A possible mechanism of anesthesia. *Exp. Neurol.* 20: 352, 1968.
7. Dilly, P. N., Wall, P. D., and Webster, K. E. Cells of origin of the spinothalamic tract in cat or rat. *Exp. Neurol.* 21:550, 1968.
8. Earle, K. M. Tract of Lissauer and its possible relation to the pain pathway. *J. Comp. Neurol.* 96: 93, 1952.
9. French, J. D., Verzeano, M., and Magoun, W. H. Neural basis of anesthetic state. *A.M.A. Arch. Neurol. Psychiat.* 69:519, 1953.
10. Goldscheider, A. *Ueber den Schmerz in Physiologischer und Klinischer Hinsicht.* Berlin: Hirschwald, 1894.
11. Hagbarth, K. E., and Kerr, D. I. B. Central influences on spinal afferent conduction. *J. Neurolphysiol.* 17:295, 1954.
12. Haugen, F. P., and Melzack, R. Effects of nitrous oxide on responses evoked in the brainstem by tooth stimulation. *Anesthesiology* 18:183, 1957.
13. Head, H. *Studies in Neurology.* London: Kegan Paul, 1920.
14. Heimer, L., and Wall, P. D. Dorsal root distribution to the substantia gelatinosa in the rat with a note on the distribution in the cat. *Exp. Brain Res.* 6:89, 1968.
15. Hillman, P., and Wall, P. D. Inhibitory and excitatory factors influencing the receptive fields of lamina 5 spinal cord cells. *Exp. Brain Res.*
16. Kerr, D. I. B., Haugen, F. P., and Melzack, R. Responses evoked in the brainstem by tooth stimulation. *Amer. J. Physiol.* 183:253, 1955.
17. Kerr, F. W. L., and Miller, R. H. The ultrastructural pathology of trigeminal neuralgia. *Arch. Neurol.* (Chicago) 15:308, 1966.
18. Lewis, T. *Pain.* New York: Macmillan, 1942.
19. Lim, R. K. S. Neuropharmacology of Pain and Analgesia. In R. K. S. Lim, D. Armstrong, and E. G. Pardo (Eds.), *Pharmacology of Pain.* London: Pergamon, 1968.
20. Livingston, W. K. *Pain Mechanisms.* New York: Macmillan, 1943.
21. Livingston, W. K. The vicious circle in causalgia. *Ann. N. Y. Acad. Sci.* 50:247, 1948.
22. Lundberg, A. Supraspinal control of transmission in reflex paths to motoneurons and primary afferents. *Progr. Brain Res.* 12:197, 1964.
23. MacCarty, C. S., and Drake, R. L. Neurosurgical

procedures for the control of pain. *Proc. Staff Meetings Mayo Clin.* 31:208, 1956.

24. McDonald, W. I. The effects of experimental demyelination on conduction in peripheral nerve: A histological and electrophysiological study. II. Electrophysiological observations. *Brain* 86:501, 1963.
25. Mark, V. H., Ervin, F. R., and Yakovlev, P. I. Stereotactic thalamotomy. *Arch. Neurol.* (Chicago) 8:528, 1963.
26. Melzack, R., and Casey, K. L. Sensory, Motivational, and Central Control Determinants of Pain: A New Conceptual Model. In D. Kenshalo (Ed.), *The Skin Senses.* Springfield, Ill.: Thomas, 1968.
27. Melzack, R., and Eisenberg, H. Skin sensory afterflows. *Science* 159:445, 1968.
28. Melzack, R., Rose, G., and McGinty, D. Skin sensitivity to thermal stimuli. *Exp. Neurol.* 6:300, 1962.
29. Melzack, R., and Schecter, B. Itch and vibration. *Science* 147:1047, 1965.
30. Melzack, R., Stotler, W. A., and Livingston, W. K. Effects of discrete brainstem lesions in cats on perception of noxious stimulation. *J. Neurophysiol.* 21:353, 1958.
31. Melzack, R., and Wall, P. D. On the nature of cutaneous sensory mechanisms. *Brain* 85:331, 1962.
32. Melzack, R., and Wall, P. D. Pain mechanisms: A new theory. *Science* 150:971, 1965.
33. Melzack, R., Wall, P. D., and Weisz, A. Z. Masking and metacontrast phenomena in the skin sensory system. *Exp. Neurol.* 8:35, 1963.
34. Mendell, L. M., and Wall, P. D. Presynaptic hyperpolarization: A role for fine afferent fibers. *J. Physiol.* (London) 172:274, 1964.
35. Mendell, L. M., and Wall, P. D. Responses of single dorsal cord cells to peripheral cutaneous unmyelinated fibers. *Nature* (London) 206:97, 1965.
36. Nafe, J. P. The Pressure, Pain, and Temperature Senses. In C. Murchison (Ed.), *Handbook of General Experimental Psychology.* Worcester: Clark University Press, 1934.
37. Nathan, P. W. Results of anterolateral cordotomy for pain in cancer. *J. Neurol. Neurosurg. Psychiat.* 26:353, 1963.
38. Noordenbos, W. *Pain.* Amsterdam: Elsevier, 1959.
39. Scheibel, M. E., and Scheibel, A. B. Terminal axon patterns in cat spinal cord. II. Dorsal horn. *Brain Res.* 9:32, 1968.
40. Schmidt, R. F., Senges, J., and Zimmermann, M. Presynaptic depolarization of cutaneous mechanoreceptor afferents after mechanical skin stimulation. *Exp. Brain Res.* 3:234, 1967.
41. Semmes, J., and Mishkin, M. Somatosensory loss in monkeys after ipsilateral cortical ablation. *J. Neurophysiol.* 28:473, 1965.
42. Sherrington, C. S. Cutaneous Sensations. In E. A. Schäfer (Ed.), *Textbook of Physiology.* Edinburgh: Pentland, 1900.
43. Sinclair, D. C. Cutaneous sensation and the doctrine of specific nerve energy. *Brain* 78:584, 1955.
44. Sweet, W. H. Pain. In J. Field, H. W. Magoun, and V. E. Hall (Eds.), *Handbook of Physiology.* Sect. 1, Vol. 1, Chap. 19, pp. 459-506. Washington, D. C.: American Physiological Society, 1959.
45. Szentagothai, J. Neuronal and synaptic arrangement in the substantia gelatinosa rolandi. *J. Comp. Neurol.* 122:219, 1964.
46. Trent, S. E. Peripheral sensory inhibition of pain with a parietal lobe lesion. *J. Nerv. Ment. Dis.* 123:356, 1956.
47. Wall, P. D. The laminar organization of dorsal horn and effects of descending impulses. *J. Physiol.* (London) 188:403, 1967.
48. Wall, P. D., and Cronly-Dillon, J. R. Pain, itch and vibration. *Arch. Neurol.* (Chicago) 2:365, 1960.
49. Wall, P. D., and Sweet, W. H. Temporary abolition of pain in man. *Science* 155:108, 1967.
50. Weddell, G. Somesthesis and the chemical senses. *Ann. Rev. Psychol.* 6:119, 1955.
51. Zotterman, Y. Touch, pain and tickling: An electrophysiological investigation on cutaneous sensory nerves. *J. Physiol.* (London) 95:1, 1939.

2

Psychological aspects of pain

H. Merskey, M.A., D.M., D.P.M.

Interest in pain never ceases. The present survey is intended to indicate some of the main current psychiatric approaches to the elucidation and treatment of pain syndromes.

SIGNIFICANCE OF PAIN

'Unprofessional persons are always accustomed to associate together the ideas of pain and danger; yet the physician well knows that the most fatal maladies are often the least painful' (Williams, 1852). The author of this remark was an astute physician who distinguished between the pains of angina pectoris and neuralgia, by which he meant what would now be called effort syndrome or psychogenic pains. Despite such views, pain is normally held to be prima facie evidence of physical disease (Stengel, 1960). To anyone trained in biology and especially in neuro-anatomy and physiology it is natural to think of pain as evidence of some physical disturbance. Yet, as Williams and Stengel have pointed out, there is much to suggest that pain is often a sign of psychological disturbance. This is particularly true if headache is included in the discussion. As a symptom, it is very common particularly in psychiatric patients; thus 6.6% of all the patients in a general practice had headache (Carne, 1967) and 8.7% of a population of army recruits undergoing selection (Weider *et al.,* 1944), while its frequency rose to 48.7% in cases rejected by the U. S. services on psychiatric grounds. For this and other reasons it has been firmly suggested (Friedman *et al.,* 1962) that most headaches are psychological in origin. Further, in considering pain as a symptom affecting any part of the body, Klee *et al.* (1959) found that 61% of a series of psychiatric patients had pain and Spear (1964) obtained similar figures. In a medical clinic Devine & Merskey (1965) found that 38% of the patients with pain and 40% of those without pain were there because of psychological illness. These findings tend to confirm what the experienced clinician has always recognized: that something which is called 'pain' is a result of emotional disturbance in at least a substantial minority of patients. A review of the literature (Merskey & Spear, 1967b) suggests that this is probably true in many different branches of medicine and surgery.

It has also long been recognized that emotional factors could abate the severity of pain or abolish it altogether, despite the presence of extensive wounds. Montaigne (1580) wrote 'We feel one cut from the surgeon's scalpel more than ten blows of the sword in the heat of battle'. Baron Larrey (cit. Chertok, 1959) observed a similar indifference to wounds by soldiers during the Napoleonic wars and comparable observations have been made by many others, either about battle (Mitchell, Morehouse & Keen, 1864) or other exciting situations (Kraepelin, 1903; Rivers, 1920). In particular, Beecher (1956) showed in a systematic study that wounded soldiers, for whom the wound represented an honourable release from danger, were far less in need of analgesics than civilians with lesions of comparable size, for whom the

Reprinted with permission of Blackwell Scientific Publications LTD. from the Postgraduate Medical Journal, **44:**297-306. Copyright 1968.
Physician in Psychological Medicine, The National Hospital for Nervous Diseases, Queen Square, London, W. C.1.

lesions represented a largely unwelcome disturbance of their normal lives. Some of the difference between soldiers and civilians may be due to different effects from injuries due to high-speed missiles as compared with surgery. There are indications that high-speed injuries are less painful than others (Livingston, 1966) but this cannot account for all the situations reported. Thus far it can be said with certainty that psychological factors quite often cause pain and frequently augment its severity. They may also serve to abate or abolish it even in the presence of extensive physical trauma. These considerations have an important bearing on what we mean by pain.

It is a commonplace experience to hear doctors talking of pain arising at nerve-endings, passing along pain fibres, travelling up the spinothalamic tracts and reaching higher centres. Walters (1963) points out, in effect, that no such thing happens. Certainly noxious stimulation affects the activity of these parts—although not perhaps so specifically as we used to think (Weddell, 1962; Noordenbos, 1959; Melzack & Wall, 1965). But pain is always a psychological event. It is something we talk about as part of our experience. As Walters indicates, the impulses in the pain fibres and tracts 'are no more the pain than the visual impulses from the retina are the perceptual fields of color and pattern that present to us when our eyes are open'. Szasz (1957), in an important theoretical discussion from the psychoanalytic aspect, takes the same view. It is therefore preferable always to talk of 'noxious stimulation' rather than painful stimulation, despite the convenience of the latter expression.

This argument may seem abstract, but ignoring it leads to trouble. It leads to doctors telling patients, who are convinced they have pain, that they do not have it because no organic disorder has been found. Most clinicians are familiar with the unfortunate and avoidable consequences of making this error. If so, they may well find it helpful to agree that the patient has an experience which to him is pain, even though no causative physical mechanism seems likely. It may be easier to do so in the light of the evidence that psychological factors are so common as causes for pain. It has accordingly been argued (Merskey, 1964; Merskey & Spear, 1967a, b) that an operational definition of pain should be adopted as follows: 'An unpleasant experience which we primarily associate with tissue damage or describe in terms of such damage, or both'. This emphasizes the relationship of pain with the experience of damage to the body and, without making any assumptions as to causes, it provides a framework whereby the statements of patients who describe bodily experiences like burning, aching, stabbing, etc., can be assessed, investigated and compared. It follows that by 'psychogenic pain' one should mean pain whose causes are mainly or wholly psychological and by 'organic pain' one means pain whose principal causes are physical. There is no necessary difference between these cases in the subjective experience which the sufferer attempts to describe. In each case it is felt as being like the experience of damage to the body. As a corollary to these views it is worth mentioning that 'mental pain' is a metaphorical expression and does not connote any experience of bodily damage. It is thus distinct from 'psychogenic pain'.

MECHANISMS OF PSYCHOGENIC PAIN

Three principal mechanisms are recognized in the psychological aetiology of pain. The first, which is relatively rare, is the occurrence of pain as a hallucination, in association either with schizophrenia or endogenous depression (Michaux, 1957; Schneider, 1959; Bleuler, 1960). Most psychiatrists have seen one or two instances of this. In schizophrenia the pain is usually one of a number of other delusional experiences, e.g. that the body is changing in size or being interfered with or that electricity or radar is being directed at the patient. Similarly, in endogenous depression any such hallucinatory pain, occurring independently of a physical mechanism, is usually part of a well-defined syndrome. Occasionally with these illnesses pain is the sole definite symptom and the diagnosis can only be made after some fresh development has occurred in the illness.

The second mechanism or group of mechanisms in psychogenic pain is represented by pain due to muscle tension where that tension itself is due to psychological causes. Another variant on the same theme is the pain of vascular distension, as in migraine, where the process can be initiated by psychological factors.

Sound evidence has been available for some years to suggest that pain often originates by such psychosomatic processes (Wolff, 1948). This evidence has not been seriously challenged. Indeed, investigators have continued to present data (Malmo & Shagass, 1949; Malmo, Shagass & Davis, 1951) that anxiety gives rise to local muscle contraction which, if persistent, causes pain. The possible chemical mediator of these processes is still in doubt (Elkind & Friedman, 1962; Wolff, 1966). Perhaps some of these mechanisms have been used too widely in explanation since demonstrable myographic differences only account for part of the variance in the experimental studies quoted, but it is easy to see how tempting this type of explanation must be, particularly when many headaches and other pains are undoubtedly relieved by reassurance, relaxation and sedatives.

The third main possible psychological mechanism is that of conversion hysteria. The concepts of hysteria and of the unconscious owe much to Freud (Breuer & Freud, 1893-95) but did not originate with him. Brodie (1837) of Brodie's abscess fame, said that 'In upper-class women' four-fifths of joint-pains were hysterical, and claimed that 'fear, suggestion and unconscious stimulation were the primary factors'. This is quite representative of other comments scattered through the literature of the last two centuries (cf. Veith, 1965).

It is of particular interest that, in the four women whom Freud described fully in his first essays on hysteria, pain was a prominent symptom. However, the actual frequency of hysteria as a cause of pain is very difficult to assess. Although the validity of the diagnosis of hysteria has been disputed (Slater, 1965) and it certainly carries hazards, there is some evidence that hysterical mechanisms are important in the development at least of persistent pain in psychiatric patients. What is of considerable importance is the idea that a pain may arise not as a result of any physiological process but by an intelligible chain of psychological events. There is also good evidence that there is a group of hypochondriacal patients whom most psychiatrists would recognize as having hysteria and in whom pain is a prominent symptom (Guze & Perley, 1963). It has to be noted that in these cases with intractable hypochondriasis the current sources of emotional conflict are sometimes few and the theory that a conflict exists has to be based upon assumptions about the patients' earlier experiences, particularly in childhood, which are not always demonstrable. But the pattern of the symptoms and the patient's personality can indicate a resemblance with those hysterical symptoms whose causes are more accessible.

Perhaps the most striking illustration of pain as a symptom solving unconscious conflicts and serving to symbolize unconscious attitudes is the couvade syndrome. This word, derived from the Basque, *couver,* meaning to sit on eggs, describes the behaviour of fathers who may act as if suffering from labour pains or lie in bed after their wives' childbirth while the women continue with their normal occupations. Such behaviour occurs in many cultures, is well known to anthropologists and was discussed in some detail by Reik (1914). It is not so attractive to the father as it may sound since many rules of abstinence may have to be observed by him. The term has also been used to cover pains and other physical complaints without organic basis which are found in expectant fathers. As such, the couvade syndrome is still known to occur in Indians of many different social levels (Bardhan, 1965a, b), in mining communities (Dennis, Henriques & Slaughter, 1965; P. Crann, personal communication, 1965) and in modern urban society (Curtis, 1955; Trethowan & Conlon, 1965). The latter authors gave a useful description of some cases and showed a significant incidence of such symptoms in a survey. The point about this syndrome, relevant to our present discussion, is again to emphasize the psychogenesis of pain as a symptom felt to occur in the body and yet not owing its existence to any physiologic mechanism. Having reiterated this possibility we can now consider the particular psychiatric diagnoses with which pain is most associated.

PAIN DUE TO PSYCHIATRIC ILLNESS

It has been indicated that schizophrenia may be accompanied by hallucinations of pain but this is rare. In several other common psychiatric illnesses pain abounds. Thus it is a frequent symptom in neurotic depression, in anxiety states and in hysteria. It does not have such a marked association with obsessional neurosis, the organic confusional states, subnormality, psychopathic personality nor, as a spontaneous symptom, with the sexual perversions.

In many instances of course the pain considered is usually transient and responds to suitable reassurance with or without sedation. Or, once it has been established that the problem is psychiatric, attention is directed away from the symptom of pain while appropriate treatment is instituted and the pain then usually resolves with the illness.

The largest series of psychiatric patients with pain has been described by Walters (1961) who reported on 430 cases seen for intractable pain. As in other series, the head and neck were the commonest site. Walters distinguished three separate ways in which psychological factors can evoke pain, as follows:

1. Psychogenic magnification of physical pain.
2. Psychogenic muscular pain (as a result of tension).
3. Psychogenic regional pain.

He recommends this last term in place of the older one of hysterical pain because these patients do not conform to the traditional picture of calm and contented hysteria. They are often depressed and anxious even though they may have some form of conversion symptom.

The writer considers this classification only partly satisfactory. The first category is acceptable but lends itself too readily to the concepts of a small, real 'organic' pain which is 'exaggerated' for psychological reasons. It must be acknowledged, however, that no more satisfactory term has been offered for this common situation which the category describes. The second category is acceptable but the third is the least satisfactory. Pain which fulfills the third set of criteria may be capable of inclusion under the other two. Walters' article is well worth attention, however, for the clinical data it contains, e.g. the finding that the descriptions of pain are often not dramatic (a point made also by Wilson, 1938, Gittleson, 1961, and Devine & Merskey, 1965). In addition, it gives a realistic and helpful picture of the way in which a combination of both general medical and psychiatric techniques of assessment is necessary and the ways in which psychiatric treatment is beneficial.

At the other end of the scale there has been a very large number of papers describing the psychodynamics and treatment of individual patients with chronic pain of psychological origin. Hart (1947) and Merskey & Spear (1967b) list most of these and discuss their implications. The authors considered generally see the condition as some form of hysteria but do not offer systematic or comparative evidence in favour of their views. They also emphasize the association of pain with resentment and guilt.

Menninger (1938) gave more evidence of the masochistic attitudes of these patients and stressed the frequency with which they underwent unnecessary operations. Greenacre (1939) made the same points in a very telling description of a single case.

A further contribution has been made by Engel (1951, 1959) who described twenty patients (nineteen of them women) with facial pain. He regarded his subjects as suffering from an hysterical conversion symptom but he emphasized that they possessed a 'masochistic' character structure, showing many varieties of self-punitive behaviour, i.e. behaviour which repeatedly placed them in unhappy situations. Like Menninger and Greenacre he stressed the frequency with which his patients underwent unnecessary operations. He also noted the gusto with which they would tolerate pain due to physical causes. This approach requires some change in the commonly held idea that psychiatric patients are more 'sensitive' to pain, even though that idea is undoubtedly partly justified. In his later paper, Engel (1959) named this type of patient the pain-prone patient. Although there is no direct comparison with other patients the volume of evidence which Engel describes supports his argument well.

In order to try and clarify which psychiatric patients were liable to pain, to obtain more data on them and to obtain some check on the foregoing theories, the writer (Merskey, 1964, 1965a, b) examined a series of 100 psychiatric patients with persistent pain and compared them with a stratified control sample of sixty-five patients who denied having pain in association with their illness. It was found that the commonest association of persistent pain in psychiatric illness was with hysteria, anxiety neurosis and neurotic depression. Although there were patients with endogenous depression and with schizophrenia who had persistent pain it was relatively less common with those diagnoses. Whilst the material was not confined like Engel's to patients with facial pain this provides systematic support for his general views. A study by Spear (1964) both confirms and complements these findings. Spear had studied psychiatric patients with and without pain but had included patients whose pain was not persistent. He, too, found pain to be associated relatively more often with diagnoses of hysteria and anxiety than with the psychoses.

PERSONALITY CHARACTERISTICS AND PAIN

It has been indicated that certain attitudes, frequently unconscious, have been attributed to patients with pain of psychological origin. These attitudes include hostility, resentment and guilt. Knopf (1935a, b) was one of the first to suggest that these traits occurred in those migrainous subjects who were liable to have their headache precipitated by psychological factors. Wolff (1948) supported these views. Largely similar attitudes have, however, been attributed not only to patients with pain in any part of the body but also to patients with asthma, eczema, dysmenorrhoea, ulcerative colitis and the other supposedly psychosomatic illnesses as well as to a number of frank psychiatric illnesses. It therefore seems desirable to know whether these particular factors are more pronounced in patients with psychogenic pain than in others. There is no doubt that they are prominent in some instances and that this is sometimes due to mutual antagonism developing between patients and doctors, as a vivid paper by Bender (1964) bears witness. Spear (1964) looked for the expression of overt or covert hostility and found no difference between psychiatric patients with pain and those without. Similarly, the writer (Mersky, 1965b) found no difference in actual acts of aggression in such groups. Merskey did find, however, that spoken expressions of resentment were more common in his patients with pain. In four out of thirty instances this resentment was directed exclusively at doctors, in nine at doctors and others impartially and in seventeen at others to the exclusion of doctors. Another study with positive results was made by Eisenbud (1937). During treatment of a man suffering from amnesia and headaches he concluded that this particular patient was unconsciously hostile to his father. Since this hostility was unacceptable to the patient's conscious mind he was liable to be made anxious and hence to develop conversion symptoms under any circumstance that might bring it to light. One such event was his father's admission to hospital and the headache this caused was relieved by abreaction under hypnosis which permitted a subsequent conscious adjustment to the problem. Eisenbud then conducted a careful series of experiments to test the hypothesis that unconscious hostility would cause headache, but not other unconscious conflict. He did this by inducing 'artificial complexes' under hypnosis. It turned out that hostile or aggressive complexes did have this effect in his patient but not erotic ones. The limited systematic evidence that is available does thus suggest that resentment and, to a lesser extent, hostility are specially relevant to the hysterical type of pain. But it is not clear whether hostility and guilt are markedly more relevant to pain than to other psychiatric and psychosomatic complaints.

Other characteristics to which pain has been related include low social class, low ordinal position in the family, frigidity, dysmenorrhoea and other psychogenic bodily complaints. In many studies, not just those concerned with pain, it has been shown that the chronic clinic attender or patient with persistent pain is of low social status—most characteristically from an economic level equivalent to social classes 3 and 4 of the Registrar-General's classification (Ruesch, 1946; Hollingshead & Redlich, 1958; Srole *et al.*, 1962; Gonda, 1962). This applies even when correction is made for selection factors as in the American epidemiological studies by Hollingshead & Redlich and by Srole *et al.*, and has been interpreted as meaning that the less sophisticated patients will tend to visit the doctor and express depression or emotional conflict in 'body language' rather than in psychological terms. Even this view has its limitations, however, for Baker & Merskey (1967) taking all forms of pain—acute and chronic—found no social class-difference in the distribution of pain in patients in a semirural general practice. As to birth order, the claim that this is relevant (Gonda, 1962) has not been confirmed (Spear, 1964). Birth-order investigation in fact, while one of the most superficially attractive topics in psychiatric research, has produced sadly conflicting results. Frigidity, however, is traditionally associated with hysteria and seems likely to be relevant (Merskey, 1965b; Kreitman *et al.*, 1965). In regard to dysmenorrhoea neither Spear nor the writer found a significant excess of this symptom in patients with psychogenic pain but other work (e.g. Kessel & Coppen, 1963) leaves little doubt that some association does exist between dysmenorrhoea and psychiatric illness and may be shown by different survey methods.

In summarizing this section it may be helpful to say that while there are numerous variations on the basic theme the most typical psychiatric patient with pain is a married woman of the working or lower-middle class, possibly once pretty and appealing, but never keen on sexual intercourse, now faded and complaining, with a history of repeated negative physical examinations and investigations, frank conversion symptoms in up to 50% of cases in addition to the pain, and a sad tale of a hard life; together with depression which does not respond to antidepressant drugs. But anyone who relies too literally on this pen-picture for the purpose of diagnosis does so at his own risk. It represents a statistical mode amongst the clinical patterns, from which actual patients will frequently diverge.

APPENDICECTOMY AND NEUROSIS

Appendicectomy and neurosis is a problem of particular interest to the surgeon. Experienced surgeons (e.g. Hinton, 1948) and gynaecologists (e.g. Atlee, 1966) are prone to emphasize the importance of psychological causes of acute abdominal pain. Hinton indeed gives the following list of its causes:

'(1) Anxiety neuroses with conversion symptoms or other psychogenic factors.

(2) Physiologic conditions such as painful ovulation.

(3) True organic diseases which require surgical care.'

Nevertheless, a history of appendicectomy has been reported as occurring frequently in patients with abdominal pain in association with neurotic illness (Crohn, 1930). Lee (1961), in a statistical study, concluded that there was an excess of such operations, especially in young women, and that some 7000-8000 unnecessary appendicectomies were performed annually in England and Wales. Harding (1962) concluded that 39.6% of a series of 1300 appendices examined histologically were completely normal, and the proportion of normal appendices removed approached two-thirds in females aged between 11 and 20 years. Wallace, Loane & Quinn (1963) obtained similar data and Ingram, Evans & Oppenheim (1965) considered that unsatisfactory results were obtained in those patients who had had normal appendices removed.

Most of this could easily have been predicted in the light of a paper by Blanton & Kirk (1947) where sixty-one patients were studied for the presence of psychological disturbance and organic pathology. Of forty-four patients with an organic pathology thirteen were emotionally disturbed. The remaining seventeen with normal appendices all had psychiatric conditions. A chisquare computation of these figures shows a significant association of neurosis and normal appendices at the level $P < 0.001$. But the thirteen neurotics with diseased appendices highlight the clinician's problem. A similar but less urgent problem has been demonstrated by Apley

(1959) in respect of children with recurrent abdominal pain. Here the experience of pain can clearly be seen to be a learnt response – often patterned on parental attitudes.

PSYCHOLOGICAL THEORIES OF PAIN

Spear (1966) points out that psychiatric work to date has led to the development of three main theories of pain. In the first it is suggested that pain is a consequence of hostility (Eisenbud, 1937; Weiss, 1947; Engel, 1951, 1956), in the second that pain arises in patients of a certain personality-type who use the complaint as a means of communication (Engel, 1958, 1959). Mention has already been made of these theories. The third approach comes from Szasz (1957) who argues that pain arises as a consequence of a threat to the integrity of the body. Here the body is regarded as an object of concern to the self. The threat may not be apparent to an outside observer and the pain will then be classed as 'psychogenic'. These theories are not mutually exclusive and are all wholly psychological, i.e. they attempt to deal with pain as a psychological event in relation to those other psychological events which cause it The theory of Szasz, in particular, utilizes the Freudian concepts of ego, id and super-ego, the ego being the part of the mind which relates both to the forces of the other two systems and to external reality. Szasz suggests that the ego perceives the body as an object and postulates that pain arises when a threat to the body is perceived, either for objective reasons or for emotional ones. The question of whether the symptom is considered organic or functional depends on the observer's assessment of the reality of the threat to the body.

Once this assessment has been made the meaning of the symptom can be considered and it is postulated that this meaning may be interpreted at three levels of symbolization. At the first level the communications are facts having to do with the sufferer's experience of the bodily symptom. At the next level pain is used as a communication which requests help. This function is always involved in any complaint of pain, the two levels being inextricably bound. Communication at the third level of symbolization is more complex and here pain can persist as a symbol of rejection, the repetition of the complaint may become a form of aggression and the continued experience of pain may serve to expiate guilt.

If these hypotheses are looked at together it would seem that Engel's views fit well as a subtheory within the system of Szasz. It has been seen that some of Engel's arguments have had factual confirmation. The same is true for Szasz's concepts. In particular it has been shown (Spear, 1966) that psychiatric patients with pain show more concern with their physical health and bodily state than others who do not experience pain as part of their illness; and this concern is wider than the single symptom of pain.

Perhaps the most important aspect of the theory of Szasz is that it emphasizes the communicative significance of pain. This is something long recognized and liable to be forgotten and re-discovered by successive generations of doctors. Further, while the reader who is unaccustomed to psychoanalytic models may have found the theory difficult to follow, it does have the merit of clarifying the logical status and semantics of pain. Anyone who has thoroughly absorbed Szasz's argument is thus less liable to make the sort of errors which Walters (1963) has criticized. As a practical corollary the theory of Szasz leads to an examination of the modes of description of pain and the function which these modes serve. Before doing so it should be mentioned that important current physiological theories of pain have been offered by Noordenbos (1959) and Melzack & Wall (1965) and that these theories can be reconciled with the psychological ones (Merskey & Spear, 1967b).

DESCRIPTIONS OF PAIN

Brain (1962) observed 'Our vocabulary for the description of pain is relatively poor and we tend to fall back on terms which describe a pain by describing the way in which it might have been produced, even though in the particular instance it has not been so produced. Thus we speak of pricking pain, stabbing pain, shooting pain, burning pain, bursting pain and so on'. The implication of damage to the body is obvious. Klein & Brown (1965) found that 58% of patients in a medical clinic used metaphors of violence to describe their pain. Descriptions of this sort are bound to be somewhat dramatic. It is often said that psychiatric patients use bizarre terms when they complain of pain. Dana (1911) gave a long list of such unusual descriptions, e.g. 'a pain in the ovary when excited, helmet sensation, sensations of the body being filled and stuffed with pricking burrs and a pricking as of pine-needles sticking out of the scalp'. As indicated in the discussion of Walters' work this view is not entirely confirmed. Thus Devine & Merskey (1965) found that only thirteen of 100 psychiatric patients with persistent pain (usually severe) gave notably bizarre descriptions of their pain and fifty-one gave very simple descriptions. The same authors noted in patients who attended a medical clinic that those with 'psychogenic' pain gave similar descriptions to those with 'organic' pain and some of the most odd descriptions were somatically strictly accurate, e.g. a patient with a rectal carcinoma spoke of a 'strong pain a few inches inside my seat—drawing the seat down as if I was going with it'. The worse a patient felt his pain to be, the more words and the more peculiar similes he used to describe it so that there was a statistically significant trend for patients who said their pain was severe to give more elaborate and complex descriptions of it than those who said their pain was mild. This after all is common sense. Severe pains will provoke far more attention than mild ones. The qualitative description of pain is thus likely to reflect the importance of the pain to the patient and how much it matters to him. It is an earnest of the degree of his concern—and not particularly likely to be a sign of its causation.

DIFFERENTIATION OF CAUSES OF PAIN

The qualitative description of pain is clearly an unreliable guide in differential diagnosis. The characteristics of pain of psychological origin which are most typical are as follows (Merskey & Spear, 1967b): Pain of psychological illness has never apparently been shown actually to rouse a patient from sleep. It is usually continuous from day to day (except at night) or else lasts upwards of 1 hr. It often involves more than one area of the body and it is commonest in the form of headache and often bilateral and symmetrical. Apart from the tendency not to disturb sleep, none of these characteristics is exclusive.

The differentiation of causes thus still depends upon clinical skill in establishing the presence of a valid physical or psychiatric diagnosis. Clearly the presence of positive physical signs (e.g. tenderness, spasm) or other evidence of physical disease is helpful. Similarly, positive evidence of psychiatric illness, the presence of the characteristics just outlined, evidence of the relevant personality traits discussed earlier and an appropriate response to psychiatric treatment may also be helpful. There are times, however, when neither physician, surgeon nor psychiatrist can find reliable evidence of a particular illness to account for a patient's pain. In these circumstances the best course is to suspend judgement, continue observation and treat the patient empirically with non-addictive analgesics.

TREATMENT

Progress both in diagnosis and treatment of chronic pain has been fostered in several centres by 'Pain Clinics' (McEwen *et al.*, 1965; Simpson *et al.*, 1965). These rely for their operation on regular consultation between several specialists, usually anaesthetists, neurosurgeons, radiotherapists and psychiatrists. Their work is evidently fruitful, as might be expected, since each of these disciplines has contributed much that is useful to the treatment of chronic pain. Anaesthetists have made a special contribution by extensive studies of the placebo response and the comparative effects of different drugs, again showing how much the abatement of fear may reduce pain. The same point is well recognized by those concerned with the care of the dying (Hinton, 1967) and of women in childbirth (Read, 1943; Chertok, 1959).

It has long been thought that hypnosis would modify or abolish pain at operation. There is reason to believe (Barber, 1958a, b) that hypnosis is not a special trance state but rather a situation in which the subject accepts the possibility of various unusual changes in his behaviour and then produces them on the suggestion of the hypnotist. Thus Barber (1963) suggests that the records of operations under hypnosis sometimes point not to an absence of pain but to an unwillingness to state that pain was experienced. Pain as an experience is not absent but is denied; and there are no greater changes in the physiological responses to noxious stimulation than can be produced by direct suggestion without hypnosis (Barber & Hahn, 1962). As a manoeuvre directed towards allaying anxiety, however, hypnosis is successful, like other methods of suggestion, in allaying even chronic pain (Dorcus & Kirkner, 1948; Butler, 1954; Barber, 1959).

Apart from these general factors the specific psychiatric treatment of pain is frequently successful. Normally this occurs where there is a well-defined condition responsive to standard psychiatric treatments, e.g. anti-depressant drugs or ECT for endogenous depression, sedation and some form of psychotherapy in neurotic illnesses. Unfortunately, where there is a well-marked persistent hypochondriacal or hysterical attitude, without marked evidence of anxiety or depression, treatment is less helpful. Despite favourable reports of the use of ECT (Von Hagen, 1957) and anti-depressant drugs (Lance & Curran, 1964; Lascelles, 1966) for chronic pain there is no really satisfactory evidence that these measures are helpful in the absence of a significant degree of anxiety or depression. Similarly, chlorpromazine which can be useful in central pain (Lassman, Moody & Gryspeerdt, 1959) or in terminal carcinoma (Saunders, 1963) is rarely useful in pain of neurotic origin. Perhaps when it is effective this is because of its action upon the reticular activating system. Occasionally, the above treatments work to the surprise of the psychiatrist, but too rarely for him who hopes to treat all psychogenic pain with drugs, so that there remains a group of patients in which the psychiatric contribution is limited to helping the patient to bear with his infirmity and the physician to bear with his patient. These usually are the hypochondriacal patients for whom the diagnosis of hysteria seems appropriate.

With regard to leucotomy for pain, similar considerations obtain as with anti-depressant drugs or ECT. It has been generally accepted for some years that leucotomy is useful if there is much anxiety, tension or depression evident. The combined use of ECT and drugs, has, however, greatly reduced the frequency with which it is considered. To relieve pain (including that of carcinoma), in the absence of anxiety or depression, leucotomy must be extensive and will then cause undesirable personality changes. This may be acceptable in terminal illness.

Treatment by stereotaxic surgery may also be appropriate and from this Cooper (1965) has made a particularly illuminating contribution to the understanding of cerebral mechanisms of pain.

EXPERIMENTAL PSYCHOLOGY

A substantial literature has accumulated on this topic showing the influence of emotions on the occurence of pain. Numerous investigations both by this method and others followed the introduction of the Hardy-Wolff-Goodell dolorimeter for heat-pain (cf. Hardy, Wolff & Goodell, 1940, 1952; Hall, 1953; Beecher, 1959; Kutscher & Kutscher, 1957; Cheymol, Gay & Duteuil, 1959a; Cheymol *et al.*, 1959b; Smith, 1963, 1966; Truchaud, 1965; Wolff *et al.*, 1966a, b; Merskey & Spear, 1967b). This is a field in which positive achievements have been made but in which opinion and emphasis has varied considerably. Dispute has particularly centred on the validity and interpretation of so called Pain Perception Thresholds and Pain Reaction Thresholds. The interested reader is referred to the references cited.

ACKNOWLEDGMENTS

I wish to thank Dr R. Gwyn Evans and Dr E. G. Oram for helpful comments.

REFERENCES

Apley, J. (1959) *The Child with Abdominal Pains.* Blackwell Scientific Publications, Oxford.

Atlee, H. B. (1966) *Acute and Chronic Iliac Pain in Women.* Thomas, Springfield.

Baker, J. & Merskey, H. (1967) Pain in general practice. *J. psychosom. Res.* **10,** 383.

Barber, T. X. (1958a) Hypnosis as perceptual cognitive restructuring: II. Post-hypnotic behaviour. *J. clin. exp. Hypnos.* **6,** 10.

Barber, T. X. (1958b) The concept of hypnosis. *J. Psychol.* **45,** 115.

Barber, T. X. (1959) Toward a theory of pain: relief of

chronic pain by pre-frontal leucotomy, opiates, placebos and hypnosis. *Psychol. Bull.* **56,** 430.

Barber, T. X. (1963) The effects of 'hypnosis' on pain. *Psychosom. Med.* **25,** 303.

Barber, T. X. & Hahn, K.W. (1962) Physiological and subjective responses to pain-producing stimulation under hypnotically-suggested and waking-imagined 'analgesia'. *J. abnorm. soc. Psychol.* **65,** 411.

Bardhan, P. N. (1965a) The fathering syndrome. *Armed Forces med. J.* **20,** 200.

Bardhan, P. N. (1965b) The couvade syndrome. *Brit. J. Psychiat.* **111,** 908.

Beecher, H. K. (1956) Relationship of significance of wound to the pain experienced. *J. Amer. med. Ass.* **161,** 1609.

Beecher, H. K. (1959) *Measurement of subjective responses. Quantitative Effects of Drugs.* Oxford University Press, New York.

Bender, B. (1964) Seven angry crocks. *Psychosomatics,* **5,** 225.

Blanton, S. & Kirk, V. (1947) A psychiatric study of 61 appendicectomy cases. *Ann. Surg.* **126,** 305.

Bleuler, E. (1960) *Lehrbuch der Psychiatrie,* 10th edn. Springer, Berlin.

Brain, Lord (1962) Presidential address in Keele & Smith (1962).

Breuer, J. & Freud, S. (1893-95) *Studies on hysteria. Complete Psychological Works of Freud.* Standard Edition, Vol. 2. Hogarth Press, London, 1955.

Brodie, B. (1837) *Lectures illustrative of certain nervous affections,* No. 2, London. Cit. Zilboorg, G. & Henry, G. W., *A History of Medical Psychology,* Allen & Unwin, London, 1941.

Butler, B. (1954) The use of hypnosis in the care of the cancer patient. *Cancer,* **7,** 1.

Carne, S. J. (1967) Headache, *Brit. med. J.* **ii,** 233.

Chertok, L. (1959) *Psychosomatic Methods in Painless Childbirth* (Transl. D. Leigh). Pergamon Press, London.

Cheymol, J., Gay, Y. & Duteuil, J. (1959a) Des différents tests proposés pour l'étude d'un analgésique. *Thérapie,* **14,** 210.

Cheymol, J., Montagne, R., Dallon, S., Paeile. C. & Duteuil, J. (1959b). Contribution au test de la stimulation électrique de la dent du lapin pour l'étude expérimentale des analgésiques. *Thérapie,* **14,** 350.

Cooper, I. S. (1965) Clinical and physiologic implications of thalamic surgery for disorders of sensory communication. I. Thalamic surgery for intractable pain. *J. neurol. Sci. (Amst.),* **2,** 493.

Crohn, B. B. (1930) The psychoneuroses affecting the gastrointestinal tract. *Bull. N. Y. Acad. Med.* **6,** 155.

Curtis, J. I. (1955) A psychiatric study of 55 expectant fathers. *U. S. Armed Forces med. J.* **6,** 937.

Dana, C. L. (1911) The interpretation of pain and the dysaesthesias. *J. Amer. med. Ass.* **56,** 787.

Dennis, N., Henriques, F. & Slaughter, C. (1956) *Coal is our Life.* Eyre & Spottiswoode, London.

Devine, R. & Merskey, H. (1965) The description of pain in psychiatric and general medical patients. *J. psychosom. Res.* **9,** 311.

Dorcus, R. M. & Kirkner, F. J. (1948) The use of hypnosis in the suppression of intractable pain. *J. abnorm. soc. Psychol.* **43,** 237.

Eisenbud, J. (1937) The psychology of headache. *Psychiat. Quart.* **11,** 592.

Elkind, A. H. & Friedman, A. P. (1962) A review of headache: 1955 to 1961. I-III. *N. Y. St. J. Med.* **62,** 1220, 1444, 1649.

Engel, G. L. (1951) Primary atypical facial neuralgia. An hysterical conversion symptom. *Psychosom. Med.* **13,** 375.

Engel, G. L. (1956) Studies of ulcerative colitis: **IV.** The significance of headaches. *Psychosom. Med.* **18,** 334.

Engel, G. L. (1958) 'Psychogenic' pain. *Med. Clin. N. Amer.* **42,** 1481.

Engel, G. L. (1959) 'Psychogenic' pain and the pain prone patient. *Amer. J. Med.* **26,** 899.

Friedman, A. P., Finley, K. H., Graham, J. R., Kunkle, C. E., Ostfeld, M. O. & Wolff, H. G. (1962) Classification of headache. Special report of the Ad Hoc Committee. *Arch. Neurol.* **6,** 173.

Gittleson, N. L. (1961) Psychiatric headache: a clinical study. *J. ment. Sci.* **107,** 403.

Gonda, T. A. (1962) The relation between complaints of persistent pain and family size. *J. Neurol. Neurosurg. Psychiat.* **25,** 277.

Greenacre, P. (1939) Surgical addiction—a case illustration. *Psychosom. Med.* **1,** 325.

Guze, S. B. & Perley, M. J. (1963) Observations on the natural history of hysteria. *Amer. J. Psychiat.* **119,** 960.

Hagen, K. O. von (1957) Chronic intolerable pain. *J. Amer. med. Ass.* **165,** 773.

Hall, K. R. L. (1953) Studies of cutaneous pain: a survey of research since 1940. *Brit. J. Psychol.* **44,** 281.

Harding, H. E. (1962) A notable source of error in the diagnosis of appendicitis. *Brit. med. J.* **ii,** 1028.

Hardy, J. D., Wolff, H. G. & Goodell, H. (1940) Studies on pain. A new method for measuring pain threshold: observations on spatial summation of pain. *J. clin. Invest.* **19,** 649.

Hardy, J. D., Wolff, H. G. & Goodell, H. (1952) *Pain Sensations and Reactions.* Williams & Wilkins, Baltimore.

Hart, H. (1947) Displacement, guilt and pain. *Psychoanal. Rev.* **34,** 259.

Hinton, J. W. (1948) The surgical significance of acute abdominal pain. *Calif. Med.* **69,** 418.

Hinton, J. (1967) *Dying.* Penguin Books, Harmondsworth.

Hollingshead, A. B. & Redlich, F. C. (1958) *Social Class and Mental Illness: A Community Study.* Wiley, New York.

Ingram, P. W., Evans, G. & Oppenheim, A. N. (1965) Right iliac fossa pain in young women; with appendix on the Cornell Medical Index Health Questionnaire. *Brit. med. J.* **ii,** 149.

Keele, C. A. & Smith, R. (1962) *The Assessment of Pain in Man and Animals.* U.F.A.W., Livingstone, Edinburgh.

Kessel, N. & Coppen, A. (1963) The prevalence of common menstrual symptoms. *Lancet,* **ii,** 61.

Klee, G. D., Ozelis, S., Greenberg, I. & Gallant, L. J. (1959) Pain and other somatic complaints in a psychiatric clinic. *Maryland St. med. J.* **8,** 188.

Klein, R. F. & Brown, W. A. (1965) Pain as a form of communication in the medical setting. Unpublished abstract.

Knighton, R. S. & Dumke, P. R. (1966) *Pain: Henry Ford Hospital International Symposium.* Churchill, London.

Knopf, O. (1935a, b) Preliminary report on personality

studies in thirty migraine patients. *J. nerv. ment. Dis.* **82,** 270, 400.

Kraepelin, E. (1903) *Allgemeine Psychiatrie,* 7th edn. Barth, Leipzig.

Kreitman, N., Sainsbury, P., Pearce, K. & Costain, W. P. (1965) Hypochondriasis and depression in out-patients at a general hospital. *Brit. J. Psychiat.* **111,** 607.

Kutscher, A. H. & Kutscher, N. W. (1957) Evaluation of the Hardy-Wolff-Goodell pain threshold apparatus and technique. *Int. Rec. Med.* **170,** 202.

Lance, J. W. & Curran, D. A. (1964) Treatment of chronic tension headache. *Lancet,* **i,** 1236.

Lascelles, R. G. (1966) Atypical facial pain and depression. *Brit. J. Psychiat.* **112,** 651.

Lassman, P. L., Moody, J. F. & Gryspeerdt, G. L. (1959) Central pain due to cerebral ischaemia. *Folia psychiat. néerl.* **62,** 34.

Lee, J. A. H. (1961) Appendicitis in young women. *Lancet,* **ii,** 815.

Livingston, W. K. (1966) Silas Weir Mitchell and his work on causalgia. *Pain: Henry Ford Hospital International Symposium* (Ed. by R. S. Knighton and P. R. Dumke), p. 561.

Malmo, R. B. & Shagass, C. (1949) Psychologic study of symptom mechanisms in psychiatric patients under stress. *Psychosom. Med.* **11,** 25.

Malmo, R. B., Shagass, C. & Davis, J. F. (1951) Electromyographic studies of muscular tension in psychiatric patients under stress. *J. clin. Psychopath.* **12,** 45.

McEwen, B. W., de Wilde, F. W., Dwyer, B., Woodforde, J. M., Bleasel, K. & Connelley, T. J. (1965) The pain clinic. *Med. J. Aust.* **52,** 676.

Melzack, R. & Wall, P. D. (1965) Pain mechanisms: a new theory. *Science,* **150,** 971.

Menninger, K. A. (1938) *Man against Himself.* Harcourt & Brace, New York.

Merskey, H. (1964) *An investigation of pain in psychological illness.* D.M. thesis, Oxford.

Merskey, H. (1965a) The characteristics of persistent pain in psychological illness. *J. psychosom. Res.* **9,** 291.

Merskey, H. (1965b) Psychiatric patients with persistent pain. *J. psychosom. Res.* **9,** 299.

Merskey, H. & Spear, F. G. (1967a) The concept of pain, *J. psychosom. Res.* **11,** 59.

Merskey, H. & Spear, F. G. (1967b) *Pain: Psychological and Psychiatric Aspects.* Baillière, Tindall & Cassell, London.

Michaux, L. (1957) Les aspects psychiatriques de la douleur somatique. In: *La Douleur et les Douleurs* (Ed. by Th. Alajouanine). Masson, Paris.

Mitchell, S. W., Morehouse, G. R. & Keen, W. W. (1864) *Gunshot Wounds and Other Injuries of Nerves.* Lippincott, Philadelphia.

Montaigne, M. E. de (1580) *Essais* (Ed. by J.-V. le Clerc), Book 1, Chap. 40, p. 374. Garnier Freres, Paris, 1865.

Noordenbos, W. (1959) *Pain: problems pertaining to the transmission of nerve impulses which give rise to pain.* Elsevier, London.

Read, G. D. (1943) *Childbirth Without Fear.* Heinemann, London.

Reik, T. (1914) Couvade and the psychogenesis of the fear of retaliation. In. *Ritual: Psychoanalytic Studies.* Hogarth, London, 1931.

Rivers, W. H. R. (1920) *Instinct and the Unconscious.* Cambridge University Press.

Ruesch, J. (1946) Chronic disease and psychological invalidism: a psychosomatic study. Psychosom. Med. Monographs No. 9. Amer. Soc. Res. psychosom. Problems, New York.

Saunders, C. (1963) The treatment of intractable pain in terminal cancer. *Proc. roy. soc. Med.* **56,** 195.

Schneider, K. (1959) *Clinical Psychopathology* (Transl. by M. W. Hamilton). Grune & Stratton, London.

Simpson, D. A., Saunders, J. M., Rischbieth, R. H. S., Rees, V. E., Burnell, A. W. & Cramond W. A. (1965) Experiences in a pain clinic. *Med. J. Aust.* **52,** 671.

Slater, E. (1965) Diagnosis of 'hysteria'. *Brit. med. J.* **i,** 1395.

Smith, R. (1963) The dynamics of pain. In: *Problems of Dynamic Neurology* (Ed. by L. Halpern). Jerusalem.

Smith, R. (1966) The use of pressure and chemical stimulation to investigate pain. *Proc. roy. Soc. Med.* **59,** 73.

Spear, F. G. (1964) A study of pain as a symptom in psychiatric illness, M. D. thesis, Bristol University.

Spear, F. G. (1966) An examination of some psychological theories of pain. *Brit. J. med. Psychol.* **39,** 349.

Srole, L., Langner, T. S., Michael, S. T., Opler, M. K. & Rennie, T. A. C. (1962) *Mental Health in the Metropolis: the Midtown Manhattan Study,* Vol. 1. McGraw Hill, New York.

Stengel, E. (1960) Pain and the psychiatrist. *Med. Press,* **243,** 23.

Szasz, T. S. (1957) *Pain and Pleasure. A Study of Bodily Feelings.* Tavistock, London.

Trethowan, W. H. & Conlon, M. F. (1965) The couvade syndrome. *Brit. J. Psychiat.* **111,** 57.

Truchaud, M. (1965) *Etude des Variations du Seuil de la Douleur sous l'Influence de l'Altitude Simulée.* Romand & Beurel, Paris.

Veith, I. (1965) *Hysteria: the History of a Disease.* Chicago University Press.

Wallace, W. F. M., Loane, R. A. & Quinn. J. T. (1963) A study of appendicectomies in Belfast in 1958. *Ulster med. J.* **32,** 199.

Walters, A. (1961) Psychogenic regional pain alias hysterical pain. *Brain,* **84,** 1.

Walters, A. (1963) The psychological aspects of bodily pain. *Appl. Ther.* **5,** 853.

Weddell, A. G. M. (1962) Observations on the anatomy of pain sensibility. In: *The Assessment of Pain in Man and Animals* (Ed. by C. A. Keele and R. Smith). Livingstone, Edinburgh.

Weider, A., Mittelmann, B., Wechsler, D. & Wolff, H. G. (1944) The Cornell Selectee Index: a method for quick testing of selectees for the armed forces. *J. Amer. med. Ass.* **124,** 224.

Weiss, E. (1947) Psychogenic rheumatism. *Ann. intern. Med.* **26,** 890.

Williams, J. C. (1852) *Practical Observations on Nervous and Sympathetic Palpitation of the Heart, as well as on Palpitation, the Result of Organic Disease,* 2nd edn. Churchill, London.

Wilson, H. (1938) Psychogenic headache. *Lancet,* **i,** 367.

Wolff, B. B. (1966) Drug studies in experimental and

clinical pain. Symp. on Assessment of drug effects in the normal human. 74th Ann. Convention of Amer. Psychol. Ass., New York.

Wolff, B. B., Kantor, T. G., Jarvik, M. E. & Laska, E. (1966a) Response of experimental pain to analgesic drugs. 1. Morphine, aspirin and placebo. *Clin. Pharmacol. Ther.* **7**, 224.

Wolff, B. B., Kantor, T. G., Jarvik, M. E. & Laska, E. (1966b) Response of experimental pain to analgesic drugs. II. Codeine and placebo. *Clin. Pharmacol. Ther.* **7**, 323.

Wolff, H. G. (1948) *Headache and Other Head Pain.* Oxford University Press, London.

3

Psychology of the pain experience*

John B. Murray

A. INTRODUCTION

Though every man can describe it, scientists have been unable to offer a successful definition of pain (2).

> The nature of pain has been the subject of bitter controversy since the turn of the century (34, p. 971).

Hardy, Wolff, and Goodell (20) suggested the term "pain experience" as a way of avoiding the confusion in measuring, defining, and investigating pain. Pain experience would include the individual's integration of all effects of noxious stimuli: *(a)* reactions to threat of pain; *(b)* reactions to noxious stimuli locally at the site of stimulation; *(c)* sensations of pain itself, with accompanying sensations—e.g., hot, cold, pressure; *(d)* reactions to the pain sensation.

Beecher (2) distinguished between the primary and secondary components of the pain experience. The primary component was the pain sensation itself; the secondary component involved the suffering, reactive aspects, and emotional responses to pain. In the same vein McGlashen, Evans, and Orne (32) pointed out that the subjective pain intensity did not necessarily reflect the level of stimulation, the extent of tissue damage, or the danger to the organism—notions that had been included in definitions of pain (2). Psychological factors—which include the meaning ascribed to the sensations, past experience, and anxiety—contribute importantly to the individual's response to pain. These psychological factors of the pain experience are the main considerations in this paper.

B. COGNITIVE ASPECTS OF PAIN

It is clear that previous experience influences the pain experience. Anticipation of pain and resulting anxiety are basic ingredients in the reaction component of the pain experience, whether the pain is pathological or experimental. Hall and Stride (19) demonstrated that subjects' attitudes influenced the amount of pain response. When the authors used the word "pain" in their instructions to the subjects of their experiment (in which a thermal stimulus was the source of pain), the subjects' anticipations were translated into greater sensitivity, or lower thresholds, for pain than those of similar subjects who had received the same thermal stimulus but with a neutral instructional set. Clark (12) confirmed these results with subjects who received electrical and mechanical pain stimuli, as well as thermal pain stimuli. Blitz and Dinnerstein (7) also demonstrated the analgesic potential of different types of instructions which encouraged reinterpretation of ambiguous experiences.

When anxiety about pain is reduced, the subjective experience of pain can be reduced. Jones, Bentler, and Petry (25) provided some of their subjects with information that reduced uncertainty about the timing or amount of pain to be endured.

Reprinted with permission of The Journal Press from The Journal of Psychology **78:**193-206. Copyright 1971.

From the Department of Psychology, St. John's University.

*Based on an address to the Continuing Education Seminar, School of Pharmacy, St. John's University, November 12, 1970.

Electric shock was the pain stimulus administered to 32 college men. The subjects had in view an electric clock and were instructed that the shock would come only at the quadrants of the clock, at the numbers 3, 6, 9, and 12. They wore earphones through which they could receive messages and had a button by which they signal for information about the timing of the next shock—whether or not it would occur in the next quadrant—and the amount of shock to be given. Amount of shock was randomized. The pain tolerance of each subject was determined before the experiment. A pain intensity scale was developed in which 5 was the maximum and intensity was scaled down in even steps to 1. Requests from the subjects for information increased whenever an interval passed in which no shock was given or when a shock of high intensity was anticipated. Answers to a questionnaire completed at the end of the experiment indicated that uncertainty concerning future pain elicited anxiety and information that reduced uncertainty reduced anxiety.

Hill, Kornetsky, Flanary, and Wikler (24) reduced anxiety by allowing their subjects to have control over the termination of the pain stimulus. Lepanto, Moroney, and Zenhausern (28) measured pain thresholds under conditions in which one phase allowed the subject to control the termination of pain stimulus and the other phase allowed the experimenter to control the termination of pain. Their data, like the results of Hill *et al.* (24), indicated that pain thresholds were significantly lower when the subject was deprived of control over the stimulus. Bandler, Madaras, and Bem (1) confirmed that the possibility of escape from a painful stimulus influenced subjects' interpretation of the painfulness of an electric shock stimulus. Ratings by the subjects of the amount of discomfort experienced during the escape and no escape trials clearly showed that discomfort ratings were lower in the escape conditions, when the subjects could push a button and turn off the pain stimulus. Galvanic skin response (GSR) was monitored on all the subjects: differences in GSR for escape and no escape conditions were not significant, and the subjects' ratings of discomfort were the exact reverse of the recorded GSR for the different experimental conditions. The subjects' ratings of discomfort were not related to internal cues after the manner of Valins' findings (48).

The subjects of Hill *et al.*'s study (24) were former drug addicts at the United States Public Health hospital in Lexington, Kentucky. The authors found that morphine diminished the pain reactions in their experiment if the anxiety level was high; but when the subjects were allowed to control the pain-producing stimulus, and anxiety was reduced, morphine had no demonstrable effect on the pain. Beecher (2) expressed the opinion that analgesic agents exerted their principal influence on the affective or reaction component of pain. Berger, Kletzkin, Ludwig, and Margolin (5) questioned whether any of the available analgesics could modify pain perception without at the same time altering the mood and consciousness of the individual. Dinnerstein and Lowenthal's subjects (15) were paid to perform a handsteadiness task under threat of electric shock. The effects of aspirin on the pain connected with the electric shock were compared with placebos; not only did the aspirin lack analgesic effects, but it apparently potentiated the subjects' responses to anxiety.

Beecher (3) observed that most American soldiers who were wounded at Anzio either denied the existence of pain or experienced so little pain that they did not want any analgesic. When brought into combat hospitals, soldiers in only one out of three cases asked for morphine for their pain. When Beecher returned to clinical practice as an anesthesiologist, he asked civilians, who in major surgery had incisions similar to the wounds received by the soldiers, whether they wanted morphine to alleviate their pain. In contrast with the wounded soldiers, four out of five claimed that they were in severe pain and needed morphine. Apparently, no direct relationship between the wound *per se* and the pain experienced existed. Perhaps, the possibility of escape, which for the soldiers meant that they were alive and need not return to battle, reduced their interpretation of the pain experience.

Evans and McGlashan (17) measured pain tolerance by means of muscle ischemia. This method of inducing experimental pain, which Beecher (4) had used, consists of a blood pressure cuff inflated above systolic pressure which occludes blood flow to the arm and causes pain. The volunteer subjects of Evans and McGlashan were required to pump a rubber bulb which displaced water. The subjects gave a signal when the sensation in their arms turned to pain. The rate of work, the amount of water displaced per second, was calculated to the point where the subjects first reported pain and again when the pain was so great that they could pump no longer. The subjects actually exerted more effort while they were experiencing pain than they did before the pain was first experienced. Interviews with the subjects indicated that they had expected the reverse to be true. As one explanation, the authors offered the possibility that the subjects pumped harder because of their increased anxiety about the increasing intensity of pain. As a second explanation, the authors thought the subjects might have pumped harder because they were trying to reach the end faster in order to be rid of the discomfort. Their results do support the common notion that pain experienced can be endured better by "bearing down" or "gritting one's teeth." Paradoxically, as the authors point out, pressing harder on the bulb to pump the water faster actually caused the pain to become more intense.

C. AFFECTIVE ASPECTS OF THE PAIN EXPERIENCE

So far it seems that the amount of pain experience need not be related to the amount of injury, and the relief of pain need not be related to the amount of analgesic agent administered. About 35 percent of over 1000 patients in 15 studies reported marked relief from pathological pain after receiving a placebo, an organically inactive substance (3). Pepper (41) remarked that his was the first article he could find on the subject of "placebos," despite centuries of use. A placebo was the term used for any medicine adopted more to please than to benefit the patient, but Pepper added that in former days, since physicians had no method of distinguishing the drugs that had true actions from those wholly inert, all medicines were considered powerful and none truly were. In incurable cases the placebo often postponed the use of sedatives or lessened the quantity that had to be given, thus helping to avoid the too quick exhaustion of opiate efficacy.

Where Pepper in 1946 had written about the placebo as a drug that had no pharmacological action but was given for its psychotherapeutic effect, Shapiro (44, p. 110) broadened the term to "placebo effect," which he spoke of as

> the psychological, physiological, or psychophysiological effect of any medication or procedure given with therapeutic intent, which is independent of or minimally related to the pharmacological effect of the medication or to the specific effects of the procedure and which operates through a psychological mechanism.

Shapiro believed that despite the scientific achievements of this century, the physician himself was the most important therapeutic agent. He recounted two episodes from 19th-century French medicine to illustrate his point: Dr. Raymond at Salpetriere in Paris treated patients by suspending them by their feet and letting the blood flow to their heads; and Dr. Haushalter at Nancy suspended patients head upwards. Both physicians obtained a similar percentage of success in treating a variety of organic and nervous diseases.

Krugman, Ross, and Lyerly (27) and Lyerly, Ross, Krugman, and Clyde (29) published studies in which they manipulated two drugs, one an energizer and the other a sedative, together with instructions to subjects that corresponded to the effects of either drug. Generally, the effects on the subjects followed the instructions given them, whether they received an energizer, sedative, or placebo.

Dinnerstein, Lowenthal, and Blitz (16) argued that placebo effects were based on the patient's comprehension of, and emotional response to, the apparent drug administration, and that both comprehension and emotional response depended largely on the instructions or suggestions given to the patient. The placebo effects thus resulted from the patient's knowledge that he had been treated plus his own interpretation of the nature of the treatment. Drugs usually are given with expressed or implied suggestions concerning some expected effect. The administration of an active drug includes many of the same variables that are involved in the placebo effect. Hence, active drugs are in part placebos, and the observed effects of drug administration are a combination of pharmacological and placebo effects. They argued that a consistent universal analgesic would require two properties: *(a)* it would produce a physiological effect that was independent of the initial physiological state of the subject, as well as of the effects of mood or expectancy; *(b)* the drug would produce a pattern of subcortical and cortical excitation and inhibition and a pattern of somesthetic stimuli that would allow only one "interpretation" by the subject. On the basis of present evidence no analgesic or tranquilizing drug had these universal qualities, and there was no certainty that highly specific drugs against pain and anxiety were even possible. If one wished to follow the action of present analgesics and tranquilizers, one would need to examine the interaction of the following factors: *(a)* the drug; *(b)* the permanent and transient physiological states and sensitivities of the subjects; *(c)* the context of treatment; *(d)* the implied and explicit suggestions accompanying drug administration; *(e)* the psychological history of the subject, which influences in turn—1) his response to the context; 2) his understanding of the suggestion; 3) his interpretation of the internal sensory changes induced by all of the variables above. Of these variables all but *(a)* and *(b)* are part of what is called the placebo effect.

Petrie (42) proposed that individuals could be ranked along a continuum from "reducers," who tended to minimize stimulus input, to "augmenters," who tended to exaggerate sensory input. Blindfolded subjects were asked to estimate the width of wooden blocks; Petrie's results suggested that "augmenters" tolerated pain least, while "reducers" accepted it best. Subjects who appeared to tolerate pain least manifested greater apprehension of pain.

Sternbach and Tursky (46) replicated research by Zborowski (52) in which he had found ethnic differences in responses to pain stimuli. Zborowski had selected four groups who varied in responsivity to pain, as follows: *(a)* Yankee—assumed to have phlegmatic, matter-of-fact, doctor-helping viewpoint; *(b)* Jewish—concerned for implications of pain, distrust palliatives; *(c)* Italian—desire pain relief; *(d)* Irish—inhibit expression of suffering, concerned about implications of pain. Following the same assumptions, Sternbach and Tursky tested housewives who answered an ad in the newspapers—15 from each of the four ethnic groups. The women were paid for their participation in the investigation. Electric shock was administered through disks on the forearm. Each subject gave two signals: first, when she became aware of any sensation; and second, when the intensity increased to unbearable pain, at which point the stimulus was shut off. The lower threshold of sensitivity was similar for women in all four groups; the upper threshold, where the pain became unbearable, differed in accord with the hypothesized ethnic differences. Italians had the lowest threshold: that is, they were least able to take pain; Yankees were more matter of fact and adapted more quickly to the stimuli. Yankees and Irish both were undemonstrative but from different attitudes; Italians and Jews were more demonstrative toward pain but again for different reasons. Though the methods differed, the results of Sternbach and Tursky appear to complement the findings of Petrie.

A recent publication of the United States Department of Health, Education, and Welfare (47, p. 3) carried this statement: ". . . some people . . . are born without any sensitivity whatsoever to pain. . . ." Such individuals can be considered extreme instances of Petrie's "reducers." Sternbach (45) reviewed the literature on "congenital insensitivity to pain" and concluded that the 17 cases reported were markedly heterogeneous in symptoms and that no case was certain in the sense of having generalized insensitivity to pain and of reaching adolescence without ever experiencing pain.

Schneider (43) commented on Sternbach's conclusions that a distinction should be preserved among insensitivity to pain, the emotional aspects of pain, and the operations of defense mechanisms of indifference to pain. Waldman (49) discussed the exclusively psychological aspects of pain. Psychogenic pain need not follow the medical model of pain, which presupposes anatomic and physiological derangements which are involuntary happenings. The psychotherapist approaches psychogenic pain from the framework that pain is purposeful rather than biologically necessary and watches for consequences of pain rather than "causes."

Comparing relative pain perception of normal and psychoneurotic subjects was the purpose of Chapman's study (11). He used heat stimulation and measured *(a)* pain perception threshold, by which he meant the subjective endpoint of beginning pain, the lowest amount of pain necessary to cause a pricking sensation; and *(b)* pain reaction threshold, the first objective evidence of wincing or withdrawal from pain stimulation. Testing 200 normal subjects, he found ethnic differences; for Jewish and Italian subjects, who were two groups identified in his study, the results were similar to Sternbach and Tursky's findings. Psychoneurotic subjects (37) were compared to normal subjects similar in sex, age, and ethnic background. The pain perception thresholds were similar for normal and psychoneurotic subjects, but the psychoneurotic subjects showed greater sensitivity to pain in terms of the pain reaction threshold. The spread between the level at which pain was perceived and the level at which wincing and withdrawal occurred was significantly less for psychoneurotic subjects than for normal subjects. Reaction to pain appeared to decrease with age among his normal subjects when they were compared in three age groupings: 10-22 years, 23-44 years, anf 45-85 years. The total number of normal subjects was 200, but no data were offered on the number in each of the age groupings. Other authors have disputed that there are differences in response to pain between normal and abnormal subjects (2).

Buss and Portnoy (8) found that strong identification with a group increased the tolerance for pain. War stories often have dramatized how men who endured danger together developed a strong and lasting bond. Buss and Portnoy administered electric shock through a finger electrode. After the pain tolerance of each subject was determined, subjects were given false norms of what comparison groups could endure in the experimental condition. The comparison groups were as follows: *(a)* Americans were told that Russians had a greater tolerance for pain; *(b)* college men were told that women could stand more pain than men; *(c)* college students were told 1) men from their rival college could stand more pain; 2) men from another college (not a rival but known to them) could stand more pain; *(d)* a control group was given no instructions.

The stronger the identification the more pain the subjects could stand beyond their established thresholds. The subjects who were given the false norms of "Russians" endured the largest amount of pain. Men to whom the false norms of women were cited withstood pain beyond their usual thresholds, but not as much as those who competed with "Russian" pain norms. College students who were put in competition with other collegians exceeded their ordinary pain thresholds: those who were told what men in a rival college could withstand endured slightly more than those to whom pain thresholds of collegians in a neighboring school were quoted. The control group, which had been given no instructions, endured the least amount of pain. According to the authors, one reason for the greater pain endurance of the subjects competing against the false norms of "Russians" was that the term "Russians" was clearly distinctive for all subjects. The second reason they offered was competition, which is a strong motivator. Such data help to explain the effects of initiation ceremonies for fraternal groups and of boot camp as used by the armed forces in building group identification.

Drs. Esdaile and Elliotson used hypnosis over 100 years ago, and the first attempts to perform surgery with hypnosis were made in France about 1821 (7). Inasmuch as hypnosis may reduce fear and apprehension, it can be valuable as an adjunct to sedatives: it may reduce tension aroused by the prospect of chemical anesthesia, and posthypnotic suggestions may minimize postoperative reactions.

Since about 20 percent of the population is not susceptible, hypnosis is not a substitute for anesthesia for all subjects (3). But chemical anesthesias may be contraindicated in some surgery—e.g., in cardiac cases where the extra burden on the circulatory system might be too great—and hypnosis might be an acceptable replacement for those who are hypnotizable. Sensitivity to pain remains, according to electromyographic studies, but in deep hypnosis the brain centers seem to ignore the messages of pain (30). Kroger and DeLee (26) described caesarian section and hysterectomy performed under hypnosis without any other sedatives or analgesics. Crasilneck *et al.* (13) employed hypnosis for painful burn surgery. They were particularly impressed with the success of hypnosis in counteracting the starvation cycle, which is so dangerous in burn cases. Under hypnosis doctors were able to stimulate not only appetite in general but also for those specific foods most needed by the patients.

Since the element of suggestion is operative both in anticipated pain and in hypnosis, the effects of hypnosis have been paralleled to the findings on placebos. McGlashan, Evans, and Orne (32) tested the hypothesis that hypnosis consisted of more than suggestion in its analgesic effects. Their 24 subjects were divided between those who were responsive to hypnosis and those essentially unhypnotizable. Ischemic muscle pain was the experimental pain stimulus. All subjects received a placebo, which was described to them as a drug that worked on the physical or cellular level. All subjects worked harder after they took the placebo, an activity that confirmed the results of the earlier study by Evans and McGlashan (17). No relationship between the placebo effect and susceptibility to hypnosis was evident; hence the authors concuded that susceptibility to hypnosis was not intrinsically correlated with placebo responsivity. Their results demonstrated that hypnotic analgesia added a potential for pain relief for susceptible subjects over and above that produced by the placebo effect. Two components appeared to be operative in hypnotic analgesia: *(a)* placebo effects of hypnosis as a method of treatment; *(b)* distortion of perception specifically induced during deep hypnosis.

Wolff, Krasnegor, and Farr (51) and Wolff and Harland (50) tested the effect on pain endurance of suggestion alone without hypnosis. They tested paid volunteers, men and women, using electric shock. After a series of trials in which the amount of shock was increased until the subjects had given the stop signal, indicating that they could stand no more, the authors invited their subjects to try once more and to imagine that they would receive $1000 if they endured the shock a little longer. They were told that they would not receive any money, but were asked to imagine that they would. The authors found slight increases in threshold and tolerance for pain on the last trial as compared with the previous trials.

Gardner, Licklider, and Weisz (18) reported that pain could be suppressed by sound. In about 5000 dental operations audioanalgesia, a procedure that combined music and noise, was effective in suppressing pain; for 65 percent of the patients, who had previously required local anesthesia or nitrous oxide in comparable operations, sound alone was effective in suppressing pain; for 25 percent of the patients the sound-induced analgesia was sufficiently effective so that no other analgesic or anesthetic agent was required; for 10 percent the audioanalgesia method was less than adequate. Other doctors used audioanalgesia for childbirth and minor operations. The patient wore headphones and had a control box which he could operate by hand. Before the operation and until the painful procedure began, the patient listened to stereo music. As soon as he anticipated pain or felt incipient pain, he turned up the intensity of noise. The doctor could judge the patient's state of anxiety by noting whether music or noise was turned on and at what intensity level. The patients reported that noise appeared to suppress pain and also masked the sound of dental drills, thereby reducing anxiety from another source. When both music and noise were turned on, the patients had to concentrate to follow the music. This introspective account of the patients seemed to say that the audioanalgesia method diverted attention from the pain.

Carlin, Ward, Gershon, and Ingraham (10) designed their investigation of the effects of auditory analgesia around the explanations of the patients. Three possible processes suggested themselves: *(a)* direct neural interaction by masking of pain impulses; *(b)* distraction (attention-attracting music and noise); *(c)* suggestion (involved in the perception of pain). The procedure used was electrical stimulation of the teeth of subjects who were patients, chosen at random, at a dental clinic. Three experimenters conducted the study; each was unaware of the experimental conditions in the other two stages. One knew which patients had the auditory analgesia; another knew the size of the electric shock; and the third knew which intensity of pain each patient had selected on a prearranged scale. The investigators obtained no evidence to support the masking, or cross-modality, explanation of the effectiveness of audioanalgesia in diminishing suprathreshold pain. Neither was there evidence that noise reduced sensitivity in the electrically stimulated tooth. There was only a hint that suggestion might raise the threshold slightly. One group of the patients had received an explanation of auditory analgesia in order to test the suggestion or placebo effect.

Though their negative results seemed to fit the placebo effect explanation of pain relief, the authors argued that the laboratory situation was artificial, as compared with the dentist's office. Also, they thought that since their subjects could focus on the tooth being tested, the influence of distraction might have been minimized. Also, the attitude of their subjects in the laboratory study might have differed from that of typical dental patients, inasmuch as the experimental subjects had limited pain, as contrasted with pain of uncertain duration and unknown severity of the actual dental condition. The effectiveness of auditory analgesia in the clinical setting of the dental office seemed likely to depend on a combination of suggestion and distraction.

In their experiments with auditory analgesia, Camp, Martin, and Chapman (9), who used radiant energy applied to the forearm, instead of painful stimulation of the teeth, found no significant differences in the intensity of pain experienced by their subjects, with and without music and noise. The authors also admitted that they had not included all aspects of the pain experience. Their stimulus probably restricted pain to the simplest sensory aspects and neglected the many aspects of threat and suffering involved in clinical pain. Similarly Marone (31) argued that audioanalgesia seemed not as effective in suppressing pain as initially demonstrated. He tested college men, with and without noise and music suppressors. Two weeks later he retested the same subjects and found significant changes in relief of pain through audioanalgesia. Repeated exposure to audioanalgesia seemed to lead to greater suppression of pain.

Beginning about 1935 brain operations, known as prefrontal lobotomies and lobectomies, were performed on severely disturbed patients as a method of last resort in hopes of making them more comfortable and tractable. These operations typically produced a state of indifference to pain, so that they were used sometimes in cases of intractable pain. The indifference to pain appeared to come about through a diminution of the prolonged disturbance that constant pain induced rather than through an absence of pain experience. Patients were still distressed by painful events and their pain threshold seemed to be lower than normal. But their pain experience did not make them feel as bad as before the operation, and they seemed less engrossed in their feelings and made fewer complaints about their situation (14).

Electrodes implanted in the brains of animals have provided the most recent source of information about pain. Miller (35) and Olds (39, 40) reported finding reward and punishment centers in the animal brain. Electrodes were implanted in the septal and hypothalamic brain areas; the electrodes ended in miniature sockets in the animal's head into which wires could be plugged. When provided with a lever by which it could administer a shock of electricity to a certain area of its brain through the electrodes, the animal acted as if it were rewarded, even choosing to press the lever in preference to food and drink. In other brain area implantations the animal acted as if punished and avoided the stimulation.

Electrodes have also been implanted in human brains (6). When electrodes were placed in the brain of patients suffering from Parkinson's disease, the patients smiled or grinned and asked for more brain stimulation. When the patients were given a button by which they could administer a shock to their own brains, they said that it "tickled" or "felt good" (36, p. 330). Patients who suffered intractable pain had brain implantations and were given a pain box, which allowed them to administer a shock to their brains. One device suppressed pain after about one hour of impulses (nine volts at a rate of 30 per second) with no irreversible damage to brain tissue (21). One advantage of the pain box was that it relieved the patient of the need for morphine-like drugs. One patient with cancer, who had required 100 milligrams of drugs every two hours, went along for three months without pain-relieving drugs once he began using the brain-stimulation device.

D. SUMMARY

Pain in its physiological aspects has been described well in recent articles by Melzack (33), Murray (38), and Hilgard (22). The term "pain experience" has been suggested as an alternative to "pain," because it includes the individual's integration of all the effects of noxious stimuli: for example, the reaction to threat of pain; sensations like heat, cold, and pressure, which accompany the sensation of pain; and physiological reactions to the pain sensation. Research on the psychological components of the pain experience has underscored the importance of cognitive and affective aspects of pain. Psychological factors, such as the meaning attributed to the pain, the age of subjects, and ethnic background, appear to contribute importantly to the individual's response to pain. Particularly relevant to the psychological aspects of pain is the use of hypnosis and audioanalgesia as anesthetics. The article reviewed studies of these "pain-killers" and investigations of a placebo effect in medical research. When psychological factors of pain are considered along with the physiological dimensions of pain, the subjective experience of pain becomes clearer, although not all the mystery of pain and suffering has been dispelled.

REFERENCES

1. Bandler, R. J., Jr., Madaras, G. R., & Bem, D. J. Self-observation as source of pain perception. *J. Personal. & Soc. Psychol.*, 1968, **9**(3), 205-209.
2. Beecher, H. K. The measurement of pain. *Pharmacol. Rev.*, 1957, **9,** 59-209.
3. ———. Measurement of Subjective Responses. New York: Oxford Univ. Press, 1959.
4. ———. Pain: One mystery solved. *Science*, 1966, **151,** 840-841.
5. Berger, F. M., Kletzkin, M., Ludwig, B. S., & Margolin, S. The history, chemistry, and pharmacology of carisoprodol *Ann. N. Y. Acad. Sci.*, 1960, **86,** 90-107.
6. Bishop, M. P. Elder, S. T., & Heath, R. G. Intracranial self-stimulation in man. *Science*, 1963, **140,** 394-396.
7. Blitz, B., & Dinnerstein, A. J. Effects of different types of instructions on pain parameters. *J. Abn. Psychol.*, 1968, **73**(3, Pt.1) 276-280.
8. Buss, A. H., & Portnoy, N. W. Pain tolerance and group identification. *J. Personal. & Soc. Psychol., 1967*, **6**(1), 106-108.
9. Camp, W., Martin, R., & Chapman, L. F. Pain threshold and discrimination of pain intensity during brief exposure to intense noise. *Science*, 1962, **135,** 788-789.
10. Carlin, S., Ward, W. D., Gershon, A., & Ingraham, R. Sound stimulation and its effect on dental sensation threshold. *Science*, 1962, **138,** 1258-1259.
11. Chapman, W. P. Measurement of pain sensitivity in normal and control subjects and in psychoneurotic patients. *Psychosomat. Med.*, 1944, **6,** 252-257.
12. Clark, J. W. Factors affecting human response to pain stimulation. Unpublished master's thesis, McGill University, Montreal, Canada, 1955.
13. Crasilneck, H. B., Stirman, J. A., Wilson, B. J., McGrainie, E. J., & Fogelman, M. J. Use of hypnosis in the management of patients with burns. *J.A.M.A.*, 1955, **158,** 103-106.
14. Deutsch, J. A., & Deutsch, D. Physiological Psychology. Homewood, Ill.: Dorsey Press, 1966.
15. Dinnerstein, A. J., & Lowenthal, M. Effects of aspirin on shock induced deterioration of hand steadiness. *Percept. & Motor Skills*, 1963, **17,** 943-946.
16. Dinnerstein, A. J., Lowenthal, M., & Blitz, B. The interaction of drugs with placebos in the control of pain and anxiety. *Perspect. Biol. & Med.*, 1966, **10**(1), 103-117.
17. Evans, F. J., & McGlashan, T. H. Work and effort during pain. *Percept. & Motor Skills*, 1967, **25**(3), 794.
18. Gardner, W. J., Licklider, J. C. R., & Weisz, A. Z. Suppression of pain by sound. *Science*, 1960, **132,** 32-33.
19. Hall, K. R. L., & Stride, E. The varying response to pain in psychiatric disorders: A study in abnormal psychology. *Brit. J. Med. Psychol.*, 1954, **27,** 48-60.
20. Hardy, J. D., Wolff, H. G., & Goodell, H. Pain—Controlled and uncontrolled. *Science*, 1953, **117,** 164-165.
21. Heath, R. G. Electrical self-stimulation of the brain in man. *Amer. J. Psychiat.*, 1963, **120**(6), 571-577.
22. Hilgard, E. R. Pain as a puzzle for psychology and physiology. *Amer. Psychol.*, 1969, **24**(2), 103-113.
23. Hilgard, E. R., Weitzenhoffer, A. M., Landes, J., & Moore, R. K. The distribution of susceptibility of hypnosis in a student population. *Psychol. Monog.*, 1961, **75,** No. 8 (Whole No. 512).

24. Hill, H. E., Kornetsky, C. H., Flanary, H. G., & Wikler, A. Studies on anxiety associated with anticipation of pain: I. Effects of morphine. *Arch. Neurol. & Psychiat.*, 1952, **67**, 612-619.
25. Jones, A., Bentler, P. M., & Petry, G. The reaction of uncertainty concerning future pain. *J. Abn. Psychol.*, 1966, **71**, 87-94.
26. Kroger, W. S., & DeLee, S. T. Use of hypnoanesthesia for caesarian section and hysterectomy. *J.A.M.A.*, 1957, **163**, 442-444.
27. Krugman, A. D., Ross, S., & Lyerly, S. B. Drugs and placebos: Effects of instructions upon performance and mood under amphetamine sulphate and chloral hydrate with younger subjects. *Psychol. Rep.*, 1964, **15**, 925-926.
28. Lepanto, R., Moroney, W., & Zenhausern, R. The contribution of anxiety to the laboratory investigation of pain. *Psychon. Sci.*, 1965, **3**, 475.
29. Lyerly, S. B., Ross, S., Krugman, A. D., & Clyde, D. J. Drugs and placebos: The effects of instructions upon performance and mood under amphetamine sulphate and chloral hydrate. *J. Abn. & Soc. Psychol.*, 1964, **68**(3), 321-327.
30. Marmer, M. J. The role of hypnosis in anesthesiology. *J.A.M.A.*, 1956, **162**, 441-449.
31. Marone, J. G. Suppression of pain by sound. *Psychol. Rep.*, 1968, **22**(3, Pt.2), 1055-1056.
32. McGlashen, T. H., Evans, F. J., & Orne, M. T. The nature of hypnotic analgesia and placebo response to experimental pain. *Psychosomat. Med.*, 1969, **31**(3), 227-246.
33. Melzack, R. Pain. In *International Encyclopedia of the Social Sciences (Vol. 11)*. New York: Macmillan & Free Press, 1968. Pp. 357-363.
34. Melzack, R., & Wall, P. D. Pain mechanisms: A new theory. *Science,* 1965 **150,** 971-979.
35. Miller, N. E. Central stimulation and other new approaches to motivation and reward. *Amer. Psychol.*, 1958, **13,** 100-108.
36. Morgan, C. T. Physiological Psychology (3rd ed.). New York: McGraw-Hill, 1965.
37. Murray, J. B. Hypnosis: A review of research. *Cath. Psychol. Rec.*, 1964, **2**(1), 9-32.
38. ———. The puzzle of pain. *Percept. & Motor Skills,* 1969, **28,** 887-899.
39. Olds, J. Self-stimulation of the brain. *Science,* 1958, **127,** 315-324.
40. ———. The central nervous system and the reinforcement of behavior. *Amer. Psychol.,* 1969, **24**(2), 114-132.
41. Pepper, O. H. P. A note on placebo. *Amer. J. Pharmacol.*, 1945, **117,** 409-412.
42. Petrie, A. Individuality in Pain and Suffering. Chicago, Ill.: Univ. Chicago Press, 1967.
43. Schneider, S. F. Some comments on "Congenital insensitivity to pain: A critique." *Psychol. Bull.,* 1964, **62**(4), 287-288.
44. Shapiro, A. K. A contribution to a history of the placebo effect. *Behav. Sci.,* 1960, **5,** 109-135.
45. Sternbach, R. A. Congenital insensitivity to pain: A critique. *Psychol. Bull.*, 1963, **60,** 252-264.
46. Sternbach, R. A., & Tursky, B. Ethnic difference among housewives in psychophysical and skin potential responses to electric shock. *Psychophysiol.*, 1965, **1,** 241-246.
47. United States Department of Health, Education, and Welfare. Pain (Pub. No. 307-707.). Washington, D.C.: Supt. of Documents, 1968.
48. Valins, S. Cognitive effects of false heart-rate feedback. *J. Personal. & Soc. Psychol.,* 1966, **4,** 400-408.
49. Waldman, R. D. Pain as fiction: A perspective on psychotherapy and responsibility. *Amer. J. Psychother.*, 1968, **22**(3), 481-490.
50. Wolff, B. B., & Harland, A. A. Effect of suggestion upon experimental pain. *J. Abn. Psychol.,* 1967, **72,** 402-407.
51. Wolff, B. B., Krasnegor, N. A., & Farr, R. S. Effects of suggestion upon experimental pain response parameter. *Percept. & Motor Skills,* 1965, **21,** 675-683.
52. Zborowski, M. Cultural components in responses to pain. *J. Soc. Iss.*, 1952, **8,** 16-30.

4

A physician looks at pain[1]

Kenneth D. Keele

Amongst the many personal tragedies that afflicted Sir James Young Simpson none to my mind is more poignant than that he who contributed so much to the relief of pain suffered so grievously from it in his own life. As well as migraine and sciatica with which he was afflicted for many years and with which he was often prostrated towards the end of his life, he suffered severely from angina pectoris which he himself called "severe rheumatism in the walls of my chest" (Shepherd, 1969). That he endured at least one cardiac infarction is revealed by the fact that he sought relief from his own brain-child, chloroform, as well as by the autopsy finding of a cardiac aneurysm and "fatty degeneration" of the heart—a term under which cardiac infarction masqueraded in 1870.

Simpson's experience demonstrates the unhappy truth that there still remains in the practice of medicine a wide spectrum of pains which we cannot yet adequately control. They lie outside the bounds of surgical anæsthesia, the dramatic success of which has too often lulled us into a false confidence and obscured the remaining pain problems, such as those of chronic, recurrent, or intermittent pain.

The current lack of interest in pain is partly due to the confusion of terminology with which the problem is bedevilled. At the end of a long life, much of it devoted to the surgery of pain, Réné Leriche's last sad words on the subject were: "We engulf in the same word all that inconveniences and worries the patient and since all this is subjective, we picture nothing at all and call it pain, a word which stifles all curiosity and hinders analytical efforts" (Leriche, 1956). A great deal of the confusion can be avoided if we remember that pain is a psychological experience. Most of us have accepted the concept of specific "pain" nerve-endings connected with "pain" tracts in the spinal cord which emanated from the work of 19th-century physiologists, most prominent of whom were Charles Bell, Johannes Muller and Von Frey. However, such neurological structures subserving pain and no other form of sensation have been dissolved during the last 20 years into a nebulous ghost of their former selves. These structures do subserve the conduction of mechanical and chemical noxious stimuli and sometimes, but by no means always, also subserve the perception of pain. In my own view, it is most important to emphasise the distinction between noxious stimulation and the experience of pain. I would like to illustrate the fundamental difference between the two by the case of little Sarah, aged 3 (Libman, 1934). This child jumped off a window-sill and fractured the first metatarsal without complaint of pain. Only when the mechanical difficulties of walking occasioned by swelling presented themselves did her parents become aware of the injury. X-ray showed profuse callus formation around the fracture. On another occasion, when her elder sister was allowed to attend a dancing class but she was not, Sar-

Reprinted with permission of the Journal of the Royal College of Surgeons of Edinburgh. **16:**15-23.
Consulting Physician, Ashford Hospital, Middlesex.
[1]Part of the proceedings of the Sir James Young Simpson Centernary Symposium, May 1970.

ah expressed her frustration by chewing her tongue: its grossly lacerated state became known to her mother only because of profuse, painless bleeding. She also painlessly chewed the flesh off her right forefinger down to the bone. Full neurological and psychological examination carried out by myself and Dr. Merskey at the National Hospital, Queen's Square, London, revealed a child of above normal intelligence with no neurological abnormality, except that she was not sensitive to the painful element of noxious stimuli of heat, pressure, electrical or chemical nature, taken to the limits of safety. Sarah thus demonstrated that a noxious stimulus for her was not the same as a painful stimulus.

How common is this insensitivity to noxious stimulation? In the case of the tissues of the body we know it is common. For example, destructive stimulation of brain or intestine is painless unlike that of the skin or meningeal arteries. So-called congenital indifference to pain has been only rarely described but is it, in fact, such a rarity? In its extreme form it probably is rare in adult life, but even insensitivity of the degree present in Sarah may fail to be detected both by parents and doctors. The behaviour of such persons in general is remarkably normal. For example, Sarah cried when her angry father slapped her bottom, though she experienced no physical pain from the punishment.

Evidence is beginning to accumulate that this extreme form of insensitivity is sometimes temporary and more common in children than in adults. To my knowledge one child has matured into normal sensitivity about the age of 8 and Sarah, during the last year, has for the first time complained of nettle stings and has been wakened by earache. This brings us to a consideration of the less marked variations of pain sensitivity (or insensitivity) present in all of us when subjected to noxious stimulation.

Libman was the first clinician to make a systematic study of the sensitivity of patients to noxious stimulation. He used a crude technique of applying finger-pressure to the styloid process of the mastoid and noted whether the patient complained of pain. On this basis he classified patients into two grades, that of "sensitive" if they found it painful and "hyposensitive" if they did not. Perhaps the greatest limitation of his test for clinical use was its lack of quantitative value. For this reason I have used a pressure algometer applied to a flat bony surface (usually the forehead) at a standard rate of pressure-increase of 1 k. per second (Fig. 1). The patient is asked to state when the pressure becomes what he would call painful. When the conditions of the test, details of which I have described elsewhere, are carefully standardised the results are reproducible within the margin of 25%. Using this method the pain threshold of 363 normal persons, mostly workers in London, was found to vary from 0.5 kg. to 6 kg., 61% lying between the range of 2-4 kg., 17% being hyposensitive and 22% hypersensitive. This distribution is similar to that found by other workers applying experimental pain-producing stimuli to unselected groups. When a general practitioner colleague, Dr. Robert Smith, applied it to 200 patients attending his surgery, he found a shift in the aggregate towards the hypersensitive side. Further study of this selected

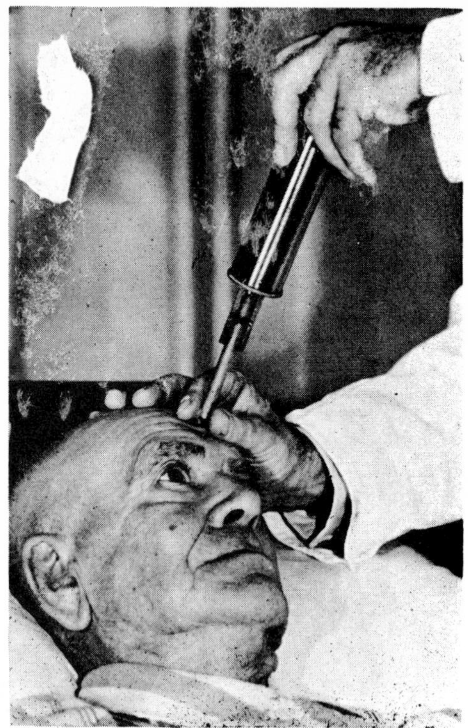

Fig. 1. Assessment of sensitivity to pressure pain using the pressure algometer.

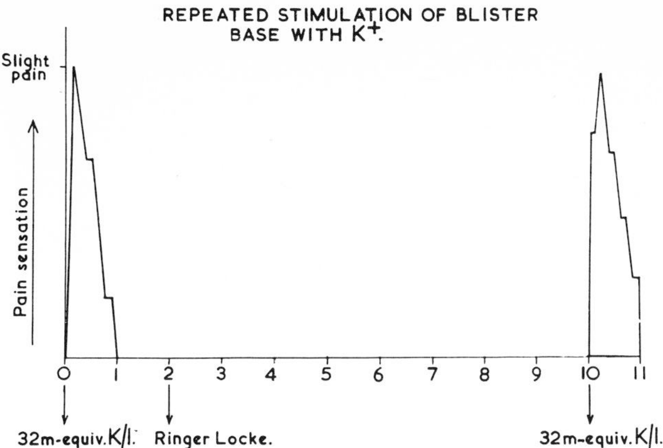

Fig. 2. Reproducible pain sensation by the application of potassium ion at a concentration of 32 mEq/l to a blister-base.

group of the population revealed to him that the hypersensitive patients on his list were those who attended most often and made the greatest demands on his time: the hyposensitive patients tended not to call in the doctor, even when they were experiencing noxious stimulation from organic disease. This finding provides food for thought particularly when one finds, among the hyposensitives, patients with acute appendicitis first presenting with general peritonitis (Smith, 1962).

Does the pain sensitivity to pressure correspond to the sensitivity to other forms of noxious stimulation? Because of a particular interest in ischæmic pain a comparison was made of the thresholds to pressure and the ischæmic pain produced in the muscles of the forearm, using a modification of Lewis's well-known test. Results showed the two to be comparable if allowance was made for the fact that some hyposensitive persons found the end-point to be fatigue rather than pain. Similar correlation was found when pressure-pain was compared with the noxious stimulation of a blister-base with solutions of potassium chloride. From these experiments it was concluded that pain sensitivity to one kind of noxious stimulus usually corresponds to sensitivity to other forms.

The use of the blister-base as a site of noxious stimulation with chemical solutions was introduced by my brother, Professor C. A. Keele. No sensation is felt when a warmed isotonic solution is applied to an open blister-base. When a pain-producing substance is applied the sensation of pain is unaccompanied by any other; it is quantitatively registered on a rotating drum. Comparison of repeated experiments reveals what a remarkably reliable experimental animal man is when his blister-base is connected directly to his central nervous system!

Many have held that it is the liberation of the potassium ion from cardiac muscle which gives rise to the pain of angina and cardiac infarction. Accordingly I made further observations with potassium solutions on the blister-base. Comparison of the sensations from potassium solutions at 8 mEq., 32 mEq. and 48 mEq. shows a graded response which when analysed suggests that the degree of pain experienced increases with the logarithm of the concentration of potassium in milliequivalents (Figs. 2, 3). This finding agrees with the Weber-Fechner law of sensation enunciated about 100 years ago. It agrees too with modern work on the sensation of brilliance of light. There is a good deal of evidence that experimental pain increases with logarithmic increase of the stimulus, or as a power function of stimulus intensity.

Another feature of experimental pain brought out by stimulation of a blister-base by the potassium ion is the development of a sensory refractory period (Fig. 4). After application of the potassium ion this period, at first absolute then relative, lasts for 5-10 minutes. In most cases it is specific for the substance used as a stimulus, *e.g.* potassium, and the application of another pain-producing substance such as bradykinin during this refractory period produces a normal pain response. It thus becomes clear that the continuous application of a noxious chemical substance produces pain followed by analgesia, not continuous pain.

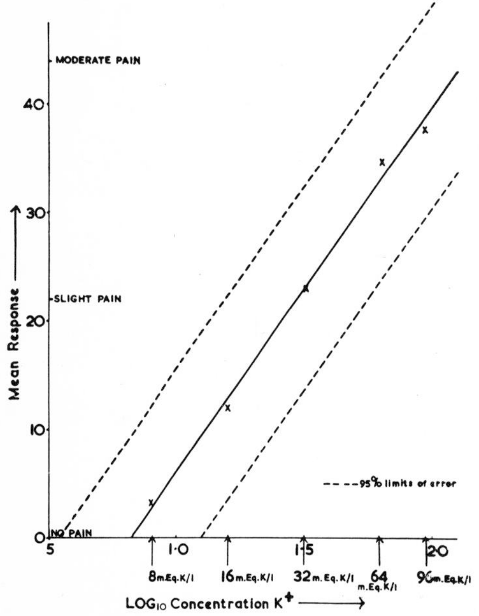

Fig. 3. The increase of pain with the application to a blister-base of the potassium ion in proportion to the logarithm of its concentration in mEq/l.

The analgesic phase may be experimentally continued indefinitely by the continued application of the potassium ion. Such a phenomenon may well be concerned with the diminution or cessation of pain in many clinical conditions which involve apparently constant pathological changes in the tissues. The waxing and waning of pain in inflammatory conditions such as abscesses, and the cessation of pain, often apparently inexplicable, in cardiac infarction may well be conditioned by a similar mechanism to that which produces the analgesic phase from potassium ion stimulation of the blister-base. The main source of potassium ion in a red infarct is hæmolysed red blood cells. A comparison of the pain produced by such hæmolysis and that of their contained potassium shows clearly that red blood cells contain other potent pain-producing substances besides potassium. A similar statement can safely be made with regard to necrosed muscle. Thus, though the potassium ion undoubtedly plays a part in the production of the pain of cardiac infarction, it is not the only factor. The release of other intracellular noxious substances such as phosphates, histamine and serotonin from platelets and the formation of plasma kinins add an unassessable quota of pain-producing substances.

The application of the potassium ion to blister-bases led directly to one of the

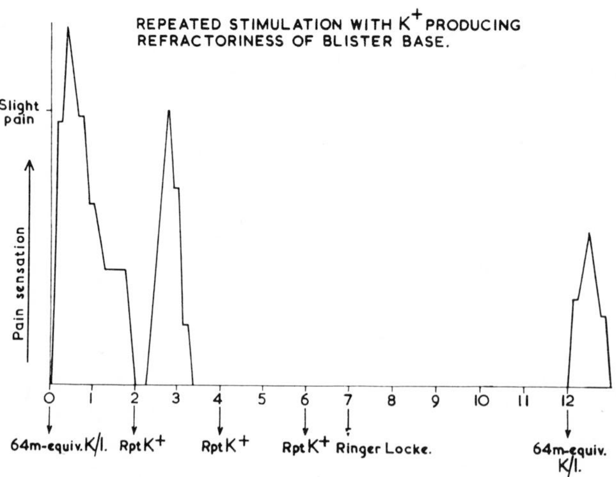

Fig. 4. The sensory refractory period to pain produced by the application of potassium ion to blister-base.

Table 1. Verbal responses to the applications of different concentrations of potassium ion to blister-bases

|———Algæsthesia———→ (from Slight 1)
|———Metæsthesia———- - - - - - - - →

	Pain scale 0		Slight 1		Moderate 2
K⁺ Concentration	↑ *8 mEq. K/l.*	↑ *16 mEq. K/l.*	↑ *32 mEq. K/l.*	↑ *64 mEq. K/l.*	↑ *96 mEq. K/l.*
Subject 1.	Nothing.	Nothing at all.	Tingling. Slight pain.	Faint burning. Slightly more painful.	
2.	Slight stinging. Not a pain. A sensation.	Stinging a little more. Not a pain. An irritation.	Sharper. Did not go off so quickly. Not a pain yet.	Sudden sting. Slight pain.	Soreness like an open cut. Unpleasant.
3.	No reaction. No sensation.	Very mild tingling. Hardly noticeable. Not a pain.	Tingling like a nettle sting. Mildly unpleasant. Very mildly painful.		Similar to the last, but more intense. Pain—yes.
4.	Slight sensation on the arm. No pain.	Slight tickle. No pain.	Slightly painful. Diminished into. something I wanted to scratch.	Something more painful.	Sting. Like a scald.
5.	Very slight pricking sensation.		Sharper prick. Little stronger than the first.	Sharper stinging pain this time.	Quite a sharp stinging pain.
6.	Nothing at all.	Slight tingling.	A tingle. Very slightly unpleasant.	Immediate tingle. Distinctly unpleasant. A pain.	

great semantic problems of the subject. What does a patient mean by pain? This arose from my personal experience of a sensation from the potassium application which although "sharp" in action was definitely not unpleasant. Was it therefore to be included under the category of "pain"? This problem was approached by applying the potassium ion in different concentrations to the blister-base of 15 subjects, tape-recording the vocabulary of their responses (Table 1). From the words they used, it became quite evident that there was a distinct field of sensation below the level described as slight pain. In this region such words as "pricking," "tingling" and "uncomfortable" were used, quite often combined with the voluntary assertion that "I would not call this pain." This stage of sensation we have come to realise as an important sensory reality demanding verbal recognition. We have called it "metæsthesia." Many examples of metæsthesia occur in everyday life: that narrow band of temperature of a hot bath in which the water is neither tepid nor too hot is the metæsthetic range of a real "hot" bath. Above this range the truly painful sensation from heat is indubitable. This can be distinguished by the word "algæsthesia." This word describes the unpleasantly painful. The stimulation of the mucous membranes of the mouth and tongue by a really "hot" curry is for some a metæsthetic experience which they want to repeat, for others it may produce algæsthesia which they do not wish to repeat. Metæsthesia may thus be neutral or pleasant in its emotional activation, algæsthesia is always unpleasant. Metæsthesia raises the problem of pleasure-pain. Witness the girl who, when asked whether the deafening music in a discotheque was painful replied: "Of course." One or two persons reported pleasurable sensations when the blister-base was stimulated by up to 16 mEq. of potassium. Perhaps one of the best examples of metæsthesia is the sensation produced by an energetic scratch of the skin, particularly in response to a slight itch. This is a noxious stimulus producing pleasurable metæsthesia, but if only a little too noxious it produces distinctly unpleasant algæsthesia. From the point of view of experimental pain, it appears that the pain threshold as ascertained by the method of Hardy Wolff and Goodell reveals the metæsthetic range of noxious stimulation. When carried out on one group of persons who, as instructed, reported the "pricking" threshold, 70% noted that they would not have described the sensation as pain. This is reminiscent of our own sensations with the potassium ion. With the pressure algometer, however, one looks for the pressure which the subject calls painful. This method reveals the algæsthetic, not metæsthetic, pain complaint threshold and this is what the patient means when he complains of pain.

The difficulty with terminology on the experimental side commonly intrudes into clinical symptomatology as, for example, when the patient answers a query as to the site of pain with the exasperating reply: "It isn't a pain, just a discomfort or ache." Such a reply commonly comes from hyposensitive persons, even with such severe pathological lesions as cardiac infarction. Once more we are reminded of the importance of the gap between the noxious stimulus and the experience of pain, the gap that is so wide in Sarah. If it had been equally wide in Sir James Young Simpson, he would not have suffered pain from his cardiac infarction and would not have required chloroform!

The basis for this statement lies in the observation of cases of cardiac infarction previously reported of which I would like briefly to cite three examples.

The first was a man of 68 sent by his general practitioner on account of mystifying dyspnœa as an isolated symptom which suggested hysteria. Examination showed left ventricular failure and the electrocardiogram revealed anteroseptal cardiac infarction, from which he made an uneventful recovery to the extent of being able to walk 6 miles without symptoms. 17 months later he returned with similar dyspnœa. The electrocardiogram showed extension of his old anteroseptal infarct, an event which was confirmed at autopsy (Fig. 5). This man was grossly hyposensitive to pressure-pain, his complaint threshold being 6.0 kg. It was this case that first suggested to me the importance of pain sensitivity in relation to the symptom pattern of cardiac infarction. It is clear that this patient was no more sensitive to cardiac infarction than Sarah was to fracture of her metatarsal.

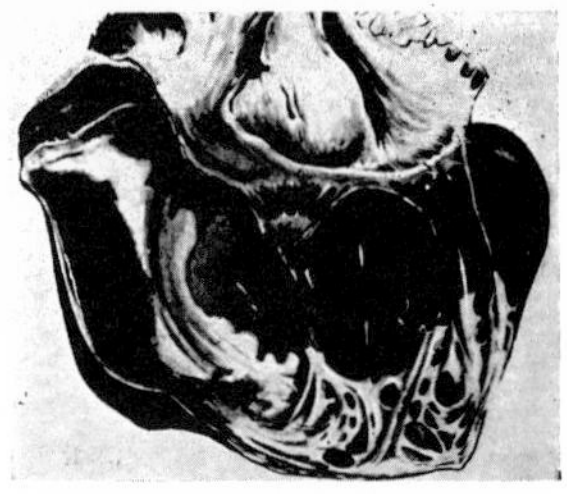

Fig. 5. Extensive anteroseptal cardiac infarction, old and recent, found at autopsy in a patient who experienced no pain.

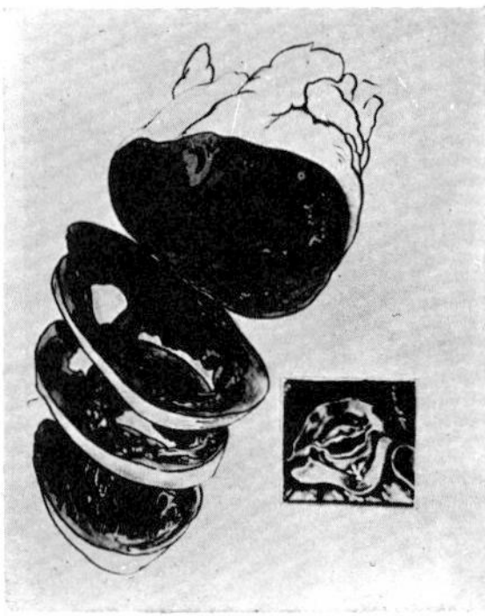

Fig. 6. Multiple areas of cardiac infarction in a man who complained only of a sensation "like a brick in the chest," and denied "pain."

In a similarly hyposensitive man with multiple cardiac infarctions, the only complaint was of a sensation "like a brick in the chest," coupled with the denial that this was pain (Fig. 6). This man can be looked upon as experiencing what I have described as the metæsthetic form of sensation in response to the noxious stimulus of cardiac infarction.

On the other hand, in a hypersensitive patient with a pressure-pain threshold of 1.5 kg. pain was so persistent, occuring repeatedly at night on dreaming, with rises of blood pressure, that eventually sympathectomy was performed and relief was obtained. He died suddenly on going out into the snow one night. At autopsy there were only several small scars of old infarcts. This man's response is reminiscent of Simpson's distress from cardiac infarction.

Such clinical observations led me to observe the relation of pain sensitivity to symptoms in a series of 74 cases of cardiac infarction. It was found that the intensity and duration of pain varied inversely with the pressure-pain complaint threshold of the patient.

In this series of patients, morphine was used as the analgesic. It was noted that the amount required was significantly correlated with the patient's sensitivity and with the duration of the pain. The morphine requirement was also significantly related to the noxious stimulus as represented by the extent of S-T segment and T-wave changes on the standard 12 lead electrocardiogram. These changes in their turn were correlated with the peak serum glutamic oxaloacetic transaminase. Unfortunately it is not possible accurately to assess the noxious stimulus in any disease to which man is heir. Cardiac infarction is exceptional in that its extent is reflected in the electrocardiograph, and this correlates with the chemical evidence of muscle destruction in the form of the liberation of transaminases. Taken together, therefore, it seems reasonable to regard them as a significant quantitative index of the noxious stimulus. If this is accepted, the pain of cardiac infarction is found to be directly related in its intensity and duration to the magnitude of the noxious stimulus and inversely to the pressure-pain threshold. The requirement of morphine was also directly related to the magnitude of the noxious stimulus and inversely to the pain threshold. Thus, elevation of the threshold of pain complaint has a similar effect on the symptom of pain to that of morphine; both reduce the pain of cardiac infarction from the distressing degree which we have called algæsthesia to the neutral sensation which we have called metæsthesia. This similarity prompts me to ask the question: does morphine act to a greater degree than has been suspected simply by raising the threshold for algæsthetic pain perception?

I have tried to show that there is a meaningful relationship between a patient's response to an experimental pressure-pain producing stimulus and the clinical pain producing stimulus of cardiac infarction. This relationship, I believe, extends to other noxious stimuli produced by disease states. It holds most firmly when the circumstances of the disease most closely resemble those of experimental pain, *i.e.* when a patient has his first experience of pain without any suspicion of its nature. Later, with education and repetition, conditioning emotional factors are built into the picture so that the simple noxious stimulus may come to form but a small factor in the complex pain edifice presented by the patient. Because of this some have claimed that experimental pain can cast no useful light on clinical pain. Patients with their first cardiac infarction and no suspicion of the diagnosis, as in the series described, show the relationship between the two types of pain, but educated patients (like doctors) with the experience of previous cardiac infarcts and much fear thereof show it far less clearly.

My theme brings me back full circle to Simpson's last tragic days of cardiac pain. His symptom pattern strongly suggests that he was sensitive to the noxious stimuli of his cardiac infarction and that he suffered greatly from it. We know, too, that he was repeatedly afflicted by migraine and sciatica throughout his life. This being so, the great achievements which characterised him sprang from a personality strong enough to overcome his sensitivity to pain. It seems to be probable that this very sensitivity to pain was at the root of his great concern with the relief of the pain of childbirth. To me this concern strongly suggests that Simpson was as sensitive to the pain of others as he was to his own. Indeed, the whole pattern of Simpson's life brings forcibly to my mind the perceptive comment of your great Gifford Lecturer, Sir Charles Sherrington, when speaking of altruism:

"Where life ranks highest, there it can suffer most. Human life has among its privileges that of pre-eminence of pain."

REFERENCES

Keele, C. A. and Armstrong, D. (1964). "Substances Producing Pain and Itch." London: Arnold.
Keele, K. D. (1954). *Lancet*, **1**, 636.
——— (1968). *Br. med. J.*, **1**, 670.
Leriche, R. (1957). *Quoted from* Alajouanine, "La douleur et les douleurs." Paris: Masson.
Libman, E. (1934). *J. Am. med. Ass.*, **102**, 335.
Shepherd, J. A. (1969). "Simpson and Syme of Edinburgh." Edinburgh: E. & S. Livingstone.
Sherrington, C. (1940). "Man on His Nature." Cambridge: University Press.
Smith, R. (1962). "The Assessment of Pain in Man and Animals." *ed.* Keele and Smith. London.

SECTION TWO

Measurement of pain

Pain measurement is both one of the most difficult and important tasks of researchers and clinicians. It affects our ability to understand the basic concepts of pain, to produce a proper clinical diagnosis, and to determine the effectiveness of medication or other means of intervention. Two points in the process of measurement have been singled out: threshold and tolerance. Threshold refers to the point where an individual first perceives the stimulation as painful; tolerance refers to the point where the individual is not willing to accept stimulation of a higher magnitude or time duration. The former is usually referred to as the sensory component of pain and has been associated mainly with physiological variables. The latter has been referred to as the reaction component of pain and is affected by psychological factors, such as attitudes and motivation (Gelfand, Gelfand, and Rardin, 1965). When the results of different studies are compared, it is important to know which pain component these studies have measured, threshold or tolerance.

A refinement in the measurement of thresholds has been the recent application of signal detection or sensory decision theory to the measurement of pain reactions (Clark, 1974). Signal detection theory is a method of sorting out a signal from noise. Applying this theory to pain thresholds, the researcher sorts the sensory component (d′) from the criterion used to judge the stimulus painful (Lx). In the assessment of a pain control technique it thus becomes possible to know whether the effects are on the basic sensory component or on the attitudinal-motivational component of pain. The report of pain by a subject or patient usually confounds both aspects—the basic sensory perception and the willingness to label this sensation painful. Craig and Weiss (Reading 25, Section five) show how social influences can increase the willingness to label even low-level noxious stimulation painful. Tursky (1975) points out that a serious drawback in the use of signal detection is the need for a large number of stimuli to evaluate a threshold. Instead, Tursky has utilized a magnitude estimation task to determine sensory perception. In this procedure the subject is asked to compare a series of equal interval stimuli (electric shock) with a standard stimulus. To assess attitudinal-motivational factors, subjects are asked to report the points at which the shock is first perceived, at which it becomes uncomfortable, at which it becomes painful, and at which it will no longer be tolerated. (The application of this procedure is illustrated in the editor's comment for Section four and in Reading 18, Section four.)

What criteria should be used for evaluating a pain stimulus? Hardy, Wolff, and Goodell (1952) and Beecher (1959) have set out a number of requirements. The stimulus should (1) be closely associated with the changes causing pain, (2) yield reproducible, quantitative measurements, (3) be controllable, (4) possess an effective range from threshold to ceiling pain, (5) cause no irreversible tissue damage, (6) evoke different qualities of pain such as burning, pricking, or aching, (7) be convenient to use, (8) yield a clear-cut sensation of pain, and (9) provide for entry at all ranges of the scale.

A large variety of pain stimuli, including chemical, mechanical, electrical, thermal, and ischemic stimuli, has been used. Each technique, it can be argued, fits the criteria of a proper pain stimulus for certain purposes. For example, Wolff and Jarvik (Reading 8) feel that pain produced by varying the concentration of saline is a good technique for producing deep pain. Other types of stimuli may be easier to use but may not be as reliable or valid for producing deep pain. Patkin (Reading 9) demonstrates that a pressure technique would be preferable for the practicing physician from the standpoint of cost, convenience, and practicality. For still further refinement, electrical stimulation might be preferred because it has the advantages of rigid stimulus control and of allowing immediate entrance at any level of stimulation without requiring that one first go through the entire range.

However, Beecher has argued that it is not possible to equate laboratory pain with clinic pain produced by pathological processes (see Reading 5). Whereas in the clinic morphine can be extremely effective in reducing pain reactions, in the laboratory the effects of morphine cannot be distinguished from those of saline. Whereas in the clinic placebos are effective with approximately 35% of patients, in the laboratory this percentage is reduced to 3.2%. The missing ingredient in the laboratory is the anxiety associated with the disease process and the threat of disfigurement or death. Reducing pain reactions in the clinic often involves reducing anxiety. The laboratory presents a different context in which the complexity of the pain response is partially ignored. Thus it may not be possible to generalize results from the laboratory to the clinic.

Sternbach (1968) has argued that the response to morphine is not the only basis for distinguishing pain measurement. In the laboratory it is also possible to create sufficient anxiety to test the effects of different procedures of pain control. In the laboratory it is possible to control the stimulus input; in the clinic it is not.

Recently even Beecher (1966) has admitted that there are laboratory procedures that he can accept. The slowly building-up pain of ischemia and the use of the Tursky, Watson, and O'Connell (1965) electrodes in electric shock stimulation have been accepted as effective pain stimuli (Smith, Parry, Denton, and Beecher, 1970).

However, other investigators have found that the pain of ischemia is not always reliable. Bloomfield and Hurwitz (1970), for example, have tested the effectiveness of aspirin in producing pain relief for ischemic pain produced by a tourniquet procedure in one group and for pain associated with an episiotomy in a second group of women. Although pain relief from the episiotomies was obtained with aspirin, no reliable results were obtained for pain produced by the tourniquets. These results emphasize the complexity of pain perception and the problems of using different pain stimuli for measuring pain reactions.

Beecher (Reading 5) and Lutterbeck (Reading 6) describe some of the procedures necessary in the clinic for adequately quantifying the effects of pain relief procedures. The first requirement is a double-blind condition where neither the patient nor the rater knows what the patient is given. The drug and the placebo are given at random; a technician administers the drug and visits the patient at two 45-minute intervals. Positive results are indicated when the patient indicates both times that his pain is half gone. The percentage of these positive results is calculated. Beecher feels that this approach works and is reproducible.

This section presents a sample of the different pain measurement procedures. At this time there is no agreement on a single best method. Some of the laboratory procedures have been transferred to the clinic and are described by Keele (Reading 4) and Patkin (Reading 9). Unfortunately, in the clinic there is still a need for a standardized, reproducible, and simple method for determining pain tolerance. Perhaps attitudinal measures will be helpful in this regard (see editor's comment for Section four). Regardless of the method to be used, it is important to carefully standardize the procedures on an adequate sample under controlled conditions. In the clinic it is easy to accept a particular approach because it seemed to predict well for one or two patients. However, after completing a rigorous test of the predictive power of a procedure based on 1 or 2 patients, the clinician can be quite shocked by how little validity this procedure has.

REFERENCES

Beecher, H. K. 1959. Measurement of subjective responses: quantitative effect of drugs, Oxford University Press, Inc., New York.

Beecher, H. K. 1966. Pain: one mystery solved, Science **151:**840–841.

Bloomfield, S. S., and Hurwitz, H. N. 1970. Tourniquet and episiotomy pain as test models for aspirin-like analgesics, Journal of Clinical Pharmacology **10:**361-369.

Clark, W. C. 1974. Pain sensitivity and the report of pain: an introduction to sensory decision theory, Anesthesiology **40:**272-287.

Gelfand, D. M., Gelfand, S., and Rardin. M. W. 1965. Some personality factors associated with placebo responsivity, Psychological Reports **17:**555-562.

Hardy, J. D., Wolff, H. G., and Goodell, H. 1952. Pain sensations and reactions, Hafner Publishing Co., New York.

Smith, G. M., Parry, W. L., Denton, J. E., and Beecher, H. K. 1970. Effect of morphine on pain produced in man by electric shock delivered through an annular-disc cellulose sponge electrode, Proceedings of the 87th Annual Convention, American Psychological Association, Washington, D. C., the Association, pp. 819-820.

Sternbach, R. A. 1968. Pain: a psychophysiological analysis, Academic Press, Inc., New York.

Tursky, B. 1975. The measurement of pain reactions: laboratory studies. In Weisenberg, M., editor: The control of pain, Psychological Dimensions, Inc., New York.

Tursky, B., Watson, P. D., and O'Connell, D. N. 1965. A concentric shock electrode for pain stimulation, Psychophysiology **1:**296-298.

5

Quantification of the subjective pain experience

Henry K. Beecher, M.D.

Part II: Psychopathology of pain, taste and time

Probably the most ancient reason for the development of the physician was the symptom of pain. Of all the ills man is subjected to, pain seems to be the one most urgently requiring treatment. Since pain has such ancient origins and connotations, this may be the reason pain and its treatment are encumbered by more folklore than anything else in medicine. The many exciting advances in specific therapeutics of recent years should not draw out attention from the fact that a very large part of the practice of medicine consists still in the relief of symptoms.

It became possible some years ago to deal with pain in a quantitative manner in terms of the percentage of individuals who present certain arbitrary criteria (i.e., pain "half gone" at both 45 and 90 minutes after a drug or placebo injection).[4,8,17,18,19,35,36] As a consequence of the quantitative approach, it has been possible to cut through and discard much of the confusing folklore in this important field. As Lord Kelvin said:

> "I often say that when you can measure what you are speaking about, and express it in numbers, you know something about it; but when you cannot measure it, when you cannot express it in numbers, your knowledge is of a meagre and unsatisfactory kind; it may be the beginning of knowledge, but you have scarcely, in your thoughts, advanced to the stage of *Science* whatever the matter may be"

For years I have been an ardent follower of this point of view.

Psychopharmacology has its roots deeply buried in sensation and in alterations in sensation produced by drugs. One could place at 200 years ago the beginnings of a modern interest in sensation with Haller's *Elementa physiologiae* (1757-1766). In this he discussed fully the senses; however, I would much prefer to place the beginnings at Charles Bell's discovery in 1811, and its confirmation 11 years later by Magendie, that there are two kinds of nerves—sensory which lead to the posterior roots of the spinal cord and motor from the anterior roots. This discovery 150 years ago ". . . reminded the physiologists that the mind's sensations were as much their business as the muscles' movements." Motor conduction could be studied a hundred years ago since the motor nerve has a muscle at its end. "At the end of the sensory nerve there was only introspection. . . ." I do not suppose anybody holds the belief that there is any such thing as a pure sensation. We have perceptions, that is, modified sensations, certainly modified at both a cortical and subcortical level, modified by drugs at sites and levels about which we know only a little.

Present gaps in fundamental knowledge need not oblige us to remain at a purely

Reprinted by permission of Grune and Stratton, Inc. from Hoch, P. H., and Zubin, J., editors: Psychopathology of perception, pp. 111-128. Copyright 1965.
From the Anaesthesia Laboratory of the Harvard Medical School at the Massachusetts General Hospital, Boston, Mass.

descriptive level. We can now proceed from descriptive words alone to numbers in many instances in psychopharmacology and I think it is urgent to do so whenever this is possible.

The beginnings of what Lord Kelvin might have called a scientific approach to these problems can be found in 1846 when Ernst Heinrich Weber became interested in separating pain from the sensation of touch. Four years later, in 1850, Fechner saw in Weber's studies on intensity of sensory experience, ". . . a way for writing quantitative relations between mind and body, or, more particularly, between sensation and its stimulus." At the moment we are not interested in whether Fechner's "logarithmic law" is the correct expression of such matters or, as Stevens believes[41] that Plateau's "power law" is the correct representation.

Before I give you practical evidence that one can indeed work with pain in quantitative terms, I should like to introduce a caution.

Since the quantification of subjective response is of first concern here, it is, in a broad sense,[41] an exercise in psychophysics. Yet those who look for what is sometimes called the "psychophysics of pain" will find no elaborate presentation of this subject. The reason is simple: enough dependable data are not as yet available. This is not to dismiss thoughtlessly the painstaking work on the "dol," an earnest attempt to establish the "psychophysics of pain" on a basis comparable to that already developed for vision and for hearing. (This work has been given a reasonably full discussion by Beecher.[9]) The failure of other careful investigators to confirm much of that work on pain leaves its precise meaning in doubt. If the psychophysics of pain is ever to be established in an orderly way, much of the material in the following pages will have to be drawn into the formulation. The complexity of the problem makes it seem unlikely that it will prove possible to describe the psychophysics of pain in a definitive manner, except perhaps in some limited experimental situations where the pain aroused may have little relation to the pain experienced in disease. A definitive psychophysics of vision, of hearing, perhaps of taste, smell, and touch, yes, for these sensations can be turned on and off by stimulus control. But the task of developing the psychophysics of significant pain would be like that of studying the "psychophysics" of emotion or of anxiety, experiences whose stimulus correlates are only to be guessed at. There is indeed reason to believe that anxiety constitutes one of the basic elements in the pain process. We are not likely to make an effective attack on the psychophysics of pain of pathological origin until a host of elusive variables have been brought under control.

Many investigators seem grimly determined to establish – indeed, too often there does not seem to have been any question in their mind – that for a given stimulus there must be a given response; that is, for so much stimulation of pain endings, so much pain will be experienced, and so on. This fundamental error has led to enormous waste. If this paper does no more than to point clearly to this, it will have succeeded in one of its major purposes. This mistake has been common in laboratories where principal attention has been devoted to techniques of producing experimental pain in man. Work presented here makes it clear that there is no simple relationship between stimulus and subjective response. It is also made evident that the reason for this is the interposition of conditioning, of the processing component, of the psychic reaction. It is evident that this component merits and must have extensive consideration. It must be taken into account not only for pain but probably for all subjective responses.

In years gone by I have been asked why one whose primary orientation is in the field of research in anesthesia should spend so much time on the problem of pain and its treatment. There is more than one good answer to this question, I believe. Rather obviously the anesthetist's entire life is concerned with the amelioration, or the avoidance, or the suppression of pain. I believe one must agree that basically – broadly – the anesthetist's interests are founded on the factors which diminish irritability. At least this is true at a cellular level. At a cellular level one must conclude that any factors which diminish the irritability of a single cell are within the anesthetist's province. Cellular irritability and the factors which determine it constitute the central problem of all biology; for that matter, they constitute the central problem of life itself.

There is another good reason why the anesthetist can quite properly be interested not only in pain and its relief but in other broadly associated fields; let me illustrate this in the following way: There are five major classes of drugs of particular interest to the pharmacologist, drugs which have as their primary purpose the alteration of subjective responses. There are sedatives and hypnotics (sleep-producing agents), analgesics (pain-relieving agents), ego depressants (used by psychiatrists to probe disturbed patients' minds) and, finally, the anesthetics. One can, by the simple expedient of administering a barbiturate, produce sedation. A small increase in the dose of the same agent and it becomes a hypnotic; further increase in the dose and analgesia is produced. A still further increase and ego depression occurs. Still more of the drug and anesthesia ensues. It is impossible for me to believe that nature is aware of boundaries between any of these pairs of arbitrarily designated conditions. Since one can by the simple expedient of increasing the dose of a given drug move from the mild state of sedation, through hypnosis, analgesia, ego depression and into profound anesthesia, it seems most likely that there are mechanisms held in common in the production of all five of these states. One would expect to find stimulating cross fertilization of ideas and new approaches to the study of anesthetics, for example, by studying hypnotics. One would expect to gain insight into ego depression by studying sedation, and so on. I shall give you some evidence for such cross fertilization from our own work over the past 20 years.

Twenty years ago we started with the supposition that pain was pain, that it varied in duration, quality and intensity but that however produced it was pretty much the same thing, varying only in the qualities just mentioned. We knew that pain had been experimentally contrived in the laboratory in many ways, by skin pricks, by electric shocks to teeth, by chemicals placed in blisters, by tourniquets, by physical pressure, by cold, by heat. In the beginning we had no doubt that all of these methods were useful, for indeed they did produce pain. That was unquestionable. So we set out to use one of the methods which had been carefully worked out by Hardy, Wolff and Goodell.[29] With our interest in quantification, this method was particularly attractive, for it presented a means of measuring accurately the amount of heat thrown on an area of the skin, usually the forehead. Since we wished to study pain in man, this seemed to be a fine approach. To cut short a long and painful period, it was a rude shock for us to find that with this beautifully worked out method we could not distinguish between a large dose of morphine (15 mg.) and 1 ml. of normal saline. Of course both of these agents were administered as unknowns to subject and to observer. (This double unknowns technique is a requirement for studies in this field.) We turned then to a man who had had a great deal of experience with this Hardy-Wolff-Goodell method and, again to shorten a long story, he was quite unable, notwithstanding his early successes with the method (when he had not worked with the double unknowns technique), to distinguish between a large dose of morphine and a little table salt in solution.

As the years have gone by, some 15 groups in England and America have now utterly failed to demonstrate any dependable relationship in man between the relief of experimentally contrived pain, called the pain threshold, and great doses of narcotic. This refers to the methods generally used at present. It may be possible in the future to devise experimental methods wherein the pain threshold will respond in dependable fashion to graded doses of narcotic. These matters have all been dealt with extensively and the proper references made elsewhere in my book.[9] This need not be documented further here.

When one takes into account the fact just mentioned of the failure of experimentally produced pain in man to respond dependably to even large doses of narcotic agents, when one places this fact alongside the universally observed fact that pain arising from disease or injury, what we shall call pathological pain from here on, *always* responds in greater or lesser degree to even small doses of morphine and similar narcotics, then one must conclude that our original assumption that pain was pain whatever its origin simply does not hold. There is some fundamental and mysterious difference between pain produced in the laboratory, even severe pain produced there, and the pain produced by disease or injury.

In fairness to Hardy, Wolff and Goodell, and other originators of experimentally produced pain studies, I should like to say at once that experimentally contrived pain surely does have its uses in man. For example, the classic work of Gasser, Erlanger, Heinbecker, Bishop, and others in which they identified pain pathways, has very often depended upon experimentally produced pain. One must add also that experimental pain in animals is a useful approach to certain kinds of important studies. The Hardy-Wolff-Goodell method works beautifully when a small quantity of heat is thrown on a rat's tail, as applied by D'Armour and Smith.[16] I suspect that all pain is to an animal serious and significant. It does not seem like a reckless assumption to assume that an animal is quite unable to distinguish between experimental pain and pathological pain. Indeed, there may be a clue in this statement to a very significant factor in the pain situation. Later on evidence will be given to indicate that the meaning of the pain sensation is the factor which determines the suffering from it. We all know that a small ache in a finger may be a trivial annoyance, easily disregarded, whereas the same duration and intensity of an ache beneath the sternum, if it connotes the possibility of sudden death from heart failure, may be a wholly unsettling experience. The implications contained in these statements are of such importance I should like to deal with them in some detail.

It long ago became apparent from study of the world's literature on pain that this subjective experience is one surrounded by many pitfalls to trap the unwary. It early became apparent that sound design of study was to be of paramount importance.

Many workers beside myself have made contributions to this area. For example, the Keeles[35,36] in England long ago understood the requirements for study here. Many important contributions have been made by colleagues in our laboratory, to name a few: Denton, Lasagna, Keats and Smith. The contributions of many others besides our own have been described in my book.[9] I should like to mention, however, in a few words the essentials of sound design in the study of the pain experience. (These remarks apply to other subjective responses as well.) As I indicated a moment ago, an individual's bias may be a crippling matter in such studies. The subject's and the observer's bias must therefore be eliminated. This is done by the use of the double blind approach where neither subject nor observer knows what has been administered in a given case. It is also essential to insert placebos into the situation, also as unknowns. The word placebo means "I shall please." A placebo is a substance inert in its ordinary biological sense, which is given to the subject with the subject's belief that it is or may be an active drug. As we shall see later on, situations can have placebo effects also, the concept of a placebo as only something that pleases has to be modified to include effects and situations produced by placebos which may be unpleasant. We must have the double blind approach, the use of placebos, randomization of the placebos and drugs studied, isolation of one subject from another so they cannot compare and discuss the effects experienced, and mathematical validation of supposed differences encountered. It is necessary to have a sufficient number of subjects, usually not fewer than 25, for work on pain. In studying postoperative wound pain, for example, one has to rely on the subject's statement that he is having pain of a given degree – none, slight, moderate or severe. In our work we chose to record whatever the fact was, severe pain for example, administer an unknown solution which might be an active drug or which might be a placebo; a neutral technician visits the patient 45 minutes later and again 90 minutes after the drug was administered. For a positive result we arbitrarily require that a patient say his pain is at least half gone on both occasions. If he says it is all gone on one occasion and not half on another, it is arbitrarily recorded as a negative result. There are many ways of approaching this problem. This one has worked well in our hands. It may seem as though the "one-half gone" decision was a difficult one to make, but actual experience has shown that patients have found this judgment easy to make and to reproduce. We then take the number of individuals in a given group whose result was "positive" and calculate their percentage. This makes it possible to fulfill Lord Kelvin's requirement of placing significant numbers in front of meaningful items. We can thus compare a new agent with a standard, usually morphine, or a placebo, in studies of pain.

You may say, what actual evidence do you have that one can deal in a quantitative manner here? I can refer you to some data obtained in this laboratory.[33] We had an outside individual make up two series of flasks, six flasks in Series A and six in Series B. We did not know what either series contained, but assumed that one series contained a pain-relieving agent. When we had completed the study, using postoperative wound pain, and broke the code, we found that both series of flasks had contained morphine. In Series A there was always 10 mg./ml. In Series B there were different concentrations of morphine in each flask. On graphing the data we constructed the two lines shown in figure 1.[33] Where the two graphs crossed, there is equivalence of analgesic action: we had equated 10 mg. morphine to 10.8, an 8 per cent error. As any statistician knows, these are not truly lines that cross but bands that cross, and one must calculate the regression lines, and this was done under the guidance of Professor Frederick Mosteller, without whom none of our work would have been possible. (As a mathematician, he has kept us from many errors.) These calculations required that we add 2 per cent more to the 8 per cent error and gives a total error of 10 per cent. We are thus able to work quantitatively in the elusive field of subjective responses. I submit that this 10 per cent error is about as accurately as one measures most objective things in man (except for perhaps chemical determinations in a sample of blood) such as blood pressure, cell counts, and so on.

Another observation which gave us reason to believe that we were working in a satisfactorily dependable manner was the reproducibility and agreement from time to time of the data obtained, not only in our own laboratory but by others. For example, Houde and Wallenstein are two of the ablest workers in this field, working usually with the pain from cancer, presumably the pain from smooth muscle and periosteum; they found also that 10 mg. morphine relieved 65 per cent of the individuals, as shown in table 1.[27,37,38] While it is true that such isolated data do not prove anything, they are contributing evidence that we were on the right track. They also gave some reason for the cautious generalization that pain from pathological origin was very much alike in that it responded in the same way to a given dose of pain-relieving agent.

Quantitative studies have led to some very practical results of a dependable sort. For example, with the great tensions in the world situation, with China fairly cut off from the Western world, we have lost that source of opium from which morphine is made. It is quite conceivable that other sources of opium, such as the Middle East and India, may become suddenly unavailable. We need have no fear that this will

Table 1. Pain relief effected by 10 mg. morphine and by a placebo in two independent laboratories

Investigators	*Studies*	*No. of patients*	*Per cent relieved*	
			Morphine 10 mg. s.c.	*Placebo*
Lasagna and Beecher	1952	66	65.8	
Postoperative wound pain	1953	56	69.3	39.0*
Houde and Wallenstein	1952-1953	67	65.0	42.0
Chronic pain in cancer patients				

*Averaged data from Lasagna, Mosteller, von Felsinger and Beecher, 1954.[38]

result in our being without adequate pain-relieving agents. For example, a considerable family of methadones,[18,19] which are made rather simply from substances common to the world of commerce, the nitriles, can be made into agents just as effective as morphine for pain relief. Several of these methadones are milligram for milligram the equivalent of morphine. Unfortunately, they are milligram for milligram equivalent to morphine in undesirable effects as well. They produce just as much depression of the respiration, just as much addiction, and so on. There is reason to believe, from our work, that the levo-iso-methadone has less nausea associated with it for an equal degree of pain relief than is true of morphine.

The quantitative approach I have just mentioned lends itself very well to a comparison of new agents designed to relieve pain. Unfortunately, pain-relieving agents must be measured against two yardsticks. There is the pain-relieving yardstick and there is the side-effect yardstick, and so what Lasagna and I[37] like to call the optimal dose of morphine, or the optimal dose of any other pain-relieving agent, is determined from placing both yardsticks where we can see them and arriving somewhat arbitrarily at the most advantageous dose of agent to use, taking into account the agent's rather accurately determined pain-relieving power per milligram and also its undesirable side effects per milligram.

It is our hope that the use of the technique referred to will make it possible eventually to find an agent which will relieve pain but not have the sometimes devastating side effects that powerful pain-relieving agents have at the present time.

AN OLD CONCEPT NEWLY APPLIED

In 1894, a philosopher, Marshall, wrote a book, *Pain, Pleasure and Aesthetics,* in which he almost made a crucial assumption.[40] He did in fact lay the background for an assumption which was made the next year by Strong.[42] This assumption said, in effect, that an experience like suffering has two major components, the original sensation and the processing component, or what I like to call the psychological reaction component. So far as I have been able to discover, neither Marshall nor Strong had any factual evidence for this concept. It seems to have been simply one of those brilliant intuitive insights which have been so rewarding in medicine over the centuries. We have been able to gain, however, considerable supporting evidence for this Marshall-Strong concept and I should like to tell you about it because this evidence has given us some rather far-reaching insights not only into the origins of pain and the control of pain but also into other subjective responses and their modification by drugs in man.

THE REACTION COMPONENT

In the immediately preceding section, I mentioned that an experience such as suffering consists of two elements, the original sensation and the reaction component. I also described, in the preceding section on "Pain," that pain as now commonly contrived experimentally does not respond in man in a dependable fashion to even large doses of narcotics. Then I made the working hypothesis that the original sensation was not the site of action of drugs such as morphine. It is surely true that there is no such thing as pure sensation, all sensations having been modified, probably at a subcortical level before they erupt into consciousness and certainly modified after erupting into consciousness by conditioning, significance, meaning. If such agents as narcotics are without effect, as seems to be the case, on the original sensation or the nearest approximation to the original sensation, then the site of action must be the reaction component. At least we can take this as a working hypothesis and then see how pertinent data relate to the concept. I should now like to present evidence that this is in truth the case, that the reaction component has vast influence on our lives. First, I should like to present in support of this thesis the effect of placebos.

PLACEBO

It was only after I had worked in this field for some years that I realized we usually had a very high average degree of effectiveness of placebos in treating postoperative wound pain and other conditions as well. Following this realization I then looked around amongst the papers of other individuals and was struck by the beautiful

Table 2. Therapeutic effectiveness of placebos in several conditions (From Beecher, 1955[5])

Condition	*Study*	*Placebo*		*Source of data*	*Number of patients*	*Per cent satisfactorily relieved by a placebo*
		Agent	*Route*			
Severe post-operative wound pain	Keats and Beecher (1950)	Saline	I.V.		118	21
	Beecher, Deffer, Fink and Sullivan (1951)	Saline	S.C.		29	31
	Keats, D'Allesandro and Beecher (1951)	Saline	I.V.		34	26
	Beecher, Keats, Mosteller and Lasagna (1953)	Lactose	P.O.		52	40 } 33
					36	26
					44	34
					40	32
	Lasagna, Mosteller, von Felsinger and Beecher (1954)	Saline	S.C.		14	50 } 39
					20	37
					15	53
					21	40
					15	40
					15	15
Cough	Gravenstein, Devloo and Beecher (1954)	Lactose	P.O.		22	36 } 40
					23	43
Drug-induced mood changes	Lasagna, von Felsinger and Beecher (1955)	Normal Saline	S.C.	Normals	20	30
				Post-addicts	30	30
Pain from angina pectoris	Evans and Hoyle (1933)	Sodium bicarbonate	P.O.		66	38
	Travell, Rinzler, Bakst, Benjamin and Bobb (1959)	"Placebo"	P.O.		19	26
	Greiner, Gold, Cattell, Travell and ten colleagues (1950)	Lactose	P.O.		27	38
Headache	Jellinek (1946)	Lactose	P.O.		199	52
Seasickness	Gay and Carliner (1949)	Lactose	P.O.		33	58
Anxiety and tension	Wolf and Pinsky (1954)	Lactose	P.O.		31	30
Experimental cough	Hillis (1952)	Normal Saline	S.C.	Many scores of experiments	1	37
Common cold	Diehl (1933)	Lactose	P.O.	Cold acute	110	35
				Subacute chronic	48	35
					1082 Total patients	35.2 ± 2.2% Average relieved

study of Evans and Hoyle[23] in England. In this pioneer and now classic study they found that the pain of angina pectoris was relieved by placebos just about as often as we later found for the pain of postoperative wounds. The paper of Evans and Hoyle marks a considerable milestone in clinical sophistication in studies of subjective responses. With this much material in hand, I then made quite a search of the literature for other comparable findings. This material is summarized in table 2, which I first presented in a paper called "The Powerful Placebo."[5] One must call attention to the fact that the data presented in table 2 are *average* figures.

I have obtained a good deal of data, some better than others, that the effectiveness of a placebo is very much greater when stress is severe than when it is not. For example, I found[7] that when pain was very severe following surgery, the usual dose of morphine relieved not the usual 65 per cent of individuals but now only 52 per cent. At the same time a placebo relieved 40 per cent. If one considers that the 52 per cent relievable by the morphine represents roughly the maximum amount of pain relievable by chemical agents, then the 40 per cent is actually 77 per cent of 52 per cent, and we see that the placebo effectiveness is twice as great as one had found on the average. When the pain diminished in severity the same dose of morphine then relieved 89 per cent of individuals, but curiously the placebo effect had fallen to 26 per cent. Twenty-six per cent of 89 per cent, is now 29 per cent compared with the earlier 77 per cent, only about one-third as much as it had been. It is true, as some have pointed out, that this may represent a special situation and one can find conflicting data. Less easily open to challenge, however, are the following data.[9] As I have pointed out, the average effectiveness of placebos when dealing with pathological pain is 35 per cent, the average effectiveness of placebos with experimentally contrived pain is only 3.2 per cent. In other words, the placebo is *10 times* more effective in relieving pain of pathological origin than it is in relieving pain of experimentally contrived origin. These data I believe, are difficult to get around; they illustrate my point. There is, it is true, a mild assumption involved here but one I do not believe anybody would have difficulty in accepting, that there is more anxiety associated with pain from disease than there is in pain experimentally contrived in the laboratory. Consider the example of the finger pain and the substernal pain mentioned above. This assumption seems to be so far removed from the possibility of adequate challenge that it need not be discussed further. When stress is severe, placebos are more effective than when stress is less or absent.

I mentioned earlier that morphine was not dependably effective in man in relieving experimentally contrived pain as usually produced, but was always effective in greater or lesser degree in relieving pain of pathological origin. Thus one can, I believe, state a new principle of drug action: some drugs are effective only in the presence of an appropriate mental state.

Much more could be said about chemical agents as placebos but before we leave this section I should like to point out that situations can also have placebo effects—the surgical situation, for example. In 1939 it was suggested, in Italy, that the pain of angina pectoris could be greatly lessened by ligation of the internal mammary arteries. Eventually this suggestion was adopted in America and rather spectacularly favorable results were obtained. Not only were the objective results impressive, the patients said they felt better and the objective evidence supported this: there was great reduction in the number of nitroglycerine pills taken, exercise tolerance was greatly increased; for example, a patient could take only 4 minutes of standardized exercise until intolerable pain stopped him and the T-waves in his electrocardiogram inverted in an ominous way. After the operation this individual could exercise for 10 minutes without pain on the exercise steps and his T-waves did not invert. Several individuals[1,15,21,24] began to wonder if this might not be a placebo effect. They went to their patients, explained the situation and told them they would like to carry out a study where the patients would not know what had been done, nor would the observers know until the study was completed. They told their patients that half of them would have the internal mammary arteries exposed and ligated and the other half would simply have them exposed but not ligated. These studies were carried out and in the case I mentioned above, the individual who had had intolerable pain after 4 minutes of exercise and who after the operation could stand 10 minutes of exercise had had only the sham operation. Many similar examples indicated that ligation had no real effect beyond that of a placebo effect. You may say, what is wrong with this? Our aim is to relieve often and to cure when we can. The difficulty in the present situation was that even though the operation was innocuous in concept, individuals with angina pectoris are in a vulnerable state—one patient died during the procedure and another had a further severe myocardial infarction. Even this simple procedure was not without real hazard. This hazard might have been tolerable if the placebo effects had been lasting, but unfortunately, placebo effects usually last from days to weeks to months at best. Thus we have here an example of a situation rather than a chemical agent acting as a placebo. We should all make a searching examination of our present procedures to see what surgical operations or medical activities at the present time may possibly be nothing more than placebo procedures.[10,11] Placebo effects however produced surely are to be construed as evidence for the existence of a powerful reaction component.

SUFFERING AND THE SIGNIFICANCE OF THE WOUND

Another type of support for the reaction component is the finding that the significance of the wound seems to have great influence on the amount of pain resulting from a given injury. In a study of men wounded in battle[3] I was astonished to find in some 215 seriously wounded men that only 25 per cent had enough pain to want anything done about it and so stated in response to a direct question which reminded them that they could have a narcotic if they wanted it. Three quarters simply did not need such help. There were 50 men in each of four groups: serious wounds of the extremities (compound and comminuted fractures or traumatic amputations), extensive soft tissue wounds, penetrated chests, penetrated abdomens, and a final group of 15 with penetrated cerebrums. Only those individuals were included in the study who were clear mentally, with normal blood pressure, not in shock. In many cases they had had no narcotic at all but in no case had they had one within 4 hours. This study was repeated in civilian life where the injury was merely a surgical wound, made under anesthesia. In this latter case the ratio was reversed. More than 80 per cent of such individuals had enough pain to want something done about it. This comparison is described in a paper on the significance of the wound.[7] The wounded soldiers were studied principally on the Anzio beachhead where shelling never stopped day or night for months and where every individual realized that the possibility of death was not a remote thing even for himself. When such men were struck down, the wound meant that the war was suddenly over for the individual; it was a ticket to the safety of the hospital and then home. In the early hours the wound seemed to be construed as a good thing. On the other hand, in the civilian experience the necessity for surgery is uniformly considered to be a disaster by normal individuals. I believe that the significance of the wound, the meaning of the wound in this case, determines the suffering therefrom. I had thought in the beginning that this was an original observation, but found this not to be the case. For example, Guthrie, writing about the Peninsular Wars in Europe in 1827, said that of two individuals suffering the same decrement from the wound, one will smile with contempt whilst the other writhes in pain.[28] Dupuytren, the leading surgeon of his time in France, said almost precisely the same thing. A small boy injured in a fist fight may have been quite severely bruised or cut and felt no pain while emotion was high. We all know that distraction can block pain, that emotion can block pain. It has always seemed puzzling to me that the wise Lord Adrian could have believed that pain dominates the central nervous system: ". . . pain messages are clearly more potent than any others . . . in capturing the attention," he said.[2] This simply is not the case. Emotion can dominate the central nervous system. One hardly needs to emphasize that fact to this group. So also can counterirritation, distraction, attention to other things—all of these can dominate the central nervous system and block the perception of pain. Pain often does not dominate. These matters reflect the power and importance of the reaction component.

• • •

All of these things, the fact that emotion can block pain, that the signifcance of the wound seemingly determines the presence or absence of suffering, the powerful action of placebos and increased effectiveness of placebos with increased stress, and the same for some active drugs—all of these things add up to strong evidence that the psychological processing of the original sensation, the reaction component, is the site of action of drugs which modify subjective responses. This also surely is the site of action of the many nonspecific forces which can modify disease and its treatment.[11]

Measurement in the field of sensations and mood presents an area of significance in human behavior. This work is relevant to the behavioral sciences. The behavioral sciences must, if they are to be soundly established, move onward from the present state which in many areas is largely one of description to one of measurement. Measurement depends upon the recognition and precise definition of variables and their relationships, and the development of tools and techniques for working with them in quantitative terms. As in all sciences eventually there must be possibility of prediction. Implicit in this not only is the necessity to recognize elements that can be measured, but to understand the existence and nature of the essential safeguards, the controls, of observations made. One goal of science is rules ("laws") and the more invariable these rules are, the better it is. We seek to predict from given situation to certain effect. In the complex field of the behavioral sciences in man, observations have, as mentioned, so far largely been descriptive. The basic purpose of these comments is to show that a quantitative approach to sensation ("feeling") is possible and rewarding. Sensation as used here and mood are often controlling factors in behavior and as such are elementary considerations in the development of the behavioral sciences.

REFERENCES

1. Adams, R.: Internal-mammary-artery ligation for coronary insufficiency, evaluation. New Engl. J. Med. *258:* 113-115, 1958.
2. Adrian, E. D.: Pain and its problems. I. The physiology of pain. Practioner *158:*76-82, 1947.
3. Beecher, H. K.: Pain in men wounded in battle. Ann. Surg. *123:* 96-105, 1946.
4. ———: Experimental pharmacology and measurement of the subjective response. Science *116:* 157-162, 1952.
5. ——— The powerful placebo. J.A.M.A. *159:* 1602-1606, 1955.
6. ———: Evidence for increased effectiveness of placebos with increased stress. Amer. J. Physiol. *187:* 163-169, 1956a.
7. ———: Relationship of significance of wound to the pain experienced, J.A.M.A. *161:* 1609-1613, 1956b.
8. ———: Measurement of Subjective Responses: Quantitative Effects of Drugs. New York, Oxford University Press, 1959.
9. ———: Increased stress and effectiveness of placebos and "active" drugs. Science 132:91-92, 1960.
10. ———: Surgery as placebo. J.A.M.A. 1102-1107, 1961.
11. ———: Nonspecific forces surrounding disease and the treatment of disease. J.A.M.A. *179:* 437-440, 1962.
12. ———, Deffer, P. A., Fink, F. E., and Sullivan, D. B.: Field use of methadone and levo-iso-methadone in a combat zone (Hamhung-Hungnam, North Korea). U.S. Forces med. J. *2:* 1269-1276, 1951.
13. ———, Keats, A. S., Mosteller, F., and Lasagna, L: The effectiveness of oral analgesics (morphine, codeine, acetylsalicylic acid) and the problem of placebo "reactors" and "non-reactors." J. Pharmacol. *109:* 393-400, 1953.
14. Boring, E. G.: Sensation and Perception in the History of Experimental Psychology. New York, Appleton-Century-Crofts, 1942.
15. Cobb, L. A., Thomas, G. I., Dillard, D. H., Meredino, K. A., and Bruce, R. A.: Evaluation of internal-mammary-artery ligation by double-blind technic. New Engl. J. Med. *260:* 1115-1118, 1959.
16. D'Amour, F. E., and Smith, D. L.: A method for determining loss of pain sensation. J. Pharmacol. *72:* 74-79, 1941.
17. Denton, J. E., and Beecher, H. K.: New Analgesics. I. Methods in the clinical evaluation of new analgesics. J.A.M.A. *141:* 1051-1057, 1949a.
18. ———, and ———: New Analgesics. II. A clinical appraisal of the narcotic power of methadone and its isomers. J.A.M.A. *141:* 1146-1148, 1949a.
19. ———, and ———: New analgesics. III. A comparison of the side effects of morphine, methadone and methadone's isomers in man. J.A.M.A. *141:* 1148-1153, 1949c.
20. Diehl, H. S.: Medicinal treatment of common cold. J.A.M.A. *101:* 2042-2049, 1933.
21. Dimond, E. G., Kittle, C. F., and Crockett, J. E.: Evaluation of internal mammary artery ligation and sham procedure in angina pectoris. Circulation *18:* 712-713, 1958.
22. Dupuytren, quoted by Lescellière-Lafosse, F. G.: Histoire de la cicatrisation, de ses modes de formation, et des considérations pathologiques et therapéutiques qui en découlent, Montpellier, France, Castel, 1836, p. 29.
23. Evans, W., and Hoyle, C.: The comparative value of drugs used in the continuous treatment of angina pectoris. Quart. J. Med *2:* 311-338, 1933.
24. Fish, R. G., Crymes, T. P., and Lovell, M. G.: Internal-mammary-artery ligation for angina pectoris; its failure to produce relief. New Engl. J. Med. *259:* 418-420, 1958.
25. Gay, L. M., and Carliner, P. E.: The prevention and treatment of motion sickness. Johns Hopkins Hosp. Bull. *84:* 470-487, 1949.
26. Gravenstein, J. S., Devloo, R. A., and Beecher, H. K.: Effect of antitussive agents on experimental and pathological cough in man. J. Appl. Physiol. *7:* 119-139, 1954.
27. Greiner, T., Gold. H., Cattell, McK., Travell, J., Bakst, H., Rinzler, S. H., Benjamin, Z. H., Warshaw, L. J., Bobb, A. L., Kwit, N. T., Modell, W., Rothendler, H. H., Nesseloff, C. R., and Kramer, M. L.: A method for the evaluation of the effects of drugs on cardiac pain in patients with angina of effort. Amer. J. Med. *9:* 143-155, 1950.

28. Guthrie, G. J.: A Treatise on Gunshot Wounds. London, 1827, p. 3.
29. Hardy, J. D., Wolff, H. G., and Goodell, H.: Pain Sensations and Reactions. Baltimore, Williams & Wilkins, 1952.
30. Hillis, B. R.: The assessment of cough suppressing drugs. Lancet *1:* 1230-1235, 1952.
31. Houde, R. W., and Wallenstein, S. L.: A method for evaluating analgesics in patients with chronic pain. Drug Addiction & Narcotics Bull., Appendix F: 660-682, 1953.
32. Jellinek, E. M.: Clinical tests on comparative effectiveness of analgesic drugs. Biomet. Bull. *2:* 87-91, 1946.
33. Keats, A. S., Beecher, H. K., and Mosteller, F. C.: Measurement of pathological pain in distinction to experimental pain. J. Appl. Physiol. *1:* 35-44, 1950.
34. Keats, A. S., D'Alessandro, G. L., and Beecher, H. K.: A controlled study of pain relief by intravenous procaine. J.A.M.A. *147:* 1761-1763, 1951.
35. Keele, C. A.: The assay of analgesic drugs on man. Analyst *77:* 111-117, 1952.
36. Keele, K. D.: The pain chart. Lancet *2:* 6-8, 1948.
37. Lasagna, L., and Beecher, H. K.: The optimal dose of morphine. J.A.M.A. *156:* 230-234, 1954.
38. Lasagna, L., Mosteller, F., von Felsinger, J. M., and Beecher, H. K.: A study of the placebo response. Amer. J. Med. *16:* 770-779, 1954.
39. ———, ———, and ———: Drug induced mood changes in man. I. Observations on healthy subjects, chronically ill patients, and "post-addicts." J.A.M.A. *157:* 1006-1020, 1955.
40. Marshall, H. R.: Pain, pleasure, and aesthetics. Macmillan, London, 1894.
41. Stevens, S. S.: Measurement and man. Science *127:* 383-389, 1958.
42. Strong, G. A.: The psychology of pain. Psychol. Rev. *2:* 329-347, 1895.
43. Travell, J., Rinzler, S. H., Bakst, H., Benjamin, Z. H., and Bobb, A. L.: Comparison of effects of alpha-tocopherol and a matching placebo on chest pain in patients with heart disease. Ann. N.Y. Acad. Sci. *52:* 345-353, 1949.
44. Wolf, S., and Pinsky, R. H.: Effects of placebo administration and occurrence of toxic reactions. J.A.M.A. *155:* 339-341, 1954.

6

Measurement of analgesic activity in man

P. M. Lutterbeck and S. H. Triay

INTRODUCTION

In a discussion of methods used in evaluating analgesics, the major problem is that of comparing experimental pain with clinical or pathological pain. Beecher (one of the authorities on this subject) suspects that to an animal all pain is serious and significant, and that an animal is quite unable to distinguish between experimental and pathological pain [5]. However, using experimental pain as a means of assessing analgesic effectiveness in man lacks meaning to the subject, whereas pathological pain is of relevance to the patient. Wolff [29], on the other hand, considers that this difference between laboratory and pathological pain has been oversimplified. Beecher [3, 25, 27] nevertheless, does not exclude the use of experimental pain and suggests that it can be related to clinical pain if it is induced slowly, such as by means of a tourniquet on the arm.

Despite periodic waves of interest in experimental pain, clinical pain has become more widely used. Numerous investigators have been guided by Beecher's technique, which demonstrates that subjective human responses can be used to measure quantitatively pathological as well as physiological clinical phenomena [4].

In considering experimental methods, the variables inherent in clinical pain must be taken into account if such methods are to constitute an advance in analgesic evaluation. Pathological pain has so many aspects that it is virtually impossible to simulate these by experimental procedures. Studies which concentrate on the peripheral manifestations fail to take into account that the major component of clinical pain is central awareness. The present trend of thought indicates that there is no substitute for pathological pain in evaluating potential analgesic drugs.

Reprinted with permission of Urban & Schwarzenberg from the International Journal of Clinical Pharmacology **6**:315-319. Copyright 1972.

CLINICAL OR PATHOLOGICAL PAIN

General considerations

1. It is generally agreed that the observation of analgesic effects in man requires full-time trained nurses as observers, this being the only reliable way of obtaining accurate clinical information [23, 24].

2. It is also recognised that the best estimates of intensity of pain are made verbally by the patients themselves [11, 16, 19].

3. The evaluation of analgesic agents is now on a satisfactory basis in that the techniques have been well worked out, to a large degree, both in theory and in practice. A new drug alleged to have pain relieving properties deserves to be studied under controlled conditions in a variety of types of pain.

Without trials in different clinical situations, one cannot tell whether an agent is generally useful (or useless) as a pain reliever, or effective (or ineffective) in certain kinds of painful states only [23].

4. Pitting the new drug against a standard drug such as morphine or aspirin is essential to the proper pigeonholing of a new agent. It is one thing to say that a drug has some analgesic effect; it is quite another to say that it is an improvement over previously available agents [23].

5. In attempting to control bias in drug assessment Modell [22] has proposed

some cardinal rules which are particularly applicable to the study of analgesics.

a) Controlled, double-blind administration is essential.

b) Psychic, symbolic and cultural implications are controlled by the administration of a placebo.

c) Extraneous factors are controlled by randomization.

An ethical question can be raised when an inert preparation is used in pain studies. This, however, is justified as it distinguishes between "organic" and "psychogenic" pain [14]. Furthermore, an inert medication may appear to relieve pain by a genuine placebo response, or may reflect insensitivity of the method of assessment [18]. A procedure to exclude placebo reactors is advisable, and the use of crossover (intrapatient) trials would minimise this factor provided that the "washout" period is sufficiently long.

CANCER

Malignant disease, as the leading cause of distressing intractable pain, readily guarantees patient availability. Patient sensitivity is sufficient to permit evaluation of relative analgesic potencies. There are, however, distinct disadvantages in using such patients. Variability in dealing with unremitting and fluctuating pain is a serious consideration. Such pain consists of two factors; the perception of painful stimuli, and the psychic modification of these stimuli. Either of these may be altered to produce relief. The patient's previous experience with analgesics and the possibility of tolerance may impede proper assessment if these are not taken into account. Mild analgesic activity may be difficult to assess as no widely acceptable standard is available.

Listed below are various aspects which determine methodology [1, 2, 12].

A) Patient selection

1. A homogenous selection of patient population should be attempted. Malignant pain can be highly variable depending on the extent of the disease and on other therapeutic measures that have been taken.

2. Patients are selected who complain of moderate or severe pain at least 3 hours after a previous analgesic has been given.

B) Trial design

1. A crossover design is more accurate and economical than interpatient trials. Dosages of morphine are compared with dosages of the test drug in a randomized crossover trial. The patient is excluded if he fails to complete a "round". (A complete "round" means that the patient receives all test drugs, each dose being given on a separate day.)

2. Assessments are made at 30 minute intervals for 4 or 5 hours or until the pain has returned to previous levels. A routine analgesic can then be given, provided two hours have elapsed after the last dose. Sleeping patients must be awakened as this state is not indicative of analgesia.

C) Evaluation

1. The patient is evaluated according to the nature and location of pain, extent of disease, prior experience with narcotics and analgesics, and ability to communicate meaningful information.

2. Pain intensity scale is useful as in the following examples:

0 = none; 1 = slight; 2 = moderate; 3 = severe.

Pain relief scale should also be included as follows:

0 = none; 1 = slight; 2 = moderate; 3 = almost complete; 4 = complete.

3. Criteria to be measured can be evaluated according to the following guidelines:

3.1 Changes in pain intensity or PID (= pain intensity difference) derived from rating of pain before medication minus the pain rating after medication.

3.2 Total effects: A measure of the area under the time-effect curve (described by plotting the hourly scores for 5 hours).

3.3 Peak effects: Calculated for change in pain intensity and pain relief (based on individual reports of maximum effect within 3 hours of drug administration).

3.4 Proportion of patients with 50% relief one and two hours after medication.

There are many other important aspects in the evaluation of a potential analgesic, but these are beyond the scope of this discussion. Nevertheless, it should be stressed that in the study of an analgesic in man emphasis must be placed upon a carefully designed and controlled investigation. Full attention must be paid to numerous details without which the trial is meaningless.

POST-OPERATIVE

Most of the comments regarding cancer pain are also relevant to the second clinical situation – post-operative pain.

This clinical entity also guarantees availability and is quite suitable for pilot or controlled studies [6, 8, 16-18, 20].

A) Patient selection

Patients should be chosen from a group with a single operative procedure, e.g. hysterectomy, prostatectomy. The site of operation should be kept uniform to ensure a homogenous population, e.g. lower abdominal surgery.

B) Trial design

1. After pre-operative medication and general anaesthesia at least 24 hours should elapse from the time the patient regains consciousness. Post-operative analgesics are usually given intramuscularly for quick relief of severe pain as well as for convenience.
2. A crossover design is again desirable in spite of rapidly changing pain, as interpatient variability makes a comparison more difficult. If a parallel group design is to be used, a large number of patients is essential. This not only extends the time to complete the trial but considerably increases the cost.
3. Placebo control is necessary in trials of this nature. The objections to placebo control are mitigated by the clear-cut negative findings with consequent discontinuation of this treatment.
4. The problem of placebo reactors must be borne in mind. It has been suggested that the potency of a placebo depends on the preceding drug. This finding must be taken into account in using crossover designs for acute studies of analgesics [13].
5. In crossover trials, the patient's preference can be considered and this would certainly be related to the incidence and severity of side effects. For example, with mild pain the patient is more apt to regard the side effects as crucial in determining his preference, whereas the converse applies with severe pain.

C) Evaluation

Pain intensity or relief scores can be handled in a similar fashion as suggested previously for cancer pain. The supine position may allow side effects such as hypotension and nausea to be missed. Again, with post-operative pain, there are other aspects which cannot be covered in this review. Such aspects are nevertheless important for a meaningful conclusion to be drawn from the accumulated data.

Although other forms of clinical pain can be assessed, e.g. musculoskeletal [7, 15], postpartum [9, 21], standardisation of methods is far less developed. The use of these other forms would require the establishment of validity and sensitivity. In the circumstances it is wiser to use the approaches which are most firmly established as sensitive for the task.

In the past, subjectivity, variation, and the absence of measurable criteria has deterred observers from using clinical or pathological pain for analgesic investigation.

However, methods have now been devised to determine analgesic potency, which have demonstrated that subjectivity is of no serious limitation provided that adequate controls are used. Individual variation in clinical pain may be greater, but not different to that found in experimental pain – and this variation can be measured and accounted for. Pathological pain can thus be measured and expressed quantitatively in terms of its relief. *Appraisal of analgesic action must be based on the capacity of the agent under trial to relieve naturally occurring pain that is a result of disease or trauma.*

EXPERIMENTAL PAIN

Following this discussion, it suffices to say that although methods are available to assess analgesics using experimental pain, none of them is widely practised. Investigators who use these methods have undoubtedly spent a great deal of time and have specialised in this particular method. It remains to be seen whether such methods will become valid tools in analgesic testing.

A) Ischaemic muscle pain

This method is based upon the inducement of pain following the inflation of a sphygmomanometer cuff applied to the upper arm. A modification of a method used by Williams [28] used a recording device attached to a metronome to register the number of minutes the hand can continue to contract [10].

B) The submaximum-effort tourniquet technique

This method which induces ischaemic muscle pain is advocated by Smith and Beecher [26, 27] and has been used as a method to ascertain its sensitivity with morphine and aspirin [25].

Although this procedure is enticing, it still begs the question whether a given drug will be effective clinically. Once it can be shown, however, that a drug possesses analgesic properties in clinical states, it would be helpful to characterise its action using this method.

C) The electrical stimulation method

Proposed by Wolff [29-31] revealed in a series of studies that pain tolerance is a more sensitive index of analgesic efficacy than pain threshold. However, this method is fraught with the reservations ascribed to experimental procedures.

REFERENCES

[1] Beaver, W. T., S. L. Wallenstein, R. W. Houde, A. Rogers: A comparison of the analgesic effects of pentazocine and morphine in patients with cancer. Clin. Pharmacol. Ther. 7 (1966), 740.

[2] Beaver, W. T., S. L. Wallenstein, R. W. Houde, A. Rogers: A comparison of the analgesic effects of profadol and morphine in patients with cancer. Clin. Pharmacol. Ther. 10 (1969), 314.

[3] Beecher, H. K.: Generalization from pain of various types and diverse origins. Science 130 (1959), 267.

[4] Beecher, H. K.: Measurement of subjective responses: Quantitative effects of drugs. Oxford University Press, New York 1959.

[5] Beecher, H. K.: Pain, placebos, and physicians. Practitioner 189 (1962), 141.

[6] Bellville, J. W., W. H. Forrest, B. W. Brown: Clinical and statistical methodology for cooperative clinical assays of analgesics. Clin. Pharmacol. Ther. 9 (1968), 290.

[7] Birkeland, I. W., D. K. Clawson: Drug combinations with orphenadrine for pain relief associated with muscle spasm. Clin. Pharmacol. Ther. 9 (1968), 639.

[8] Denton, J. E., H. K. Beecher: New analgesics I. Methods in the clinical evaluation of new analgesics. J. Amer. med. Ass. 141 (1949), 1051.

[9] Gruber, C. M., et al.: The use of postpartum patients in evaluating analgesic drugs. The effectiveness of dextropropoxyphene, codeine, and meperidine when administered orally with acetylsalicylic compound and alone. Clin. Pharm. Ther. 2 (1961), 429.

[10] Hampel, H.: Analgesimetrie am Menschen. Arzneimittel-Forsch. 18 (1968), 1166.

[11] Houde, R. W., et al.: Clinical Pharmacology of analgesics 1. A method of assaying analgesic effect. Clin. Pharm. Ther. 1 (1960), 163.

[12] Houde, R .W., S. L. Wallenstein, W. T. Beaver: Evaluation of analgesics in patients with cancer. In: L. Lasagna (Ed.): International Encyclopedia of Pharmacology and Therapeutics, Section 6, Volume 1, Clinical Pharmacology, p. 59. Pergamon Press, 1966.

[13] Kantor, T. G., A. Sunshine, E. Laska, M. Meisner, M. Hopper: Oral analgesic studies: Pentazocine hydrochloride, codeine, aspirin, and placebo and their influence on response to placebo. Clin. Pharmacol. Ther. 7 (1966), 447.

[14] Keele, K. D.: The pain chart. Lancet II (1948), 6.

[15] Lamphier, T. A.: A comparison between propoxyphene hydrochloride (Darvon) and chlorphenesin carbamate (Maolate) in musculoskeletal disorders. Curr. ther. Res. 11 (1969), 234.

[16] Lasagna, L.: The clinical measurement of pain. Ann. N. Y. Acad. Sci. 86 (1960), 28.

[17] Lasagna, L.: The evaluation of analgesic compounds in patients suffering from postoperative pain. In L. Lasagna (Ed.): International Encyclopedia of Pharmacology and Therapeutics, Section 6, Volume 1, Clinical Pharmacology, p. 51. Pergamon Press 1966.

[18] Loan, W. B., J. W. Dundee: The clinical assessment of pain. Practitioner 198 (1967), 759.

[19] Loan, B. W., J. D. Morrison, J. W. Dundee: Evaluation of a method for assessing potent analgesics. Clin. Pharmacol. Ther. 9 (1968), 765.

[20] Loan, B. W., J. D. Morrison, J. W. Dundee: Evaluation of a method for assessing potent analgesics. Clin. Pharmacol. Ther. 9 (1968), 765.

[21] McQuitty, F. M.: Relief of pain in labour. J. Obstet. Gynaec. Brit. Cwlth 74 (1967), 925.

[22] Modell, W.: The protean control of clinical pharmacology. Clin. Pharm. Ther. 4 (1963), 371.

[23] Parkhouse, J., et al.: The clinical dose reponse to aspirin. Brit. J. Anaesth, 40 (1968), 433.

[24] Parkhouse, J., et al.: Postoperative analgesia with Cl-572. Canad. med. Ass. J.99 (1968), 887.

[25] Smith, G. M., H. K. Beecher: Experimental production of pain in man: sensitivity of a new method to 600 mg of aspirin. Clin. Pharmacol. Ther. 10 (1968), 213.

[26] Smith, G. M., et al.: An experimental pain method sensitive to morphine in man: the submaximum effort tourniquet technique. J. Pharm. exp. Ther. 154 (1966), 324.

[27] Smith, G. M., E. Lowenstein, J. H. Hubbard, H. K. Beecher: Experimental pain produced by the submaximum effort tourniquet technique: further evidence of validity. J. Pharmacol. exp. Ther. 163 (1968), 468.

[28] Williams, M. W.: Ischemic arm pain and nonnarcotic analgesics. Toxicol. appl. Pharmacol. 1 (1959), 590.

[29] Wolff, B. B., T. G. Kantor, M. E. Jarvik, E. Laska: Response of experimental pain to analgesic

drugs I. Morphine, aspirin, and placebo. Clin. Pharmacol. Ther. 7 (1965), 224.

[30] Wolff, B. B., et al.: Response of experimental pain to analgesic drugs II. Codeine and Placebo. Clin. Pharm. Ther. 7 (1966), 323.

[31] Wolff, B. B., et al.: Response of experimental pain to analgesic drugs III. Codeine, aspirin, secobarbital, and placebo. Clin. Pharm. Ther. 10 (1969), 217.

7

Measurement of the pain threshold determined by electrical stimulation and its clinical application

S. L. H. Notermans, M.D.

Part I. Method and factors possibly influencing the pain threshold

Investigations of the sensory threshold to stimulation of the skin have become increasingly intensive during the last sixty years.[1,2]

Electrical stimuli were selected in this investigation to determine the pain threshold because of the following advantages of this method:

1] It is a simple way in which an exactly measurable and, therefore, reproducible stimulus can be applied over various regions of the body and can easily be expressed in physical terms (milliamperes).

2] It has the least chance of damaging the tissues.

3] It produces an easily recognizable and easily definable "pricking pain" sensation.

The clinician needs to measure the pain sense quantitatively instead of relying on his subjective impression obtained with the help of his so-called "neurologic pin."

In this study, we define pain threshold in the same way as Bonica,[3] that is, as the lowest electrical current—expressed in milliamperes—which at a fixed frequency and impulse duration first evokes a sensation of (pricking) pain.

The purpose of this study was to develop a practical and reliable method for clinically determining pain thresholds of the skin, particularly in patients with disturbances of pain sensation.

Specifically, this study attempted to establish those characteristics of a reproducible electrical stimulus necessary to measure and standardize the pain threshold of the skin.

The following problems also were investigated: [1] the relationship and characteristics of an electrical stimulus required for its being exactly reproducible as pain threshold stimulus, [2] factors which might influence the pain threshold, [3] possible variations of the pain threshold in the course of time (in the same individual), [4] the pain threshold of different parts of the body surface, [5] possible variation of the pain threshold in different individuals, and [6] the influence of diseases of the nervous system on the pain threshold.

The electrical method with square wave impulses has many advocates as noted by Björn,[4] Sigel,[5] Chemnitius and associates,[6-8] and Blake and associates.[9]

Harris and Blockus[10] described this method as being perhaps one of the most suitable for future use because it is very simply applied and constant reproducibility of the stimulus is possible.

A survey of the literature regarding electrical stimulation of the skin indicates that control of voltage alone is quite unsatisfactory. In this study, it is stressed that in electrical skin stimulation, the applied voltage does not represent the exact pain threshold, since the stimulating current in

Reprinted with permission of the author from Neurology **16:**1071-1086. Copyright 1966, The New York Times Media Company, Inc.
From the University Hospital, Department of Neurology, Oostersingel 59, Groningen, the Netherlands.

each case depends upon varying skin resistance.

Constant current impulses must be used, whereby the intensity of the stimulating current is independent of the skin resistance. Therefore, a constant current source was used, so that at every moment the intensity of the stimulating current remained the same.

Because the most important aspect of threshold measurement in this study was its clinical applicability, other stimuli such as thermal, chemical, and mechanical ones were not used, for the following reasons.

The thermal method as described by Hardy, Wolff, and Goodell[11-13] is impractical because one cannot easily blacken out the patient's entire body skin with India ink as required for this method and because one is not quite certain that the actual amount of heat has a linear relationship to the intensity of the stimulus applied.

Goetzl and associates[14] explained that the total amount of heat within the receptive field may also depend on local vasodilatation which renders the temperature variable. So, the exact intensity of the actual heat stimulus cannot be reliably reproduced.

The main objection against clinical application of the chemical method is injury to the skin. Furthermore, one cannot vary the stimulus intensity by small measurable amounts, and the chemical stimuli do not immediately reach their maximum intensity because of chemical properties, concentration of the chemical agents, and the permeability of the skin in the stimulated area.

The mechanical method described by Keele,[15] among others, has the disadvantage that there are always "touch" or "push," or both, sensations apart from the pain sensations; thus, one has great difficulty in describing or distinguishing clearly measurable and reproducible pain thresholds. For practical purposes, the intensity of mechanical stimuli is not constant because the desired peak is reached gradually and usually at an inconstant rate as described by Goetzl, Burrill, and Ivy.

APPLIED METHOD

Apparatus. For stimulating with a square wave current, we used a Tektronix type 310 oscilloscope and a multivibrator stimulator (Figs. 1 and 2). (A more detailed diagram of the stimulating apparatus can be obtained from the author.) The frequency could be varied from 0.5 to 1,500 cps, and the impulse duration range varied from 0.01 msec. to 100 msec. The stimulating current is immediately readable and can vary from 0 to 8 ma. (the apparatus itself was accurately calibrated to within 0.05 ma.). One could also control the exact stimulating current in a constant number of impulses at any value desired.

The stimulating electrode has a conical stainless steel tip with a radius of 1 mm. which is fixed to the site of stimulation. The electrode weighing approximately 3 gm. hangs vertically from a frame and is adjusted until the tip rests securely on the skin site chosen for stimulation (see Fig. 2).

Electrode paste was used as the conducting medium. The indifferent electrode is a plate of aluminum, which is placed in

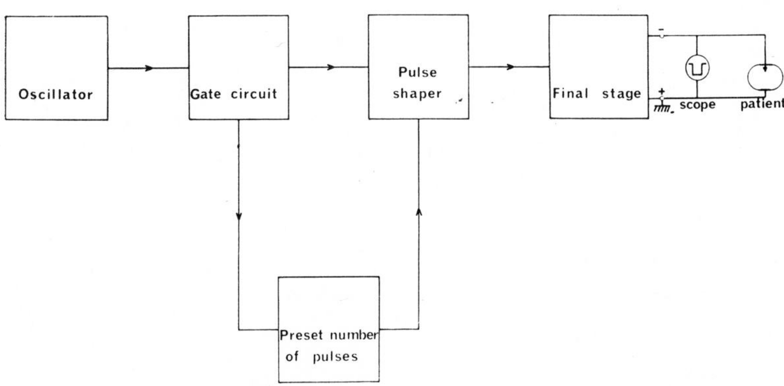

Fig. 1. Block diagram. Detailed diagram of the stimulating apparatus.

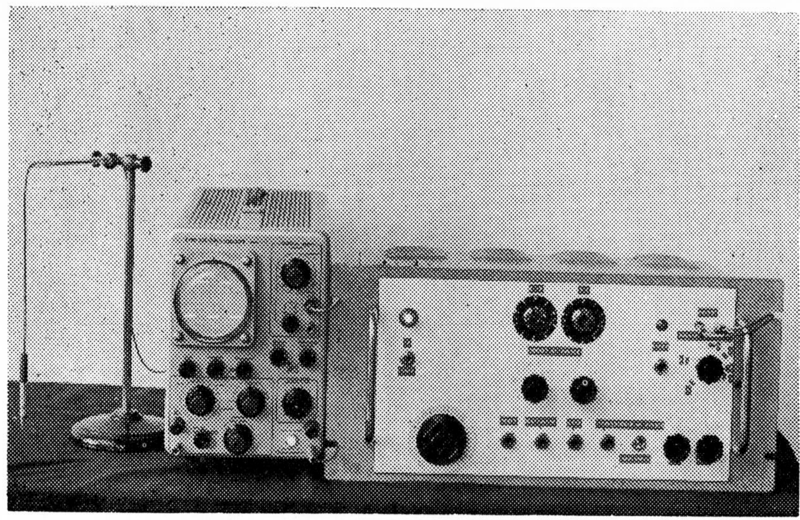

Fig. 2. Photograph of the used apparatus.

such a position that if the apparatus is defective the current cannot pass through the heart. As a safety precaution, the apparatus is so constructed that the current automatically stops when it exceeds a certain value.

To determine the threshold accurately, the intensity of the current is increased stepwise by a fixed known number of impulses at a time (20 impulses at a time was found suitable, as shown in Fig. 5).

Technique. The subjects were placed in such a way that they could not see the testing apparatus. The method of instruction was standardized as follows: "This is an apparatus using electrical current for investigation of sensitivity to pain. You are to say 'stop' or 'ow' or anything you like, as soon as you experience a painful sensation like a pinprick." It is especially emphasized that the subject is not to bear the pain as long as he can but to indicate the first moment he perceives a painful sensation. After this instruction, the stimulating electrode and ground plate are fixed to the body. To gain the subject's confidence, the stimulus is first applied to the dorsum of his hand, so he may experience the painful sensation and need be in no fear of it.

Procedure. The stimulus current is raised slowly to just that level at which the subject gives a sign that he perceives "pain" for the first time. Then the apparatus is switched over to give a series of 20 impulses at a time, and again the threshold is measured while the current is raised, each time by 0.05 ma. Each recorded threshold is the average of at least 3 measurements. As a control, we also give "false impulses" with the stimulating current held at zero.

All the experiments were carried out in the same room at a nearly constant temperature of 23° C.

RESULTS

The study of the relationship of induced pain to characteristics of electrical shock stimuli was based on pain threshold measurements on 30 neurologically normal subjects.

Effect of frequency. The pain thresholds for these subjects were measured at different frequencies (Fig. 3). When frequencies less than 10 cps were used, the sensations of all subjects were first described as tapping or pulsating rather than painful in nature. As the stimulating current was increased, these sensations became more painful and were often described as being very unpleasant but were definitely not described as pricking pain. The subjects could not describe an exact "threshold sensation" and the obtained values varied greatly. With frequencies of above 400 cps, the subjects often first described sensations of "vibrating" or "tickling" but again did not experience a constant "pain-prick" sensation. It was found that more reliable threshold sensations associated with a "pain-prick" feeling seemed to be experienced at frequencies from 30 to 200 cps. For practical purposes, a frequency of 50 or 100 cps was chosen.

Effect of pulse duration. We kept the frequency constant at 50 cps and varied the duration from 0.1 to 15 msec. With an impulse duration at 1 msec. or less, the subjects perceived "vibratory" sensations and tickling sensations around the stimulation site, and they could not exactly describe a constant "pain" threshold sensation.

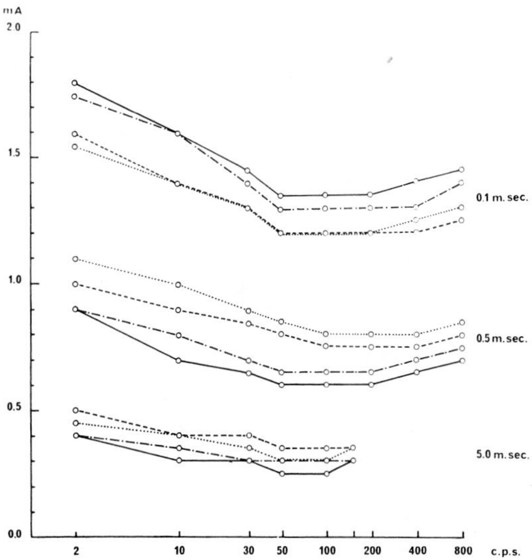

Fig. 3. Ordinate: Pain threshold in ma.; abscissa: frequency in c.p.s.; at different impulse duration (4 pp).

With an impulse duration of more than 10 msec. the sensations were always of a "burning" and "unbearable" nature. Fig. 4 shows that the pain threshold descends rapidly when the impulse duration becomes longer and that the thresholds established with an impulse duration of 5 msec. give nearly the same values as measured with longer impulse duration. For routine investigation, an impulse duration of 5 msec. was chosen which gives a very constant pain threshold value as shown in Table 1.

Effect of the number of impulses. It is also advisable to standardize the number of impulses. The frequency and the impulse duration of the stimulus current of the apparatus were fixed at 100 cps and 5 msec., respectively, and the number of impulses varied. As Figure 5 shows, at 20 impulses or more, the threshold value did not alter significantly. If less than 10 impulses were administered, it was difficult for the subject to indicate a constant pain threshold at all.

Reliability. Estimates of the reliability of pain thresholds were made in 12 individuals using fixed electrodes and a gradual

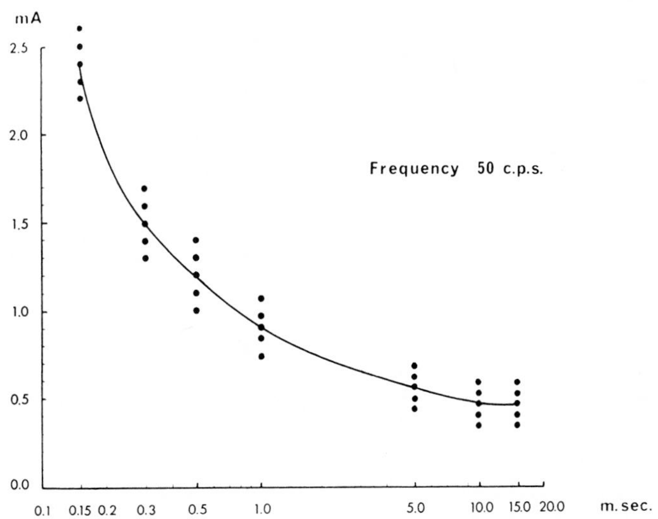

Fig. 4. Pain threshold plotted against the impulse duration.

Table 1. Variation in pain threshold values of 12 normal persons established on the dorsal surface of the middle finger

Subject (age in years)	*Mean pain threshold value in ma.*	*Highest and lowest threshold measured in ma.*	*Number of pulses*	*Range in ma.*
Male				
32 year	0.43	0.40-0.45	40	0.05
34 year	0.39	0.35-0.40	40	0.05
30 year	0.50	0.48-0.54	40	0.06
35 year	0.45	0.42-0.50	40	0.08
37 year	0.40	0.38-0.43	40	0.05
27 year	0.50	0.48-0.55	40	0.07
Female				
20 year	0.42	0.39-0.45	40	0.06
21 year	0.60	0.50-0.65	40	0.15
22 year	0.65	0.60-0.70	40	0.10
27 year	0.42	0.40-0.45	40	0.05
27 year	0.48	0.45-0.52	40	0.07
22 year	0.55	0.50-0.58	40	0.08

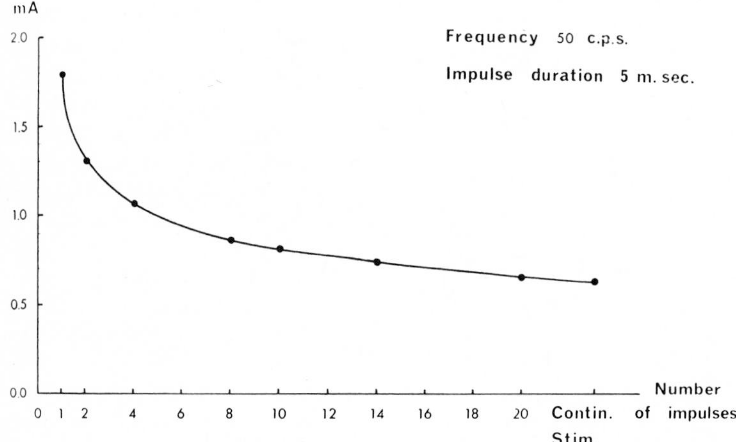

Fig. 5. Pain threshold plotted against the number of impulses at each measurement.

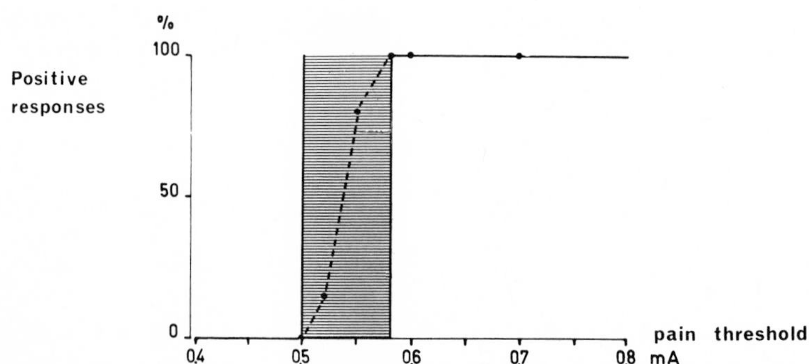

Fig. 6. Abscissa: pain threshold values in ma. Ordinate: positive responses of pain experience at threshold values.

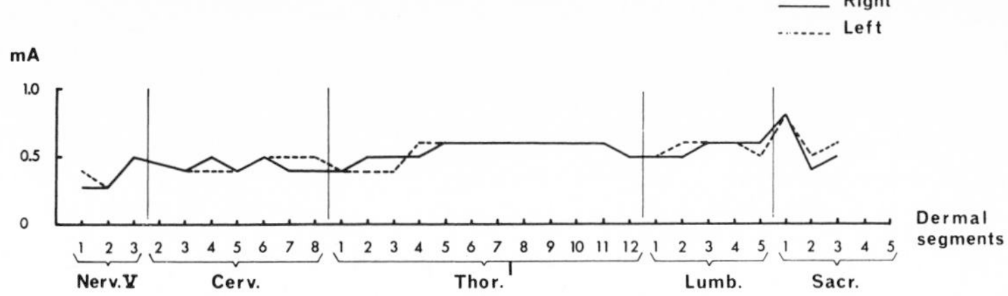

Fig. 7. Pain threshold of different segments of the whole body in a normal individual.

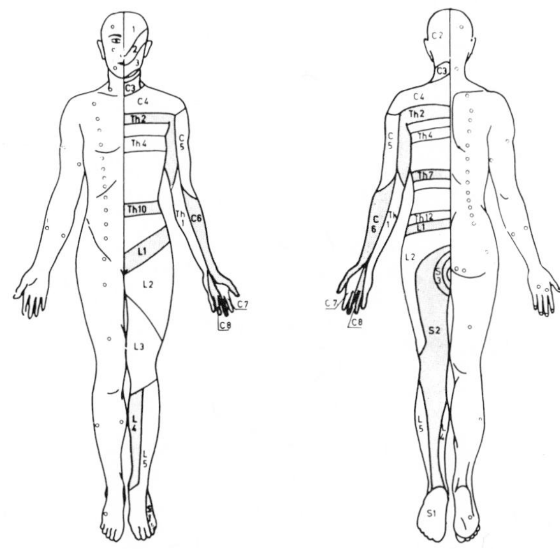

Fig. 8. Dermal segmentation. The circles represent the stimulating points for pain threshold determination.

increase of the stimulus current. Every measurement was repeated 40 times with a minimal interval of twenty seconds. Table 1 shows the results. The same procedure applied to these individuals using a series of 20 impulses at a time gives the same nearly constant threshold values as those shown in Table 1. Figure 6 shows the mean spread of the threshold in the same individual over 40 measurements. The conclusion can be drawn that, using the above described method with a fixed electrode, a good reproducible and measurable pain threshold can be established. From our experience, it appears that the mean pain threshold is about 0.5 ma. (± 0.05 ma.).

Figure 7 shows the thresholds in milliamperes of one individual measured on all dermatomes. It is noted that the pain threshold is quite constant over the entire body. It should be emphasized that it is important to check with the patient from time to time during the investigation about whether the sensation he is using to indicate his pain threshold is in truth a pain-prick sensation. So, we hope to avoid wrong interpretations, by using the verbal report of the individual as a parameter for measuring the thresholds.

Results of analyzing the factors which might influence the pain threshold measurement. The control series was composed of 64 persons medically fit for sport, and their pain thresholds were measured over the entire body as Figure 8 shows. On every dermatome, the threshold was measured at 3 different places at a distance of 2 cm. from one another. Figure 8 gives the mean threshold values per body segment for men and women. The standard deviation is calculated according to the formula:

$$\sigma = \sqrt{\frac{\epsilon(x - \bar{x})^2}{n - 1}},$$

where σ = standard deviation, x = measured pain threshold, $\bar{x}$ = mean pain threshold, and n = number of measurements.

The spread of the pain threshold values for both men and women in this control series follows a consistent pattern. Each individual appeared to have a nearly constant "threshold sensation" expressed in pain threshold values as Figure 7 shows.

The measured pain threshold values varied from one person to another over a range of nearly ± 50% from the mean value. The pain threshold was always lower than 1 ma. in normals. In a total of 4,000 measurements, the difference in value of the pain threshold between corresponding places on the left and right sides of the body of the same individual was never more than 0.1 ma. with a mean threshold of 0.55 ma. We called a value pathologic if

Table 2. Pain threshold in milliamperes established on the dorsal surface of the middle finger and on the forehead

Time of day (hours)	*Male (38 years)*	*Male (33 years)*	*Male (29 years)*	*Male (31 years)*	*Male (43 years)*	*Male (35 years)*	*Male (27 years)*	*Male (34 years)*	*Female (34 years)*	*Female (30 years)*
9:00	0.30	0.40	0.60	0.45	0.30	0.30	0.45	0.60	0.60	0.50
11:00	0.30	0.40	0.60	0.40	0.30	0.30	0.45	0.60	0.70	0.50
12:30	0.30	0.40	0.60	0.40	0.25	0.30	0.45	0.50	0.60	0.55
14:00	0.30	0.30	0.60	0.40	0.25	0.30	0.40	0.50	0.60	0.55
16:00	0.25	0.40	0.50	0.40	0.25	0.30	0.35	0.50	0.75	0.50
18:00	0.25	0.30	0.50	0.40	0.25	0.30	0.35	0.50	0.75	0.50
20:00	0.25	0.30	0.50	0.35	0.25	0.25	0.35	0.50	0.75	0.50
22:00	0.25	0.30	0.50	0.40	0.25	0.25	0.35	0.50	0.70	0.55
9:00	0.30	0.30	0.40	0.40	0.25	0.40	0.40	0.50	0.80	0.40
11:00	0.30	0.40	0.40	0.40	0.25	0.30	0.40	0.40	0.80	0.40
12:30	0.30	0.30	0.45	0.35	0.25	0.30	0.35	0.50	0.70	0.45
14:00	0.30	0.30	0.40	0.35	0.25	0.40	0.40	0.50	0.70	0.45
16:00	0.35	0.30	0.40	0.35	0.25	0.35	0.30	0.50	0.80	0.40
18:00	0.35	0.40	0.40	0.35	0.25	0.40	0.40	0.40	0.60	0.40
20:00	0.30	0.40	0.40	0.35	0.25	0.35	0.30	0.50	0.70	0.45
22:00	0.30	0.30	0.40	0.30	0.25	0.30	0.30	0.50	0.70	0.40

Table 3. Pain threshold values of 10 healthy persons established in the course of 4 months. In total the threshold was measured 40 times at each person.

Subject (sex, age in years)	*Pain threshold in ma.*	*Number of measurements* — *Left* — *Middlefinger*	*Left* — *Ringfinger*	*Right* — *Middlefinger*	*Right* — *Ringfinger*	*Forehead*
Male 33	0.3	0	2	8	2	11
	0.3	7	24	24	23	26
	0.4	28	12	8	13	3
	0.5	5	2	0	2	0
Male 35	0.3	12	6	9	4	3
	0.4	20	20	23	19	27
	0.5	6	10	7	13	8
	0.6	2	4	1	4	2
Male 27	0.3	4	2	6	2	0
	0.4	12	10	24	12	5
	0.5	22	27	9	23	31
	0.6	2	1	1	3	4
Female 20	0.4	0	0	0	0	11
	0.5	0	2	0	2	24
	0.6	3	8	4	13	5
	0.7	13	22	19	18	0
	0.8	20	7	15	7	0
	0.9	4	1	2	0	0
Female 28	0.4	0	0	0	0	2
	0.5	4	2	3	5	13
	0.6	8	10	12	6	22
	0.7	20	19	18	21	2
	0.8	8	9	7	8	0
Female 30	0.3	11	12	10	12	16
	0.4	24	26	24	20	24
	0.5	5	2	6	8	0
Female 21	0.3	3	4	3	4	0
	0.4	12	18	19	20	8
	0.5	19	12	14	13	30
	0.6	6	6	4	3	2
Female 26	0.4	2	2	1	2	10
	0.5	26	30	9	10	26
	0.6	10	7	24	22	4
	0.7	2	1	6	6	0
Female 26	0.4	0	0	0	2	8
	0.5	0	2	0	12	22
	0.6	4	21	3	18	6
	0.7	8	14	11	6	4
	0.8	20	3	17	2	0
	0.9	8	0	9	0	0
Female 22	0.4	0	0	0	0	12
	0.5	0	0	0	0	22
	0.6	12	12	6	3	6
	0.7	18	20	14	7	0
	0.8	8	7	17	24	0
	0.9	2	1	3	6	0

there was more than a 30% difference between the left and right side for the pain threshold measured on corresponding body segments or if the values are above 1 ma., or both.

As Figures 7 and 9 show, the pain threshold is nearly uniform over the entire body. Most individuals show the lowest values in the face and neck. On the other hand, these values were often relatively high on foot sole and palm. One could not obtain reliable threshold values on these parts of the body, perhaps because of local "callus" formation.

Diurnal variation. Pain thresholds in 10 controls were established in the course of a day as shown in Table 2. We did not find any significant diurnal variation, the values being nearly constant (see Figure 10). Also, we measured daily pain thresholds in the same 10 individuals over the course of four months. Figure 11 shows the results in 3 persons, and in Table 3 we have recorded all the measurements. The conclusion seems justified, that in the course of time there is but little variation (less than 20%) in pain threshold values in the same individual.

Attention and simultaneous stimulation. One might expect that diversion or distractions of the subjects' concentration independent of the way in which it was affected would always have an influence on the value of the pain threshold. We are dependent on the cooperation of the subject with regard to his verbal reporting. Accordingly, we have also determined the pain threshold in a series of 10 controls, with and without distraction of their concentration. In the first series of experiments, a manometer cuff was placed around a bar and the subject was instructed to inflate the cuff to 300 mm. Hg using his free hand. In the meantime, we established his pain threshold on the other hand in the manner previously described. We always obtained by this method much higher threshold values than without the distraction (see Table 4).

In another series of experiments, the threshold was measured on the left hand of a subject, whilst at the same time a cuff placed on his right arm was blown by the operator until an evident pain sensation was evoked. That is, the subject received nearly simultaneously two different pain sensations in different parts of his body. Table 4 shows an increase of the pain threshold values from nearly 40 to 50% as indeed one would have expected.

Attitude of the subject. In the literature, many authors have described the influence of the "attitude" of the individual on the value of the pain threshold (Hall,[16] Clausen and associates,[17] Clark and Bindra,[18] Wolff and Goodell,[19] Keats and Beecher,[20]

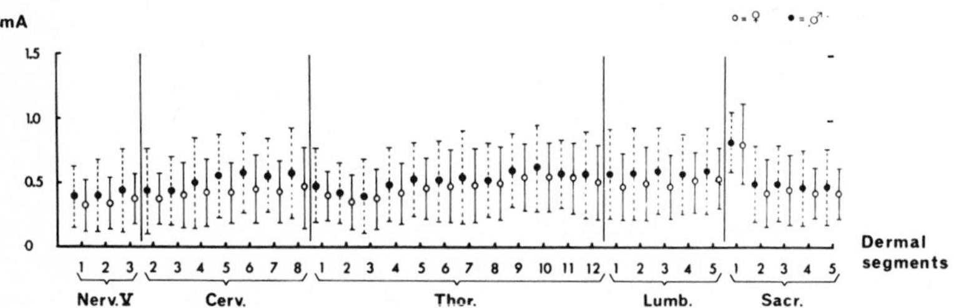

Fig. 9. Mean pain thresholds over the whole of the body in 64 individuals. The lines give the standard deviation.

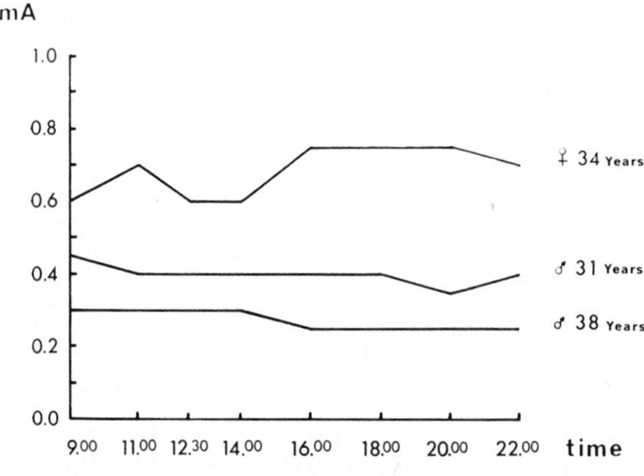

Fig. 10. Diurnal variation.

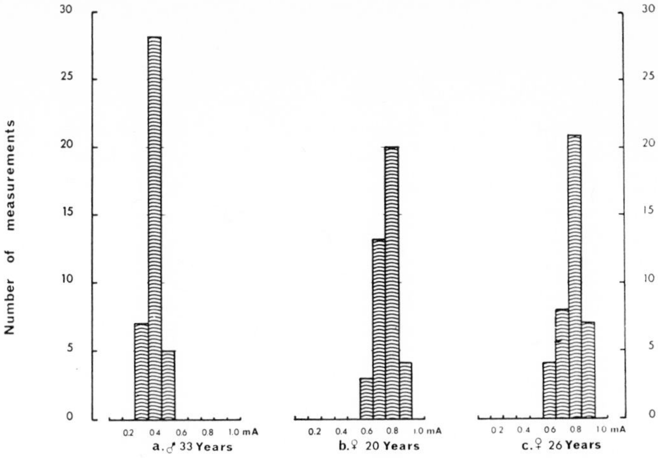

Fig. 11. Pain threshold in milliamperes over a period of four months. Total of 40 measurements for each person.

Table 4. Determination of pain threshold in 10 controls

Subject (sex, age in years)	*Pain threshold without pain sensation elsewhere (ma.)*	*Pain threshold with determined pain sensation elsewhere (ma.)*
Male 33	0.40	0.70
Male 31	0.40	0.60
Male 27	0.50	0.70
Male 22	0.60	0.90
Female 28	0.45	0.80
Female 26	0.50	0.70
Female 30	0.40	0.65
Female 22	0.60	0.90
Female 27	0.60	1.00
Female 20	0.30	0.60

Wikler,[21] Hill and associates,[22] and Wolff and Wolf[23]). However, it should be noted that all these authors have used the heat radiation method of Hardy and associates.[11] Chapman,[24] on the other hand, did not find any difference.

Using electrical stimulation, we also did not find any great influence from the "attitude" of the subject. However, one tries to prevent the likelihood of error by giving exact, extensive, and standardized instructions, which are important to remove any possible feeling of "fear" of the applied method. Most individuals have a tendency to give an early and unduly verbal report of pain because of fear of the expected so-called "pain" sensation. We have investigated the possible influence of "attitude" of the subject on the pain threshold, by measurement of these thresholds in 30 healthy medical students: 21 males and 9 females. In each student, we measured the threshold in two different ways. In the first experiment the students received only minimal instruction as follows: "This is a method of testing your sensitivity to electrical stimulation with this electrical apparatus. It will not hurt you." In this instruction we expressly avoided the word "pain." Furthermore, we explained what we expected from the subject, namely, that he should describe all the sensations felt during electrical stimulation on the dorsum of his hand. It appeared, from analyzing the comments of the students in this series, wherein they for the first time mentioned the sensations of painful experiences, that the values were almost exactly the same as those established by the originally described method. We concluded that with our technique for determining pain threshold, the values were not greatly affected by the attitude of the subjects.

Other factors—such as training, fatigue, sex, and age—also did not appear to have much influence on the threshold values in our series. Thus, our results agree with Schumacher,[25] Chapman and Jones,[26] Clausen and King, [27] Swartz,[28] and Hardy and associates,[12] who also did not find any

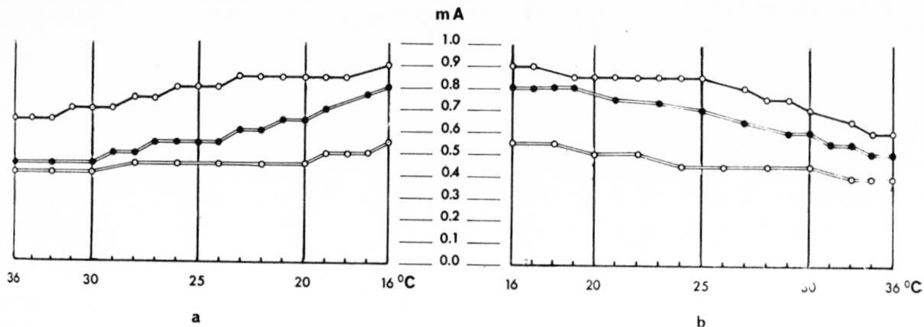

Fig. 12. Pain threshold in relation of skin temperature in 3 persons.

real influence from these factors on their threshold values.

Influence of the skin temperature. To investigate the influence of skin temperature on the pain threshold, the pain threshold was measured at different skin temperatures in 10 students. In this series of experiments, the threshold was determined on the dorsum of the distal phalanx of the middle finger. The temperature was measured with an electrical universal thermometer, type T E 3 (Elektrolaboriet, Copenhagen). At first, the hand of these persons was warmed to about 33 to 34° C., using an ordinary infrared lamp, and then the hand was cooled to 16° C. The cooling procedure was as follows: the hand of the subject was placed on a block of ice, and every two minutes the skin temperature and the pain threshold were measured.

It appeared that only with a drop of 10° C. did the threshold increase by about 30% of the original value and at 16° C. the increase was about 50%.

Figure 12 shows the course of the pain threshold in relation to skin temperature in 3 of the 10 persons. The other people showed a similar picture.

Thus, we concluded that the influence of the skin temperature on the pain threshold was minimal and that the values appeared to be rather constant, provided the temperature of the experimental room was maintained between 20 and 25° C. In our experiments, the room temperature was always about 23° C.

DISCUSSION

A survey of the previous literature reveals that no one has succeeded in discovering objective criteria for the "pain feelings" of any patient, if such a thing in fact is possible, and therefore an exact method for measurement of "experienced pain sensations" is also lacking. Blood pressure, heart rate, respiration rate, electroencephalogram, and galvanic skin response have been used in vain. The biggest problem is that none of these criteria are specific measurements of "pain feelings" and, therefore, do not give constant results as is often mentioned in the literature (Benjamin and Ivy,[29] Wolff and associates,[30] Andrews,[31] Furer and Hardy,[32] Edwards,[33] Clausen and associates,[17] and Barber[34]). All these authors have remarked that these criteria could not be used as "pain indicators" because often they appeared to measure "pain expectation" rather than the "pain feeling" itself and, moreover, never gave constant results. Perhaps, this is due to the problem surrounding the concept of the word "pain" itself, of which hitherto no one has succeeded in giving a generally accepted definition. But, nevertheless, "pain" is and remains a universal experience of mankind and everyone knows what is meant by it.

Thus, pain is a subjective matter, clearly "known to us by experience and described by illustration."[35] We are in agreement with Hall[16] who said: "Pain may be studied as a sensation in one experiment, as a perception and as involving attitudes in another, and as related to emotional behaviour in a third." One should emphasize that pain does not mean the same as "unpleasantness." As Edwards[33] said: "The distinction between pain and unpleasantness is fundamental to present-day thinking on the subject of pain. The word pain is now used to refer to a perception, like a tone or a color, rather than an affective state or a performance in a choice situation."

In this study, "pain sensation" is characterized as a pain perception and the verbal report of the patient is used as the criterion, as many authors have done previously.[11,33,35-37]

The problem often is that to investigate the "pain feeling" of patients, one needs an adequate and measurable pain stimulus, and the most suitable pain stimulus is one that does not harm the patient. A pain stimulus does not need to "hurt" the patient, as was mentioned by Goetzl,[14] Bishop,[38] Beecher,[2] and Weddell.[39]

An ideal method, which must be clinically applicable for determining pain sensibility disturbances in patients with nervous disorders, must also avoid causing skin lesions.

An electrical stimulus was chosen as the most suitable stimulus, for the following reasons:

1. It is a simple way in which a stimulus, well-quantifiable in physical terms, can easily be applied over the entire body surface.
2. There is only the barest chance of skin damage at threshold stimuli, so that the stimulus may be repeated as often as desired.
3. There is constancy of the pain threshold values as shown by our results in a series of experiments on individual patients. Thus, every patient acts as his own control.
4. It is possible to vary the intensity of the stimuli by increasing the current gradually or step by step to any desired value. Thus, one can measure the threshold value accurately.
5. It gives an easily recognizable and therefore reproducible "pain threshold prick sensation." Thus, we had the same experience as many other investigators who described the electrical stimulus as giving a good recognizable "pricking pain sensation" (Bishop,[40] Mueller,[41] Uttal,[42] and Gerard[43]).

We choose the electrical stimulus as the best method to determine pain threshold in order to obtain an objective impression in possible "pain" disturbances on the basis of our experimental results and of those of previous investigators. Significant deviations in the pain threshold values are indicators of possible pathologic disorders of sensibility as Kramer,[44] Fender,[45] and Quensel[46] have mentioned and as our own results show.

Before 1940, currents generated by an induction coil were often used for electrical stimulation of the skin and sensory nerves, as first employed by Helmholtz[47] and after him by many investigators until well into this century (see Goetzl[14]). A special disadvantage of this method is the inconstancy of the current which is not uniform and depends on the distance apart of the induction coils, so that one never knows the exact intensity of the stimulus. Other experimenters have tried condenser discharges to determine pain thresholds.[44-46]

However, Lanier[48] pointed out that with this method, also, thresholds were not uniform or constant, but perhaps the major disadvantage of this method is that the discharge is strongly dependent on skin resistance. Bishop[40,49,50] stimulated with an electrical spark. The disadvantage of this method is that one could not use it for clinical purposes because of the great danger of skin lesions.

At present, the most suitable method for electrical stimulation is to use square wave pulses, ordinarily with voltage sources as outlet points (Koch,[51] Hauck and Neuert,[52] Haimann and Schenk,[53] Björn,[4] Harris and Blockus,[10] Sigel,[5] Dawson,[54] Lipsitt and Levy,[55] Chemnitius,[7,8] Feirstein and Miller,[56] and Ekman and associates[57]).

Most of these authors, however, reported pain threshold values expressed in volts. But, it should be emphasized that voltage alone is not representative of the pain threshold because by this method one does not know the exact stimulus current, since it also depends on the skin resistance (see also Hill and associates[38]). This fault can be overcome by measuring the stimulus current directly on the stimulating point, as we did (see Fig. 1).

The current is held constant and continuously measured as the oscilloscope indicates. Thus, one needs an adjustable current source, in order to have constant current impulses, whereby the intensity of the stimulating current is independent of the skin resistance and variable at will.

In considering the factors which could possibly influence the pain threshold, as mentioned before, the following should be noted.

Concerning "diurnal variation" in pain threshold values, there is no agreement in the literature. Macht[59] and Hardy, Wolff, and Goodell[12] did not find any influence at all, whilst, on the contrary, Grabfield and Martin,[60] Jores and Frees,[61] and Chapman and Jones[26] did. They observed that the pain threshold values obtained by their method were higher in the afternoon and evening than in the morning. However, in my own experiments, as Figure 10 shows, I did not find any significant or constant influence on the pain threshold value from diurnal variation.

The same discrepancy in the literature exists concerning the importance of the influence of the passage of time on pain threshold values. Hardy and associates[11] are sure that the pain threshold is constant over the course of time as their experiments show. The same conclusion was drawn by Schumacher and associates[25] and Miller.[62] All of them used the radiant heat method for measuring pain threshold. On the other hand Macht[59] and Lanier[48] found that with electrical stimulation the pain threshold could vary over an extremely wide range. But we are in agreement with Hardy and associates and found a nearly constant pain threshold when measured in the same individual with our own method of electrical stimulation. The maximal variation was less than 20% of the mean value.

Concerning the factors of "attention" and "simultaneous stimulation," as mentioned in many publications, "distraction" has always been found to exert a great influence on threshold values (see Clausen and King[27] and Wolff and Goodell[19]). Also, "simultaneous stimulation" has a significant influence as Hardy[12] remarks. It gives an evident rise in the pain threshold of at least 35%. The same observations were made by Parsons and Goetzl[63] and also Wynn[64] and Berlin and associates.[65]

Concerning the factor of "sex differences," most investigators had the same experience as our results indicate. They did not find any significant correlation between pain, threshold values, and sex. In our case, although the curve in Figure 8 is suggestive of a possible slight tendency toward lower threshold values in females, this difference, however, was not significant. Also, see for instance Schumacher and associates,[25] Chapman and Jones,[26] Hardy and associates,[66] Clausen and King,[27] and Swartz.[28] On the contrary, however, Kennard[67] and Hall and Stride[68] did find a lower pain threshold in women than in men. Kennard[67] thinks it is culturally determined, because: "men are not supposed to cry out to pain as quickly and easily as are women."

Concerning the factor "age" in pain threshold, we also did not find a real relationship. The age of our control subjects varied from 10 to 65 years. Chapman and Jones[26] mentioned that in older age there is a tendency toward a decrease in pain threshold values, and the same conclusion was drawn by Clausen and King[27] and Hall and Stride.[68] We did not find any real influence of age on the pain threshold value, which was in agreement with Hardy, Wolff, and Goodell.[11,12]

Concerning the factor of "training" and "fatigue," our experience was that one sometimes observed some influence. So, a greater constancy of pain threshold values after training was found occasionally. In the experimental series of our control groups, as mentioned before in the results, the experience was that the values of those individuals, who in the course of four months had daily pain threshold determinations, were almost constant in the last three months of measuring and showed only a little decrease in value, namely, about 0.1 ma. (15 to 20%). In the literature, Schumacher and associates[25] did not find a real difference between controls and trained subjects; also, Hardy, Wolff, and Goodell[12,69] had the same experience. But Miller,[62] Clausen and King,[27] and Kutscher and Kutscher[70] did find some influence of training on the pain threshold values, even when measured by the radiation method. In the routine clinical practice, one can avoid making faulty measurements by good prior instruction and by stimulating beforehand on the dorsum of the hand.

Concerning "fatigue," Chapman and Jones[26] noted a tendency in an eight-hour experiment toward decreased pain threshold values of about 10% of the original threshold value which they attributed to "mental" fatigue. We also did not find a great influence as was established by our control series of 10 healthy subjects in determining the threshold over the course of one day (Fig. 10).

Concerning "temperature," it is important to mention that in the past Von Frey[71] found an increase of pain threshold with cold. Especially be measuring with the heat radiation method one could expect a real effect from body temperature (Birren and associates[72]).

Thus, Buettner[73] and Benjamin[74] concluded that pain caused by heat was dependent on the subcutaneous temperature, as also mentioned by Wertheimer and Ward.[75]

Our results show that when the temperature of the room is constant between 20 and 30° C. the pain threshold value as measured by electrical stimulation is nearly constant regardless of skin temperature.

Thus, if we summarize the conditions for an ideal pain stimulus, it appears that the described method meets all requirements. The electrical stimulus is reproducible and simple to apply. The stimulus intensity is easy to quantify and to express in physical terms. The stimulus evokes at threshold level a good recognizable "pricking pain sensation." which one can easily distinguish from other possible sensations, and the pain stimulus did not give a macroscopic skin lesion, even when the stimulus was twice the threshold value.

CONCLUSION

1. A difference of the pain threshold of more than 0.2 ma. between corresponding innervation areas (dermatome areas) has to be considered as pathological. In percentages, this works out at a difference of at least 30% or more. Pain thresholds of more than 1 ma. are also to be regarded as pathological.
2. The values of the pain threshold in the same individual are fairly uniform over the entire body surface.
3. Diurnal variation has not been found.
4. In the course of a few months, the pain threshold in the same person proves to vary no more than 15 to 20%.
5. Distraction, as well as simultaneous stimulation of other parts of the body, causes a large increase in the pain threshold.
6. With fear, there is an inclination toward a lower threshold.
7. The attitude of the subject may play a role in the measurement of the pain threshold. This makes it necessary to give standardized instructions for the test.
8. Training has only a little influence on the pain threshold.
9. With fatigue, there is a tendency toward a slight decrease in the threshold.
10. One may assume that, in general, the pain threshold shows no clear sex differences.
11. Age has no distinct influence on the value of the threshold.
12. The influence of the skin temperature on the threshold, established by means of electrical stimulation, is small. Only after cooling of the skin surface to below 20° C. was there a clear increase in the level of the threshold observed.

SUMMARY

Determination of pain thresholds proved to be a suitable method for the detection and definition of disorders of pain sensitivity in patients. Application of electrical current gave reliable, reproducible, and, therefore, quantifiable results. By a pain threshold stimulus is meant the smallest intensity of an electrical current, expressed in milliamperes, which at a certain frequency and duration of stimulus evokes a pain sensation. Essential to the method is the use of a constant current device, so that the intensity of the stimulating current is independent of skin resistance. Pulse frequency was variable from 0.5 to 1500 cps and impulse duration from 0.01 to 100 msec. The modifying influence of a number of factors was measured, such as location of the stimulus, temperature of the skin, sex, age, attention, training, fatigue, and so on. The method proved valuable for diagnostic purposes in neurological patients.

REFERENCES

1. Beecher, H. K.: The measurement of pain. Prototype for the quantitative study of subjective responses, Pharmacol. Rev. 9:59, 1957.
2. Beecher, H. K.: Measurement of Subjective Responses, Quantitative Effects of Drugs. New York: Oxford University Press, 1959.

3. Bonica, J. J.: The management of pain. Philadelphia: Lea & Febiger, 1953.
4. Björn, H.: Elektrisk Retnig av Tänder och dess Tilläapning inom Tandlärkarkonsten. Svensk tandläk T. 39:625, 1946.
5. Sigel, H.: Prick threshold stimulation with square wave-current: A new measure of skin sensibility. Yale J. Biol. Med. 26:145, 1953.
6. Chemnitius, K. H., and Hofmann, H.: über ein neue Methode zur Analgesiemessung an Mensch und Tier. Wissenschaft. Ztschr. Friedrich-Schiller Univ. Jena 4:323, 1955.
7. Chemnitius, K. H., and Machnik, G.: Messung der Algesie mit Hilfe elektrischer Reize. I. Grundsätzliches. Elektromedizin 5:66, 1960.
8. Chemnitius, K. H., Kramer, H. H., and Machnik, G.: Messung der Algesi mit Hilfe elektrischer Reize. II. Anwendung veschiedener Rechteckströme. Elektromedizin 5:73, 1960.
9. Blake, L., Graeme, M. L., and Sigg, E. B.: Grid shock test for analgesic assay in mice Med. exp. (Basel) 9:146, 1963.
10. Harris, S. C., and Blockus, L. E.: The reliability and validity of tooth pulp algesimetry. J. Pharmacol. exp. Ther. 104:135, 1952.
11. Hardy, J. D., Wolff, H. G., and Goodell, H.: Studies on pain. A new method for measuring pain threshold: observations on spatial summation of pain. J. clin. Invest. 19:649, 1940.
12. Hardy, J. D., Wolff, H. G., and Goodell, H.: Pain Sensations and Reactions. Baltimore: Williams & Wilkins Co., 1952.
13. Hardy, J. D., Wolff, H. G., and Goodell, H.: Pricking pain threshold in different body areas. Proc. Soc exp. Biol. (N.Y.) 80:425, 1952.
14. Goetzl, F. R., Burrill, D. Y., and Ivy, A. C.: A critical analysis of algesimetric methods with suggestions for a useful procedure. Quart. Bull. Northw. Univ. med. Sch. 17:280, 1943.
15. Keele, K. D.: Pain sensitivity tests, the pressure algometer. Lancet 1:636, 1954.
16. Hall, K. R. L.: Studies of cutaneous pain: a survey of research since 1940. Brit. J. Psychol. 44:279, 1953.
17. Clausen, J., Gjesvik, A., and Urdal, A.: Changes in galvanic skin resistance as indication of pain threshold. J. genet. Psychol. 49:261, 1953.
18. Clark, J. W., and Bindra, D.: Individual differences in pain threshold. Canadian J. Psychol. 10: 69, 1956.
19. Wolff, H. G., and Goodell, H.: The relation of attitude and suggestion to the perception of and reaction of pain. Ass. Res. nerv. Dis. Proc. 23: 434, 1943.
20. Keats, A. S., and Beecher, H. K.: Pain relief with hypnotic doses of barbiturates and a hypothesis. J. Pharmacol. (Kyoto) 100:1, 1950
21. Wikler, A.: Recent experimental studies on pain and analgesia. Neurology (Minneap.) 3:656, 1953.
22. Hill, H. E., Belleville, R. E., and Wikler, A.: Studies on anxiety associated with anticipation of pain. II. Comparative effects of pentobarbital and morphine. Arch. Neurol. Psychiat. (Chic.) 73: 602, 1955.
23. Wolff, H. G., and Wolf, S.: Pain, 2nd ed. Oxford: Blackwell Scientific Publications, 1958.
24. Chapman, W. P.: Measurements of pain sensitivity in normal control subjects and in psychoneurotic patients. Psychosom. Med. 6:252, 1944.
25. Schumacher, G. A., Goodell, H., Hardy, J. D., and Wolff, H. G.: Uniformity of the pain threshold in man. Science 92:110, 1940.
26. Chapman, W. P., and Jones, C. M.: Variations in cutaneous and visceral pain sensitivity in normal subjects. J. clin. Invest. 23:81, 1944.
27. Clausen, J., and King, H. E.: Determination of the pain threshold on untrained subjects. J. Psychol. 30:299, 1950.
28. Swartz, P.: Pain scaling and the influence of sex and personality on the pain response. Thesis, University of Rochester, New York, 1951.
29. Benjamin, F. B., and Ivy, A. C.: Electroencephalographic changes associated with painful and nonpainful peripheral stimulation. Proc. Soc. exp. Biol. (N.Y.) 72:420, 1949.
30. Wolff, H. G., Hardy, J. D., and Goodell, H.: Studies on pain. Measurement of the effect of ethyl alcohol on the pain threshold and on the "alarm" reaction. J. Pharmacol. exp. Ther. 75:39, 1942.
31. Andrews, H. L.: Skin resistance changes and measurements of pain threshold. J. clin. Invest. 22:517, 1943.
32. Furer, M., and Hardy, J. D.: The reaction to pain as determined by the galvanic skin response. Ass. Res. nerv. Dis. Proc. 29:72, 1950.
33. Edwards, W.: Recent research on pain perception. Psychol. Bull. 47:449, 1950.
34. Barber, T. X.: Toward a theory of pain: Relief of chronic pain by prefrontal leucotomy, opiates, placebos and hypnosis. Psychol. Bull. 56:430, 1959.
35. Lewis, T.: Pain, New York: Monograph 1942.
36. Hardy, J. D., Wolff, H. G., and Goodell, H.: Experimental evidence on the nature of cutaneous hyperalgesia. J. clin. Invest. 29:115, 1950.
37. Michelson, J. J.: Subjective disturbances of the sense of pain from lesions of the cerebral cortex. Ass. Res. nerv. Dis. Proc. 23:86, 1943.
38. Bishop, G. H.: Personal communication, 1956. (cit. Beecher, H. K., 1957).
39. Weddell, G.: Studies related to the mechanism of common sensibility. Advances in Biology of Skin, vol. 1. Cutaneous Innervation. Edited by W. Montagna. Oxford: Pergamon Press, 1960, p. 112.
40. Bishop, G. H.: Neural mechanisms of cutaneous sense. Physiol. Rev. 26:77, 1946.
41. Mueller, E. E., Loeffel, R., and Mead, S.: Skin impedance in relation to pain threshold testing by electrical means. J. appl. Physiol. 5:746, 1954.
42. Uttal, W. R.: Cutaneous sensitivity to electrical pulse stimuli. J. comp. physiol. Psychol. 51:549, 1958.
43. Gerard, R. W.: The physiology of pain. Ann. N.Y. Acad. Sci. 86:6, 1960.
44. Kramer, F.: Elektrische Sensibilitätsuntersuchungen mittels Kondensatorentladungen. Ztschr. Elektrologie Röntgenkunde 10:89, 217, 1908.
45. Fender, F. A.: A precision device for faradic stimulation. Science 89:491, 1939.
46. Quensel, W.: Über die Faserspezifität im sensiblen Hautnerven. Pflügers Arch. ges. Physiol. 248:1, 1944.
47. Helmholtz, H. von: Über die Dauer und den Ver-

lauf der durch Stömesschwankungen inducierten elektrischen Ströme. Poggendorff's Annalen Physik und Chemie 83:505, 1851.
48. Lanier, L. H.: Variability in the pain threshold. Science 97:49, 1943.
49. Bishop, G. H.: Responses to electrical stimulation of single sensory units of skin. J. Neurophysiol. 6: 361, 1943.
50. Bishop, G. H.: The skin as an organ of senses with special reference to the itching sensation. J. invest. Derm. 11:143, 1948.
51. Koch, H. Eine Röhrenanordnung zur Erzeugung pulsierender Gleichströme variabler Frequenz, Intensität und variabele Unterbrechungsverhältnisses. Pflügers Arch. ges. Physiol. 231:169, 1933.
52. Hauck, A., and Neuert, H.: Untersuchungen über die Hautsensibilität. I. Die Schmerzschwellen bei elektrischer Reizung des sensiblen Nerven. Pflügers Arch. ges. Physiol. 238:574, 1937.
53. Haimann, E., and Schenk, E. W.: Untersuchungen über die Hautsensibilität. Über Schmerzsummation und die Veränderungen der Schmerzschwellen nach Insulin und Alkohol. Pflügers Arch. ges. Physiol. 238:584, 1937.
54. Dawson, G. D.: The relative excitability and conduction velocity of sensory and motor nerve fibers in man. J. Physiol. (Lond.) 131:436, 1956.
55. Lipsitt, L. P., and Levy, H.: Electrotactual threshold in the neonate. Child Develop. 30:547, 1959.
56. Feirstein, A. R., and Miller, M. E.: Learning to resist pain and fear: effect of electric shock before versus after reaching goal. J. comp. physiol. Psychol. 56:797, 1963.
57. Ekman, G., Frankenhauser, M., Levandei, S., and Mellis, I.: Scales of unpleasantness of electrical stimulation. Scand. J. Psychol. 5:257, 1964.
58. Hill, H. E., Flanary, H. G., Kornetsky, C. H., and Wikler, A.: Relationship of electrically induced pain to the amperage and the wattage of shock stimuli. J. clin. Invest. 31:464, 1952.
59. Macht. D. I., Herman, N. B., and Levy, C. S.: A quantitative study of analgesia produced by opium alkaloids, individually and in combination with each other in normal man. J. Pharmacol. exp. Ther. 8:1, 1916.
60. Grabfield, G. P., and Martin, E. G.: Variations in the sensory threshold for faradic stimulation in normal human subjects. I. The diurnal rhythm. Amer. J. Physiol. 31:300, 1912-1913.
61. Jores, A., and Frees, J.: Die Tagesschwankungen der Schmerzempfindung. Dtsch. med. Wschr. 63: 962, 1937.
62. Miller, L. C.: A critique of analgsic testing methods. Ann. N.Y. Acad. Sci. 51:34, 1948.
63. Parsons, C. M., and Goetzl, F. R.: Effect of induced pain on pain threshold. Proc. Soc. exp. Biol. (N.Y.) 60:327, 1945.
64. Wynn, W. H.: Counter-irritation. Practitioner 158:185, 1947.
65. Berlin, L., Goodell, H., and Wolff, H. G.: Studies on pain. Relation of pain perception and central inhibitory effect of noxious stimulation to phenomenon of extinction of pain. Arch. Neurol. Psychiat. (Chic.) 80:533, 1958.
66. Hardy, J. D., Wolff, H. G., and Goodell, H.: The pain threshold in man. Ass. Res. nerv. Dis. Proc. 23:1, 1943.
67. Kennard, M. A.: Responses to painful stimuli of patients with severe chronic painful conditions. J. clin. Invest. 31:245, 1952.
68. Hall, K. R. L., and Stride, E.: The varying response to pain in psychiatric disorders: a study in abnormal psychology. Brit. J. med. Psychol. 27: 48, 1954.
69. Hardy, J. D., Wolff, H. G., and Goodell, H.: Pain—controlled and uncontrolled. Science 117: 164, 1953.
70. Kutscher, A. H., and Kutscher, H. W.: Evaluation of the Hardy-Wolff-Goodell pain threshold apparatus and technique. Review of the literature. Int. Rec. Med. 170:202, 1957.
71. Frey, M. Von: Die Gefühle und ihr Verhältnis zu den Empfindungen. Beiträge zur Physiologie des Schmerzsinnes. Ber. Verhandl. Königl. Sächs Gesells. Wissensch. Z. Leipzig, Math.-Phys. Kl. 46:185, 283, 1894.
72. Birren, J. E., Casperson, R. C., and Botwick, J.: Pain measurement by radiant heat method. Individual differences in pain sensitivity, the effects of skin temperature, and stimulus duration. J. exp. Psychol. 41:419, 1951.
73. Buettner, K.: Effects of extreme heat and cold on human skin. I. Analysis of temperature changes caused by different kinds of heat application. J. appl. Physiol. 3:691, 1951.
74. Benjamin, F. B.: Pain reaction to locally applied heat. J. appl. Physiol. 4:907, 1952.
75. Wertheimer, M., and Ward, W. D.: The influence of skin temperature upon the pain threshold as evoked by thermal radiation—a confirmation. Science 115:499, 1952.

8

Quantitative measures of deep somatic pain
Further studies with hypertonic saline

B. B. Wolff and M. E. Jarvik

In a previous study published in this journal, Wolff *et al.* (1961) described a psychophysical technique for the measurement of the deep somatic pain threshold in man, based on earlier work by Lewis & Kellgren (1939). Wolff *et al.* (1961) injected 0.1 ml hypertonic saline of various concentrations into the human gastrocnemius muscle through sixteen needles, and they demonstrated the mean pain threshold for ten normal subjects to be 2.3% NaCl. They also found that volume and pressure of saline were important variables in the production of pain. However, one of the basic requirements for a satisfactory psychophysical technique for measurement of a sensory threshold is that a relatively large number of stimulations around threshold value should be given to a subject in order to arrive at an accurate estimate of his mean threshold. The gastrocnemius muscle is relatively small and does not permit the introduction of a large number of needles for measurement of the deep somatic pain threshold, and thus a larger skeletal muscle was needed for our technique. The gluteus medius was thus chosen, although initially some hesitation was displayed about using it, as this muscle is known to be relatively insensitive to pain (Kellgren, 1937). Nevertheless, after a series of preliminary trials, the gluteus medius proved to be a satisfactory muscle, and this paper describes several studies with our standard method of measuring the deep somatic pain threshold.

Reprinted with permission of Blackwell Scientific Publications Ltd. from Clinical Science and Molecular Medicine. **28**:43-46. Copyright 1965.
From the Department of Medicine, New York University Medical Center, New York (B. B. Wolff), and the Department of Pharmacology, Albert Einstein College of Medicine, New York (M. E. Jarvik).

EXPERIMENT 1

In a preliminary study with four subjects, two men and two women, the possible effects of volume or pressure as deep somatic pain producers in the gluteus medius were investigated. A small area of skin overlying the gluteus medius muscle was anaesthetized intradermally with 1 ml of 1% procaine hydrochloride on each side. One 25 G 1½ in. needle was inserted through the anaesthetized bleb into the muscle. A 3 ft length of sterile polyethylene tubing (Clay-Adams, No. PE 20) was attached to the Luer-Lock of the needle and led to a Statham P23AC strain gauge transducer, which was connected to a Grass model 5B polygraph via a model 5P1 low-level DC pre-amplifier. Another 2 ft length of polyethylene tubing led from the second Luer-Lock of the Statham transducer to a 20 ml hypodermic syringe. The system was filled with sterile isotonic saline, and volumes of respectively 1, 2, 5, 10 and 20 ml were injected into the gluteus medius at different pressures, obtained by simply varying the force of pushing the plunger through the syringe. The amount of pressure applied in each case was recorded on the moving paper of the Grass polygraph and varied from 40 to 400 mmHg/cm², the latter pressure being the maximum possible in the system.

None of the four subjects reported painful sensations even for the maximum volume of 20 ml isotonic saline injected at the maximum pressure of 400 mmHg/cm². The subjects were generally not aware of having been injected when the smaller volumes of 1 and 2 ml were used. They did feel the injections of the larger volumes, however, although the latter were not usually accompanied by pain, but referred to as cold, wet or odd sensations or as pressure.

These results suggest that for the gluteus medius muscle, isotonic saline when injected in volumes up to 20 ml or with pressures up to 400 mmHg/cm² does not produce pain. These findings for the gluteus medius are thus in contrast to those for the gastrocnemius in which relatively small volumes and pressures were found to be significant pain producers (Wolff *et al.*, 1961). It is true, of course, that our results for the gluteus medius and those for the gastrocnemius are based on different subjects, and thus care must be taken in attempting to make direct comparisons between these muscles. Furthermore, as the number of subjects in this experiment was so very small, although adequate for our specific purpose, it should be explained that in some other pilot trials, not reported here, all of these four subjects did feel pain when stimulated with even very small volumes of hypertonic saline. Thus the possibility that by chance selection all four subjects may have been pain insensitive did not occur.

EXPERIMENT 2

In some preliminary trials, which among others also included the four subjects from Experiment 1, it had been established that volumes as small as 0.2 ml of *hypertonic* sodium chloride injected into the gluteus medius produced deep somatic pain. The results of Experiment 1 also indicated that a volume as small as 0.2 ml of *isotonic* saline is most unlikely to produce pain. Therefore, with 0.2 ml pain would appear to be due to the hypertonicity and not the volume. Furthermore, we considered 0.2 ml to be a safe volume of hypertonic saline to use with human subjects, as any resulting tissue damage would be negligible. It was thus decided to run a pilot study to investigate the likely range of the deep somatic pain threshold in the gluteus medius and to see if the technique previously used with the gastrocnemius (Wolff *et al.*, 1961) may also be applied to the gluteus medius in order to develop an adequate psychophysical method for measuring the deep somatic pain threshold. In this pilot study we were primarily interested in obtaining a rough estimate of the spread of the pain threshold for a diverse group of individuals and thus used (a) relatively large intervals between saline concentrations, (b) a wide age range, and (c) both healthy subjects and patients with rheumatoid arthritis. The latter group contained individuals who had suffered from chronic clinical pain, which might possibly have influenced their experimental deep somatic pain threshold.

Subjects

Twelve subjects, six men and six women, aged from 24 to 59 years, of whom half were healthy volunteers (three men and three women), and the other half were patients with rheumatoid arthritis (three men and three women). The latter were free of clinical pain and had received no medication on the day of examination. The healthy volunteers were grossly similar in age and intelligence with the patients, but they tended to have a slightly higher educational level.

Method

Six areas of skin overlying the gluteus medius muscles—three on each side—were anaesthetized with intradermal procaine hydrochloride injections. Through each anaesthetized area four needles (25 G, 1½ in.) were inserted intramuscularly in rosette fashion in such a manner that the tips of the needles were about 1 in. apart in the muscle. A total of twenty-four needles was applied, the cutaneous anaesthesia preventing any pain due to this procedure, except for a momentary pricking pain in two instances. Injections of 0.2 ml saline were made at 2-min intervals, using a different concentration and needle each time. Each needle was utilized once only. Prior to the actual experiment, sterile solutions of six different saline concentrations had been prepared, consisting of 0.9 (i.e. isotonic), 2.0, 4.0, 6.0, 8.0 and 10.0% NaCl. In advance of the actual investigation it had been planned to use a balanced randomized blocks design, which would determine the saline concentration to be given as well as the order of injections. This experimental design allocated equal numbers of injections of each saline concentration in a random order of both concentration and needle, except that each rosette would receive not more than one injection of saline of a given concentration. This design thus allowed four complete series, each of six injections at different concentrations. However, as it was not known in advance which of the saline concentrations would produce pain in a given subject, it was decided that the first series of injections would be in an ascending order of concentrations rather than randomized. This served as a precautionary measure to avoid inflicting unnecessary pain. Should it be found that the lower concentrations from 2.0 to 6.0% NaCl already produce pain then it was planned not to give the highest (i.e. 10.0% NaCl) concentration, but to change the design to five series, except that the first (ascending and exploratory) series would also omit 8.0% NaCl, as only twenty-four (and not twenty-five) needles were available. In actual fact, this latter design was used so that all subjects received five randomized series of injections of each five different concentrations, except for the first ascending series, and hence 8.0% NaCl was the highest concentration employed, the 10.0% NaCl being discarded.

The subject's verbal responses during and following each saline injection were recorded and classified into three categories, namely (a) 'pain', when the subject reported the presence of a burning or dull aching sensation in the muscle, developing after a minimum latency of 15 sec following injection and persisting for at least 20 sec; (b) 'doubtful', when the subject reported any kind of pain sensation during or immediately following an injection, which persisted for only a few seconds, as this was considered a mechanical artifact due to accidental movement of the needle during injection; and (c) 'no pain', when the

Table 1. The deep somatic pain thresholds produced by hypertonic saline injections into the gluteus medius

Subject	*Age (yr)*	*Pain thresholds expressed in % NaCl weight/volume*					
		Series					
		1	*2*	*3*	*4*	*5*	*Mean*
A. Men							
(1) Normals							
1	32	2.0	4.0	4.0	2.0	4.0	3.2
2	27	2.0	2.0	2.0	2.0	2.0	2.0
3	46	6.0	4.0	6.0	6.0	6.0	5.6
(2) Patients							
4	59	6.0	4.0	2.0	4.0	4.0	4.0
5	24	2.0	2.0	2.0	2.0	2.0	2.0
6	38	4.0	4.0	4.0	4.0	4.0	4.0
		All men (S_1 to S_6)					3.5
B. Women							
(1) Normals							
7	28	2.0	6.0	6.0	4.0	6.0	4.8
8	49	4.0	4.0	4.0	4.0	4.0	4.0
9	31	2.0	2.0	2.0	2.0	2.0	2.0
(2) Patients							
10	30	4.0	6.0	6.0	4.0	6.0	5.2
11	49	2.0	4.0	4.0	2.0	4.0	3.2
12	56	2.0	4.0	2.0	4.0	2.0	2.8
		All women (S_7 to S_{12})					3.7
		Mean					3.6
		Median					3.6
		Standard deviation					1.25

subject perceived no pain or remained unaware of having been stimulated. The technique was always performed as a single-blind procedure with the subject's gluteal region screened from his view and without his knowledge of when and how he had been stimulated and what concentration was used. A subject's pain threshold was defined as the lowest concentration of saline which produced a pain response in any complete series of injections.

Results

Table 1 shows the deep somatic pain thresholds for all subjects for each series, as well as the individual and group mean thresholds. Individual pain thresholds ranged from 2.0 to 6.0% NaCl, and the subjects' mean thresholds varied from 2.0 to 5.6% NaCl. The group mean threshold was found to be 3.6% NaCl with an identical median. There were no significant sex differences in thresholds (i.e. $P > 0.05$). It will also be noted from Table 1 that five

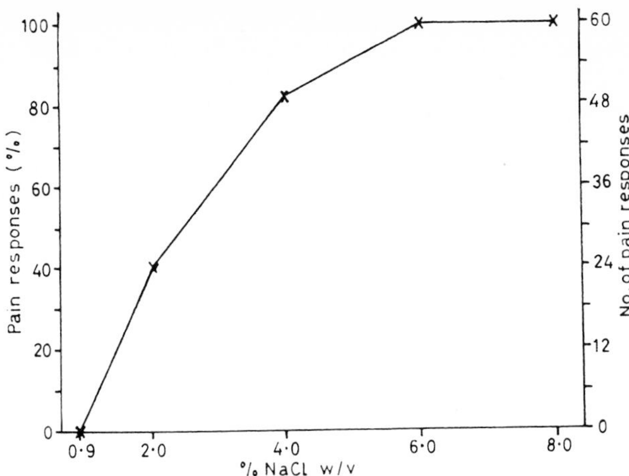

Fig. 1. The frequencies of pain responses at each sodium chloride concentration (five responses per subject at each concentration).

subjects gave identical pain threshold responses for each series of injections, five other subjects differed by only one step (i.e. by 2.0% NaCl) between their threshold responses, and only two subjects differed by two steps (i.e. 4.0% NaCl) between their threshold responses.

Fig. 1 clearly indicates that the pain response is an increasing function of the stimulus (i.e. sodium chloride concentration). There were no pain responses at isotonicity, twenty-four (i.e. 40%) pain responses at 2.0% NaCl, forty-nine (i.e. 82%) pain responses at 4.0% NaCl, and at 6.0 and 8.0% NaCl all responses were painful (i.e. 100%).

Conclusion

These results support our hypothesis that this injection method could be developed into a satisfactory psychophysical technique for the determination of the deep somatic pain threshold. On the basis of these 288 stimulations of twelve subjects (i.e. twenty-four per subject) it would appear that the hypothetical absolute deep somatic pain threshold for the human gluteus medius may lie somewhere between 0.9 and 6.0% NaCl, with 3.6% NaCl as the mean for these twelve subjects. There were no significant (i.e. $P > 0.05$) differences in the mean pain thresholds between normals and patients. This is, therefore, a practical and workable range for threshold determinations, especially as the duration of the pain responses at the upper threshold limit (i.e. 0.6% NaCl) did not exceed 4 min. The sensory quality of the pain responses was usually described as a diffuse, dull ache, with a latency of about 20 sec and of gradually increasing and decreasing pain intensity. The qualitative nature of the pain sensation in the gluteus medius thus resembles that for the gastrocnemius. A direct quantitative comparison of these two muscles is not possible, however, as different groups of subjects were used. Nevertheless, our results do suggest tentatively that the gastrocnemius may be more sensitive to pain than the gluteus medius, because the mean pain threshold of 3.6% NaCl (Table 1) for the gluteus medius is higher than that of 2.3% NaCl for the gastrocnemius (Wolff *et al.*, 1961). The latter result is enhanced by the fact that the volume of saline used in this experiment was twice that used previously for the gastrocnemius. These findings are consistent with Kellgren's (1937) results.

EXPERIMENT 3

Purpose

To standardize our intramuscular hypertonic saline method for use with the gluteus medius muscle with a variety of different subjects, and to investigate its reliability. Furthermore, to study the effects of sex and age upon the deep somatic pain thresholds.

Subjects

Thirty-six subjects (fifteen men and twenty-one women), aged from 19 to 61 years (median age 30.5 years), participated in this study. Twenty-one subjects (seven men and fourteen women), with a median age of 46.0 years, were chronic arthritic patients; twelve with rheumatoid arthritis, five with ankylosing spondylitis, two with psoriatic arthritis and two with osteoarthritis. Table 2 lists their age distributions. The patients were consecutive admissions of the Arthritis Service of Bellevue Hospital, and they were hospitalized for elective corrective surgery or for intensive physiotherapy. No patient was tested during an acute phase of his disease, and on the day of examination the patients had received no medication and they were free of clinical pain. Their socio-economic level varied from very low to middle class. The remaining fifteen subjects (eight men and seven women) were healthy adults, paid volunteers, and their ages ranged from 21 to 38 years (median age of 23.0 years), as shown in Table 2. They represented a variety of occupational and socio-economic levels, except the lowest.

The normal subjects as a group were significantly younger than the patients (Table 2). This age difference is not surprising, because the normal subjects were not matched on any variable with the patients as a wide sample range was desired. The only precaution taken was to avoid an age bias between the two sexes, and this was achieved within reason as shown in Table 2.

Table 2. Measures of central tendency and dispersion of age for all subjects and for the various sub-groups

Subjects		*Age (yr)*			
		Mean	*Median*	*SD*	*Range*
All Ss	($N=36$)	35.1	30.5	13.3	19-61
Patients	($N=21$)	42.6	46.0	13.0	19-61
Normals	($N=15$)	24.6	23.0	4.6	21-38
Men	($N=15$)	35.1	27.0	15.2	21-59
Women	($N=21$)	35.1	31.0	13.2	19-61

Patients *vs.* Normals: Difference is significant ($P < 0.001$).

Method

The skin overlying the gluteus medius muscle was anaesthetized in eight areas, four on each side, as before by intradermal injections of 1 ml of 1% procaine hydrochloride. Four needles (25 G, lengths varying from 1 to 2 in., depending on the amount of adipose tissue) were again inserted into the muscle through each bleb, resulting in a total of thirty-two needles, sixteen on each side. Each needle received a code number, arranged in such a manner that the subject could not guess which needle or location was referred to, and additional 'false' code numbers were also provided for non-existing needles and locations to serve as pseudo stimuli. Sterile isotonic and hypertonic saline solutions, the latter ranging in concentration from 1.5 to 10.0% NaCl in steps of 0.5% NaCl, were provided, and each saline concentration was written on a separate card. Every subject was instructed in advance to shout 'now' immediately when he felt any kind of pain, ache or hurting sensation in his buttock; then to rate this pain along a 10-point scale of pain intensity, based on his subjective judgement; to describe the quality of the sensation; to indicate any changes in intensity and quality; and finally to report its cessation. Two experimenters (E_1 and E_2) participated. E_1 (the first author) called out instructions to E_2 (the second author or another physician) by referring simply to the code number or pseudo code. This informed E_2 which specific needle to use. At the same time E_1 produced one of the cards with the appropriate saline concentration written on it, placing it behind a screen hiding it from the subject. E_2 thus knew what concentration of sodium chloride to inject and which needle to use. The calling of the code number by E_1 was deemed a useful feature as it alerted the subject that he was about to receive a stimulation. This was considered an advantage by us as it prepared the subject to focus his attention on his gluteal region, which, as usual, was totally screened from his view. To overcome subjective bias and to check the subject's veracity as well as his suggestibility, occasional pseudo stimuli were interspersed with the real, coded stimuli, and E_2 would thereupon go through the motions of injecting another test solution but would actually only touch one of the needles gently. This, therefore, was a single-blind technique in which the subject was warned about a forthcoming stimulation (i.e. injection), but otherwise the subject had no idea where and how he would be stimulated.

The experimental design was the method of limits with ascending and descending series of saline concentrations, starting from isotonicity and raising the tonicity in 0.5% NaCl steps until the first pain threshold (i.e. the first 'pain' response) was reached. Two additional adjacent steps of saline were given and then the descending series was started by decreasing the concentration until a 'no pain' response was obtained. The design was such that each series contained injections of saline two steps below and two steps above each threshold. Thus a minimum of six series (three ascending and three descending) was possible. Occasional injections of isotonic saline were given to serve as a placebo (i.e. painless stimulus) to investigate the subject's placebo reaction. In order to qualify as a definite pain response the subject had to report a painful sensation of at least number 1 intensity (or above), which either had to have a latency between 10 and 45 sec with a minimum duration of 15 sec, or which had to start immediately following injection and which had to persist for a minimum duration of 25 sec. A pain response during or immediately following an injection and lasting less than 25 sec was termed a doubtful response and was considered primarily due to mechanical artifacts. This new criterion of pain response was considered superior to that used in previous experiments, as it had been observed empirically that occasionally a hypertonic saline injection would produce an immediate sharp pain sensation which gradually changed into the more usual pain sensation of a diffuse dull ache after some seconds (usually after about 15-30 sec).

The order of needles to be used followed a randomized blocks design, except that each rosette could receive not more than one injection of a given saline concentration. Each needle was used once only. The subject's responses were timed and recorded verbatim. Each subject's mean pain threshold was calculated as the average of the six ascending and descending thresholds.

Results

Table 3 indicates the mean deep somatic pain threshold for all subjects to be 3.0% NaCl. The mean pain threshold for the patients of 3.3% NaCl was significantly higher with $P < 0.05$ than that of 2.5% NaCl for the normals. This threshold difference is further accentuated by the medians of respectively 2.0 and 3.0% NaCl. The men had a slightly higher mean threshold than the women (3.2 compared to 2.8% NaCl), but this was not significant. However, the difference in the median thresholds between the sexes was much larger. The range of thresholds was approximately similar for all sub-groups, as were the standard deviations.

In view of these results it was decided to investigate the possible effect of age upon the pain threshold. All subjects were divided into three sub-groups, namely normals (which was a young sub-group), young patients and old patients (Table 4). There were only eight patients who corresponded in age with the normals, while

Table 3. Measures of central tendency and dispersion of the deep somatic pain thresholds for the various sub-groups

	Deep somatic pain threshold (% NaCl)			
Subjects	*Mean*	*Median*	*SD*	*Range*
All Ss ($N=36$)	3.0	2.9	1.2	1.0-5.0
Patients ($N=21$)	3.3	3.0	1.2	1.5-5.0
Normals ($N=15$)	2.5	2.0	1.0	1.0-4.8
Men ($N=15$)	3.2	3.5	1.3	1.0-5.0
Women ($N=21$)	2.8	2.5	1.1	1.5-5.0

Patients *vs.* Normals: Difference is significant ($0.05 > P > 0.02$).

Table 4. Measures of central tendency and dispersion of the deep somatic pain thresholds for normals, young patients and old patients

	Deep somatic pain threshold (% NaCl)			
Subjects	*Mean*	*Median*	*SD*	*Range*
Normals (21-38 yr) $(N=15)$	2.5	2.0	1.0	1.0-4.8
Young patients (19-39 yr) $(N=8)$	2.8	2.3	1.4	1.5-5.0
Old patients (40-61 yr) $(N=13)$	3.6	4.0	1.1	2.0-5.0

Difference:
Normals *vs*. Young patients: Not significant.
Normals *vs*. Old patients: Significant $(0.02 > P > 0.01)$.
Young patients *vs*. Old patients: Not significant.

Table 5. Analysis of variance of the deep somatic pain thresholds of normals, young patients and old patients

Source	*S.S.*	*df*	*MS*	*F*
Between groups	8.00	2	4.00	3.33*
Within groups	39.75	33	1.20	
Total	47.75	35		

$^*P < 0.05$.

thirteen patients were considerably older. Table 4 (footnote) indicates that there was a significant pain threshold difference ($P <$ 0.02) between the normals and the older patients, but not between the young and old patients. This lack of significance for the latter difference is probably largely a function of the small N of the young patients' sub-group. The normals and young patients had similar mean pain thresholds (2.5 and 2.8% NaCl), but the older patients had considerably higher thresholds (mean = 3.6% NaCl) with the medians showing even larger differences.

In addition, a simple analysis of variance was performed on the pain thresholds of these sub-groups and it was found that there was a significant difference between groups (rather than within groups) with $P <$ 0.05, as shown in Table 5.

The next step consisted of correlating the deep somatic pain thresholds with age, and as shown in Table 6 there was a small but significant relationship at the 5% level of confidence for all subjects for these two variables ($r = 0.37$). This could suggest that the older an individual the higher tends to be his pain threshold. However, when these subjects are divided into their various sub-groups it will be seen from Table 6 that only the men actually contribute to

Table 6. Deep somatic pain thresholds: split-half reliabilities and product-moment correlations with age

Subjects	*N*	*Split-half reliabilities*	*Product-moment correlations with age*
All subjects	36	0.62**	0.37*
Men	15	0.58*	0.58*
Women	21	0.69**	0.18
Patients	21	0.72**	0.29
Normals	15	0.35	–0.14

$^*P < 0.05$.
$^{**}P < 0.01$.

this significant relationship, because they demonstrated a much higher correlation of 0.58. There was no real correlation between age and threshold for either the women or the normals. For the latter the lack of correlation is not surprising as the normals represented a very homogeneous group in terms of age. On the other hand, the women represented a very diverse age group.

The deep somatic pain thresholds were subjected to tests of their split-half reliability (i.e. comparison of the first half with the second half of the trials per subject). Table 6 indicates that for all subjects the split-half reliability was 0.62, significant at the 1% level of confidence. The patient sub-group yielded the highest reliability ($r = 0.72$), whereas strangely enough the normals gave a low and insignificant reliability ($r = 0.35$). The split-half reliabilities for both men and women were significant.

Conclusion

Some rather interesting findings were obtained in this detailed study with thirty-six subjects. The mean pain threshold of all subjects was found to be 3.0% NaCl with a threshold range from 1.0 to 5.0% NaCl, which is a reasonable range for psychophysical studies. There was a difference of 0.8% NaCl between the mean pain thresholds of patients and normals (Table 3), significant at the 5% level of confidence. Furthermore, normals and patients differed very significantly in age, the former being considerably younger than the latter.

Analysis of the data suggested that age does seem to bear a significant relation to the pain threshold, but that interestingly men and not women were responsible for this significant correlation between age and threshold. This sexual difference cannot be explained in terms of age, as both men and women had approximately similar age distributions (Table 2). The present results would thus seem to suggest that as a man becomes older his deep somatic pain threshold increases (Table 6), but that for a woman there is not such a corresponding change with age.

There are relatively few published studies which have as their *primary* aim the investigation of the effect of age upon the pain threshold. A recent specific study is one by Schludermann & Zubek (1962), who compared the effect of age upon the radiant heat pain threshold of 171 male subjects. These investigators found that pain sensitivity declines significantly in the late fifties, and that the mean pain threshold of their older subjects, aged 60 years and over, was significantly higher than those for the younger age groups. These workers only used men in their study and thus their results are supported by our present findings. Two decades ago, Chapman & Jones (1944) also demonstrated that the radiant heat pain threshold increased with age. They used sixty out of 200 normal subjects and held race and sex constant, but it is not clear from their paper if men, women or both were used.

The split-half reliabilities of the pain thresholds are relatively low in this study (Table 6). This is chiefly due to the normal sub-group, whose reliability was only 0.35 as compared to 0.72 for the patients, this large difference in reliability being significant with $P < 0.02$). It is difficult for us to explain the lower reliability for the normal sub-group as our impression has been that our standard modification of the Lewis-Kellgren technique is quite reliable and it is indeed odd that the fifteen normal subjects in this study yield such a poor reliability. It was thus decided to investigate this point specifically in the next experiment.

EXPERIMENT 4

Purpose

To reinvestigate both the split-half and the long-term retest reliabilities of the deep somatic pain thresholds produced by hypertonic saline injections into the gluteus medius muscle.

Subjects

Thirteen subjects (six men and seven women), aged from 21 to 56 years with a median age of 27 years. Eight subjects (four men and four women) were healthy volunteers, and five subjects (two men and three women) were patients with chronic rheumatoid arthritis. The latter, as usual, were not in clinical pain or under medication during the experiment.

Method

The procedure for inducing deep somatic pain in the gluteus medius muscle was exactly the same as described in the previous study (Experiment 3). In other words, our standard modification of the Lewis-Kellgren saline method was employed, using thirty-two needles and eight rosettes of four needles each.

All subjects were retested with the same technique after intervals ranging from a minimum of 3 to a maximum of 28 days with a median of 14 days. The same two Es were used each time, E_1 always being the first author and E_2 being the second author.

Results

Table 7 shows that the split-half reliability was 0.96 for the first testing session. Actually, seven subjects demonstrated no variability whatever on either half of the test, their ascending and descending pain thresholds always remaining constant, and the other six subjects only evidenced very slight variability. This accounts for the very high split-half reliability. Only one

Table 7. The split-half and retest reliabilities of the deep somatic pain thresholds for thirteen subjects

	Deep somatic pain threshold (%NaCl)			
	Mean	*Median*	*SD*	*Range*
Split-half				
A. First half	2.9	–	–	–
B. Second half	2.9	–	–	–
Retest				
X. First test	2.9	3.0	1.06	1.5-4.8
Y. Second test	2.7	2.0	1.21	1.0-5.0

Reliabilities:
Split-half: $r_{ab} = 0.96$; $P < 0.001$.
Retest: $r_{xy} = 0.79$; $0.01 > P > 0.001$ (Median time interval = 14 days).

subject had a difference in thresholds exceeding 0.5% NaCl between the first and second half (i.e. 2.5 and 1.8% NaCl).

Table 7 indicates that the mean pain threshold was 2.9% NaCl for the first test, and for the retest it was 2.7% NaCl. The retest reliability was found to be 0.79, which is significant at the 1% level of confidence. The median time interval between the first and second tests was 2 weeks. Four subjects had identical thresholds on both tests, and only three subjects demonstrated a pain threshold difference of 1.0% NaCl or larger, in spite of the apparent larger difference suggested by the median pain thresholds.

Conclusion

The high split-half and retest reliabilities obtained in this study are very satisfactory and suggest that our standard modification of the Lewis-Kellgren method is adequately reliable. It is of interest that the present split-half reliability of 0.96 is considerably higher than that of 0.62 (or 0.72 for patients) obtained in the previous study with thirty-six subjects (i.e. Experiment 3). At first glance it might appear that the reliability based on a larger number of subjects would be more accurate than that obtained with fewer subjects, but it is believed that in this case it is not really so. There are four probable explanations for this opinion. In Experiment 3, different physicians (i.e. E_2s) were employed, varying both in skill and experience with this technique, whereas in the present experiment the same physician was used. The personal errors of both Es (E_1 and E_2) were thus held constant. Secondly, both E_1 and E_2 had obtained considerable experience with this technique by the time of this experiment, and the experimental error was thus probably much less than in the earlier studies. The two most common experimental errors are (a) use of the wrong saline concentration, and (b) the injection of the saline into the incorrect needle. It is considered that in the present experiment these type of errors had virtually been eliminated. Thirdly, in this study the first author (E_1) always encouraged the subject to be as definite as possible in his responses and to attempt to resolve doubtful responses into either definite pain or no pain responses. Therefore, very few doubtful responses appeared in the final records, and the pain threshold responses were more clear-cut than in the previous studies. Finally, the present subjects, both normals and patients, were probably more cooperative and careful in their verbal responses than the previous subjects. All subjects had been informed in advance that after some days, usually 2 weeks, a retest would be given to check their pain responses, and they all agreed to this without hesitation.

DISCUSSION

When our present findings are compared with those published previously by Wolff *et al.* (1961), they could suggest that the human gluteus medius is less sensitive to pain than the gastrocnemius in terms of reaction to volume, pressure and concentration of sodium chloride solutions. However, this is only by inference as a direct comparison cannot be made because different groups of unmatched subjects were used. Kellgren's (1937) earlier results, showing the gluteus medius to be a relatively insensitive muscle, tends to support this conclusion.

In these experiments the sample mean deep somatic pain thresholds for the gluteus medius varied from 2.9 to 3.6% NaCl. Individual (i.e. per series) thresholds ranged from 1.0 to 6.0% NaCl, although the subjects' mean thresholds showed a smaller range from 2.0 to 5.6% NaCl. In another recently published study on the variations in cutaneous and deep somatic pain sensitivity (Wolff & Jarvik, 1963), we found the mean deep somatic pain threshold of the gluteus medius for twenty subjects to be 4.0% NaCl. These various results suggest that the mean deep somatic pain threshold of the gluteus medius for the general population may lie somewhere between 3.0 and 4.0% NaCl.

The split-half reliability of our standard modification of the Lewis-Kellgren hypertonic saline technique was found to be 0.96 in the last experiment, although it varied from 0.72 to 0.35 for respectively patients and normal subjects in Experiment 3. It would appear that it is important for both experimenters (E_1 and E_2) to be experienced in the use of this method and to restrict the subject's verbal responses as much as possible to 'pain' and 'no pain' reports before good reliability results can be obtained. In Experiment 3 in which the reliability was found to be considerably lower than in Experiment 4 it was assumed that more errors occurred as several E_2s participated, some of whom had no experience whatever with this technique, and in addition many more 'doubtful' responses were obtained, as the subjects were not specifically requested to choose between 'pain' and 'no pain' if at all possible. This explanation tends to be supported by the reliability of 0.95 obtained in our other recently published study, quoted above, where both experimenters were experienced and where the stricter subjective response criterion as in Experiment 4 was applied (Wolff *et al.*, 1963). The possibility that the difference in split-half reliability may be a function of either disease (i.e. pain experience) or age is unlikely, as in Experiment 4 both patients and healthy subjects with a reasonably wide age range were used. The long-term retest reliability of this technique is also satisfactory as it was found to be 0.79 after a median time interval of 14 days (Experiment 4).

It is considered that these experiments have demonstrated our standard modification of the Lewis-Kellgren method to be an objective and satisfactory psychophysical technique for the measurement of the deep somatic pain threshold. No definite assumptions are made at present as to the likely value or use of our technique for measuring supra-threshold pain or pain tolerance levels. Tentatively, however, we feel that our technique is not suitable for such suprathreshold measurements. Firstly, high sodium chloride concentrations frequently tend to yield severe pain of long duration, the long time factor especially making repeated measurements impracticable. Secondly, we have observed that occasionally intramuscular injections of 10.0% NaCl do not yield a pain response at all. This lack of pain following injections of solutions with a high sodium chloride concentration occurs sufficiently frequently that we plan to investigate this phenomenon in greater detail in the future. This phenomenon may be related to Rhode's (1921) findings that local anaesthesia results within 1-2 min following injections of 5.0 and 10.0% NaCl, but not after lower hypertonic and isotonic saline injections.

Our findings suggesting that age has an effect upon the pain threshold support those of Schludermann & Zubek (1962) and of Chapman & Jones (1944). The former used men only, but it is not clear from Chapman & Jones' paper if men, women or both were used. Our results are particularly interesting as we found that age had a significant effect on the pain thresholds of men only and not on those for women. It is difficult at present to state a reason for this apparent sex difference, but obviously this point requires more detailed investigation.

It had been pointed out earlier in this paper that a satisfactory pyschophysical technique requires the administration of a relatively large number of stimulations in order to obtain an adequate mean sensory threshold, whatever sense modality is involved. The gluteus medius, being a large muscle, permits the introduction of thirty-two needles, which is a reasonably large number to allow adequate stimulation for psychophysical experimentation. The adequacy of our standard technique with thirty-two stimulations is demonstrated by the satisfactory reliability when experienced experimenters are employed.

In conclusion, it is important to state the significance and value of this type of study. Firstly, it is of considerable interest from the point of view of basic research in psychophysiology to establish the hypothetical absolute deep somatic pain threshold for a specific body locus with a standard psychophysical technique, just as it has been of importance in other areas of sensation, such as for the auditory or the visual thresholds. Secondly, our standard technique may serve as a prototype for investigating deep somatic pain under experimental conditions. There are many ways of inflicting pain upon man and animals, but the value of an experimental technique is in its validity and reliability. Thirdly, it is hoped that our standard technique may eventually have practical applications, such as testing the analgesic efficiency of certain drugs. Finally, this technique may perhaps permit future comparison of experimental with clinical pain.

ACKNOWLEDGMENTS

This study was made possible largely by the receipt of Research Grant No. AM-2920 from the National Institute of Arthritis and Metabolic Diseases, United States Public Health Services. We wish to thank Professor Currier McEwen, Chairman, Rheumatic Diseases Study Group, for his constant advice and encouragement, and Dr Thomas G. Kantor, Department of Medicine, for his many helpful suggestions. We are indebted to the physicians of the Rheumatic Diseases Study Group for their generous co-operation. We are grateful to the Lederle Laboratories Division of the American Cyanamid Corporation, New York, for supplying the special hypertonic saline solutions. Some of this study was mentioned in an unpublished doctoral thesis submitted to the University of Edinburgh in 1963 by the first author.

REFERENCES

Chapman, W. P. & Jones, C. M. (1944) Variations in cutaneous and visceral pain sensitivity in normal subjects. *J. clin. Invest.* **23,** 81-91.

Kellgren, J. H. (1937) Observations on referred pain arising from muscle. *Clin. Sci.* **3,** 175-190.

Lewis, T. & Kellgren, J. H. (1939) Observations relating to referred pain, visceromotor reflexes and other associated phenomena. *Clin. Sci.* **4,** 47-71.

Rhode, H. (1921) Untersuchungen über lokalanästhetische Wirksamkeit bei Antipyreticis. Opiumalkaloiden und Salzen. *Arch. exp. Path. Pharmak.* **91,** 173-217.

Schludermann, E. & Zubek, J. P. (1962) Effect of age on pain sensitivity. *Percept. mot. Skills,* **14,** 295-301.

Wolff, B. B. & Jarvik, M. E. (1963) Variations in cutaneous and deep somatic pain sensitivity. *Canad. J. Psychol.* **17,** 37-44.

Wolff, B. B., Potter, J. L., Vermeer, W. L. & McEwen, C. (1961) Quantitative measures of deep somatic pain: Preliminary study with hypertonic saline. *Clin. Sci.* **20,** 345-350.

9

Measurement of tenderness with the description of a simple instrument

Michael Patkin, M.B., B.S. (Melb.), F.R.C.S. (Eng.), F.R.C.S. (Edin.), F.R.A.C.S.[1]

Tenderness is one of the few signs of clinical medicine which is not measured or recorded in terms of number. It is represented as a scalar quantity, in such terms as very slight, mild, moderate, marked, and exquisite. Although the same pathological process gives tenderness which varies from one individual patient to another, some importance is attached to its absolute level. In some situations, such as deciding whether to operate upon patients with peritonitis or possible intraabdominal bleeding, great reliance is placed on a change in the level of tenderness.

For such reasons, it would seem useful to attempt to measure tenderness in terms of the amount of force, applied gradually, that it takes to cause pain to the patient.

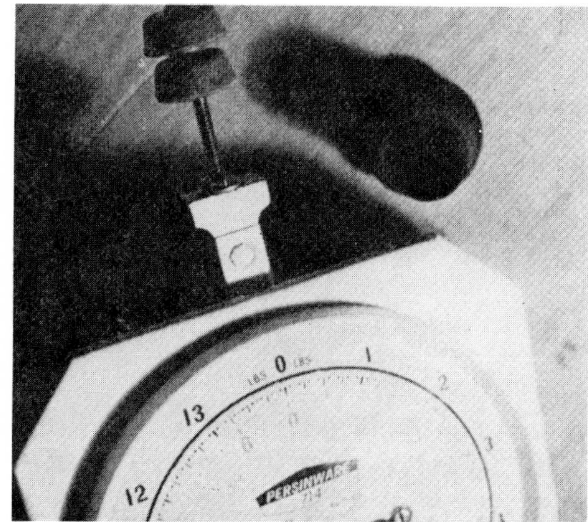

Fig. 1. Components of the "tenderness meter".

TECHNIQUE

In an ordinary, spring-operated kitchen weighing scale, the pan is replaced by a long bolt and some rubber disks carrying a large rubber knob, actually a rounded tip for a chair leg, measuring 4 cm in diameter (Figure 1). This "tenderness meter" can be put together in a hardware shop in a few minutes. The scale setting must be adjusted so that a zero reading is shown with the instrument upside down and the rubber tip just starting to exert downward pressure on a horizontal surface.

In actual use, the instrument is held upside down by one hand. Its weight is gradually allowed to be taken up by that part of the abdomen or other part of the patient's body being tested, and pressure is gradually applied over a period of 10 or 20 seconds (Figure 2). The patient is asked to say when he feels pain as a result of the increasing pressure in such terms as "tell me as soon as you feel it just starting to hurt".

When this occurs, the reading on the scale is noted, at what might be usefully, if crudely, termed the "ouch point".

An alternative method of use (Figure 3) is to place one hand on the patient's abdomen in the normal posture for palpation,

Reprinted with permission from The Medical Journal of Australia **1**:670-672. Copyright 1970.

From Dungog and District Hospital, New South Wales.

[1]Honorary Medical Officer.

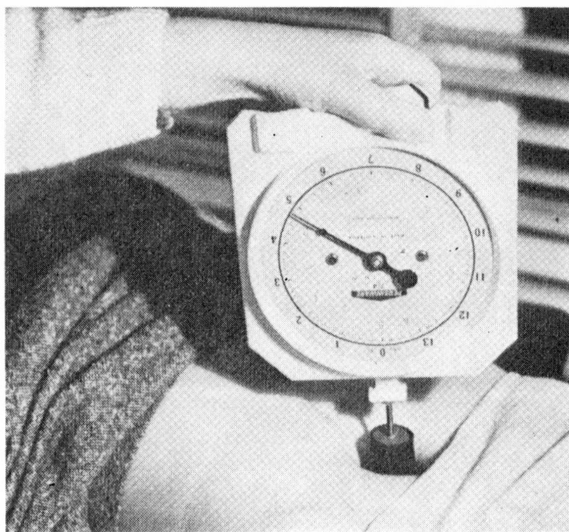

Fig. 2. Measuring tenderness.

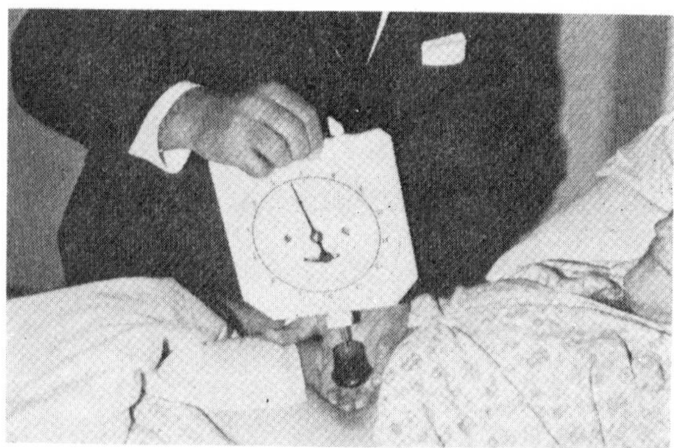

Fig. 3. Measurement of tenderness with passive use of the hand.

and to apply the knob of the tenderness meter to the backs of the fingers so that its force is transmitted passively. The latter method allows more than just the visual appreciation of muscle guarding. No difference has been noted in the measurements obtained by the two methods.

CLINICAL EXPERIENCE

Case 1. A plump man, aged 30 years, had a two-day history of appendicitis, confirmed later at operation. He had tenderness on pressure of 3½ lb weight (1,600 gm) at McBurney's point. The further away from this point on the abdominal wall, the greater the force required to elicit tenderness (Figure 4). Repeated measurements showed some alterations, which remained stable on a third examination. This could be attributed to a shift of bowel and inflammatory exudate, similar to that invoked to explain the mechanism of Rovsing's sign.

Case 2. A boy, aged nine years, was admitted to hospital at Dungog after a fall from a horse, during which his abdomen was hurt. Initial examination showed no more than slight tenderness in the left hypochodrium on manual palpation. Between two and two and a half hours after admission, his pulse rate rose from 100 to 120 beats per minute. On account of a rare accident, telephone communication from sister to doctor broke down temporarily. On her own initiative, the sister made use of the tenderness meter, which happened

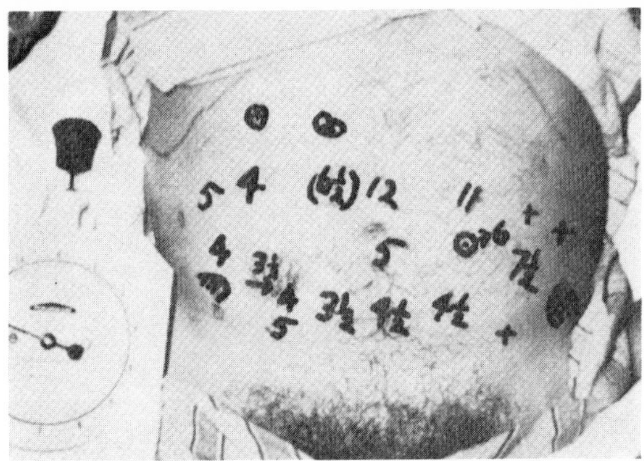

Fig. 4. Preoperative findings in a case of appendicitis.

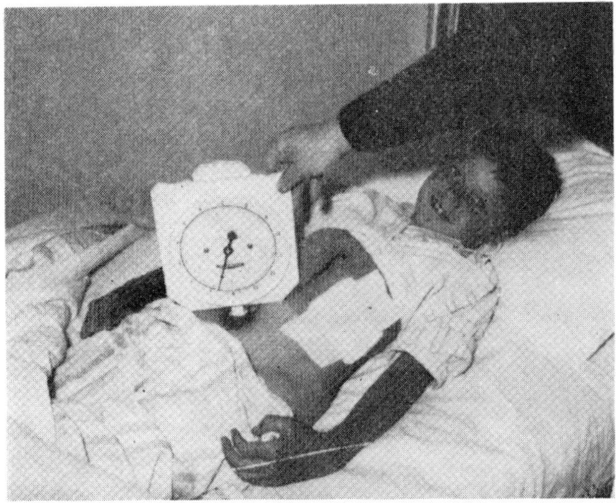

Fig. 5. Postoperative measurement of tenderness after splenectomy (Case 2).

Table 1. Measurement of tenderness and pulse rate (Case 2)

Hours after admission	*Pulse rate (beats per minute)*	*Minimum force to elicit pain*
0	92	
0.5	98	
1	100	
1.5	98	
2	100	
2.5	120	
3	116	2 lb 12 oz (1,250 gm)
3.5	122	2 lb (900 gm)
4	120	
4.5	118	Transfer to theatre

to be within the hospital. She noted maximum tenderness to be under the left hypochondrium, elicited by a pressure of 2 lb 12 oz (1,250 gm). Thirty minutes later, it took only 2 lb (900 gm) to elicit the same tenderness (Table 1).

At operation a little later, between 200 and 300 ml of intraperitoneal blood was found, and a ruptured but otherwise normal spleen was excised. Daily postoperative measurements of tenderness showed an interesting and gradual reversion to normality, in accord with common-sense experience (Figure 5).

Measurements on a number of other patients showed that marked or "acute" tenderness corresponded to a pressure of 1 lb to 2 lb (500 to 1,000 gm, approximately), moderate tenderness to a pressure of 4 to 5 lb (about 2,000 gm), and slight tenderness to a pressure of 6 to 8 lb (3,000 to 4,000 gm). Tenderness of a skin boil was elicited with pressures of only a few grammes.

These personal levels were found to correspond closely to those of several surgical colleagues, who were asked to apply pressure corresponding to what they considered to be mild, moderate, or marked tenderness. Presumably these figures agreed because of proprioceptive impulses learned by doctors from a common pool of patients and symptoms.

DISCUSSION

This brief experience hints at the possible value of a simple and cheap instrument which can be used to measure tenderness. It may be of help in making earlier decisions in such conditions as diverticulitis not responding sufficiently well to conservative treatment, a retroperitoneal tear of the duodenum not declaring itself clearly, or peritoneal irritation from other causes. Objective trials in a busier surgical centre than Dungog would be needed to form any reliable opinion on this possibility.

The apparatus can be used by a trained nursing sister, in the absence of a doctor, much as if the pulse or the temperature was being measured. It may be used when the care of a patient is transferred from one doctor to another many miles away, or when a patient is far from medical help, as on a ship at sea or in a space craft.

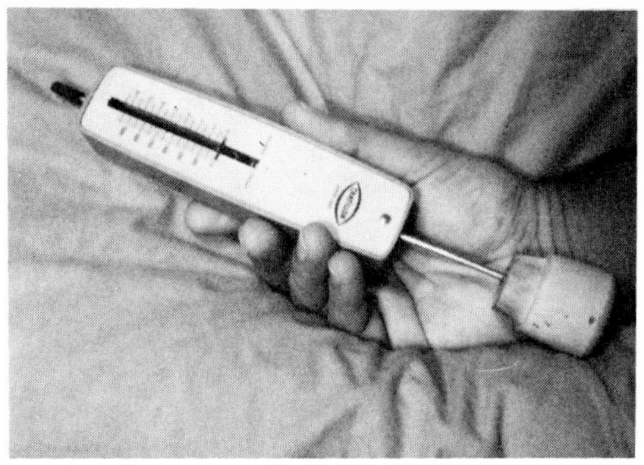

Fig. 6. Apparatus as improved since publication of this reading.

The "tenderness meter" described is cumbersome, and hardly likely to be carried like a stethoscope in the pocket or a thermometer in the bag. There are compact engineering instruments the size of a large pencil, known as "push-pull" gauges, which can measure the same range of force, and which would be much more convenient. Their price, unfortunately, is 10 times that of the kitchen scale illustrated.

ACKNOWLEDGEMENTS

I am grateful to Sister Margaret Smith (now Mrs R. Jones, of Dungog), who demonstrated so effectively that measurement of tenderness by a trained nurse was perfectly feasible, and who used her initiative to such good effect. I remain deeply indebted to Dr Henry Smith, of Morpeth, who travelled far over country roads to administer a perfect anæsthetic to the patient described in Case 2.

FURTHER ADDENDUM

Since publication of the above paper, an improved apparatus has been made from an inexpensive Chatillon push-pull gauge, on which the hook has been cut off and replaced by a rubber crutch tip on a perforated wooden plug (Figure 6).

SECTION THREE

Social and psychological correlates of pain perception

The problem of concern in this section is: What are the characteristics of people who respond more strongly and less strongly than others to pain stimuli? Attempts to answer this question emphasize once more the great complexity of the reaction to pain. It is difficult to draw definite conclusions from much of the available data.

Several points should be kept in mind as one evaluates the results of these studies. One must consider whether these studies are referring to pain threshold (the point where the sensation of pain is first perceived) or to pain tolerance (the point where the person no longer wishes to receive any more stimulation or go any higher. Most studies, for example, do not find sex differences for threshold but do for tolerance. The kind of pain stimulation being used is significant. Variations in these studies include cutaneous pain from electric shock, the relatively slowly arising pain of cold water, the even slower and more intense pain of muscle ischemia, and the deep pain of mechanical pressure. That differences between different types of stimulation exist is known. What is not always clear from the literature is the nature of these differences. Beecher's preference is to use ischemic pain because it is affected by morphine. (see the editor's comment for Section two). Another example can be found in Hilgard's reading (Reading 26, Section six), in which hypnosis is shown to be differentially effective in changing physiological reactions for ischemic and cold water pain.

One must also consider how these data are to be utilized. The differences obtained in these studies and the conclusions drawn from them are based on comparisons of groups; for example, women have a lower pain tolerance than men (see Readings 11 and 16). If a woman were chosen at random, it would be fair to say that it is probable that she would have a lower pain tolerance in comparison with a man chosen at random. It would not be fair, however, to conclude that a particular woman, Mrs. Jones, therefore has a lower pain tolerance than a man chosen at random. That is, on the basis of statistical significance between groups of subjects, it is usually not possible to predict for a specific woman. This point has been illustrated by Weisenberg (1972). Table 1 is based on fictitious data that show a difference statistically significant at the 0.001 level of confidence. It might be concluded that there is a greater pain tolerance for individuals in personality group A than in group B.

How can this be used by the practitioner who is treating Jimmy Smith? Can he

Table 1. Percentage of high and low pain tolerance scores as a function of the personality group

	Pain tolerance		
	Low	*High*	*Total*
Personality group			
A	20%	80%	100%
B	60%	40%	100%

merely assume that since Jimmy is from group B he has a low pain tolerance? This would be an unfair assumption based on the data in Table 1, for 40% of the group B sample did have a high pain tolerance. Furthermore, it is not clear from these data what type of pain tolerance is involved. Nor is it clear from these data what the circumstances of pain tolerance are. Does high pain tolerance mean reward, such as group approval? Does high pain tolerance mean punishment, such as less anesthetic for a procedure? Often the circumstances can be more powerful than the personality predisposition.

It is important to learn how to utilize group data. One approach is to think of such results as probability statements even in some gross manner. Rather than starting with an equal probability for each group, knowing that 8 out of 10 group A's and only 4 out of 10 group B's have high pain scores is of greater benefit. It is a starting hypothesis that can be of value in treatment.

Furthermore, in trying to find the variables that contribute to these differences one learns a great deal about the pain reaction and how it can be modified. For example, Ryan and Kovacic (Reading 15) found that contact athletes are able to tolerate pain more than noncontact athletes. They offer several possible explanations that lend themselves to experimental testing. Verification of these explanations would increase our ability to control pain even without knowledge of athletic participation.

There are other circumstances where choices are often made on an arbitrary basis. Yet, a given choice can be of help to many people if it is correct and can result in little harm to others if it is not. Murray and Hagen (Reading 13), for example, have found that the left hand and foot are more sensitive to pain and have a lower pain tolerance than the right hand and foot. Where there is an arbitrary choice it would seem reasonable therefore to choose the right hand and foot over the left ones, when applying a painful procedure, such as venipuncture.

From a statistical viewpoint one should also note the effect of sample size. When small samples are used (less than 30 subjects), it is possible to raise legitimate questions concerning generalization. However, the results are probably due to a relatively large difference between groups (assuming the results are reliable and not due to chance).

When the sample is large, there is less of a question concerning the ability to generalize the findings. However, there is an increased possibility of magnifying even small differences that may not always be meaningful.

The results in Reading 16 are based on 41,119 patients, a significant sample. All other things being equal, the procedures used were working in favor of finding differences between groups. The remarks made here are not intended to invalidate these results but merely to point out the care needed in interpreting and utilizing such data.

REFERENCE

Weisenberg, M. 1972. The transformation of behavioral science knowledge into health practice. In Teaching behavioral sciences in schools of medicine: behavioral science perspectives in medical education, vol. 3, U. S. Public Health Service, Rockville, Md., pp. 409-442.

10

How children perceive pain

Nancy V. Schultz

"Pain (pān), n.-bodily or mental suffering or distress."[1] Such cold words – so devoid of feeling – yet they mean so much to the person who is *in* pain. One person may accept pain almost gratefully, as punishment for misdeeds; another, hysterically, beyond comprehension; and someone else, happily, glad to be alive. Children often experience pain fearfully, not understanding what is happening to them. Regardless of how it is experienced, pain causes change.

Pain alters the person feeling it – physiologically, (via nerve pathways) by changing one's posture, gait, heart rate, or blood pressure; or psychologically and emotionally by causing restlessness, anxiety, hostility, anger, anguish, or despair. Whatever its degree, pain always causes change, change causes stress, and stress increases pain. Thus a vicious circle evolves and is perpetuated. Somewhere, somehow, this circle must be broken.

Many theories about pain have been advanced and it is well for nurses to understand the physiological reasons for pain.[2] However, these theories are worthless unless they are integrated with other knowledges, applied and tested in our work with patients and families, and lead to practical relief for the sufferer. Rather than concentrate exclusively on the family's coping mechanisms or the theories about pain, nurses should also apply principles of growth and development – that is, the behavior and characteristics of people at various age-stages of development. It was for this reason – to improve my nursing care of children – that I elected to learn more about the attitudes and perception of pain of ten- and eleven-year-old children and relate that information to normal growth and development.

Much of the past research on normal growth and development of children, especially in social development, is becoming outdated. Children are changing with the times; they are now better informed because of our more sophisticated communication facilities; they are made more aware of the frailties of human beings by television programs and newspaper headlines. We are a child-centered society, and books are written about, for, and by them. Finally, they are often treated as pseudoadults, under the name of permissiveness, and thus are talked to, reasoned with, and consulted.

Regardless of the fact that culturally, economically, and socially children are reared differently and are of different creeds, colors, and races, there are still many commonalities among those in the same age-stage of development – an important consideration in planning the care of children in pain. My reason then, for conducting a survey of their perception of pain was to understand some of the commonalities in the way children in the same age-stage of development have experienced it or perceived it.

Reprinted with permission of The American Journal of Nursing Co. from Nursing Outlook **19**:670-673.

From the Nassau Community College Department of Nursing, New York University, New York.

HOW, NOT WHY

I wanted to find out *how* children at a fixed age-stage of development view pain, rather than *why* they react to it as they do. I believed that if we could learn, before a child is admitted to a hospital, how he might react to pain just because he *is* three, five, eight, or ten, we could begin to give him support immediately and with more understanding. Although this is only the first step in finding out *why* a particular child feels pain as he does, it would at least give us a lead in understanding the fears, fantasies, guilts, and anger that children experience when unexplained change (in this case, pain) occurs. Further, such knowledge would help us see him compassionately through an otherwise traumatic experience.

All children change as they progress from one stage of development to another. Though considered normal, these changes are often viewed as stress situations or crises. However, there is pattern and orderly progression—both physiologically and psychologically—in the child's maturation. The time it takes for a child to develop at each level depends on both environment and heredity, but he still develops, whatever the rate. The milestones that have been identified in normal growth and development data do serve as a guide for recognizing retardation in growth. It is therefore my assumption that we can realistically use these same data as a guide for anticipating certain reactions of children to pain.

THE STUDY

The study group consisted of 74 ten and eleven-year-old boys and girls from a public grammar school in a town of upper-middle- middle- and lower-middle-class families. The children were both black and white, although the majority were white.

Since I could not interview each child, I constructed a list of questions I thought them capable of answering. The only vital statistics I asked for were age and sex and they were unsigned. The children were told that only I would read their answers. It was explained to them that I was a nurse who worked with children, and that I was interested in their reactions so that I could better help children who are in pain. They seemed eager to cooperate and all of them answered the following questions:

1. Have you ever been in the hospital?
2. Why were you in the hospital?
3. List three things that have happened to you that made you feel pain.
4. Underline no more than *two* of the following: When I have pain I feel afraid, brave, nervous, like crying but I don't, like crying and I do.
5. What does pain mean to you? Write everything that comes to your mind about pain.

The first two questions were asked mainly to secure data for use in future study; there may be a relationship between a child's perception of pain and his reaction to it if he has been hospitalized in the past. His perception may be hazy if he has blocked a bad experience, or clearer if he was successfully helped to cope with it. This topic requires much more study than I could give it in this survey.

From the third question I had hoped to gain some idea of what types of experiences with pain the children had had and whether their reactions, as expressed in answers to the question, had occurred concomitantly with the pain or injury they had sustained.

I asked Question 4 to test my theory that children in the nine-to-eleven-year-old group, especially, have strong feelings that they have learned to control and that therefore do not show in their behavior. Their answers strengthened my belief that they do need support and reassurance, and that because their behavior doesn't overtly point this out, we often overlook these children and comfort those who cry or scream.

The reason for asking Question 5 is self-evident. I wanted to find out how ten- and eleven-year-olds view pain, rather than

Table 1. Number and type of behavior responses to pain by ten- and eleven-year-old boys and girls

Behavior responses	*Boys* 11 yrs.	*Boys* 10 yrs.	*Girls* 11 yrs.	*Girls* 10 yrs.
Total	19	19	17	19
Brave	14	7	2	2
Nervous or afraid	15	13	All	All
Wants to cry and does	1	1	1	5
Wants to cry but won't	12*	16	10	9

*Nine of these also answered brave and three answered nervous.

why, and I think I was fairly successful. The answers ranged from purely physiologic to anxiety-ridden psychologic, with a few surprising ones in between.

FINDINGS

Briefly, 39 of the 74 children had been hospitalized at some time. However, judging from the answers only, without sophisticated correlation and a larger sample, previous hospitalization did not seem to have much effect on the children's answers to Question 4. There were still only eight out of the 74 who said that when they felt pain they wanted to cry and did (see table). The number of responses to Question 4 was double the total number of children in each age group, since two responses were given by all but two.

These findings are interesting, but not surprising. Often the boys answered *brave,* but also *nervous* or *afraid,* an interesting combination. The first answer of *brave* seems to express what nurses and society expect, and the last two constitute a compromise he allows himself—as long as he doesn't cry—because "only babies cry," or "big boys don't cry."

SOCIETY'S EXPECTATIONS

Mussen and Kagan state that boys in middle childhood are expected to be strong, assertive, and courageous (14 out of 19 eleven-year-old boys, and seven out of 19 ten-year-old boys answered *brave*)[3]. As they grow older they are expected to supress fear and control expression of emotions in times of stress (only two out of 38 boys said they wanted to cry). Yet, these authors assert girls are allowed to express fear, hurt feelings, and general emotional upsets. All of the 36 girls in this study admitted to being *afraid* or *nervous,* and only four felt *brave.*

I believe that the reason only six girls said they would cry, and more than half that they wanted to cry but wouldn't, rests in the fact that at this age children are struggling to become independent; they hate to feel infantile.[4] This may be the answer, but another possibility is that the girls didn't answer honestly or that when they actually came face to face with pain it would be another story. Nevertheless, this is how they viewed themselves, and is a significant indicator of the lengths that ten- and eleven-year-olds often go to in order to hide their feelings from us.

The mere contrasts in choices picked by the children, for example, *brave* and *afraid, brave* and *won't cry, afraid/nervous* and *want to cry but won't,* should show us the conflict these children are in when experiencing pain. This in itself is worth intervention and understanding.

Question 5 sought to elicit what pain means to ten- and eleven-year-old children. So that my theory of commonalities may be more meaningful, I have grouped the responses under some of the major "normal" behavioral manifestations and developmental processes of this age group.

FEAR INCREASES PAIN

Fear of death is one aspect of the perception of pain that ten- and eleven-year-old children experience. It may be increased when the child is hospitalized, and such fear probably increases pain.[5] Because this age group fears physical harm, their reaction is based more on their fear than on the pain experienced.[6] In answer to the question: What does pain mean to you? Some of the replies were: "It hurts. It hurts inside." "I feel like screaming." "The doctor." "I think I'm going to die." "Getting shots. Getting injections." "It hurts so much it kills ya." "Like a hammer beating into me." "When something hurts real bad you get in shock." "I think it's serious but it never is."

In his textbook, *Pediatrics,* Barnett states that among children of this age "fear of bodily injury is universal, and slight injuries might elicit disproportionate reactions of distress and fear. They're proud of their scratches and bruises, but also tend to exaggerate every minor body damage."[7] The survey findings bear this out, but the reality remains that, because this is how these children view pain, this is what we have to work with.

It's helpful to know that their reaction to pain and fear of bodily damage are exaggerated, so that we do not either medicate these children unnecessarily, or ignore them because we feel they're being "babies" and making a "big deal" about nothing. Rather, we should realize that this is normal behavior for this age group, and try to group them with children their own age so they can complain to each other and share experiences.

Also, we need to spend time listening and reassuring them because their pain and fear are real. In light of the responses given, it would appear that some of our palliative measures—injections for pain, for example—are likely to cause more suffering and fear than the original pain. Oral medications would be wiser to use at these times.

Fear has many facets, as can be seen from some of the responses that were more abstract and dealt with pain and fear on another level. I was surprised at the following descriptions of pain that I think are justifiably critical of the sterotypes many of us have of ten- and eleven-year-olds. Pain is:

> Being nervous (girl, ten years old).
> Not growing up healthy (boy, eleven years old)
> Being afraid (boy, eleven years old).
> When you scream for help and nobody comes (girl, eleven years old; had been hospitalized).
> Going through the hospital with everyone looking at you (boy, ten years old).
> When something hurts you and you can't get help (girl, eleven years old; had been hospitalized).

These statements contain implications for nursing intervention. How many times have we heard a child this age call for a nurse and be told to wait till the nurse stopped a toddler's crying, or finished her charting. It never before hit me so forcefully that these children would feel so abandoned. After counting responses and finding that 64 out of 74 children connected pain with being afraid or nervous, I would say that "fear is pain."

ANXIETY AND ANGER

Mussen and Kagan state that all children in middle childhood have problems with anxiety, frustration, and conflict.[8] They believe, however, that these problems will be transient and limited in severity if the child's parents provide good role models, are warm and accepting, and are consistent and flexible in their disciplinary techniques, yet not overbearing. Nurses can take a few cues from this when working with children in pain, especially in the hospital setting where they might work with a child over an extended period of time.

One difficulty in understanding anxiety at this age is that the real sources of the child's concern are not expressed.[9] This, of course, can be seen in responses to Question 4, yet some of the children managed to put this elusive feeling of anxiety in relation to pain into words in stating pain is:

> Something you have no control of.
> You think it will never end.
> Something that hurts and you can't stop it.
> When you get nervous, you sweat, and feel tense; moaning.

What better source of anxiety than something you can't control! The mere fact that in their struggle for independence these children have to deal with something they cannot control is a problem in itself, without the added distress of physical pain. They practically tell us they can't help themselves, so it's clear that intervention is necessary. In light of their dependence-independence struggle, we can best intervene by helping them to help themselves control their pain. When their pain is lessened, their independence will be strengthened.

How we help each child will, of course, depend on the patient, and this, in turn, will depend on how the nurse uses her knowledge of his life style, of his parents' reactions to pain, and of how he has coped with pain in the past.

Ten- and eleven-year-olds may also be angry at themselves for being ill.[10] They are very "school conscious" and worry about poor grades and failing. Authorities on growth and development point this out, but how often do we meet this need when the child is in the hospital? Of course, some hospitals employ tutors, but it often takes a long time to arrange for this service. Provisions for tutoring should be made, if necessary, on admission, especially if the child has an orthopedic, or other condition that will keep him confined for weeks. Even when a hospital stay is short, the child should be kept informed of what his class is doing. Parents can help in this latter case but nurses can do their part by giving them time to do homework in a quiet place, and by supporting them. Rarely is this done, probably because the need isn't recognized. In agreement with this need, some children said they viewed pain as, "getting a failing mark," "getting a bad report card."

If such statements identify situations that are viewed as pain or as being painful, it becomes our responsibility to help the child faced with this reaction. The recognition that such situations can be painful will give us a clue as to why the hospitalized child is sometimes destructive, belligerent, and hostile. When we realize that children this age might be angry at themselves for being ill, perhaps we can cease being punitive and begin to be more understanding. This alone, by lessening some of the anger and anxiety, will mitigate this painful experience. Thus we see—once again—that to a 10- or 11-year-old child, pain is not always the result of physical injury.

DRIVE AND ENERGY

Fourth- and fifth-graders are usually full of energy and very interested in group sports and activities, especially physical ones.[11] One 11-year-old boy said, "The worst thing about pain is that you can't play football or any other kind of sport"; and a 10-year-old boy wrote, "When I broke my arm I worried that I wouldn't be able to pitch again." This says a lot. Often children view pain as a hindrance to their wants and needs, as well as a physical or psychological trauma. This is another facet of pain perception that an understanding of normal growth and development can help us to deal with.

Obviously, we can't get a game of football going in the playroom, but we can refrain from chastising children who get restless and mischievous in the hospital setting. We can do such positive things as allowing older children roommates who are their own age. Peer companionship is much needed by the mid-childhood group.

We can let them stay up later than the younger patients and have exclusive use of the playroom for their discussions and games. We can accept the offer of some parent to make a gift to the unit, and ask for an electric football or baseball game, rather than the eternal high chair that is usually donated. With a little application, we could probably think of other positive and ingenious ways of meeting these children's need for activity, but, most important, we must be aware of their feelings and their normal developmental needs.

Middle childhood is a critical period during which conscience develops at a rapid rate. Piaget feels that the period between ages eight and eleven is one of progressive equalitarianism. "If a responsible parent, because of his parental warmth and love, is a rewarding figure for the child to identify with and model himself after, adoption of the parent's standards is more likely to occur, and violations of these standards then become painful. . . ."[12] Some of the children viewed pain from a purely psychological point of view, thus showing the beginning of the development of mature levels of thinking. The children who took this view were all eleven years old, whereas most of the ten-year-olds discussed or described pain in physical terms. Both of these outlooks were "normal" for the children's ages, with those eleven showing increasing awareness of a more elusive type of pain—that caused by injury to one's feelings. Some of these responses regarding pain were:

> If you do something wrong you feel bad.
> Getting scolded.
> When someone you love does something to hurt you.

Implications for nursing intervention for the relief of pain in this context are obvious. All that is required of us is that our attitudes be warm, accepting, and nonjudgmental, and that we treat the children like the feeling, thinking, persons they are. We must remember that children have feelings that can cause them pain or add to it. What is required of us is little more than practicing the golden rule. It may not always be easy to do, but it is important both to the children and to ourselves that we do it. We must be careful not to make judgments or create stereotypes, and we must be careful not to inflict pain through methods we use to alleviate it.

CONCLUSIONS

One theme emerges from this presentation—the nurse who would understand a child's reaction to pain must constantly look at the total, everchanging child in relation to his pain. This is how it must be if we would truly see a child as an open system, constantly interacting with his environment. We have seen that when one "system" is disturbed, it often disturbs the equilibrium of the others, since we are not just an assemblage of parts but, rather, highly organized, patterned individuals, moving unidirectionally.[13]

As we view the life processes of man, we see how the constant interaction between man and his environment is constantly changing him and being changed by him. Since I believe that change causes stress, that stress causes or can be caused by pain, and that pain causes or can be caused by change, I also believe that nurses must begin to view the normal processes a child goes through as the painful experiences that the child perceives them to be.

Pain isn't just a broken leg, or an injection; it is also growing, changing, being scolded, failing in school, and not having visitors. If we are to be truly helpful in alleviating a child's pain, we must first understand how he perceives pain and, second, we must learn to anticipate what might be a painful experience to a child of a certain age and take measures either to prevent or lessen it.

REFERENCES

1. Barnhart, C. L., ed. *American College Dictionary.* New York, Random House, 1962, p. 870.
2. Guyton, A. C. *Textbook of Medical Physiology.* 3rd ed. Philadelphia, W. B. Saunders Co., 1966.
3. Mussen, P. H., and others. *Child Development and Personality.* 3rd ed. New York, Harper and Row, Publishers, 1969, p. 504.
4. Marlow, Dorothy R., and Sellew, Gladys. *Textbook of Pediatric Nursing.* 2d ed. Philadelphia, W. B. Saunders Co., 1965, p. 507.
5. *Ibid.*,p. 524.
6. *Ibid.*, p. 522.
7. Barnett, H. L. *Pediatrics.* 14th ed. New York, Appleton-Century-Crofts, 1968, p. 263.
8. Mussen, and others, *op. cit.,* p. 515.
9. *Ibid.*, p. 516.
10. Marlow, *op. cit.,* p. 521.
11. Blake, Florence G. *Child, His Parents, and the Nurse.* Philadelphia, J. B. Lippincott Co., 1954, p. 361.
12. Mussen, and others, *op. cit.,* p. 513.
13. Rogers, Martha E. *Introduction to the Theoretical Basis of Nursing.* Philadephia, F. A. Davis Co., 1970.

11

Sex difference in pain tolerance and pain apperception

S. L. H. Notermans and M. M. W. A. Tophoff

INTRODUCTION

There is no agreement in the literature about sex differences in relation to sensitivity to pain. Whereas some publications state that women have a greater sensitivity to pain than men, *(5, 7, 10, 18, 20)* other authors, on the contrary, have denied this and did not find any evidence of variation in pain reactions between the two sexes *(3, 4, 8, 9, 19)*.

Most of these above-mentioned authors, however, have reached their conclusions from the values of pain threshold measurements and not from maximum pain tolerance.

In our own investigations on this subject we also found no significant differences in pain threshold values between men and women *(12)*.

In this paper we intend to reexamine the question of sex differences in pain sensitivity, but now in relation to maximum pain tolerance. In this study we define maximum pain tolerance as the lowest electrical current—expressed in milliampères—which at a fixed frequency and impulse duration, evokes an intolerable sensation of pain in the subject.

There are investigations in relation to maximum tolerance of pain mentioned in the literature, which specially are concerned with the 'apperception' factor of pain *(15, 16)*. According to Petrovich *(15, 16)* this factor plays an important role in pain experience and tolerance. He found that when illustrations of painful situations were shown to women, they tended to identify them in terms of greater severity than did men *(16)*. In this paper we also intend to check this aspect of pain experience.

METHOD

(a) Subjects

In this investigation two different groups of subjects were used:

(1) Fifty patients admitted to the Psychiatric Department of the State University of Groningen: 25 males, 25 females, ranging in age from 18 to 65 years. Males and females were comparable as to age and education. Excluded were psychotic patients because of their incapacity to cooperate in this experiment.

(2) Forty-seven normal subjects: students, 23 males and 24 females, ranging in age from 18 to 28 years, who were medically fit for sport and neurologically normal. These subjects also were comparable as to age and education.

(b) Pain stimulation

In order to measure the maximum pain tolerance of the subject we used an electrical stimulus with square wave current, as is described in detail in a previous study *(12)*. The stimulating electrode was always placed on the dorsal side of the right middlefinger on the terminal phalanx, 1 cm proximal to the fingernail border. The sub-

Reprinted with permission of the Elsevier Scientific Publishing Co. from Psychiatria, Neurologia, Neurochirurgia **70**:23-29. Copyright 1967.

From the Neurological Department (Head: Prof. Dr. J. Droogleever Fortuyn), Psychiatric Department (Head: Prof. Dr. W. K. van Dijk), Psychological Department (Head: Dr. P. E. Boeke), State University, Groningen (The Netherlands).

Table III. Comparison of PAT-scores from all male and female subjects

	Male			*Female*			
Subjects	*Number of cases*	*Mean of PAT scores*	*S.D.*	*Number of cases*	*Mean of PAT scores*	*S.D.*	*t*
Intensity							
A. Psychiatric patients	25	65.68	9.20	25	64.65	10.69	0.05
B. Normals	23	68.77	6.28	24	68.08	9.71	−0.004
Duration							
A. Psychiatric patients	25	65.16	8.58	25	60.92	12.04	0.22
B. Normals	23	59.21	9.62	24	60.75	9.65	0.08

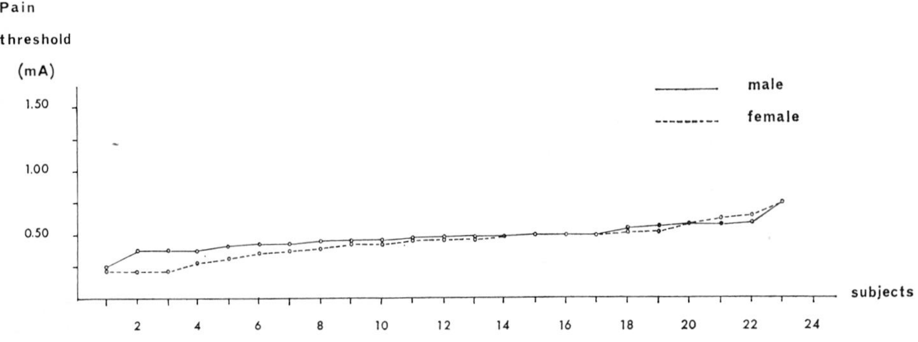

Fig. 2. Average Pain Thresholds in the normal sample.

Table III reveals clearly that we could not demonstrate significant differences. Nor does it indicate a trend as to the PAT-scores of males and females of both our groups of subjects, either in the Intensity scores or in the Duration scores.

In Fig. 2 is presented the individual average pain thresholds in the normal sample, to show once more that there is no sex difference.

In Fig. 2 are plotted the average Pain Thresholds in mA, for the male subjects (solid line) and the female subjects (dotted line). Subjects were ranked in the above described manner as to their mean Pain Threshold. Clearly is illustrated the fact, that with stimulation at pain threshold level no sex difference can be found (see also Notermans *(12)*) and that the pain threshold is relatively constant in subjects of both sexes. Our results, as presented in Fig. 2, agree with the findings of others *(3, 4, 8, 9, 19)*.

Summarizing our results, we can claim to have established a significant sex difference in the PTT: men can tolerate pain better than women in an experimental situation. This finding holds not only for our sample of normal subjects, but also for the groups of psychiatric patients. In accordance to the reports of Notermans *(12)* our results indicate that there is no significant sex difference in pain threshold as such. Furthermore the great reliability of the PTT-method is demonstrated. On the other hand, we could not confirm the findings of Petrovich *(15)* concerning sex difference in Pain Apperception.

DISCUSSION

The results prove that indeed there is a real difference in pain tolerance between men and women. It must however be emphasized once more, that in this experiment the significant difference in pain perception was only found in relation to the maximum tolerance of pain and not to pain threshold level. Schumacher *(17)* and Hardy *et al.* *(9)* also came to the same conclusion, using the radiant heat method in relation to the pain threshold. They also could not find any significant sex differences by stimulating at pain threshold levels. On the other hand Lipsitt *(11)* and Bell *(2)* described sex differences with electrical stimulation of neonates. In regard to maximum pain tolerance, Petrie *(13)* found, as we do, that there is a sex difference.

We found a great inter-individual variation in pain tolerance threshold in our subjects. Indeed many other authors (Beecher, *1*), have pointed out that reactions to pain vary greatly from one individual to another. Petrie *(14)* considered that this should not be regarded as exceptional when one looks for instance at the great differences in visual sensibility between blindness and normal vision. He suggests that in the same way sensitivity for pain can vary in degree (Petrie, *13*).

The difference between the Pain Apperception Test and our pain stimulation method obviously is to be found in the totally different stimulus-situations and procedures in these two ways of measurement. Pain in the PAT concerns imaginative and projected pain, while with the stimulation method there is a real pain stimulus with a real pain sensation, though in the experimental setting of a laboratory. The sex difference in maximum pain tolerance possibly can be explained by postulating that men – at least in an experimental pain situation – incline much more than women towards 'being firm', by which attitude the unpleasant stimulus can be tolerated much longer. This inclination perhaps seems to be culturally determined, as Kennard *(10)* also states that 'men are not supposed to cry out to pain as quickly and easily as are women'.

Besides the fact that sex of the subject is an important variable in pain tolerance, there must be other variables, which play a role in the great inter-individual differences in pain tolerance threshold, such as are illustrated in Fig. 1. In the literature the source of these differences is sought mainly in personality variables or personality dimensions as neuroticism and extraversion. These variables will be the subject of a later study.

SUMMARY

In a study to assess sex differences in maximum pain tolerance and the predisposition to experience pain, a reliable electrical pain stimulation method and the Pain Apperception Test were employed. Two different groups of subjects, psychiatric patients and normals, including males and females, were studied. Results showed a significant sex difference in pain tolerance in both groups of subjects, indicating that, in an experimental pain situation, men can tolerate pain better than women. As to the Pain Apperception Test, differences between males and females could not be demonstrated.

REFERENCES

1. Beecher, H. K., *Measurement of Subjective Responses*, Oxford University Press, New York, 1959.

2. Bell, R. G. and Costello, N. S., Three tests for sex differences in tactile sensitivity in the newborn, *Biol. Neonat. (Basel)*, 7 (1964) 335-347.

3. Chapman, W. P. and Jones, C. M., Variations in cutaneous and visceral pain sensitivity in normal subjects, *J. clin. Invest.*, 23 (1944) 81-91.

4. Clausen, J. and King, H. E., Determination of the pain threshold on untrained subjects, *J. Psychol.*, 30 (1950) 299-306.

5. Critchley, M., Some aspects of pain, *Brit. med. J.*, 2 (1934) 891-896.

6. Guilford, J. P., *Fundamental Statistics in Psychology and Education*, McGraw-Hill, New York, 1956.

7. Hall, K. R. L. and Stride, E., The varying response to pain in psychiatric disorders: a study in abnormal psychology, *Brit. J. Psychol.*, 27 (1954) 48-60.

8. Hardy, J. D., Wolff, H. G. and Goodell, H., The pain threshold in man, *Proc. Ass. Res. nerv. ment. Dis.*, 23 (1943) 1-15.

9. Hardy, J. D., Wolff, H. G., Goodell H., *Pain Sensations and Reactions*, Williams and Wilkins, Baltimore, 1952.

10. Kennard, M. A., Responses to painful stimuli of patients with severe chronic painful conditions, *J. clin. Invest.*, 31 (1952) 245-252.

11. Lipsitt, L. P., Electrotactual threshold in the neonate, *Child Develop.*, 30 (1959) 547-554.

12. Notermans, S. L. H., Measurement of the pain threshold determined by electrical stimulation and its clinical application, Part 1 (Method and factors possibly influencing the pain threshold), *Neurology (Minneap.)*, 16 (1966) 1071-1086.

13. Petrie, A., Some psychological aspects of pain on the relief of suffering. *Amer. N. Y. Acad. Sci.*, 86 (1960) 13-27.

14. Petrie, A., Collins, W. and Solomon, P. H., The tolerance for pain and for sensory deprivation, *Amer. J. Psychol.*, 73 (1960) 80-90.

15. Petrovich, D. V., The Pain apperception test: An application to sex difference, *J. clin. Psychol.*, 15 (1959) 412-415.

16. Petrovich, D. V., The pain apperception test: Psychological correlates of pain perception, *J. clin. Psychol.*, 14 (1958) 367-374.

17. Schumacher, G. A., Goodell, H., Hardy, J. D. and

Wolff, H. G., Uniformity of the pain threshold in man, *Science*, 92 (1940) 110-112.

18. Sherman, E. D., Sensitivity to pain, *Canad. med. Ass. J.*, 48 (1943) 437-441.

19. Swartz, P., *Pain Scaling and the Influence of Sex and Personality on the Pain Response*, Thesis, University of Rochester, N.Y., 1951.

20. Wilder, R. M. J., Sensitivity to pain, *Proc. Mayo Clin.*, 15 (1940) 551-554.

12

The cutaneous pricking pain threshold in old age

P. Procacci, G. Bozza, G. Buzzelli and M. Della Corte

THE CUTANEOUS PRICKING PAIN THRESHOLD IN OLD AGE

Aging in human skin has been extensively studied, and a recent symposium [Montagna, 1965] covered many aspects including morphology, biophysics, biochemistry and physiology. Anatomical changes in the sensory receptors were noted by Winkelmann [1965] who suggested that it would be worthwhile studying the physiology of skin sensation in relation to age.

In fact, studies of sensation in relation to touch and pressure began with the work of Ronge [1943/1944] who showed that there was a decline in the number of Meissner's corpuscles with advancing age. The tactile sensitivity of the cornea, where there are only free nerve endings, was found to decrease with age by Jalavisto *et al.* [1951]. Vibration sense was found to diminish in the toes (but not the fingers) with advancing age by Cosh [1953] while Poole [1956] showed that ischaemic paresthesiae from compression of the limbs could be produced more readily in younger than in older subjects. Further differences in the quality of the sensation caused by ischaemia in old people were noted by Galletti *et al.* [1959].

None of these studies however concern only the sensation of the skin itself. Deeper structures were always involved. Sensation in the skin alone can, however, be studied in relation to pain. Pain can be induced mechanically, electrically and by chemical and thermal stimuli. Galletti *et al.* [personal communication] studied the reaction of the skin to CO_2 snow and other chemicals. They showed a diminished pain response in older subjects.

Pain sensation is best examined by determining the threshold at which pain begins. The stimulus required to produce this can be accurately measured. Beyond this point the intensity of pain is more subjective and harder to estimate.

Pain threshold can most conveniently be studied by exposing the skin to radiant heat. Chapman and Jones [1944] showed a rise in pain threshold with age but Hardy *et al.* [1952] denied this and for several years their opinion prevailed [Bonica, 1953; White and Sweet, 1955]. However, Sherman and Robillard [1960] re-examined the problem and found a lower pain threshold in younger subjects. They also observed that women had a lower threshold than men. Few of the previous studies were done with sufficient subjects for statistical analysis and this led us to examine the problem further using a new method [Della Corte *et al.*, 1965].

METHOD

In our algometer radiant energy produced by a projection lamp is focused by a condensing lens on a skin surface previously blackened with ink. The duration of exposure to the lamp is controlled by a shutter and timed with a stop watch. The end point, or pain threshold, occurs when the subject first experiences a pricking

Reprinted with permission from Gerontologia Clinica **12:**213-218 (Karger, Basel 1970).
Istituto di Patologia Speciale Medica e Metodologia Clinica, Istituto di Fisica Medica, Università delgi Studi, Firenze (Italy).

sensation. Both the intensity (I) and the time (t) can be varied at will. Intensity is measured with a special radiometer.

THEORETICAL CONSIDERATIONS

Let us assume that the skin is formed by an external layer (A) and by an internal one (B). Layer A contains the receptors giving origin to the pricking sensation when the skin is exposed to heat. This layer whose primary characteristics can be considered constant absorbs radiant heat.

Layer B which separates layer A from the deeper structures is rich in blood vessels and from a thermal point of view is non homogeneous. It absorbs part of the heat transmitted by radiation to layer A but the extent to which it does so is affected by its blood supply.

THRESHOLD ENERGY

These considerations led us to introduce a new concept, threshold energy (TE) [Della Corte *et al.*, 1965]. TE expressed in $mcal/cm^2$ is the energy per surface unit of layer A required to stimulate the receptors to a sense of pain. TE is derived from the ratio of 2 expressions $\lambda (T - T_0)$ and $\lambda 1 c\rho$, where 1 is the thickness, c the specific heat and ρ the density of layer A, while $(T-T_0)$ is the difference between the threshold temperature of the pain receptors T and the temperature of the skin surface T_0. λ is a constant which characterizes the efficiency of the heat dispersion process. Threshold energy is given by the formula

$$TE = 1\, c\, \rho (T - T_0).$$

THE PRESENT INVESTIGATION

The object of the present study was to compare the threshold energy in a group of young subjects with a group of older subjects covering a wide age span.

The subjects. The young subjects, 165 male and 93 female, were between 18 and 28 years of age. They included students from the university, cadets from the Army Medical School and student nurses. All were healthy and free of skin disease or any condition likely to cause pain.

The older subjects, 135 male and 132 female were between 50 and 90 years of age. They came from an old people's home in Florence. They were free of pain and in good condition physically and mentally. They were divided into three groups according to age (table I).

Table I

Age in years	*Number of cases*	*Mean value of TE (mcal/cm²) ± SD*
Men		
18–28	165	924 (± 18)
50–59	29	962 (± 51)
60–69	55	941 (± 29)
70 and over	51	981 (± 37)
Women		
18–28	93	829 (± 12)
50–59	22	842 (± 55)
60–69	22	888 (± 60)
70 and over	88	926 (± 24)

Method. The tests were performed at room temperature (18-20° C), taking particular care that no sweating occurred in the skin areas under observation. The pain threshold was determined by exposing the subject to a stimulus of known intensity and noting the time which elapsed before a pricking sensation was felt. The apparatus was as described above.

We fixed 9 increasing values for the stimulus intensity (I) and measured the time (t) needed to reach the pain threshold in 9 adjacent areas on the volar surface of each forearm. Our previous work had shown that the pain threshold was the same in all these areas.

We thus obtained 9 pairs of values for I and t in each subject. From these we deduced the parameters required to calculate the threshold energy (TE) and the standard deviations. The calculations were programmed and performed on a IBM 1620 computer.

Results. The results show that TE (and therefore the cutaneous pricking pain threshold) increases with age in both men and women. Threshold differences between men and women previously noted in younger subjects were found to persist in the older subjects. The TE values were lower in women at all ages (table I).

As the threshold energy is derived from the ratio of the expressions $\lambda (T - T_0)$ and $\lambda 1\, c\, \rho$, we have tabulated these figures and have found that these also increase with advancing age (table II).

Table II

Age in years	$\lambda\ (T-T_0)$	$\lambda\ 1\ c\ \rho$
Men		
18–28	46.47	0.0539
50–59	46.90	0.0500
60–69	48.90	0.0531
70 and over	50.62	0.0557
Women		
18–28	37.43	0.0463
50–59	39.68	0.0482
60–69	43.80	0.0511
70 and over	45.17	0.0512

DISCUSSION

Our study shows that with advancing age there is a progressive increase in the threshold of the skin to pricking pain. Why should this be so?

Anatomy suggests some possible reasons. Histologically in ageing skin the corpuscular end organs are reduced in number and modified in structure [Cauna, 1965; Winkelmann, 1965]. On the other hand free nerve endings which must be considered the fundamental receptors of pain sensation do not apparently undergo any changes either in distribution or structure as far as we can tell with present methods [Cauna, 1965].

Other skin structures also change with ageing. The epidermis becomes thinner having fewer cell layers. The ridges become shallower and papillary bodies are reduced in number [Oberste-Lehn, 1965]. The smaller vessels show few striking changes, but the sub epidermal plexus of capillaries form shallow arches instead of loops [Christophers and Kligman, 1965].

Our mathematical results also throw light on the problem. We found that the values for the expressions $\lambda\ (T-T_0)$ and $\lambda/1\ c\ \rho$ increased with age (table II). This result could be due to an increase in the value of λ, the multiplying factor of both expressions characterising the heat dispersal process. A decrease in skin thickness would facilitate the increased dispersal of heat via the blood supply and an increase in the value of λ expresses this fact.

On the other hand since the expression for threshold energy: $TE = 1\ c\ \rho\ (T-T_0)$, does not include the factor λ, we must look elsewhere for the reason why TE increases with age. Mathematically, an increase in TE could be due to an increase in the value of the product 1 c ρ. But, we can assume that the specific heat (c) and the density (ρ) do not change with age, and we know that the skin thickness (1) gets less and not more as the patient grows older. The value for 1 c ρ must therefore get less with age and we must look at the other half of the expression $(T-T_0)$, that is the difference between the receptor threshold temperature T and the skin surface temperature T_0, for the explanation. The most reasonable hypothesis is that an increase in TE is due to an increased difference between T and T_0. In our earlier studies [Della Corte *et al.*, 1965] we found that the skin surface temperature under our experimental conditions was around 33° C and did not vary appreciably with age. We can, therefore, conclude that the factor which leads to the observed increase in TE is an increase in T, the threshold temperature of the receptors.

One further point deserves comment. It is possible that age increases the threshold of the nervous structures which conduct and integrate sensation and causes delay in the patient's response. We have not investigated this ourselves, but Birren [1959] and Anderson [1959] have both shown that there is no delay in the response of old people to simple stimuli. Such delays only occur when old people have to respond to successive stimuli and are required to perform serial tasks.

SUMMARY

The cutaneous pricking pain threshold was measured in 258 subjects ranging from 18 to 28 years and 267 from 50-90 years of age. The threshold was determined by means of a thermal algometer using a newly devised method. The cutaneous pricking pain threshold was observed to increase progressively with advancing age. Threshold values are lower in women than in men. The mathematical analysis of the experimental data suggests that two different factors are involved in the increase in the cutaneous pain threshold in old age: (i) an increase in the dispersion of the thermal energy absorbed; (ii) an increase in the threshold of the cutaneous receptors giving origin to the pain sensation.

REFERENCES

Anderson, J. E.: Fourth round-table discussion; in Birren, Imus and Windle The process of aging in the nervous system (Blackwell, Oxford 1959).

Birren, J. E.: Sensation, perception and modification of behavior in relation to the process of aging; in Birren, Imus and Windle The process of aging in the nervous system (Blackwell, Oxford 1959).

Bonica, J.: The management of pain (Lea & Febiger, Philadelphia 1953).

Cauna, N.: The effects of aging on the receptor organs of the human dermis; in Montagna Advances in biology of skin, vol. 6 (Pergamon Press, Oxford 1965).

Chapman, W. P. and Jones, C. M.: Variations in cutaneous and visceral pain sensitivity in normal subjects. J. clin. Invest. *23*:81 (1944).

Christophers, E. and Kligman, A. M.: Percutaneous absorption in aged skin; in Montagna Advances in biology of skin, vol. 6 (Pergamon Press, Oxford 1965).

Cosh, J. A.: Studies on the nature of vibration sense. Clin. Sci. *12:* 131 (1953).

Della Corte, M.; Procacci, P.; Bozza, G. and Buzzelli, G.: A study on the cutaneous pricking pain threshold in normal man. Arch. Fisiol. *64:* 141 (1965).

Galletti, R.; Procacci, P. e Vecchiet, L.: Sul comportamento della funzione sensitiva delgli arti superiori nell'età senile. G. Geront *7*:7 (1959).

Hardy, J. D.; Wolff, H. and Goodell, H.: Pain sensation and reactions (Williams & Wilkins, Baltimore 1952).

Jalavisto, E.: Orma, E. and Tawast, M.: Ageing and relation between stimulus intensity and duration in corneal sensibility. Acta physiol. scand. *23:* 224 (1951).

Montagna, W.: Advances in biology of skin, vol. 6 (Pergamon Press, Oxford 1965).

Oberste-Lehn, H.: Effects of aging on the papillary body of the hair follicles and on the eccrine sweat glands; in Montagna Advances in biology of skin, vol. 6 (Pergamon Press, Oxford 1965).

Poole, E. W.: Ischaemic and post-ischaemic paraesthesiae. Normal responses in the upper limb with special reference to the effect of age. J. Neurol. Neurosurg. Psychiat. *19:* 148 (1956).

Ronge, H.: Altersveränderungen in der Anzahl Meissnerscher Nervendkörper in der Haut. Zbl. Haut-GeschlKr. *70:* 534 (1943/44).

Sherman, E. D. and Robillard, E.: Sensitivity to pain in the aged. Canad. med. Ass. J. *83:* 944 (1960).

White, J. C. and Sweet, W. H.: Pain. Its mechanism and neurosurgical control (Thomas, Springfield 1955).

Winkelmann, R. K.: Nerve changes in aging skin; in Montagna Advances in biology of skin, vol. 6 (Pergamon Press, Oxford 1965).

13

Pain threshold and tolerance of hands and feet

Frank S. Murray and Barbara C. Hagan

A previous study (Murray & Safferstone, 1970) concerning the relationship between pain threshold and tolerance and hand preference produced evidence that the left hand was more sensitive to pain than the right hand for both sinistral and dextral subjects. Of the 41 subjects in that experiment, 3 had a sinistral hand preference. It was suggested that the greater sensitivity of the left hand might be accounted for in terms of the bilateral asymmetry of the brain. If this were the case, the left foot should also show greater sensitivity to pain than the right foot.

The purpose of the present investigation was twofold: *(a)* to determine if sensitivity and pain of the left hand was supported when an equal number of sinistral and dextral subjects were tested; and *(b)* to determine whether this phenomenon could be demonstrated with the feet as well as with the hands.

METHOD

Subjects

Twenty female students at Randolph-Macon Woman's College volunteered to participate in this experiment. These subjects were chosen on the basis of handedness: 10 sinistral and 10 dextral. A questionnaire administered after the experiment confirmed handedness.

Apparatus

Two thermostat-controlled water baths were used. The temperature of the adapting bath was 32° C. (± 1.0°), approximately the normal temperature of the hand (Kenshalo & Nafe, 1963). The cold-water bath to induce pain had a constant temperature of 2° C. (Wolf & Hardy, 1943).

Procedure

The procedure followed was identical to that used by Murray and Safferstone (1970) except that both hands and feet were tested in the present study. For all subjects, 10 trials with the feet were run first, followed by 10 trials with the hands. Preliminary observation had indicated a great disparity in pain perception between the feet and hands, and it was felt that the greater sensitivity of the hands might affect the subjects expectation of perception in the feet if the hands were tested first. The same left-right sequence as determined randomly by the experimenter was used for the hands and the feet of a particular subject. If, on Trial 1, the right foot was submerged, the left foot was submerged on Trial 2, and this pattern of alternation was continued for the remaining eight trials; this same presentation sequence was repeated for the 10 trials with the hands. A trial began by submerging 1 foot (to the ankle) or hand (to the wrist) in the adapting bath for 2 min., during which time the subject was asked at 30-sec. intervals to estimate the temperature of the water on a 200-point scale divided into 10-point intervals, ranging from −100 (extremely cold) through O (neutral) to +100 (extremely hot). At the end of the 2-min. period, the subject immediately placed her foot (hand) in the cold-water bath. The pain threshold was recorded when the subject first indicated "pain" and the tolerance

From the Journal of Comparative and Physiological Psychology **84:**639-643.

From the Department of Psychology, Randoph-Macon Woman's College, Lynchburg, Virginia 24504.

measure was determined by the entire duration the subject was able to maintain her foot (hand) in the cold-water bath saying "stop" and removing her foot (hand). If the subject had not said "stop" at the end of 3 min., the trial was terminated. This occurred with 2 subjects, 1 dextral and 1 sinistral. After a 15-sec. intertrial interval, the procedure was repeated with the alternate foot (hand) and the experiment continued until there had been a total of 20 trials, 5 with each foot and 5 with each hand. After Trial 20, the subject completed a questionnaire consisting of the following questions:

1. With which hand do you write? L R
2. With which hand do you hold a tennis racquet or play ping-pong? L R
3. With which hand do you eat? L R
4. With which hand do you iron? L R
5. Are you right or left handed? L R

If the subject had the same response to at least 2 of the first 4 questions, besides answering the fifth question with a similar response, then that reply wes determined to be the subject's handedness.

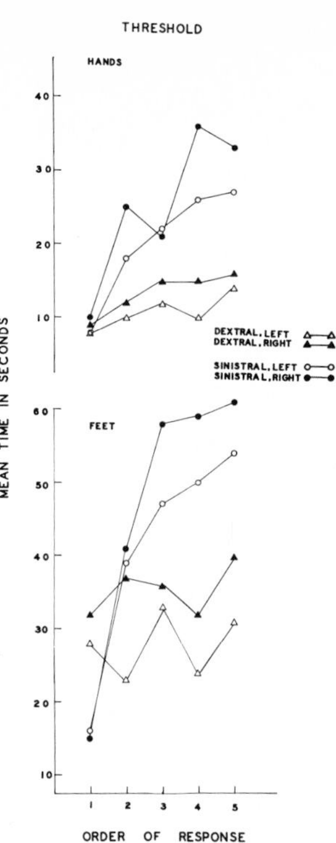

Fig. 1. Mean time in seconds for thresholds of pain for hands and feet plotted over order of response.

RESULTS

The results show that the left hands and feet had a significantly lower threshold and tolerance for pain than the right hands and feet for both sinistral and dextral subjects. In addition, the sinistral subjects were found to have higher threshold and tolerance levels for both hands and feet than the dextral subjects, and the feet of both groups were found to be less sensitive to pain than the hands. However, those differences were not statistically significant. The results of the adaptation trials indicated a tendency towards higher temperature judgments as the number of trials increased. The 2 subjects who were told to remove their hands or feet from the cold-water bath at the end of 3 min. on some or all of the 20 trials were included in the data analyses.

Threshold

The mean thresholds for pain in seconds for the 10 dextral subjects were 10.81 for the left hand, 13.63 for the right hand, 27.83 for the left foot, and 35.21 for the right foot. The mean thresholds for the 10 sinistral subjects were 19.99 for the left hand, 24.76 for the right hand, 41.21 for the left foot, and 46.71 for the right foot. The mean thresholds for the dextral and sinistral subjects for order of placing their hands and feet in the cold-water bath are shown graphically in Figure 1. The differences in sensitivity both between left and right hands and between sinistral and dextral subjects are clearly represented in this figure. The greater sensitivity of the feet of the sinistral subjects initially can perhaps be explained by the fact that the judgments were first made with the feet in the adapting bath for 2 min., and this "anchored" the first judgments of pain to the cold water. However, an anchoring or contrast effect can not be the complete answer, since dextral subjects did not show a similar effect.

An analysis of variances for repeated measures (Winer, 1962) revealed statistical significance between hands ($F = 6.24$, $df = 1/18$, $p < .05$) and over order of responding for hands ($F = 5.37$, $df = 4/72$, $p < .05$). No significant difference was obtained for handedness. In a similar analysis for feet, a

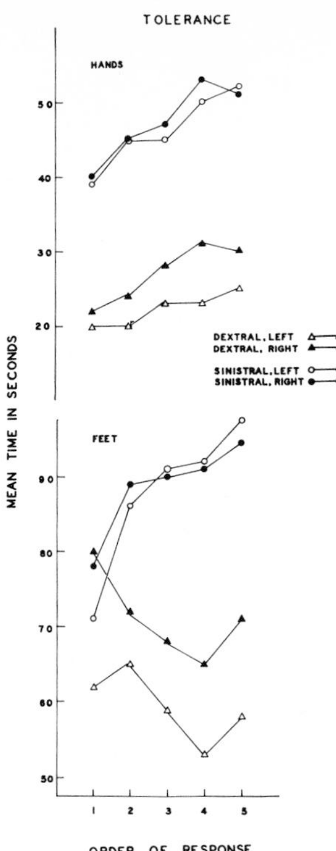

Fig. 2. Mean time in seconds for tolerance of pain for hands and feet plotted over order of response.

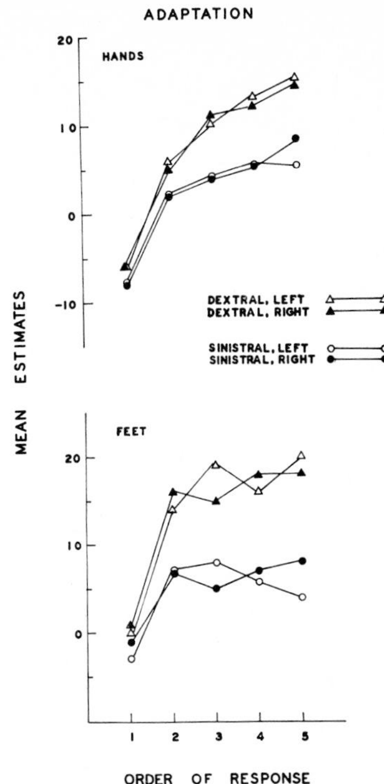

Fig. 3. Mean adaptation judgments for hands and feet plotted over order of response.

significant difference in order of responding was also obtained ($F=4.50$, $df=4/72$, $p<.05$) as well as a significant Handedness × Order of Responding interaction ($F=3.39$, $df=4/72$, $p<.05$).

Tolerance

The mean tolerances for pain in seconds for the 10 dextral subjects were 22.16 for the left hand, 27.19 for the right hand, 59.75 for the left foot, and 71.50 for the right foot. For the 10 sinistral subjects, the mean tolerances were 46.32 for the left hand, 46.99 for the right hand, 87.33 for the left foot, and 88.67 for the right foot. As was found in regard to pain thresholds, tolerance was significantly greater for the right hand and right foot for both sinistral and dextral subjects, but the sinistral subjects had a higher tolerance than the dextral subjects. These results are shown in Figure 2, in which the mean tolerance in seconds is graphed over the order of response.

Analysis of variances indicated statistical significance between hands ($F<5.79$, $df=1/18$, $p<.05$) and over order of response for hands ($F=5.26$, $df=4/72$, $p<.05$). A significant Handedness x Order of Response interaction for feet was also found ($F=4.08$, $df=4/72$, $p<.05$). Again, no significant differences were obtained for handedness.

Adaptation

Analysis of variance was computed using the mean of the 4 adaptation judgments on each trial for each subject for the order of response with both the hands and the feet. Statistical significance was obtained over response with both the hands and the feet. Statistical significance was obtained over order or response for both the hands and the feet (hands: $F=20.77$, $df=4/72$, $p<.05$; feet: $F=6.38$, $df=4/72$, $p<.05$). These results indicate that subjects tended to give judgments of higher temperature with increasing order of response. The dextral subjects tended toward higher temperatures than the sinistral for both hands and feet. These results can be seen in Figure 3, in which mean adaptation judgments are graphed over order of response.

DISCUSSION

The results of this study indicated greater sensitivity of pain for the left hands and the left feet of the sinistral and dextral subjects. These results support those of Murray and Safferstone (1970) with dextral subjects and indicate that a greater left-hand sensitivity is also present in sinistral subjects. Furthermore, the present study lends evidence to the idea that bilateral asymmetry in the brain may account for the differences in pain sensitivity by showing that the greater left sensitivity can also be demonstrated with the feet.

This study also demonstrated that the feet are less sensitive to pain than the hands. The temperature in the cold-water bath was kept at a constant 2° C. when both the hands and the feet were being tested. If a more extreme (colder) temperature had been used for the feet, lower threshold and tolerance levels would probably have been obtained. A colder temperature for the feet might also have resulted in greater differences between the sinistral and dextral subjects. The feet have been shown to have higher thresholds for pressure (Woodworth & Schlosberg, 1954, p. 274), higher concentrations of warm and cold spots, and greater distribution of pain "points" (Geldard, 1972, pp. 325-345) than the hands; and in view of the present results, it seems reasonable to postulate a higher pain threshold for feet also.

A positive relationship was found between adaptation, threshold, and tolerance, as can be seen by comparing Figures 1 and 2 with Figure 3. It appears that with increased responding there is a tendency towards higher temperature judgments and lower pain sensitivity.

The present results neither support nor invalidate the so-called "callus" hypothesis which states that the preferred hand is tougher and less sensitive because of greater use. For the dextral subjects, the right hand did show less sensitivity to pain, which would follow from the callus hypothesis. This was not the case, however, for the sinistral subjects; the right hand still showed a lower sensitivity, which is not what would be expected. One possible explanation can be found in the subjects' answers to the hand-preference questionnaire. Although all 20 subjects clearly qualified as having either a sinistral or dextral preference under the established criteria, 6 of the 10 sinistral subjects indicated their right hand for 1 or 2 of the first 4 questions, whereas only 2 of the dextral subjects indicated use of the left hand. It seems likely that hand preference is not as clearly defined for the sinistral subjects as for the dextral subjects. Further study using more sinistral subjects seems desirable to answer this question fully.

REFERENCES

Geldard, F. A. *The human senses.* (2nd ed.) New York: Wiley, 1972.

Kenshalo, D. R., & Nafe, J. P. Cutaneous vascular system as a model temperature receptor. *Perceptual and Motor Skills,* 1963, **17,** 257-258.

Murray, F. S., & Safferstone, J. F. Pain threshold and tolerance of right and left hands. *Journal of Comparative and Physiological Psychology,* 1970, **71,** 83-86.

Winer, B. J. *Statistical principles in experimental design.* New York: McGraw-Hill, 1962.

Wolf, S., & Hardy, J. D. Studies on pain, observations on pain due to local cooling, and on factors involved in the "cold pressor" effect. *Research Publication of the Association for Nervous and Mental Disease,* 1943, **23,** 123-142.

Woodworth, R. S., & Schlosberg, H. *Experimental psychology.* (2nd ed.) New York: Holt, Rinehart & Winston, 1954.

14

Note on pain reactivity and family size

Donald R. Sweeney[1] and Bernard J. Fine

Several investigators have attempted to relate adult pain reactivity to quantitative and qualitative pain experiences in childhood. Frequently, the nature of such early pain experiences has been inferred from family structure variables such as birth order and family size. In general, the results of these studies have been equivocal.

Collins (1965) found higher pain tolerance in young men with higher protection scores and lower independence scores on a childhood history questionnaire. Firstborn and/or only children are thought to be more protected and dependent (Schachter, 1959). Theoretical extrapolation yields a prediction that *higher* pain tolerance would be found in firstborn and only children and also in members of smaller families where there would be proportionately more firstborn and only children. The latter relationship is supported by the results of Gonda (1962) who found that a significantly greater number of neurological patients from large families had chief complaints of pain as compared with those from small families. Schachter (1959) reported *lower* pain tolerance in firstborn and only children than in later borns; neither Gelfand (1963) nor Collins and Stone (1964) could replicate this finding. However, it is supported by combining the results of Ryan and Kovacic (1966), who found lower pain tolerance in nonathletes than in contact-sport athletes, and of Nisbett (1968), who reported that firstborns were under-represented among contact-sport athletes. The purpose of the present study was to examine further the relationship between family size, birth order and responses to a pain-inducing stimulus.

Method. As part of a larger study (Fine & Sweeney, 1968) 52 soldiers were given a battery of psychological and psychophysiological tests. Information on family structure and early background was obtained by means of a questionnaire. Pain was induced by immersion of *S*'s right hand in a thermostatically controlled water bath set at 4° C. Duration of exposure was 10 min., but *S*s were not so informed, being told only that they could withdraw their hands if pain became intolerable. *S*s rated pain intensity every 30 sec. during immersion using a 7-point numerical scale for which verbal descriptors ranging from "no pain" to "almost unbearable pain" were also provided. Hand skin temperature was monitored using a thermocouple attached to the posterior surface of the fifth digit.

Reprinted with permission of author and publisher: Sweeney, D. R., & Fine, B. J. Note on pain reactivity and family size. Perceptual and Motor Skills, 1970, **31**, 25-26.

From the U. S. Army Research Institute of Environmental Medicine, Natick, Mass. 01760.

[1]Now at University of Rochester Medical Center.

[2]For example, responses to the question "Would you come back again soon to participate in an identical study?" (referring not only to the hand immersion study but to an entire week of experimentation) indicated that 32 out of 33 non-withdrawers would return, whereas 10 out of 19 withdrawers so indicated ($\chi^2 = 12.54$, $p < .01$). In addition, withdrawers were less intelligent on the WAIS ($\chi^2 = 4.07$, $p < .05$), indicating to us that they might not have understood the purposes of the study as explained to them and were, therefore, less motivated to perform well. Of the 19 *S*s who withdrew, 7 of the 10 who said that they would return were "late withdrawers;" 7 of the 9 who would not return were "early withdrawers." The "late withdrawers" may have withdrawn because of pain rather than lack of motivation. However, their pain responses do not support this conclusion. We, therefore, consider withdrawal to be motivational primarily until shown to be otherwise. A number of personality measures were found to be related to withdrawal but no coherent pattern could be established.

Results. Data were from the 33 *S*s who underwent the full 10-min. immersion period (non-withdrawers). Independent interview data had shown that a high proportion of the 19 withdrawers was characterized by dissatisfaction with the role of *S* and, consequently, by low motivation to participate, which was confounded with pain reactivity in an unknown way.[2] Pain reactivity was defined as the numerical sum of the ratings in the first two immersion minutes, during which pain reaches its peak intensity. Beyond 2 min., some *S*s exhibit a reflex vasodilation which tends to reduce pain intensity, some *S*s a reflex vasodilation which appears unrelated to pain intensity, and some *S*s do not exhibit any reflex vasodilation and may or may not change in pain reactivity. This confounding of reflex vasodilation with pain-intensity ratings suggested the 2-min. criterion. The 33 *S*s were divided into high, medium and low pain-reactivity subgroups who were then compared for differences in birth order and family size. Table 1 demonstrates a significant association between family size and pain reactivty, *S*s from smaller families exhibiting higher pain reactivity. The strength of this relationship was also estimated by computing a Spearman rank difference correlation coefficent, .50 ($p <$ .01). Birth order was analyzed in the same way, its association with pain reactivity not reaching a statistically significant level although the trend was in the direction of increased pain reactivity for firstborns. Since birth order and family size are not independent, perhaps a larger sample might have yielded a statistically significant relationship. At any rate, the results appear to run counter to the data of Gonda (1962), and, if it is accepted that members of larger families become more independent at earlier ages, there is also disagreement with the results of Collins (1965).

Table 1. Family size in three pain reactivity groups

Children in family	*High pain*	*Medium pain*	*Low pain*
1-3	9	6	3
4 or more	2	4	9
		$\chi^2 = 7.64$, $df = 2$, $p < .05$	

REFERENCES

Collins, L. G. Pain sensitivity and ratings of childhood experience. *Perceptual and Motor Skills,* 1965, 21, 349-350.

Collins, L. G., & Stone, L. A. Family structure and pain reactivity. *Journal of Clinical Psychology,* 1966, 21, 672-673.

Fine, B. J., & Sweeney, D. R. Personality traits and situational factors and catecholamine excretion. *Journal of Experimental Research in Personality,* 1968, 3, 15-27.

Gelfand, S. The relationship of birth order to pain tolerance. *Journal of Clinical Psychology,* 1963, 19, 406.

Gonda, T. A. The relationship between complaints of persistent pain and family size. *Journal of Neurology, Neurosurgery, and Psychiatry,* 1962, 25, 277-281.

Nisbett, R. E. Birth order and participation in dangerous sports. *Journal of Personality and Social Psychology*, 1968, 8, 351-353.

Ryan, E. D., & Kovacic, C. R. Pain tolerance and athletic participation. *Perceptual and Motor Skills,* 1966, 22, 383-390.

Schachter, S. *The psychology of affiliation.* Stanford: Stanford Univer. Press, 1959.

15

Pain tolerance and athletic participation

E. Dean Ryan and Charles R. Kovacic

From observation of everyday experiences in athletics it would be expected that ability to withstand pain should be related to participation in certain types of athletic events. In many sports such as football or boxing, the ability to withstand pain appears to be essential to successful performance, while in sports such as tennis or golf, the ability to withstand pain would be less important. Thus, it is not inconceivable that an individual's ability, or inability, to tolerate pain may well determine the category of participation he selects. An individual with a high pain threshold might be oblivious to bumps and bruises received in a football game, whereas the individual with a low pain threshold might avoid such contact.

Although this hypothesis seems plausible, several factors may seem contradictory of such a simple relationship. First, under certain conditions adaptation to pain occurs, i.e., a stimulus that on first presentation produces a pain reaction will upon repeated presentation fail to elicit the pain response (Beecher, 1959; Stone & Dallenbach, 1936). Second, in general the relationship between pain threshold and pain tolerance is rather low (Beecher, 1959; Gelfand, 1964). Third, many factors influence the amount of pain an individual will tolerate, i.e., fear, anxiety, desire for group membership (Lambert, *et al.,* 1969; Beecher, 1959).

Gelfand (1964) and Wolff (1964) have hypothesized that pain tolerance is more highly loaded with psychological than physiological components, while the reverse is true of pain threshold. If this is correct, the relationship between pain threshold and the selection of athletic activities might reflect basic physiologic differences, while the relationship between pain tolerance and selection of activities might reflect environmental differences.

This study was designed to investigate the proposed relationships between pain response and athletic participation. Specifically, pain threshold and pain tolerance were studied in three groups of *S*s, contact, non-contact, and non-athletes.

METHOD

Subjects

A questionnaire was administered to male university students in ROTC classes. They were asked about their likes, dislikes, hobbies, recreational activities, etc. On the basis of these answers three groups of 20 *S*s each were selected. Group I was composed of *S*s who had participated in contact sports (football, boxing, or wrestling) during high school or college, Group II of *S*s who had participated in non-contact sports only, such as golf or tennis, and Group III of *S*s who had not participated in varsity athletics of any kind. The fact that the study was related to athletic performance was kept from *S*s. Testing was done by a graduate student who had no official connection with the Department of Physical Education or athletics.

Apparatus

Three methods to deliver controlled pain were used. Radiant heat was used to measure pain threshold, while gross pressure and muscle ischemia were used to measure pain tolerance. Because it has been shown

Reprinted with permission of author and publisher: Ryan, E. D., & Kovacic, C. R. Pain tolerance and athletic participation. Perceptual and Motor Skills, 1966, **22,** 383-390.
From the University of California, Davis.

that beyond a certain point great increases in heat result in no perceptibly greater pain, radiant heat was used only for threshold measurements (Clark & Bindra, 1956). The two measures of pain tolerance were selected on the *a priori* assumption that gross pressure was representative of the bumps and bruises received in contact sports, while muscle ischemia was representative of the pain associated with severe muscle fatigue.

Radiant heat (pain threshold). An adaptation of the D'Amour-Smith technique was used (Beecher, 1959). A 500-w prefocus projection lamp served as the heat source. The light was focused by means of a projector system condensing lens through a fixed aperture, 1 in. in diameter, on *S*'s forehead. A shutter that *S* could control by means of a switch was mounted between the light and the aperture. When the shutter was opened a Standard Electric timer was activated, and when closed, the radiation was cut off, and the timer stopped. As a result, radiation exposure could be measured precisely. In this instance, the measure of pain threshold was the time lapse between the opening and closing of the shutter.

Gross pressure (pain tolerance). An adaptation of Poser's mechanical stimulator was used (Poser, 1962). A plastic, aluminum tipped, football cleat was secured to a curved fiber plate and fitted to the leg. The cleat was placed against the anterior border of the tibia, midway between the ankle and the knee. The sleeve of a standard clinical sphygmomanometer was used to secure the cleat firmly in place. Cleat pressure against the tibia was obtained by inflating the armlet at a slow, constant rate (approximately 5 mm Hg/sec.) until *S* indicated verbally that he was no longer willing to endure the pain. The data were recorded in mm Hg.

Muscle ischemia (pain tolerance). *S* sat with the elbow of his preferred arm resting on a table. The arm was flexed at approximately a 90° angle to avoid the accumulation of blood in the distal part. A sphygmomanometer cuff was applied to the upper arm and the pressure elevated to 300 mm Hg. *S* flexed his fingers to form a fist and then extended his fingers at the rate of once per second. The rhythm was kept by the use of a metronome. The number of times the hand opened and closed was recorded (Beecher, 1959).

Design

Two sessions were devoted to testing. The first session was used to measure pain threshold and grip strength while the second measured pain tolerance. At the first testing session two trials on a hand dynamometer were given in order to check the possible relationship between grip strength and number of contractions in the muscle ischemia test. *S* was told that the experiment was designed to study various factors associated with pain and that the object of the first test was to measure when pain was first noticed and not how much pain could be tolerated. This point was emphasized a second time. *S* was seated in front of the radiant heat lamp and his forehead was blackened with lampblack to ensure total absorption of heat radiation. *S* was instructed that he would first experience a warm sensation, followed by heat, and then pain. He was instructed to close the shutter when the first sharp stab of pain was evident. A preliminary trial on the hand was administered to familiarize *S* with the apparatus and allay possible fear. Immediately therafter, *S*'s forehead was placed against the aperture and the test administered, with *S* operating the switch. A second trial was given 1 min. later.

Prior to the beginning of testing in the second session *S* was told that pain tolerance was the factor being tested, wherein he should make an effort to stand as much pain as possible. The pressure cleat was applied and *S* was informed that pressure to the leg would be increased gradually and terminated when he could stand no more. After the first trial *E* commented that the score was quite a bit lower than the average of the group tested, and *S* was asked to take the test a second time, doing better if possible. The cleat was lowered 1 in. and the second trial was given.

The pressure cuff was then applied to the arm and *S* was instructed to go as long as possible counting "one and two and one and two and" with each opening and closing of the hand. This prevented *S* from counting the actual number of times the hand was extended. At the conclusion of the first trial *E* commented that, as with the pressure cleat *S* was again somewhat lower than average, and was asked to repeat the test.

RESULTS

Of the 60 *S*s originally selected for the experiment, only 55 were actually tested as two *S*s from Group I, one *S* from Group II, and two *S*s from Group III failed to appear for either test. In addition, 11 *S*s were unavailable for testing at Session 1 and one *S* was unavailable for Session 2. All data were used for each, however, resulting in a different *N* for each test. The Pearson product-moment correlation coefficient was used for all correlations.

A simple analysis of variance was used to test the difference between groups under the several conditions, and when significant differences were found the Duncan test was used to determine which means were different. The reciprocals of the original data for pain threshold were used due to heterogeneity of variance in the raw data ($\chi^2 = 16.62$, 2 *df*). In each of the other comparisons variance was homogeneous. The data for all comparisons are summarized in Table 1.

Pain threshold

The immediate test-retest reliability of the pain threshold was .75 ($N = 43$). To get as stable a threshold measure as possible the mean of Trials 1 and 2 was used for analysis. There were no significant differences among the three groups ($F = 3.08$, $df = 2/41$).

Pain tolerance

Pressure. The immediate test-retest reliability of cleat pressure pain tolerance was .95 ($N = 55$). On the first trial there was a highly significant difference among groups ($F = 41.00$, $df = 2/52$), with the Duncan test indicating that each group differed significantly from the others. Group I (the contact athletes) tolerated most pain, the nonathletes tolerated least, with the non-contact athlete between the two. For the second trial, after being told they had done poorly, the pattern was the same ($F = 79.61$, $df = 2/52$).

The effect of instructing each individual that he had done poorly on the first pain test was analyzed by computing the change from Trial 1 to Trial 2. There was a significant difference between groups ($F = 22.39$, $df = 2/52$), with the contact athletes showing an increase on the average of 28.61 mm Hg, the non-contact athletes an increase on the average of 9.21, and non-athletes a decrease of 11.06 mm Hg on the second trial.

Muscle ischemia. The immediate test-retest reliability was .87 ($N = 55$). On Test 1 there was a significant difference between groups ($F = 27.40$, $df = 2/52$), with the Duncan test indicating that the two groups of athletes did not differ in their pain responses, but both of these groups differed from the non-athletes. On Trial 2 there was a significant difference between

Table 1. Means ± standard deviations, and *F*s for experimental groups

Test	*Group I (CA)* *M* ± *SD*	*Group II (NCA)* *M* ± *SD*	*Group III (NA)* *M* ± *SD*	*F*
Pain threshold	2.96 ± 00.10*	3.18 ± 00.86*	2.50 ± 00.04*	3.08
Pain tolerance				
Pressure I	232.28 ± 44.86	86.32 ± 47.38	113.39 ± 20.98	41.00†
Pressure II	257.67 ± 36.27	95.63 ± 46.07	102.33 ± 25.85	79.61†
Diff.	28.61 ± 23.33	9.21 ± 12.68	11.06 ± 15.89	22.39†
Pain tolerance				
Ischemia I	174.54 ± 39.33	175.79 ± 24.83	113.00 ± 25.28	16.47†
Ischemia II	220.76 ± 38.70	191.92 ± 26.13	102.50 ± 36.39	48.30†
Diff.	43.61 ± 27.07	17.36 ± 18.48	−11.45 ± 21.32	26.87†
Adj. ischemia I	174.15	175.62	113.43	7.76†
Ischemia II	213.82	189.62	110.15	19.29†

*Transformed, using reciprocal of original data.
†$p = .01$.

groups ($F = 67.22$, $df = 2/52$), with the Duncan test indicating that all three groups differed significantly from each other: contact athletes tolerated most pain, non-contact athletes next, and non-athletes tolerated least.

An analysis of change from Trial 1 to Trial 2 indicated a significant difference among the three groups ($F = 26.87$, $df = 2/52$), with the same pattern as cleat pressure. The contact athletes increased an average of 43.61 contractions, the non-contact athletes increased an average of 17.36, and the non-athletes decreased 11.45 contractions.

Because differences in the muscle ischemia could have been due to individual differences in grip strength, an analysis of covariance was performed, holding grip strength constant. Group adjusted mean scores are shown in the last lines of Table 1. While the mean scores were changed slightly, results of the analysis of covariance did not differ from those of the simple analysis.

Relation between pain threshold and pain tolerance. Table 2 indicates a low but statistically significant relation between pain threshold and pain tolerance, regardless of the method of measurement. In each instance the product-moment correlation between the sum of both trials on pain threshold and cleat pressure was .38, and when corrected for attenuation, .45. The correlation between pain threshold and ischemic pain tolerance was .35, and when corrected for attentuation, .44. The relationship between the two measures of pain tolerance, on the other hand, was higher. The correlation between the sum of both tests on cleat pressure and ischemic pain scores was .82, and when corrected for attenuation $r = .86$.

DISCUSSION

Examination of the results indicates a definite relationship between an *S*s willingness, or ability, to tolerate pain and the type of athletic activity in which he chooses to participate. The contact athlete, i.e., the football player or wrestler, will tolerate more pain than the athlete who participates only in non-contact sports such as tennis or golf, and both groups of athletes are willing to tolerate more pain than the non-athlete. In addition, after being told that his initial effort was poor, the contact athlete showed marked improvement on a second attempt, while the non-contact athlete improved some, but the non-athlete tolerated less pain than on the first attempt.

The question of cause and effect—whether a boy learns to tolerate pain because he engages in contact sports, whether he engages in contact sports because he can more easily tolerate pain (either for physiological or psychological reasons), or whether the two covary with a third but unexplored source—is, of course, unanswered by these data. If the hypothesis is true that pain threshold is associated with physiological components, then the results of this experiment suggest that differences between activity groups are psychological in nature and probably the result of cultural or environmental influences. There are, however, a number of possible explanations for these results, some with a psychological slant, others more physiological in nature.

Zborowski (1952) has suggested that two culturally determined attitudes, pain expectancy and pain acceptance, are important to differences in pain response. Pain expectancy is anticipation of pain as being unavoidable in a given situation, while pain acceptance is characterized by a willingness to experience pain. As an example, labor pain is generally expected as part of childbirth in all cultures. In one culture, the pain is not accepted and various means are used to alleviate it, while in another the pain is accepted, and little or nothing is done to relieve it. It may be that the differences found in this study are due to differences in "pain acceptance." The contact athletes, and to a lesser extent the

Table 2. Correlations between pain threshold and pain tolerance level

		1	*2*	*3*
1 Pain threshold	(thermal)	.75*‡	.38†	.36†
2 Pain tolerance	(cleat)	.38†	.95*‡	.82‡
3 Pain tolerance	(muscle)	.36†	.82‡	.87*‡

*Immediate test-retest reliability.
†$p = .05$.
‡$p = .01$.

non-contact athletes, have frequently been in situations where pain was unavoidable. Through parental or peer pressure it is possible that the ability to tolerate pain has been associated with "manliness" by the athlete and as such is socially valued. The non-athletes, on the other hand, have much less often been in situations where pain was unavoidable and thus have not associated ability to tolerate pain with socially desirable traits or characteristics.

Another possibility may be that because of repeated experiences with pain, the contact athlete will be more realistic in his evaluation of the significance of pain and thus will fear pain less than the non-athlete. It has been pointed out that the significance of the pain experience is important in determining how "painful" the experience appears to be. An ache beneath the sternum, in connoting the possibility of sudden death from heart failure can be a wholly upsetting experience, whereas the same intensity and duration of ache in a finger is a trivial annoyance easily disregarded (Beecher, 1959). It is possible that contact athletes, having had previous experience with the two types of pain used in the test, were fully aware that the pain experienced was not of a harmful nature. The non-athletes, because of little experience with this type of pain, had no way of knowing whether or not the cleat might break a bone or puncture the skin. The differences on the second trial can be explained the same way. The contact athlete, having experienced the initial pain, would as a result of previous experience have some reference point and be aware that the stimulus was not going to do physical damage. The non-athlete, on the other hand, having limited experience with painful stimulation, would be less apt to know how "serious" the pain actually was, and thus, due to apprehension, tolerate less on the second trial.

The most intriguing explanation stems from the work of Petrie and her associates (Petrie, 1960; Petrie, McCulloch, & Kazdin, 1962; Petrie, Collins, & Soloman, 1960). Their studies indicate that certain individuals tend consistently to reduce the intensity of their perceptions subjectively, while others tend to constantly augment the intensity of their perceptions. Pain and suffering are related to these contrasted perceptual types. The reducers tolerate pain well, the augmenters poorly. Petrie suggests that the reducer's tolerance for pain is partially due to his tendency to reduce the perceptual intensity of the stimulation. Thus an intermittent change in the intensity of a pain wave may cause later pain to appear less severe. In addition, the reducers have been shown to be more extroverted (Eysenck, 1957) and less tolerant of sensory deprivation (Petrie, Collins, & Soloman, 1960). All of the characteristics associated with the reducer, i.e., tolerance of pain, intolerance of sensory deprivation and extroversion, are actually common to groups of athletes. It may be that the subjective reduction of sensory stimulation is associated with the choice of activities in which a child engages. If, indeed, the reducers suffer from lack of stimulation, as suggested by Petrie, *et al.* (1962), then they would need change, movement, speed, and possibly body contact, rather than more sedentary pursuits. Athletics could be the child's answer to sensory deprivation, with the ability to tolerate pain an added incentive to participate in contact sports.

Although any one of the three *a priori* hypotheses could partially account for the results of this experiment, all are incomplete. The problem of cause and effect in the relationship between pain tolerance and athletic participation deserves further consideration.

REFERENCES

Beecher, H. K. *Measurement of subjective responses; quantitative effects of drugs.* New York: Oxford Univer. Press, 1959.

Clark, J. W., & Bindra, D. Individual differences in pain thresholds. *Canad. J. Psychol.*, 1956, 10, 69-76.

Eysenck, H. J. *The dynamics of anxiety and hysteria.* London: Routledge & Kegan Paul, 1957.

Gelfand, S. The relationship between experimental pain tolerance and pain threshold. *Canad. J. Psychol.*, 1964, 18, 36-42.

Lambert, W. E., Libman, E., & Poser, E. G. The effect of increased patience of a membership group on pain tolerance. *J. Pers.*, 1960, 38, 350-357.

Petrie, A. Some psychological aspects of pain and the relief of suffering. *Ann. N. Y. Acad. Sci.*, 1960, 86, 13-27.

Petrie, A., Collins, W., & Soloman, P. The tolerance for pain and for sensory deprivation. *Amer. J. Psychol.*, 1960, 73, 80-90.

Petrie, A., McCulloch, R., & Kazdin, P. The perceptual characteristics of juvenile delinquents. *J. nerv. ment. Dis.*, 1962, 134, 415-421.

Poser, E. G. A simple and reliable apparatus for the measurement of pain. *Amer. J. Psychol.* 1962, 75, 304-305.

Stone, L. J., & Dallenbach, K. M. The adaptation of areal pain. *Amer. J. Psychol.*, 1936, 48, 117-125.

Wolff, B. B. The relationship of experimental pain tolerance to pain threshold: a critique of Gelfand's paper. *Canad. J. Psychol.*, 1964, 18, 248-253.

Zborowski, M. Cultural components in response to pain. *J. soc. Issues,* 1952, 8, 16-30.

16

Pain tolerance

Differences according to age, sex and race

Kenneth M. Woodrow, MD, Gary D. Friedman, MD, A. B. Siegelaub, MS, and Morris F. Collen, MD

Differences in patients' pain tolerance have been a continuing source of interest and concern to their physicians. Some individuals appear to bear severe pain with surprising equanimity, while others react to more moderate pain with apprehension and emotional turmoil.

A test of pain tolerance was included in the routine multiphasic health examination of more than 40,000 subjects in the hope that the findings would be clinically useful. While the clinical value has yet to be demonstrated, rather clear-cut differences in pain tolerance according to age, sex and race were noted. These differences may reflect important cultural and biologic variability in pain reaction.

SUBJECTS

The subjects were the 41,119 persons who presented themselves for the Automated Multiphasic Screening (AMS) examination at the San Francisco or Oakland multiphasic testing laboratories between January 1 and December 31, 1966. More than 99% were members of the Kaiser Foundation Health Plan. The majority of patients who apply for the AMS examination do so of their own accord; only 13.1% are referred by doctors.

The demographic characteristics of the study population are shown in Table 1. Race was determined by observation of the subject's skin color. The educational categories in the table indicate the highest level of attainment but do not imply graduation.

METHODS

The pain tolerance test was given as a routine part of the AMS examination (1). The seated subject placed his heel on the

Table 1. Demographic characteristics of population examined for pain tolerance

41,119 Subjects	*%*
Age	
< 20	2.3
20-29	12.9
30-39	18.7
40-49	27.0
50-59	22.4
60-69	12.7
70+	4.0
Sex	
Male	42.3
Female	57.7
Race	
White	82.9
Black	13.1
Oriental	4.0
Education	
Elementary	10.9
High school	29.1
Trade or business	12.3
College, 1-2 years	16.3
3-4 years	13.3
Postgraduate	15.2
Unknown	2.9

Reprinted with permission of the American Psychosomatic Society from Psychosomatic Medicine **34**:548-556. Copyright 1972.
From the Department of Psychiatry, Stanford University Medical Center (Dr. Woodrow), Stanford; and the Department of Medical Methods Research, the Permanente Medical Group (Dr. Friedman, Mr. Siegelaub and Dr. Collen), Oakland, Calif.
Supported in part by a grant from the Kaiser Foundation Research Institute; and USPHS Grant HS 00288 from the National Center for Health Services Research Development.

floor with the Achilles tendon positioned between two motor-driven rods whose tips measure 1/4″ × 3/8″. The subject was then instructed as follows, without use of the word "pain": "This is a pressure tolerance test. This test is to determine the amount of pressure which you can take on your ankle tendon. I will increase the pressure and stop it as soon as you tell me to. This test cannot injure you in any way. Try to stand it as long as you can."

The instrument, custom-built for about $200, produces deep pain (with some cutaneous contamination), is easily standardized, functions rapidly (average test time is 30 seconds) and requires minimal staff training.

Pain tolerance was studied for possible relation to age, sex and race.

Each pain tolerance test experience may affect the reaction to subsequent tests by alleviating or increasing apprehension and anxiety. Thus, any test of reliability or reproducibility of the instrument itself may be confounded by changes in the mental state of the patient. Nevertheless, some estimate of reliability was obtained by examining differences in response by the same subjects from one examination to the next. Changes in pain tolerance over time in individuals were studied by comparing the first three examinations of 14,046 subjects who had been examined at least three times during a 4-year period. The mean interval between the first and second examinations was 14.3 months, with a standard deviation of 4.0 months. Between the second and third the mean was 14.5 months, with a standard deviation of 4.0 months. Only 21 subjects (0.15%) had undergone their first and second examinations at intervals of less than 6 months, and 17 (0.12%) had taken the second and third examinations at intervals of less than 6 months. Of the 41,119 subjects tested in 1966, 44% had had previous AMS examinations.

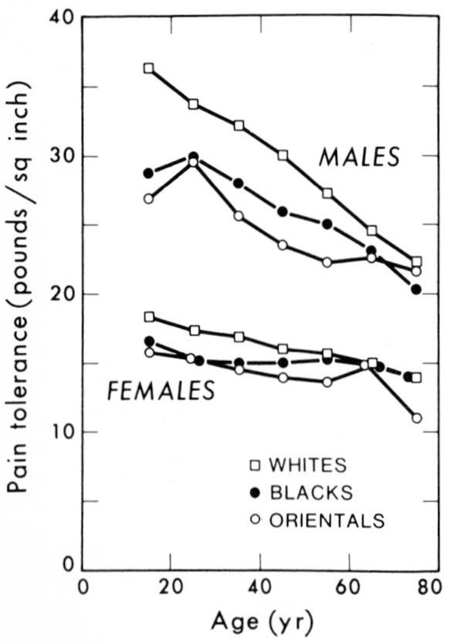

Fig. 1. Differences in pain tolerance according to age, sex, and race.

RESULTS

There were consistent and statistically significant differences in pain tolerance according to age, sex and race (Figure 1 and Table 2).

Age

The age trend observed in a cross-section of the study population as a whole was based on the first test for 56% of the subjects. Pain tolerance decreased with increasing age for both sexes. In males the age trend was fairly smooth, with those age 60 and over showing about two-thirds to three-fourths the pain tolerance of those under 30. In females the decrease with age was also steady but less marked.

Sex

Men tolerated more pain than did women (Figure 2). Six percent of men could endure pain above the upper limit of the test – 50 pounds/sq inch. Even the oldest men had a higher average pain tolerance than the youngest women. The mean pain tolerance of all men was 28.7 pounds/sq inch; the mean for all women was 15.9 pounds/sq inch. The difference was highly significant ($P < .001$). In addition, pain tolerance varied less among women than among men.

Race

Racial differences were consistent in both sexes but were less marked than were differences by age and sex. Whites showed the highest average pain tolerance (males 29.2, females 16.1 pounds/sq inch); Blacks were second (male 26.5, females 15.2

Table 2. Mean pain tolerance in pounds per square inch according to age, sex and race

	Age							*Total*
	<20	*20-29*	*30-39*	*40-49*	*50-59*	*60-69*	*70+*	
Male								
White								
Number	319	1565	2801	3844	3394	1948	735	14,606
Mean	36.29	33.77	32.14	30.03	27.26	24.58	22.33	29.21
SD	10.59	11.23	10.90	10.19	9.53	8.93	8.18	10.60
Black								
Number	50	249	452	728	422	139	17	2057
Mean	28.82	29.95	28.04	25.97	25.01	23.17	20.35	26.54
SD	11.19	10.54	9.42	8.57	9.46	8.86	6.74	9.46
Oriental								
Number	11	73	227	244	144	44	6	749
Mean	26.91	28.62	25.26	23.53	22.31	22.59	21.67	24.30
SD	9.63	10.99	9.82	8.40	7.77	9.25	10.09	9.24
Female								
White								
Number	440	2697	3164	4873	4566	2863	868	19,471
Mean	18.42	17.35	16.90	16.01	15.67	14.96	13.93	16.07
SD	7.32	6.41	6.17	5.50	5.21	4.88	4.43	5.68
Black								
Number	108	576	742	1103	617	172	18	3336
Mean	16.62	15.20	15.13	15.11	15.35	14.73	14.06	15.20
SD	5.97	5.01	4.84	4.81	4.92	4.34	3.96	4.89
Oriental								
Number	13	159	311	290	87	37	3	900
Mean	15.85	15.31	14.52	13.97	13.64	14.81	11.00	14.42
SD	5.49	4.90	4.94	4.67	3.74	6.83	0.00	4.86

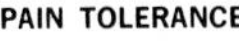

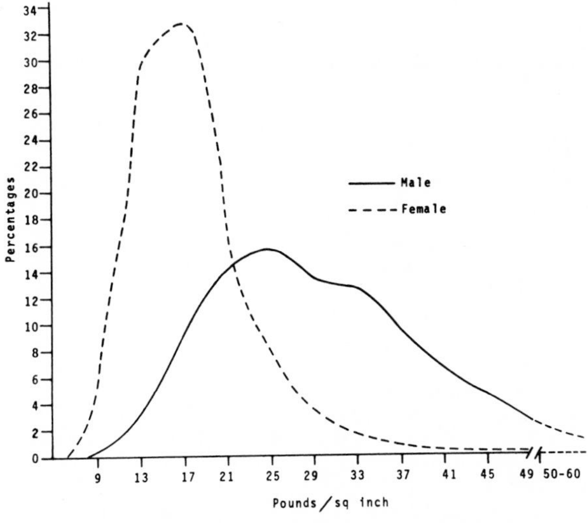

Fig. 2. Pain tolerance distributions for men and women.

Table 3. Pain tolerance in pounds per square inch in the same subjects examined three times

		First examination		*Second examination*		*Third examination*	
	No.	*Mean*	*SD*	*Mean*	*SD*	*Mean*	*SD*
Men	5963	28.7	7.8	29.2	10.2	30.1	9.8
Women	8083	19.5	6.4	16.9	6.1	17.8	6.1
Total	14046	23.4	8.3	22.1	10.2	23.1	10.0

pounds/sq inch); and Orientals were lowest (males 24.3, females 14.4 pounds/sq inch). All differences between racial groups were significant ($P < .001$). Both race and age differences in pain tolerance were more marked in men than in women.

Changes with time in the same individuals

Table 3 shows the means and standard deviations of pain tolerance values on three consecutive examinations for men and women. The total group shows very little change over the years. The overall mean dropped from 23.4 to 22.1 pounds/sq inch between the first and second examinations but then rose to 23.1 pounds/sq inch on the third. However, the changes in men differed from those in women. Pain tolerance in men rose slightly, on the average, with each successive examination. This is opposite in direction to the decrease noted with age in a cross-section of the population. In women the situation was more complex. The mean fell by 2.6 pounds/sq inch between the first and second examinations but then rose 0.9 pounds/sq inch between the second and third.

The correlation coefficients between the results of the first and second examinations were .51 and .48 for men and women, respectively. Between the second and third examination they were .69 and .56 for men and women, respectively.

DISCUSSION

Pain is a topic of widespread scientific interest. Its ramifications have been examined by psychiatrists, psychologists, anesthesiologists, pharmacologists and others who have contributed to a vast, unwieldly literature. Some order and perspective has been brought to the subject by such workers as Merskey and Spear (2) and Sternbach (3) in their thorough and lucid reviews.

Since Libman's work in 1934 (4), investigators have experimented with many instruments capable of producing deep and superficial pain. Of the various mechanical, electrical, chemical and thermal techniques used for investigation, only thermal and mechanical methods seemed to yield reproducible results; the others have been largely discarded. The most popular device, the Hardy, Wolff and Goodell dolorimeter, used a focused light source directed at a black spot on the forehead (5). It gave good reliability and quantification but had two major shortcomings from a clinical standpoint. The instrument was hard to standardize, and more important, the "heat-spot" technique was a measure of *superficial* pain rather than *deep* pain. The difficulty with using a superficial pain stimulus, such as thermal radiation, is that this type of pain is not relieved by morphine any better than by a placebo (6). Thus, it differs from most clinical pain.

To circumvent these problems, experimenters (7-11) employed a wide variety of pressure devices, which improved reliability and standardization. (The submaximal effort tourniquet technique, inducing ischemic pain, had not been reported at the time this project was started.) The instrument employed in our studies similarly applied calibrated pressure, but the pressure is applied to the Achilles tendon instead of to the skin of the forehead or arm. Measurement of deep pain was selected primarily because we assumed that deep pain was more significant clinically than superficial pain. So far, however, our pain tolerance test results have not been shown to be correlated with clinical pain.

Pain tolerance versus pain threshold

Once a particular method of pain induction is selected, one must decide whether to measure pain threshold, pain tolerance or both. Pain threshold is that level of stimulus at which the subject first recognizes pain or discomfort. Pain tolerance is that greater level of stimulus at which the subject requests stimulus cessation.

Some workers (12) have found pain threshold and pain tolerance highly correlated (correlation coefficient = 0.72) and have suggested that the factors contributing to individual differences for threshold and tolerance are largely the same. The more convincing data of Benjamin (13) and Gelfand (14) indicate that pain threshold and pain tolerance are probably not highly related.

In an excellent summary of the differences between pain threshold and pain tolerance, Merskey and Spear (15) concluded that "pain threshold is more dependent on physiological factors, and pain tolerance on psychological factors." Petrie (16) reported that the pain threshold remains unchanged after prefrontal lobotomy and may also remain constant after pain-relieving drugs, although pain tolerance increases in both situations.

We selected pain tolerance rather than pain threshold, because we felt the former had greater clinical utility. Medical attention is sought more on the basis of intolerance of pain and discomfort than on pain recognition.

Induced versus endogenous pain

The issue of whether induced pain felt by "well" subjects in a experimental situation can accurately refelct endogenous clinical pain is a troubling one. Beecher is one of the most articulate proponents of the view that experimental pain cannot be compared with clinical pain, and he supports his argument by showing that most experimental pain is useless in assaying the potency of analgesic medication (6). He notes that the symbolic quality of pathologic pain is crucially important in the assessment of analgesic efficacy. We agree with this point but believe that such differences as we have found in reaction to induced pain may be of value in other areas of concern to the medical practitioner. However, confirmation of such clinical utility remains absent at the present time.

In studying our results we looked carefully for components in the testing situation which might be responsible for the differences in pain tolerance we found. Beecher has compiled an extensive list of factors which may influence experimental pain perception (17). Included in this list are such variables as nausea, skin temperature, anxiety, room temperature, fatigue and diurnal variation, most of which do not seem immediately relevant to our study, principally because of the randomization resulting from our very large sample size.

The physical setting was constant and nonthreatening. As perceived by the authors the pain tolerance phase did not seem to arouse any more apprehension or negative reactions than the other aspects of the multiphasic testing. Previous work (18) has shown how the personality of the interviewer can influence anxiety and hostility, and secondarily, pain tolerance (17). Therefore, technician personality might influence pain tolerance in a relatively small sample. But given the size of our sample and the nonsystematic interscheduling of patients and technicians, personality appears to be an unlikely determinant of observed differences in pain tolerance. We have concluded, therefore, that differences in pain tolerance in our study are due to underlying differences in our subject groups. The extent to which these differences in pain tolerance are culturally determined or biologically determined is still unknown.

Group differences in pain tolerance

Age. Probably the most important finding in our study is that pain tolerance decreases with increasing age. This is true for both sexes, and for White, Black and Oriental people. This finding is contradictory to all previous studies (19-23) except one (24).

There appears to be a discrepancy between the general decrease in pain tolerance with age and the increase in pain tolerance noted on repeated examinations of men. It seems likely that this increase is due to adaptation to the test situation.

We believe that the explanation for the difference between our observation of decreasing tolerance with age, and the observations of others, lies in the means of measuring pain tolerance employed in the different studies. When pain tolerance is measured by radiant heat, it increases with age. When measured by pressure on the Achilles tendon, it decreases with age.

It appears, therefore, that with increasing age, tolerance to cutaneous pain increases and tolerance to deep pain decreases. If correct, this concept may prove helpful in understanding and relieving pain clinically. Much has been written about differential systems of pain perception. Pain has been divided into epicritic and protopathic, fast and slow, superficial and deep, somatic and visceral, A-gamma (smallest myelinated) and C (unmyelinated) conducted. If there are opposite changes with aging in two different pain perception systems, it is quite possible that more effective analgesia could be developed on the basis of these differences.

Sex. In a recent review Notermans and Tophoff (25) noted wide disagreement in the relationship of pain sensitivity to sex. They cited five publications which stated that senstivity to pain is greater in women then in men, and five publications which reported no differences between the sexes in pain sensitivity. Interestingly, there is virtually no experimental evidence to back the widely held notion that women are more tolerant of pain then men.

One explanation for the sex differences in pain tolerance might be a desire on the part of male patients to impress a young appealing female technician. With this in mind, we reviewed our records and found that during the test year eight female technicians were employed—five Black, two White and one Philippine. Their age range was from 28 to 60, with a mean age of 41. When the personnel supervisor was asked if any of the technicians were likely to elicit a "show-off" response, the answer in seven instances was "no" and in one "possibly." It thus appears that the sex-appeal factor was not a significant determinant in the higher pain tolerance of men.

In published studies it is often difficult to separate sex differences in pain threshold, labeled as "pain perception," "sensitivity," and "verbal report of pain," from sex differences in pain tolerance, "pain reaction point." While a majority of authors have concluded that men have somewhat higher pain thresholds than women, there is much disagreement concerning this point (25). However, when pain tolerance is measured, the evidence is more consistent: men tolerate more pain than women (25, 26). This agrees with our own findings.

Race. In contrast to the numerous studies detailing the association of pain tolerance to sex and age, there are very few studies of racial and ethnic differences in pain tolerance. Chapman and Jones (27) found that "Jewish and other Mediterranean races" had lower pain tolerance than Caucasions of "Northern European stock" and that their pain tolerance levels closely corresponded to those of the Negro. Micmac Indians were reported by Sherman (28) to have higher pain tolerance than patients who came to his office with a variety of organic and functional illnesses. Sherman and Robillard (20) found that pain tolerance in a combined population of Jewish and French subjects was lower than in a comparable Candian Anglo-Saxon group.

Merskey and Spear (11), using a pressure device over the tibia and forehead, found no difference in pain tolerance between male White students and male Afro-Asian students. Chapman and Jones (27) found the pain tolerance of Negro subjects to be below that of Caucasians as measured with the Hardy-Wolff-Goodell heat appartus; but this study is marred by failure to specify the sex of the subjects. No differences were found in the ability of Negro and White women to tolerate obstetric pain (29).

It would appear that, with the exception of the findings of Chapman and Jones (27), there has been no experimental evidence to show that Blacks have a lower pain tolerance than Whites. The uniformity of our findings within every age group and for both sexes (the single exception being women over 70) considerably reduced the chance that our observation was an artifact.

The possiblity that the racial differences were due to socioeconomic factors was explored. Pain tolerance was studied in all racial groups, subdivided by educational attainment, in a mid-age sample (40 to 49 years) of 10,671 subjects. The racial differ-

Table 4. Pain tolerance according to education, sex and race in subjects age 40 to 49

	Education						
				College			
	Elementary	*High school*	*Trade school*	*1-2 yr*	*3-4 yr*	*Post-graduate*	*Total*
Male							
White							
Number	229	910	420	578	605	1006	3748
Mean	29.2	30.1	29.7	30.0	30.9	29.9	30.1
SD	9.8	10.2	10.1	10.2	10.4	10.2	10.2
Black							
Number	136	228	118	96	53	37	668
Mean	25.3	26.4	26.0	26.5	27.1	25.9	26.1
SD	8.2	8.3	8.3	9.7	8.4	10.0	8.6
Oriental							
Number	17	40	32	42	67	36	234
Mean	20.2	24.1	24.5	22.6	24.1	22.6	23.4
SD	5.1	9.5	9.3	7.9	9.1	6.4	8.4
Female							
White							
Number	315	1581	740	787	539	766	4728
Mean	15.4	15.9	15.7	15.8	16.9	16.6	16.0
SD	4.9	5.2	5.2	5.4	6.4	5.9	5.5
Black							
Number	186	381	147	155	73	77	1019
Mean	15.7	15.1	14.6	14.3	15.7	14.9	15.1
SD	5.3	4.5	4.2	5.0	4.9	5.0	4.8
Oriental							
Number	22	107	40	50	27	28	274
Mean	13.3	13.8	13.5	14.3	13.5	14.8	13.9
SD	4.5	4.7	3.8	5.2	4.2	3.9	4.5

ences in pain tolerance were observed at all levels of educational attainment (Table 4), and educational level was not related to pain tolerance in any consistent manner. Although we found no consistent relationship between educational level and pain tolerance, it should be noted that Schuldermann and Zubek (21) reported higher socioeconomic status associated with higher pain threshold.

The discovery that Orientals have lower pain tolerance than Whites and Blacks is a new finding so far as we could determine from the English language literature. (In our study no distinction was made between Japanese and Chinese.) It is intriguing to speculate whether this deviation from the popular stereotype of the "stoic Oriental" can be ascribed primarily to biologic differences or to cultural factors such as minority status (29, 30).

SUMMARY

This analysis of the pain tolerance scores of 41,119 subjects who took the Automated Multiphasic Screening examination during 1 year showed that, on the average: a) Pain tolerance decreases with age; b) Men tolerate more pain that women; and c) Whites tolerate more pain than Orientals, while Blacks occupy an intermediate position. When the results of this study are compared with earlier work, it appears that with increasing age, tolerance to cutaneous pain increases and tolerance to deep pain decreases.

REFERENCES

1. Collen MF: Periodic health examinations using an automated multitest laboratory. JAMA 195:830-833, 1966.
2. Merskey H, Spear FG: Pain: Psychological and Psychiatric Aspects. London, Billière, Tindall & Cassell, 1967
3. Sternbach RA: Pain: A Psychophysiological Analysis. New York, Academic Press, Inc, 1968
4. Libman E: Observations on individual sensitiveness to pain: with special reference to abdominal disorders. JAMA 102:335-341, 1934
5. Hardy JD, Wolff HG, Goddell H: Pain Sensations and Reactions. Baltimore, Williams & Wilkins Co. 1952

6. Beecher HK: The measurement of pain in man, Pain. Proceedings of the International Symposium on Pain. Edited by A Soulairac, J Cahn, J Charpentier. New York, Academic Press, Inc, 1968, pp 207-208
7. Hollander E: A clinical gauge of sensitivity to pain. J Lab Clin Med 24:537-538, 1939
8. Pelner L: The determination of sensitivity to pain: a simple clinical method. J Lab Clin Med 27:248-251, 1941
9. Gluzek LJB: Dolorimetry: A quantitative method of measuring pain and deep sensibility. Ohio State Med J 40:49-50, 1944
10. Clutton-Brock J: The cerebral effects of overventilation. Br J Anaesth 29:111-113, 1957
11. Merskey H, Spear FG: The realiability of the pressure algometer. Br J Soc Clin Psychol 3:130-136, 1964
12. Clark JW, Bindra D: Individual differences in pain thresholds. Canad J Psychol 10:69-76, 1956
13. Benjamin FB: Effect of aspirin on superthreshold pain in man. Science 128:303-304, 1958
14. Gelfand S: The relationship of experimental pain tolerance to pain threshold. Canad J Psychol 18: 36-42, 1964
15. Merskey H, Spear FG: (2) p 142
16. Petrie A: Individuality in Pain and Suffering. Chicago, University of Chicago Press, 1967, p 21
17. Beecher HK: Measurement of subjective responses, Quantitative Effects of Drugs. New York, Oxford University Press, 1959, pp 136-156
18. Gottschalk LA: Some psychoanalytic research into the communication of meaning through language: The quality and magnitude of psychological states. Br J Med Psychol 44 (Pt 2): 131-147, 1971
19. Lambert WE, Libman E, Poster EG: The effect of increased salience of a membership group on pain tolerance. J Pers 28:350-357, 1960
20. Sherman ED, Robillard E: Sensitivity to pain in the aged. Canad Med Assoc J 83:944-947, 1960
21. Schludermann E, Zubek JP: Effect of age on pain sensitivity. Percept Motor Skills 14:295-301, 1962
22. Hall KRL, Stride E: The varying response to pain in psychiatric disorders: a study in abnormal psychology. Br J Med Psychol 27:48-60, 1954
23. Sherman ED, Robillard E: Sensitivity to pain in relationship to age. J Am Geriatr Soc 12:1037-1044, 1964
24. Collins LG, Stone LA: Pain sensitivity, age and activity level in chronic schizophrenics and in normals. Br J Psychiatr 112:33-35, 1966
25. Notermans SLH, Tophoff MMWA: Sex differences in pain tolerance and pain appreception. Psychiatr Neurol Neurochir 70:23-29, 1967
26. Petrie A: (16) p 146
27. Chapman WP, Jones CM: Variations in cutaneous and visceral pain sensitivity in normal subjects. J Clin Invest 23:81-91, 1944
28. Sherman ED: Sensitivity to pain (with analysis of 450 cases). Canad Med Assoc J 48:437-441, 1943
29. Winsberg B, Greenlick M: Pain response in Negro and white obstetrical patients, J Health Soc Behav 8:222-227, 1967
30. Zoborowski M: Cultural components in responses to pain. J Soc Issues 8 (No. 4): 16-30, 1952

SECTION FOUR

Cultural influences on pain perception

The reactions of several cultural and ethnic groups to pain have been studied under a variety of conditions, both in clinical and laboratory settings. Wolff and Langley (Reading 17) present a fairly comprehensive review of the research undertaken in this area. Among the groups studied are the Italians, Irish, Jews, and Yankees (Zola, 1966; Zborowski, 1969; Sternbach and Tursky, 1965), blacks (Chapman and Jones, 1944; Merskey and Spear, 1964; Woodrow, Friedman, Siegelaub, and Collen [Reading 16, Section three]; Weisenberg, Kreindler, Schachat and Werboff, 1975), Eskimos and Indians (Meehan, Stoll, and Hardy, 1954), Puerto Ricans (Weisenberg and others, 1975), and an assortment of anthropological studies of groups around the world (Wolff and Langley, Reading 17).

Major differences between these groups seem to be related to what is commonly referred to as the reaction or tolerance component of pain rather than to the discrimination of the pain sensation. This finding is illustrated in the study of the cultural reactions to pain by Sternbach and Tursky (1964). Yankee, Irish, Jewish, and Italian women were asked to respond in two different ways to electric shock stimulation.

On one task they were asked to specify several points by means of the method of limits. The lower threshold was referred to as the point when the subject became aware of the stimulus, and the upper threshold was referred to as the point when "you tell us you don't want any more." Some subjects were coaxed to accept a higher level of shock. No ethnic group differences were obtained for the lower threshold level, but significant group differences were obtained for both upper thresholds—with and without coaxing. The Italians tolerated the least amount of shock and their reactions differed significantly from those of the Yankee and Jewish subjects. The Irish subjects were at the low end of the tolerance scale and did not significantly differ from other groups.

Subjects were then presented with a magnitude estimation task requiring them to assign appropriate numbers to a series of nine different stimulus intensities in comparison with a standard shock labeled "ten." *No* ethnic groups differences were obtained.

Tursky and Sternbach (Reading 18) and Sternbach and Tursky (1965) have demonstrated that differences in cultural attitudes can affect psychophysical and autonomic functioning. Yankees, defined as Protestants of British descent who have a phlegmatic, matter-of-fact orientation toward pain showed the fastest rate of adaptation to electric shock of diphasic palmar skin potentials. Irish subjects, described as inhibiting their expression of suffering and concern for pain, consistently showed lower palmar skin resistance. The present-time orientation of the Italian subject was found in the positive correlation between upper pain threshold and heart rate (those with the highest threshold had the highest heart rate). The opposite was seen in Jewish subjects, who were future oriented in the clinic but not in the laboratory; they showed a negative correlation between upper threshold and heart rate (those with the highest upper thresholds had the lowest heart rates).

According to a theory of social comparisons (Festinger, 1954), differences in social-cultural reactions to pain are not all unexpected. Basically, the theory states that there exists a drive to test the validity of a person's judgment and opinions of the outside world. When outside sensory means for evaluation are reduced, the individual turns toward his social environment for validation of his judgments. Since pain is a private, ambiguous situation, comparison with others helps to determine what reactions are appropriate. Is it permissible to cry? Must one "grin and bear it"? When is it permissible to ask for help? When is it appropriate to mask the pain with analgesics?

People learn to express their reactions by observing the reactions of others. One chooses models who are similar to oneself, whereas one rejects those who are too divergent (Bandura and Whalen, 1966).

The first important source of comparison is the family, which transmits the cultural norms to its children. As Shoben and Borland (1954) have shown in their study of fears of dental care the experiences and attitudes of one's family are the most important factors determining whether one will react with anxiety to dental treatment, avoid it for a long time, and be uncooperative in the chair.

Underlying attitudes and anxiety reactions seem to be the major sources of the cultural differences in pain tolerance. Zola (1966) and Zborowski (1969) for example, found their major cultural differences in attitudes toward pain. In a study of black, white and Puerto Rican dental patients, Weisenberg, Kreindler, Schachat, and Werboff (1975) found that the use of 4 variables in a multiple discriminant analysis (2 anxiety and 2 attitudinal) were adequate to permit correct groupings of 18 out of 24 Puerto Ricans, 12 out of 25 blacks, and 16 out of 24 whites.

Stressing attitudinal and anxiety differences as major mediating mechanisms between cultural groups implies that variables that influence these mediators would also influence pain reactions. This approach has been competently demonstrated by Craig and Weiss (Reading 25, Section five). It suggests the desirability of greater efforts at achieving a fuller understanding of how behavior and attitude change principles affect pain reactions.

The interaction process between experimenter and subject is another important element usually neglected in pain research. One cannot help but wonder, for example, if Chapman and Jones (1944) would have concluded that blacks have low pain tolerance if they had used a black experimenter. Wisburg and Greenlick (Reading 19) found no differences between black and whites. In a clinical study of whites, blacks, and Orientals tested for deep pain tolerance (Woodrow, Friedman, Siegelaub, and Collen, Reading 16), it was found that whites tolerated the greatest amount of pain and Orientals the least. This finding is most surprising in view of the well-known stereotype of the stoic Oriental. Once more, one wonders how the conditions of testing and the tester influenced the outcome. Would the same results have been obtained with an Oriental tester? Does tolerating more pain imply that less anesthetic will be used in later medical procedures?

From the clinical standpoint, an easily used, standarized independent measure of pain is badly needed. The search has led to many different methods, from radiant heat to eye blink tests. None has been widely adopted. The search has been essentially for a measure to discriminate degrees of pain sensation. The pain reaction, however, is composed of both the perception of pain sensation and the motivational affective-cognitive component. Even though an independent measure of pain sensation is missing, it might still be possible to use attitudinal and anxiety measures to discover the type of reaction component anticipated. It is likely, therefore, that research designed to discover which measures of attitudes and anxiety would be most appropriate for a given treatment would be extremely valuable in clinical decision making.

These are but a few of the ways in which knowledge of cultural reactions can be used for understanding and controlling pain. They are of interest from a theoretical point of view as well as from a treatment point of view; they can point to the variety of methods that can be used in dealing with pain.

REFERENCES

Bandura, A., and Whalen, C. K. 1966. The influence of antecedent reinforcement and divergent modeling cues on patterns of self-reward, Journal of Personality and Social Psychology **3**:373-382.

Chapman, W. P., and Jones, C. M. 1944. Variations in cutaneous and visceral pain sensitivity in normal subjects, Journal of Clinical Investigation **23**:81-91.

Festinger, L. 1954. A theory of social comparison processes, Human Relations **7**:117-140.

Meehan, J. P., Stoll, A. M., and Hardy, J. D. 1954. Cutaneous pain threshold in native Alaskan Indian and Eskimo, Journal of Applied Psychology **6**:297-400.

Merskey, H., and Spear, F. G. 1964. The reliability of the pressure algometer, British Journal of Social and Clinical Psychology **3**:130-136.

Shoben, E. J., and Borland, L. 1954. An empirical study of the etiology of dental fears, Journal of Clinical Psychology **10**:171-174.

Sternbach, R. A., and Tursky, B. 1965. Ethnic differences among housewives in psychophysical and skin potential responses to electric shock, Psychophysiology **1**:241-246.

Weisenberg, M., Kreindler, M. L., Schachat, R., and Werboff, J. 1975. Pain: anxiety and attitudes in Black, White and Puerto Rican patients, Psychosomatic Medicine **37**:123-135.

Zborowski M. 1969. People in pain, Jossey-Bass, Inc., Publishers, San Francisco.

Zola, I. K. 1966. Culture and symptoms: an analysis of patients' presenting complaints, American Sociological Review **31**:615-630.

17

Cultural factors and the response to pain
A review

B. Berthold Wolff and Sarah Langley

The response to pain is certainly an important component of human behavior and thus deserves study by anthropologists. It is, therefore, with distinct disappointment that one searches the literature for material on the influence of culture on the form of response to pain. Tangential references to pain are often found in anthropological studies, but there appears to be a dearth of published reports specifically concerned with cultural factors and the human pain response.

Pain is the most common symptom of disease or injury as well as the most frequent aversive stimulus for manipulation of behavior. Physicians are concerned with the alleviation of pain, while educators, psychologists, and sociologists have studied the deterrent effects of pain in child development, on adult behavior, and in penology. Furthermore, aversive and noxious stimuli, especially electric shock, are administered almost routinely in most experimental psychological laboratories, although it is curious that usually the resultant pain sensation is not directly studied.

In medicine and physiology, philosophical theories of pain have existed for thousands of years and are still met in hedonistic attitudes and in psychoanalysis. Systematic scientific studies of pain probably did not begin until Schiff in 1858 made the definitive formulation that pain deserves to be placed in a sensory category of its own, later confirmed by Funke (1879). A great impetus for the study of pain was the discovery of pain sensitive points in the skin by Blix (1884) and Goldscheider (1884). Since then neuroanatomists and neurophysiologists have been actively engaged in pain research. However, their investigations have been focused on somatic rather than behavioral aspects of pain. Apart from nonexperimental theorizing by philosophers and psychoanalysts, usually utilizing some variation of the hedonistic pleasure-pain principle, there have been few experimental behavioral studies of pain until comparatively recently. Modern systematic behavioral studies commenced with the work of Hardy, Wolff, and Goodell (1940, 1952). Their work utilized psychophysical principles, but they were not primarily concerned with the study of cultural and psychological factors on pain sensation and reaction. Beecher (1959) strongly criticized Hardy, Wolff, and Goodell as he considered that they did not take into account the psychological aspects and subjective nature of pain.

Beecher has played a very important role in modern American clinical pharmacology by repeatedly emphasizing the importance of double-blind procedures[2] and use of placebo in the study of analgesic drugs (1959). Clinical pharmacologists are thus well aware of placebo effects in analgesic assays. Nevertheless, current pharmacological studies on the whole fail to take cognizance of cultural and psychosocial effects, such as the patient's cultural group membership, socioeconomic class and expectation of treatment (Wolff 1967).

Reproduced by permission of the American Anthropological Association from the American Anthropologist 70 (3) 1968.
From the Department of Medicine and the Rheumatic Diseases Study Group, New York University.

The research investigator is more concerned with the physical nature and somatic basis of pain than with psychosocial and cultural components. The practicing physician, on the other hand, tends to be aware of psychosocial and cultural components in the human pain response; his clinical observations have made him realize that there are ethnic and cultural differences in patients' responses to pain. However, the paucity of adequately controlled experimental studies in this area is remarkable. In fact, with few exceptions, our knowledge of cultural and psychosocial differences in the human pain response is based on empirical rather than experimental evidence.

The Pain Group of the Department of Medicine of New York University Medical Center has been investigating behavioral mechanisms of human pain for some years. Initially, the group developed objective psychophysical techniques for measuring cutaneous and deep somatic pain (Wolff and Jarvik 1964, 1965), and for evaluating analgesic drugs (Wolff, Kantor, Jarvik, and Laska 1966). More recently the group has studied the effects of certain psychological variables, such as suggestion, upon pain (Wolff, Krasnegor, and Farr 1965; Wolff and Horland 1967). An impressive fact, emerging from investigations involving a large number of healthy individuals and patients with arthritis, has been the difference in the pain response due to ethnocultural factors. This difference resembled that observed by clinicians among patients in pain. A review of publications dealing with the effect of cultural variables on pain was, therefore, begun. Initially, this review focused on experimental studies published in scientific journals within the general areas of medicine, physiology, and psychology. We were astonished to observe that in the field of experimental algesimetry there is almost a complete lack of published papers discussing cultural factors. Thus, the literature search was extended to the field of anthropology, but here the yield was even poorer. Consequently, we decided to assemble the few isolated published experimental studies into this review paper. Our purpose is twofold; namely, to inform other investigators of the current status of work in this area, and, more hopefully, to stimulate interest among anthropologists in the experimental study of human pain.

Chapman (1944) and Chapman and Jones (1944) compared the pain responses of 18 Southern Negroes with those of 18 Americans of North European ancestry (not otherwise specified), matched for age and sex, employing the Hardy, Wolff, Goodell (1940) radiant heat technique with stimulation of the forehead. They found that Negroes had a lower pain perception threshold (i.e., point at which pain begins) than the North Europeans, indicating that they are more sensitive to pain. Even more interesting was their finding that Negroes had a much lower pain reaction threshold (i.e., point at which the subject winces and tends to withdraw) than the North Europeans. Thus Negroes were able to tolerate much less pain and the range between their perception and reaction thresholds was much smaller than that for the North Europeans. Chapman and Jones in the same study investigated the role of skin pigmentation and concluded that the difference in pain responses between Negroes and North Europeans was unlikely to be due to pigmentation. These investigators also studied 30 Russian Jewish and Italian subjects (not specified in what proportion) and found that they tended to have pain perception and reaction thresholds similar to those of the Negroes, being much lower than those of the North Europeans. The Negroes, however, did not complain, while the subjects of Mediterranean ancestry complained loudly at pain reaction threshold. Chapman and Jones's overall conclusion was that differences exist in pain sensitivity and pain tolerance due to ethnic factors.

Meehan, Stoll, and Hardy (1954) compared 26 Alaskan Indians from Fort Yukon, 37 Eskimos from the Endicott Mountains and 32 whites from the Ladd Air Force Base. They also used the Hardy, Wolff, and Goodell radiant heat technique, but stimulated the back of the hand, instead of the forehead, measuring only the pricking pain threshold (i.e., point at which a pricking sensation is first noticed). They found that the whites and the Indians had similar, but the Eskimos higher, pain thresholds. However, after applying a conversion formula to correct for skin temperature, they found that the whites had the highest and the Eskimos the lowest pain thresholds, but these differences were not statistically significant. Meehan et al., in another study, used a modification of the radiant heat technique and with it compared 4 whites to 16 Eskimos. Once again they found the differences in pain threshold after temperature correction to be insignificant. They concluded, therefore, that there were no significant differences in pain threshold between these three ethnic groups.

In a recent study in England, Merskey and Spear (1964) compared the pain reactions of 28 white and of 11 Afro-Asian male medical students. They used the pressure algometer, a simple mechanical device for experimental pain induction by pressure, which is placed against a hard, bony surface, such as the shin or forehead. Pressure is gradually exerted until the required pain responses have occurred. They found that there were no significant differences between the white and Afro-Asian students in the verbal report of pain (i.e., pain threshold), the pain reaction point (i.e., when the subject stated that it hurt a lot), and the reaction interval (i.e., the difference between the verbal report to pain and the pain reaction point). Merskey and Spear concluded that there were no significant differences in the pain response between white and colored medical students of the same sex.

Sternbach and Tursky (1965) studied pain and skin potential responses to electric shock in 60 housewives, divided into four ethnic groups of 15 women each. "Yankees" were Protestants of British descent whose parents and grandparents were born in this country, most were from old New England families. All other groups consisted of women whose parents came to the U. S. as immigrants. The Irish and Italian groups were Roman Catholic, and the latter came mainly from Southern Italy and Sicily. The Jews were either Orthodox or Conservative and the majority came from Eastern European countries. There were no significant differences between groups for a variety of physical variables, such as age, height-weight ratio, etc. All groups fell into the same social "middle class" on the Hollingshead scale (i.e., class III), but the difference between Hollingshead scores of "Yankees" and Jews, on the one hand, and Irish and Italian, on the other, was significant at the 5 percent level. Each subject participated in an interview during which relevant personal information was collected. Several weeks later each woman returned to the laboratory for measurements of her pain responses and autonomic reactivity. Electrical stimulation was administered to the dorsal surface of the left forearm from a constant current source, and skin potentials were recorded from the right palm. Sternbach and Tursky found consistent differences among the groups, both at pain threshold and pain tolerance levels, but these reached significance only at pain tolerance. Italian women differed significantly both from "Yankee" and from Jewish women. At pain tolerance levels, the "Yankees" had the highest mean scores, followed by the Jews and then the Irish, with the Italians producing the lowest mean scores. There were no significant differences between the groups in stimulus magnitude estimation, but "Yankees" produced a significantly more rapid and greater decrease in skin potential than the other three groups. Sternbach and Tursky concluded that attitudinal differences among these four subcultures accounted for the psychophysical and autonomic differences. "Yankees" tended to have a matter-of-fact attitude toward pain, while the Italians showed a present-time-orientation in respect to pain and thus focused on the immediacy of the pain. The Jewish housewives, being future-oriented, were not dismayed by the experimental pain and thus tended to resemble the "Yankee" and Irish groups, the latter being undemonstrative with respect to pain. Sternbach and Tursky utilized Zborowski's (1952) hypothesis to arrive at their conclusions. Zborowski's study will be discussed later.

Lambert, Libman, and Poser (1960) studied the effects of religious affiliation rather than of ethnic group on pain tolerance. They used the Hollander (1939) technique, which induces pressure pain by means of a blood pressure cuff into which hard rubber blocks have been sewn. This cuff is placed around the forearm and gradually inflated. The resulting pain responses are measured as pressure in millimeters of mercury. Lambert et al. used 80 female students, 40 Jewish and 40 Protestant, between 18 and 23 years of age. Each group was subdivided into an experimental and a control subgroup of 20 subjects each and given two administrations of the pain-inducing technique. In the first administration, which served as a base with similar experimental conditions for all groups, it was found that the mean pain tolerance scores for the Jewish groups were somewhat, but not significantly, lower than those for the Protestant groups. In the second, the experimental Jewish subgroup was informed that Jews could not tolerate pain as well as Protestants, while the experimental Protestant subgroup was told that Protestants could not tolerate as much pain as Jews. The original instructions were repeated for the two control subgroups. It was found that on the second trial the experimental Jewish subgroup significantly increased its mean pain tolerance, whereas neither the Jewish controls nor the two Protestant subgroups showed significant changes in their pain tolerance. Lambert et al. interpreted these results as indicating that Jews try to become more like the majority group when they are made aware of differences, whereas this is not true of Protestant groups.

In a second study, Lambert, et al. used 160 female undergraduate students (80 Jews and 80 Protestants), and two experimenters, one of whom was obviously Jewish and the other obviously Protestant. The subjects were divided into three subgroups of 30, 30, and 20 respectively with the latter serving as controls. The first experimental subgroup was told that Jews (or Christians) could take less pain than Christians (or Jews), whereas the second experimental subgroup was told that Jews (or Christians) could take more pain than Christians (or Jews). The authors used the term "Christian" to emphasize a distinction between Jews and Christians that did not appear to have been present in their first study when they used the term "Protestant."

Lambert et al. again found no significant differences between all six subgroups on the first trial. On the second trial the experimental Jewish subgroup, which had been told that Jews take less pain than Christians, again increased its pain tolerance significantly. However, the second experimental Jewish subgroup, previously informed that Jews take more pain than Christians, did not significantly increase its mean pain tolerance. On the other hand, both experimental Protestant subgroups (i.e., those told that Christians take less and those told that Christians take more pain than Jews) significantly increased their mean pain tolerance. The two control subgroups showed no significant changes between first and second trials.

The researchers concluded that Jews tend to increase their pain tolerance when told that Jews take less pain than non-Jews (i.e., the majority group), but are quite satisfied with the *status quo* when told that Jews can take more pain. On the other hand, when a religious difference is made explicit to Protestants they strive to increase their pain tolerance, even if they "know" that supposedly they can take more pain to start with. These results suggest that even if there are no basic ethnic differences in terms of pain response between groups, cultural factors, such as those relating to religious affiliation if made explicit, can impose a differential pain response pattern between Jewish and Protestant groups of the same sex, education, and socio-economic status.

Poser (1963) extended these studies, using a total of 88 subjects, divided into Jewish and Roman Catholic groups. The Jews were subdivided into 22 Jewish students born in Canada and 22 Jewish immigrants, and the Catholics were similarly classified into two subgroups, each with 22 subjects. He also used a Jewish and a Roman Catholic experimenter and employed the Hollander technique. Poser's measure of pain tolerance this time was the difference between pain tolerance and pain threshold, which Wolff (1964) terms "pain sensitivity range" (PSR). With a Jewish experimenter the Jewish students had a significantly lower mean PSR than the Roman Catholic students. Similarly, the Jewish immigrants had a significantly lower mean PSR than the Roman Catholic immigrants. However, with a Roman Catholic experimenter, there was no significant difference between Jewish and Roman Catholic immigrants, the former having a lower mean PSR. Furthermore, the effect of a Jewish experimenter as compared to a Roman Catholic experimenter was significant only for the Jewish students. An analysis of variance indicated the ethnic origin of the subject to be a very significant factor with the ethnic origin of the experimenter being a significant second factor. However, citizenship and interactions were found to be nonsignificant. Poser concluded that there were cultural differences that are much more marked for immigrant groups than for native Canadians who were able to follow the behavior pattern of the majority group if made aware either explicitly or implicitly of ethnic differences.

These few studies appear to be the only published reports in which experimenters skilled in the application of experimental pain-inducing techniques specifically investigated the possible effect of ethnic or cultural factors on the pain response. It appears to be quite clear from the studies by Lambert, Libman and Poser (1960), Poser (1960) and Sternbach and Turksy (1965) that cultural factors in terms of attitudinal variables, whether explicit or implicit, do indeed exert significant influences on pain perception.

However, the results from the other studies reported here are inconclusive from an ethnocultural standpoint. The early study of Chapman and Jones (1944) does indicate ethnic group differences in the pain response between Southern Negroes and Americans of North European stock, but Meehan, Stoll, and Hardy (1954) obtained no significant differences between Alaskan Indians, Eskimos and whites. Since both groups of investigators used the radiant heat technique, their different findings can not be attributed to differences in method. However, Meehan et al. corrected their data for skin temperature, while Chapman and Jones did not. It is thus possible that had the latter also corrected for skin temperature, they might not have found significant differences. In any case, these two teams of investigators used different ethnic groups, and consequently their results would not be comparable even if skin temperature corrections had been applied to all data. It is thus not possible to draw any conclusion as to whether or not ethnic differences in pain response are detectable with the radiant heat method. Merskey and Spear (1964), using a completely different pain-inducing technique, found no significant differences in pain threshold and pain tolerance between the white and Afro-Asian medical students. Their study is important as they controlled for socioeducational level.

Care must be taken in evaluating these experimental results. Merskey and Spear's study is experimentally sound, but unfortunately they were able to compare only a very small number of subjects from an ethnocultural standpoint. Similarly, Chapman and Jones, in order to match Negroes and Northern Europeans for sex and age, had to reduce the number to 18 each, although they started with a total of 200 subjects, consisting of 130 Northern Europeans, 25 American Negroes, 15 Ukrainians, and a miscellaneous group of 30 Jews and persons of Mediterranean ancestry. Furthermore, the fact that Chapman and Jones did not correct their results for skin temperature poses another problem. There is a possibility that skin temperature varies among ethnoracial groups. If so, pain responses obtained with a thermal method, such as the radiant heat technique, should be corrected for temperature. Johnson and Corah (1963) obtained significant differences in basal skin resistance between 120 white and 54 Negro children as well as between 21 Negro and 21 white adults. This suggests that there may be basic differences for certain physiological skin variables between different groups.

Meehan, Stoll, and Hardy used a sophisticated formula for correcting skin temperature, yet their experimental conditions were completely different for their three ethnic groups as they themselves point out. The Eskimos were tested as a whole group in a tent at a temperature of 5° C with distraction to the subjects due to noise and conversation. Furthermore, an interpreter had to be used and it is not certain if the Eskimos fully understood the instructions. The Alaskan Indians, some of whom also required an interpreter, were tested individually in a heated room. The white control subjects were tested in small groups of 4 and 5 in a heated room. Thus, from a strictly scientific point of view these results are not directly comparable, thus making generalizations risky.

Similarly, from the standpoint of the anthropologist, the validity of Meehan, Stoll, and Hardy's study is doubtful, as there was a distinct possibility that the white group was mixed in cultural background. The implied equation of race and culture, while doubtless unintentional, is, of course, invalid (Boas 1940; Benedict 1940). Their results indicated no significant differences in temperature-corrected pain thresholds for Indians, Eskimos, and whites; and they concluded that behavioral differences among these three groups are culture-bound.

Therefore, none of these experimental pain studies allows a definitive conclusion as to whether or not there exist basic differences in pain response among ethnic groups. On the other hand, there is strong experimental evidence that attitudinal factors tend to influence the pain response of different cultural groups.

The paucity of published studies in anthropology dealing specifically with pain has been mentioned previously. Apart from the many indirect and tangential references, Zborowski's (1952) study appears to be the only one in anthropology pertinent to the theme of this review. Zborowski distinguished between self-inflicted, other-inflicted, and spontaneous pain. He defined self-inflicted pain as deliberately self-inflicted, such as self-mutilation, whereas other-inflicted pain is that incurred in culturally accepted and expected activities, such as fights, sports, war, etc. Spontaneous pain denotes that resulting from disease or injury.

It would seem that Zborowski created conceptual and semantic difficulties for himself by attempting to distinguish between "pain" as a basically physiological phenomenon and the "pain experience," which has emotional components. This distinction between the physiological and psychological components of pain has been made frequently (e.g., Beecher 1959), possibly because there is still no generally acceptable all-inclusive scientific definition of pain (Lewis 1942; Beecher 1959). However, it appears to us that conceptually pain sensation and pain experience are at different connotative levels. The pain experience is a higher order concept than pain sensation and would seem to include the latter. Semantically, it would have been more meaningful to use the terms pain sensation and pain reaction instead of pain and pain experience. It is unfortunate that there exists no general terminology for pain, thus frequently leading to confusion in the literature, especially when different studies are compared (Wolff 1964). We would like to suggest that, in any case, it is not too rewarding for the behavioral scientist to attempt to differentiate between physiological and psychological components of pain, but to recognize that both components contribute to pain, pain reaction, pain experience, or whatever terms are used. It is, of course, very true that pain response parameters differ in their loadings of physiological and psychological components (e.g., Gelfand 1964). The behavioral scientist should concern himself with evaluating the effects of affective, autonomic, cognitive, cultural, psychosocial, and similar factors on the pain response and thereby add to our understanding of pain.

Zborowski (1952) studied clinical pain qualitatively in 103 subjects (87 hospitalized patients and 16 of their healthy relatives or friends), but restricted his main comparisons to 26 "Old Americans," 24 Italians and 31 Jews. Zborowski indicated that the hospital staff tended to uphold the "Old American" tradition in which pain is reported but few emotional side reactions are permitted. Hospital staff members stated that both Italians and Jews tended to overreact to pain, to be emotional about pain, and to complain excessively. Zborowski disagreed with this rather simple description of pain response in Italians and Jews. He found that Italians tend to call for immediate relief of pain by any means, such as drugs, and are happy when pain is alleviated. On the other hand, whereas Jews also seek relief of pain, they are skeptical or suspicious of the future and tend to keep complaining even after their pain has been diminished. Zborowski concluded, therefore, that Italians are present-oriented, and when in pain demonstrate present-oriented apprehension. Jews are future-oriented, and when in pain present future-oriented anxiety. "Old Americans" are also future-oriented but, unlike Jews, tend to be rather optimistic. When in pain, the "Old Americans" tend to withdraw socially, while both Jews and Italians prefer the social company of their relatives. Zborowski drew the following two conclusions: (1) similar reactions to pain demonstrated by members of different ethnocultural groups do not necessarily reflect similar attitudes to pain, and (2) reactive patterns similar in terms of their manifestations may have different functions in various cultures.

Zborowski's concern was less with recording differences in overt behavior among his groups than in preparing an analysis of the traits in each culture that contribute to the observed patterns. His approach is thus basically functional, paralleling that of Linton (1945) in the area of mental disorders, as is reflected in the latter's conclusion that similar patterns do not necessarily have the same function.

Opler (1961), expanding on Zborowski's findings, suggested that the excessive response to pain by Italian patients, male and female, may be due at least in part to a general preoccupation with bodily function and body image. He concluded that, by contrast, the stoicism of the Irish may stem in part from a tendency to pride themselves on disregarding the physical self.

In comparing well-matched male schizophrenic patient groups, Opler (1959) found that while the Irish are inclined to be nondisruptive, docile, given to fantasy and well-organized delusional systems, the Italian group tended to be more overtly emotional, unpredictable, and even assaultive.

It would appear from these studies that the response to pain for a given cultural group, such as the Italian, is similar irrespective of the underlying disease. Therefore, any attempt to delineate cultural factors in the pain response should be made within the wider context of cultural attitudes toward sickness and health. It is possible that religious attitudes, insofar as they influence the perception of the physical self, may also color the pain response.

An exploration of ethnographic literature suggests that there already exists an impressive array of data on cultural attitudes toward illness, but that it is unfortunately scattered. This is particularly true of material written prior to 1950. After this date, there appear a number of studies more or less directly concerned with attitudes toward medicine and health, especially in the so-called underdeveloped areas of the world, although many of these are more sociological than anthropological in their general orientation.

An effort was made to see if additional ethnographic material could be found. A missionary priest (Morice 1901:20-21), writing of the Déné, an Athabascan tribe of inland Alaska, stated that these people could tolerate extreme pain calmly and remarkably well for brief periods, provided it was accompanied by the hope of fast relief or recovery. He added, however, that prolonged discomfort was very poorly tolerated. An informant of ours, a registered nurse with a background of ten years practice among the Alaskan Eskimos, gives parallel information for this group, stating that when a favorable outcome is anticipated, pain is well tolerated, but that when the prognosis of the disease or injury is unknown, tolerance is notably poor. This supports the suggestion of Meehan, Stoll, and Hardy (1954) that the slightly lower temperature-corrected pain threshold obtained for the Eskimo was probably due to lack of understanding by them of the testing procedure.

An attempt has been made to show that although there is a wealth of anthropological material in which pain is discussed, there is nevertheless a paucity of studies in which both the pain response and cultural factors are directly and experimentally controlled. The few experimental pain studies that do exist suffer from anthropological naivety, while the anthropological reports lack experimental control of pain.

It is not being suggested that medical scientists become experts in cultural anthropology. What is being suggested is that the techniques of cultural anthropology can profitably be applied by those who would understand such aspects of human behavior as response to pain. Some knowledge of a patient's cultural matrix can, in all probability, provide the researcher with insight into the general form of that individual's behavior. In short, it can have both predictive and interpretive value. There is thus a need for the cultural anthropologist to combine forces with the medical scientist in order to add to our knowledge about the human pain response.

NOTES

[1]This work was supported in part by United States Public Health Service Grant NB-05788 and in part by Vocational Rehabilitation Administration Grant RD-1733-P. We wish to thank Dr. Ruth S. Freed for her helpful suggestions.

[2]Double-blind procedures consist of an experimental design in which all drugs, including placebo, are coded and neither the patient receiving the drug nor the physician or nurse administering the drug know or can recognize the specific drug being used.

REFERENCES CITED

Beecher, H. K. (1959) Measurement of subjective responses: quantitative effects of drugs. New York: Oxford University Press.

Benedict, R. F. (1940) Race, science, and politics. New York, Viking Press.

Blix, M. (1884) Experimentelle Beiträge zur Lösung der Frage über die specifische Energie der Hautnerven. Zeitschrift für Biologie 20:141-160.

Boas, F. (1940) Race, language, and culture. New York, Macmillan.

Chapman, W. P. (1944) Measurements of pain sensitivity in normal control subjects and in psychoneurotic patients. Psychosomatic Medicine 6:252-257.

Chapman, W. P., and C. M. Jones (1944) Variations in cutaneous and visceral pain sensitivity in normal subjects. Journal of Clinical Investigation 23:81-91.

Funke, O. (1879) Der Tastsinn und die Gemeinge fühle. *In* Handbuch der Physiologie der Sinnersorgane. L. Hermann, ed. 3:297.

Gelfand, S. (1964) The relationship of experimental pain tolerance to pain threshold. Canadian Journal of Psychology 18:36-42.

Goldscheider, A. (1884) Die specifische Energie der Gefühlsnerven der Haut. Monatschrift für praktische Dermatologie 3:283.

Hardy, J. D., H. G. Wolff, and H. Goodell (1940) Studies on pain. A new method for measuring pain threshold: Observations on the spatial summation of pain. Journal of Clinical Investigation 19:649-657. 1952 Pain sensations and reactions. Baltimore, Williams & Wilkins.

Hollander, E. (1939) A clinical gauge for sensitivity to pain. Journal of Laboratory and Clinical Medicine 24:537-538.

Johnson, L. C., and N. L. Corah (1963) Racial differences in skin resistance. Science 139:766-767.

Lambert, W. E., E. Bibman, and E. G. Poser (1960) The effect of increased salience of a membership group on pain tolerance. Journal of Personality 38: 350-357.

Lewis, T. (1942) Pain. New York, Macmillan.

Linton, R. (1945) The cultural basis of personality. New York, Appleton-Century-Croft.

Meehan, J. P., A. M. Stoll, and J. D. Hardy (1954) Cutaneous pain threshold in the native Alaskan Indian and Eskimo. Journal of Applied Physiology 6: 397-400.

Merskey, H., and F. G. Spear (1964) The reliability of the pressure algometer. British Journal of Social and Clinical Psychology 3:130-136.

Morice, A. G. (1901) Déné Surgery. Transactions of the Canadian Institute 7:15-27.

Opler, M. K. (1959) Culture and mental health. New York, Macmillan. (1961) Ethnic differences in behavior and health practices. *In* The family: a focal point for health education. I. Galdson, ed. New York, New York Academy of Medicine.

Poser, E. G. (1963) Some psychosocial determinants of pain tolerance. Read at XVIth International Congress of Psychology, Washington, D.C.

Schiff, J. M. (1858) Lehrbuck der Physiologie 1:228.

Sternbach, R. A. and B. Tursky (1965) Ethnic differences among housewives in psychophysical and skin potential responses to electric shock. Psychophysiology 1:241-246.

Wolff, B. B. (1964) The relationship of experimental pain tolerance to pain threshold: A critique of Gelfand's paper. Canadian Journal of Psychology 18: 249-253. (1967) Some behavioral mechanisms of human pain. *In* Symposium IX: Pharmacology of Pain, IIIrd International Pharmacological Congress, 1966. London, Pergamon Press (In Press).

Wolff, B. B., and A. A. Horland (1967) Effect of suggestion upon experimental pain: a validation study. Journal of Abnormal Psychology 72:402-407).

Wolff, B. B. and M. E. Jarvik (1964) Relationship between superficial and deep somatic thresholds of pain with a note on handedness. American Journal of Psychology 77:589-599. (1965) Quantitative measures of deep somatic pain: Further studies with hypertonic saline. Clinical Science 28:43-56.

Wolff, B. B., T. G. Kantor, M. E. Jarvik, and E. Laska (1966) Response of experimental pain to analgesic drugs. II. Codeine and placebo. Clinical Pharmacology and Therapeutics 7:323-331.

Wolff, B. B., N. A. Krasnegor, and R. S. Farr (1965). Effect of suggestion upon experimental pain response parameters. Perceptual and Motor Skills 21:675-683.

Zborowski, M. (1952) Cultural components in responses to pain. Journal of Social Issues 8:16-30.

18

Further physiological correlates of ethnic differences in responses to shock

Bernard Tursky and Richard A. Sternbach

In a previous paper (Sternbach and Tursky, 1965) we reported that subcultural differences in attitudes toward pain, reflected in standardized interviews, had correlates in psychophysical and autonomic measures. Yankee, Irish, Jewish and Italian housewives participated in threshold, magnitude estimation, and physiological reactivity studies of responses to electric shock. In the paper cited we reported that significant differences in upper pain thresholds, and in the adaptation of diphasic palmar skin potentials, were consonant with attitudinal differences toward pain among the groups as verbalized by the subjects in the interviews. Briefly, these attitudinal differences were: Yankees have a phlegmatic, matter of fact orientation toward pain; Jews express a concern for the implication of pain and distrust palliatives; Italians express a desire for pain relief and the Irish inhibit expression of suffering and concern for the implications of the pain.

The present report is concerned with a further analysis of the autonomically innervated variables, exploring differences among the ethnic groups in their physiological response measures: The hypothesis being tested is that differences in subjects' sets, acquired by virtue of ethnic membership, will be associated with differential autonomic response patterns in a situation designed to maximize the influence of the sets. Specifically, attitudes toward pain will become salient in an experiment in which subjects receive electric shocks, and when these culturally-determined attitudes are elicited they will modulate autonomic responsivity in the situation. This hypothesis was derived from earlier studies on effects of instructional sets (Sternbach, 1964, 1965).

METHODS AND PROCEDURE

The selection of subjects, the variables on which they were matched, and the operational definition of their ethnic membership was described previously (Sternbach and Tursky, 1965). Briefly, Irish, Jewish, and Italian subjects were those who were born and reared in this country, of parents who emigrated from Europe. Yankee subjects were Protestants of British descent whose parents and grandparents were born in this country. All subjects were housewives with at least one child of school age. There were 60 subjects, 15 from each group. In some of the analyses shown below, however, different numbers were used when data were incomplete.

The experimental session was conducted in a well lighted, air-conditioned soundproof room with subject seated in a reclining chair. Verbal contact was maintained by means of a two-way communication

Reprinted with permission of the Society for Psychophysiological Research from Psychophysiology 4:67-74.

From the Massachusetts Mental Health Center (B. Tursky); and the Department of Psychiatry, University of Wisconsin (R. A. Sternbach).

This investigation was supported in part by U. S. Public Health Service Grant MH0412 from the National Institute of Mental Health, M. Greenblatt principal investigator, and in part by an NIMH Special Fellowship, 5 F3 MH-15, 670 to R. A. S.

We thank Michael Ross, Linda M. Levey and Daniel Kalikow for their assistance.

system and E could observe the subject through a one-way window. Electrical stimulation was delivered through an annular disc electrode on the treated dorsal surface of the left forearm with a 60 cps constant current source, and impedance of the electrode-skin circuit was maintained at 5000 ± 500 ohms (Tursky and Watson, 1964; Tursky, Watson, and O'Connell, 1965).

The dependent variables recorded were: heart rate, palmar skin potential, palmar skin resistance, face temperature, and respiration. Heart rate (HR) was picked up by standard EKG electrodes and recorded tachometrically as beat-to-beat variation. Skin potential (GSP) and skin resistance (GSR) level and response measures were picked up by silver-silver chloride electrodes placed on the palm and dorsal aspect of the forearm of each arm (O'Connell and Tursky, 1960; O'Connell, Tursky, and Orne, 1960), and recorded as DC measures. The temperature measure (FaT) employed a VECO 32A11 thermistor transducing cheek temperature to a change in resistance whose level was calibrated in degrees C. Respiration was picked up by a strain gauge respirometer; this variable was used to monitor changes in the other systems associated with sudden respiratory changes, and was not in itself used as a response measure.

The experimental session consisted of seven periods.

(1) First rest. A fifteen min period in which the subject was told to relax.

(2) Level setting. A variable length period during which the subject received a series of increasing intensity shocks. The subject was instructed to identify her lower threshold (the level at which subject first became aware of sensation) and then the upper threshold (the level at which the subject asks that the stimulation be stopped). Some subjects had to be coaxed to reach a criterion level (of 7 ma). This Motivated Threshold Level was the highest level reached (above 7 ma) by those who were coaxed.

(3) Second rest. Five min rest period.

(4) Repeated stimuli. A fifteen min period of reptitive 7 ma, 1 sec shocks, delivered at 30 sec intervals.

(5) Third rest. A two min rest period.

(6) Magnitude estimation. A variable length magnitude estimation period.

(7) Fourth rest. A two min rest period.

DATA PROCESSING

All physiological measures were recorded simultaneously on a modified Offner Type D EEG Recorder and on a Sanborn Ampex Model 2000 FM magnetic tape recorder. The visual record was used to supplement programmed elimination of artifactual responses. Data from the tape were processed through an automatic data processing system (Tursky, Shapiro, and Leiderman, 1966).

A sampling rate of 1 sample per sec was used to digitize all periods except period 4 (repeated stimuli), where it was changed to 3 samples per sec to obtain a better measurement of response amplitude. Mean and variance were calculated from these samples for each half min subperiod throughout all periods. Discrete response measures were extracted for each trial in period 4. These were: a measure of the level (Pre) previous to the onset of the stimulus; the maximum (Max) and minimum (Min) reading during the ten sec period following the stimulus. From these data three response measures were computed.

1) Max minus Pre = Negative response
2) Pre minus Min = Positive response
3) Max minus Min = Total response

RESULTS

Mean level for HR, GSP, GSR, and FaT for the four groups for each period for the entire session are shown in Fig. 1. An analysis of variance for each measure for the entire session shows that GSR level differentiates among the groups. It is apparent from inspection of Fig. 1 that the Irish subjects' lower skin resistance contributes most of the difference, which is highly significant ($F = 7.09$, $p < 0.001$). Differences among the groups on the other measures are not significant.

A separate analysis of variance was done for each period. The consistent differences in FaT levels (Italian subjects lowest) which appeared only as a trend in the overall session analysis, reach significance in period 2 ($F = 2.95$, $p < 0.05$). This result, as well as the overall difference in GSR, is shown in Fig. 1.

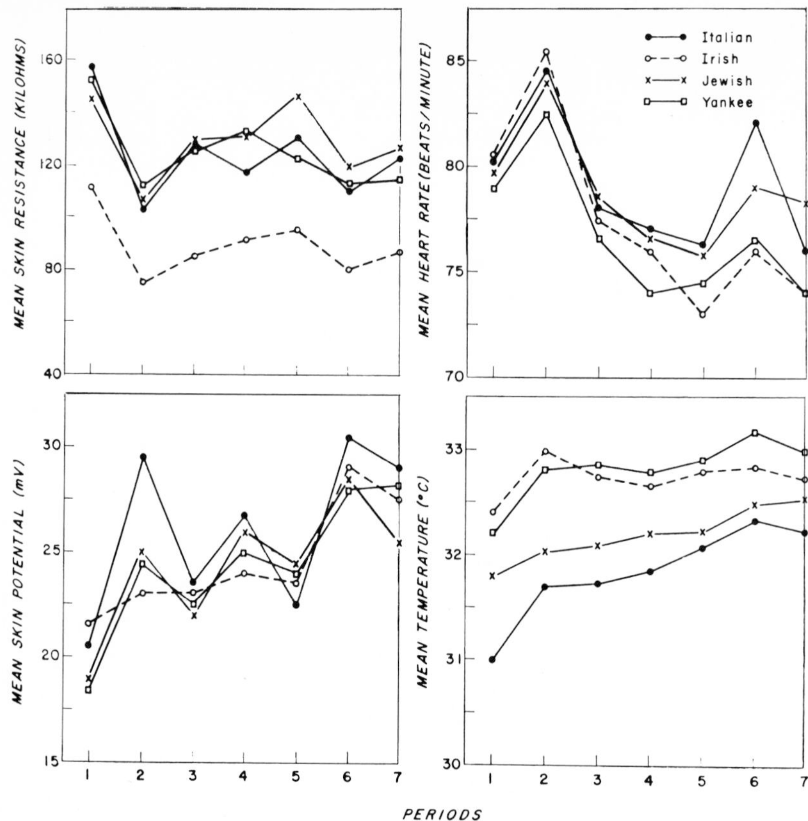

Fig. 1. Mean levels of palmar skin resistance, heart rate, palmar skin potential, and face temperature for the four ethnic groups for each of the seven experimental periods. Response values shown are single means for each period.

In period 4 where 30 shocks were presented at half min intervals, a repeated measurement analysis of variance was computed (Winer, 1962) and the following group over time differences were found for the three measures. Total response (Max − Min) showed a clear difference between groups ($F = 10.0$, $p < 0.001$). The positive response (Pre − Min) showed the same trend ($F = 4.35$, $p < 0.05$). The negative response (Max − Pre) however, does not differentiate among groups ($F = 2.37$, $p < 0.25$). These measures are shown in Fig. 2.

A further analysis of the data is the Spearman rank order correlation matrix shown in Table 1. These correlations are between each of the three levels of intensity, Lower threshold, Unmotivated upper threshold, and Motivated upper threshold, and mean levels of GSP, GSR, and HR for the entire experiment; the temperature variable was not included in this analysis.

No motivated upper threshold data are presented for the Yankee subjects because, as described in the earlier report, too few of them require coaxing to accept the higher shock strengths.

It may be seen in Table 1 that upper thresholds are negatively correlated with GSP for Irish subjects, significantly and positively correlated with GSR for Yankee subjects, significantly and negatively correlated with HR for Jewish subjects, and positively correlated with HR for Italian subjects.

Some of the reversals in signs of the coefficients also differentiate among the groups of subjects. For example, the near-significant negative correlations between GSP and average threshold for the Italian subjects change to positive correlations with their motivated upper threshold, and the quantitative changes are quite large. Similarly with the Irish subjects' HR cor-

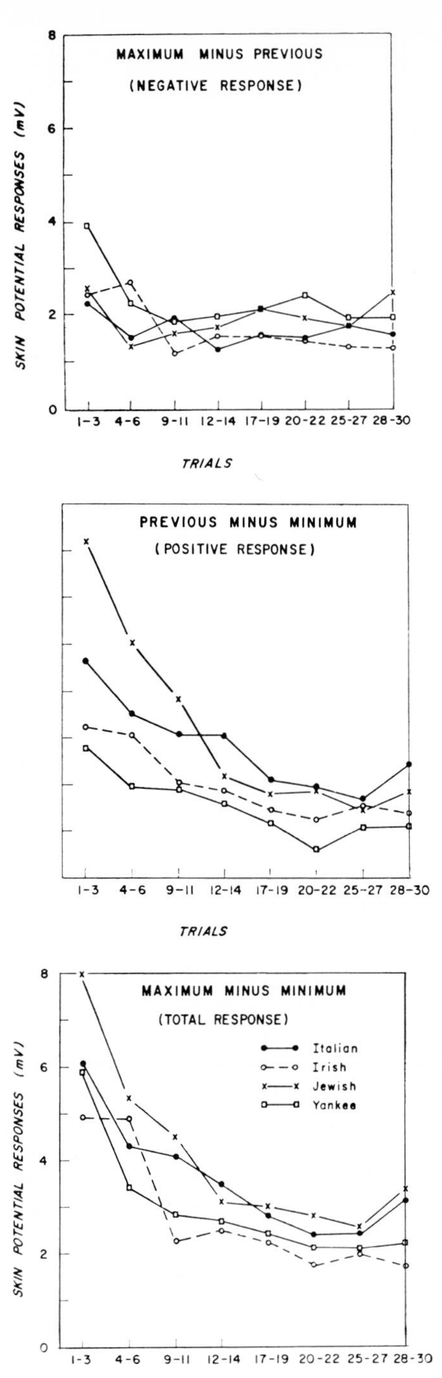

Fig. 2. Palmar skin potential responses for the four ethnic groups during period 4. Curves shown are smoothed, as plotted points are selected from moving averages of three for clarity of presentation. The Max-Min (total) and Pre-Min (negative) responses differentiate the groups.

Table 1. Spearman rank order correlation between level of shock intensity and the mean levels of HR, GSP, and GSR for the four ethnic groups

	GSP				*GSR*				*Heart rate*			
	Yankees	*Jewish*	*Irish*	*Italian*	*Yankees*	*Jewish*	*Irish*	*Italian*	*Yankees*	*Jewish*	*Irish*	*Italian*
Average lower threshold	−0.34	−0.31	0.10	−0.50	0.36	−0.03	0.02	−0.19	0.25	0.44	0.35	0.45
Unmot. upper threshold	−0.39	−0.04	0.13	−0.22	0.72*	−0.24	0.11	0.15	0.49	0.07	0.25	0.26
Motivated upper threshold		−0.06	−0.54	0.06		−0.06	0.01	0.03		−0.68*	−0.24	0.61

relations: the large positive correlations of HR and both average and unmotivated upper thresholds change to negative correlations with the motivated upper thresholds; the quantitative differences, if taken by themselves, would constitute highly significant correlations.

DISCUSSION

In our previous report we indicated that the Italian subjects' significantly lower upper thresholds for shock was consonant with and predictable from what is known of the ethnic differences in value systems and attitudes toward pain. The same was true for the more rapid adaptation of the Yankee subjects' diphasic GSP during the repetitive shock presentations in period 4. To these differences may now be added the Irish subjects' consistently lower palmar skin resistance; this is associated with their considerable anxiety which they feel constrained not to verbalize or express overtly, a phenomenon predicted from their interviews (Sternbach and Tursky, 1965).

Two other variables clearly distinguish among the ethnic groups, although the differences are not readily understandable on cultural grounds. One is the consistently lower face temperature of the Italian subjects. The other is the greater GSP responsiveness to period 4 shocks shown by the Jewish subjects, a phenomenon which surprised us; we would have predicted it for the Italians among the expressive subjects, or the Irish among the undemonstrative subjects.

It is interesting to note that these differences in responsivity were demonstrated on the total (Max − Min) and positive (Pre − Min) responses and not on the negative (Max − Pre) response. The positive and negative skin potential responses have long been known to be different (Forbes, 1936; Wilcott, 1957) and to indicate two different levels of neural activity. Edelberg (1963) demonstrated a response specificity for these measures. The results of the present experiment indicate that the (negative) skin potential response can be used to differentiate groups in a repetitive stimulus situation.

The differences shown in the correlation matrix are intriguing. The relationships among thresholds and response systems clearly differentiate among the groups, and so do the changes in sign of the coefficients. Among the significant correlations, it is seen that for the Irish subjects, those with lower motivated thresholds tend to have the higher skin potentials, a result consistent with their "silent suffering" attitude toward pain. The Yankees show significant positive correlations between unmotivated thresholds and GSR: those with the highest thresholds have the highest skin resistance, a finding consistent with their "take it in stride" attitude towards pain, and also represented in their more rapid adaptation of the diphasic GSP potential. The Jewish subjects show significant negative correlations between upper thresholds and heart rate; that is, those with the highest thresholds have the lowest heart rate. This is consistent with their attitude of "searching for the meaning" of the pain. We had predicted that "in our laboratory situation, where the stimuli carried no implication of future impairment, no activation of this concern would be expected for the Jewish group" (Sternbach and Tursky, 1965), a phenomenon supported by the present finding. The Italian subjects on the other hand who have a present time orientation toward pain or, as previously stated, a focusing on the immediacy of the pain itself (Zborowski, 1952) showed a strong positive correlation between upper thresholds and heart rate, that is, those with the highest thresholds had the highest heart rates.

While it is clear that the physiological differences among the ethnic groups reported here parallel what we know of their sets toward pain, emotional expressiveness, doctors and laboratories, etc., it is also true that we cannot rule out possible genetic differences in autonomic responsivity. Our selection procedure (first generation Americans except for Yankees, who were at least third generation) virtually insured our drawing from four discrete genetic pools. A kind of indirect support for this view comes from the patterns of correlations and changes in the sign of correlation coefficients, which are suggestive of a form of "ethnic specificity" in response hierarchies, and which might imply inborn differences. But this is a tenuous relationship. Much more impressive is the close association between direction of attitudinal and autonomic responses, an association which argues for early childhood conditioning in the home rather than a genetic determination.

We feel it is important to add a cautionary note to this discussion of response differences among the ethnic groups. We found great intragroup variability. In some analyses, trends toward mean differences failed to reach significant levels because of large within-group variances. Whatever the possible genetic-cultural interactions contributing to the responses which do differentiate among the groups, it is clear that there is often great overlap among them due to individual differences. Therefore we cannot make predictions about an individual's autonomic response pattern based solely on his ethnic membership.

Furthermore, to place these findings in context, we do not view the demonstration of subcultural differences as important or useful in themselves. Rather, they respresent another instance of the influence of sets on autonomic functioning. Previously we demonstrated the role of explicit (instructional) sets which may occur in the laboratory (Sternbach, 1964, 1965). The present studies illustrate the influence of implicit sets, which subjects bring with them to the experiment. We believe that such influences, which cannot be avoided, sufficiently affect physiological processes as to require special techniques for assessment and control, such as those suggested by Orne (1962). Thus, these findings should alert us to the kinds of "extraneous" variables which may distort or subtly influence or greatly increase the variance of the results in our experimental procedures, often without the experimenter's awareness.

REFERENCES

Edelberg, R. Electrophysiological characteristics and interpretation of skin potentials. USAF School of Aerospace Medicine, TDR-63-95, Nov. 1963.

Forbes, T. W., and Bolles, M. Marjorie. Correlation of the response potentials of the skin with "exciting" and "non-exciting" stimuli. *J. Psychol.,* 1936, *2*:273.

O'Connell, D. N., & Tursky, B. Silver-silver chloride sponge electrodes for skin potential recording. *Amer. J. Psychol.,* 1960, *73*:302-304.

O'Connell, D. N., Tursky, B., & Orne, M. T. Electrodes for the recording of skin potential. *Arch. gen. Psychiat.,* 1960, *3*:252-258.

Orne, M. T. On the social psychology of the psychological experiment: with special reference to demand characteristics and their implications. *Amer. Psychologist,* 1962, *17*:776-783.

Sternbach, R. A. The effects of instructional sets on autonomic responsivity. *Psychophysiology,* 1964, *1*: 67-72.

Sternbach, R. A. Autonomic responsivity and the concept of sets. In N. S. Greenfield & W. C. Lewis (Eds.), *Psychoanalysis and Current Biological Thought.* Madison: Univer. of Wisconsin Press, 1965, Pp. 215-226.

Sternbach, R. A., & Tursky, B. Ethnic differences among housewives in psychophysical and skin potential responses to electric shock. *Psychophysiology,* 1965, *1*:241-246.

Tursky, B., Shapiro, D., & Leiderman, P. H. Automatic data processing in psychophysiology: a system in operation. *Behav. Sci.,* 1966, *11*: 64-70.

Tursky, B., & Watson, P. D. Controlled physical and subjective intensities of electric shock. *Psychophysiology,* 1964, *1*:151-162.

Tursky, B., Watson, P. D. & O'Connell, D. N. A concentric shock electrode for pain stimulation. *Psychophysiology,* 1965, *1*:296-298.

Wilcott, R. C., Darrow, C. W., & Siegel, A. Uniphasic and diphasic waveforms of the skin potential response. *J. comp. physiol. Psychol.,* 1957, *50*:217.

Winer, B. J. *Statistical principles in experimental design.* New York: McGraw-Hill, 1962. Pp. 319-337.

Zborowski, M. Cultural components in responses to pain. *J. soc. Issues,* 1952, *8*:16-30.

19

Pain response in Negro and white obstetrical patients*

B. Winsberg and M. Greenlick

The role of sociocultural factors in pain expression and evaluation has received little investigation. This study investigates these factors by assessing: (1) the impact of cultural factors on patients' responses to obstetrical pain, and (2) the consistency of pain evaluations by people occupying different professional roles.

It has been frequently stated that modes of expression differ among different cultures and intracultural groups.[1] If this is the case it would seem reasonable that personnel involved in patient care might evaluate the response from analagous pain differently, depending upon their sociocultural derivation. The clinician should be aware of these possible differences so he can minimize the patients' suffering with as little medication as possible, since the restricted use of analgesia reduces the potential dangers which follow over-sedation in many medical and surgical situations.

In the special case of obstetrics, for example, increasing analgesia tends to minimize patient suffering, but may, at the same time, increase the dangers to mother and child. The effective handling of this clinical dilemma requires the judicious use of analgesia. This can only be achieved when effective rapport is established between the patient and the involved medical care personnel. If the patient's level of distress is communicated in terms which may be misinterpreted, the consequences can be greater risk and/or increased patient discomfort.

Hardy, Wolff and Goodell,[2] using a technique of comparing painful stimuli (dolimetrics), concluded that the experience of pain in the various stages of labor is quantitatively similar, although the reaction to that pain is relatively dissimilar. The reaction to childbirth depends partly on pain, but to a greater extent on other factors. They conclude that the intensity of the pain experienced by the patient could not be reliably evaluated on the basis of her reaction nor correlated with her apparent distress. Therefore, it can be assumed that the differences in response to obstetrical pain would be determined by whatever

From the Children's Psychiatric Hospital, Ann Arbor, Mich. (B. Winsberg), and the Kaiser Foundation Hospital, Portland, Ore. (M. Greenlick).

*Appreciation is extended to W. A. Anderson, M.D., Chief of Obstetrics, Wayne County General Hospital, Eloise, Michigan, and to Dr. Anderson's staff for their cooperation; and to Mrs. K. Block, Senior Research Assistant, Medical Care Research Unit, Kaiser Foundation Hospital, for her efforts in compiling the data and preparing the manuscript for this project.

[1]William Caudill, "Effects of Social and Cultural Systems in Reaction to Stress," *Social Science Research Council Pamphlet*, No. 14, 1958; W. La Barre, "Cultural Basis of Emotions and Gestures," *Journal of Personality*, 16 (1947), pp. 49-68; Leo Simmons, "Cultural Patterns in Childbirth," *American Journal of Nursing*, 52 (1952), pp. 989-991; R. I. Simons, "Involution Psychosis in Negroes," *Archives of General Psychiatry*, 13 (1965), pp. 148-155; M. M. Vitols, H. G. Waters and M. H. Keeler, "Hallucinations and Delusions in White and Negro Schizophrenics," *American Journal of Psychiatry*, 120 (1963), pp. 473-477; Mark Zborowski, "Cultural Components in Response to Pain," *Journal of Social Issues*, 8(1952), pp. 16-30.

[2]J. D. Hardy, H. G. Wolff and H. Goodell, "Studies on Pain," *Journal of Clinical Investigations*, 27 (1948), p. 380.

cultural, psychological and biological factors generally determine response to pain.

Beecher,[3] in an early article, arrived at a similar conclusion. Analyzing the pain responses of patients with battlefield wounds, he concluded that the physiologic pain reactions were similar among different soldiers but that the expressive modes were different. He assumed that similar wounds produced quantitatively similar pain.

Zborowski[4] studied reaction to pain among four ethno-cultural groups—Jewish, Italian, Irish and "Old American"—basing his conclusions on clinical observations and interviews with 103 patients in a New York City hospital. He concluded that there were differences in pain expression among these groups dependent upon their ethnocultural background. Zborowski's study however was self-admittedly tentative and incomplete. On the other hand, after studying pain response during childbirth among the people of 80 primitive groups, Freedman[5] concluded that the pain response of these groups is similar to that of Europeans and Americans. This finding would appear to contradict Zborowski.

METHOD

This study attempted to investigate the above problem by asking two specific questions:

(1) Do white and Negro obstetrical patients of similar social class respond differently to the pain of childbirth?

(2) Are there differences in the evaluation of the pain response of white and Negro obstetrical patients by people occupying the different staff positions in an obstetrical department?

In order to answer these questions, the responses of all patients admitted to the O.B. unit of Wayne County General Hospital in Michigan during a three-month period were evaluated by all attending personnel. It was assumed that if cultural differences were important in pain response, they would dictate differences between the response patterns of Negro and white patients. Wayne County General Hospital appeared to be an appropriate setting for this study. Nearly equal numbers of white and Negro mothers delivered at this hospital and they were of equivalent lower or lower-middle social class, since most were medically indigent.

Three components of pain response were evaluated by the physician, the nurse, and the aide independently immediately following the termination of labor of each patient delivered during the study period. Only normal spontaneous deliveries were included in the study. The components evaluated were amount of pain, response to pain, and cooperation. The personnel were asked to make the evaluation independently and as soon after the completion of labor as possible. The specific items used in these evaluations were:

I. What was the degree of pain that the patients felt?
   1. Very severe pain
   2. Severe pain
   3. Average pain
   4. Mild pain
   5. Very mild pain

II. How did the patient respond to her pain?
   1. Very excitedly
   2. Excitedly
   3. Average
   4. Calmly
   5. Very calmly

III. How cooperative was the patient?
   1. Very cooperative
   2. Cooperative
   3. Average
   4. Uncooperative
   5. Very uncooperative

In a separate questionnaire, the patient was asked to evaluate the intensity of her pain experience. Information about the patients' age and race were recorded from her medical record.

RESULTS

The design resulted in 365 successive normal spontaneous deliveries being included in the sample. Of these births 207 (56.7%) were to white mothers and 158 (43.3%) to Negro mothers. The age distributions, shown in Table 1, were similar although the Negro mothers were slightly

[3]H. K. Beecher, "Pain in New Wounded in Battle," *Annals of Surgery,* 123 (1946), p. 96.

[4]Zborowski, *op. cit.*

[5]Lawrence Zelic Freedman and Vera Masius Ferguson, "The Question of 'Painless Childbirth' in Primitive Cultures," *American Journal of Orthopsychiatry,* 20 (1950), pp. 327-363.

Table 1. Age distribution of Negro and white patients in sample

Age	*White*	*Negro*	*Total*
Below 15	0	3	3
15-19	48	49	97
20-24	63	39	102
25-29	34	21	55
30-34	19	8	27
35-39	11	7	18
40 and above	2	2	4
Total	177	129	306
N.A.	30	29	59
	207	158	365
Mean	23.9	22.4	23.3
Median	22	21	22

Table 2. Distribution of questionnaires by personnel completion

Physician	*Nurse*	*Aide*	*Patient*	*N*	*%*
X	X		X	106	29.0
X	X	X	X	95	26.0
X	X	X		36	9.9
X	X			35	9.6
X			X	33	9.0
			X	22	6.0
X				12	3.3
	X		X	8	2.2
	X	X	X	4	1.1
	X			4	1.1
	X	X		2	0.5
X		X	X	2	0.5
X		X		1	0.3
. .	. .	. .	. .	5	1.4
320	290	140	270	365	99.9
(87.7%)	(79.5%)	(38.4%)	(74.0%)		

Number with:

Both physician and nurse	272 (74.5%)
Both physician and patient	236 (64.7%)
Either physician or nurse and patient	248 (67.9%)

Table 3. Distribution of questionnaires by personnel completion, Negro and white patients

	Negro	*%*	*White*	*%*
M.D.	140	88.6	180	87.0
Nurse	123	77.8	167	80.7
Aide	56	35.4	84	40.6
Patient	111	70.3	159	76.8
Total	158		207	

Table 4. Distribution of Negro and white patients by personnels' and patients' evaluation of patients' pain (question 1)

	White		*Negro*	
Physician	N	%	N	%
1 (Very severe pain)	2	1	2	1
2 (Severe pain)	14	8	12	9
3 (Average pain)	142	79	106	76
4 (Mild pain)	21	12	17	12
5 (Very mild pain)	1	1	2	1
	180	101	139	99
Nurse	N	%	N	%
1	1	1	0	0
2	16	10	16	13
3	128	77	93	76
4	20	12	13	11
5	2	1	1	1
	167	101	123	101
Aide	N	%	N	%
1	3	4	0	0
2	6	7	7	13
3	61	73	40	73
4	12	14	8	15
5	1	1	0	0
	83	99	55	101
Patient	N	%	N	%
1	26	16	17	15
2	52	33	38	35
3	62	39	44	40
4	17	11	8	7
5	3	2	3	3
	160	101	110	100

younger. The mean age of the white mothers was 23.9 years and the median 22.0 years, while the Negro mean was 22.4 years and the median 21.0 years.

Table 2 gives the distribution of personnel completeness of the questionnaire and shows that the physicians completed 87.7 percent of all questionnaires, the nurses 79.5 percent and the aides only 38.4 percent. The patients responded to 74.0 percent of their questionnaires. Both a physician and a nurse evaluation appeared on 74.5 percent of the questionnaires. The completion rates were approximately equal by race as shown on Table 3.

Tables 4, 5, and 6 show the distribution of Negro and white patients by the personnel's evaluation of the patients' pain, behavior, and cooperation, respectively. Two conclusions appear obvious. *There are no observed Negro and white differences in pain response; and the involved personnel tend to evaluate the patients in the same way.* Statistical tests (Chi-square) were applied to each set of data where any differences could possibly be surmised, but

Table 5. Distribution of Negro and white patients by personnels' evaluation of patients' response to pain (question 2)

	White		*Negro*	
Physician	N	%	N	%
1 (Very excitedly)	12	7	15	11
2 (Excitedly)	51	28	27	19
3 (Average)	84	47	58	42
4 (Calmly)	30	17	35	25
5 (Very calmly)	3	2	4	3
	180	101	139	100
Nurse	N	%	N	%
1	11	7	6	5
2	30	18	34	28
3	82	49	53	43
4	38	23	25	20
5	6	4	5	4
	167	101	123	100
Aide	N	%	N	%
1	9	11	5	9
2	11	13	10	18
3	35	42	21	38
4	23	28	18	33
5	5	6	1	2
	83	100	55	100

Table 6. Distribution of Negro and white patients by personnels' evaluation of patients' cooperation (question 3)

	White		*Negro*	
Physician	N	%	N	%
1 (Very cooperative)	23	13	24	17
2 (Cooperative)	79	44	61	44
3 (Average)	53	29	33	24
4 (Uncooperative)	21	12	17	12
5 (Very uncooperative)	4	2	4	3
	180	100	139	100
Nurse	N	%	N	%
1	27	16	6	5
2	77	46	34	28
3	42	25	53	43
4	17	10	25	20
5	4	2	5	4
	167	99	123	100
Aide	N	%	N	%
1	18	22	11	20
2	37	45	19	35
3	23	28	14	25
4	4	5	10	18
5	1	1	1	2
	83	101	55	100

Table 7. Mean values of personnels' evaluation of Negro and white patients on pain response, and cooperation

	Physician	*Nurse*	*Aide*	*Patient*
Pain: (Range 1.0–very severe to 5.0–very mild)				
White	3.0 (180)	3.0 (167)	3.0 (83)	2.5 (160)
Negro	3.0 (139)	3.0 (123)	3.0 (55)	2.5 (110)
Response: (Range 1.0–very excited to 5.0–very calm)				
White	2.8 (180)	3.0 (167)	3.0 (83)	
Negro	2.9 (139)	2.9 (123)	3.0 (55)	
Coopreation: (Range 1.0–very cooperative to 5.0–very uncooperative)				
White	2.5 (180)	2.4 (167)	2.2 (83)	
Negro	2.4 (139)	2.9 (123)	2.5 (55)	

Table 8. Number of patients in sample, mean age, and mean parity by severity of pain evaluation by physician

Physicians' pain evaluation	*N*	*Mean age*	*Mean parity*
Severe or very severe	36	21.3	2.3
Average	65	22.5	2.7
Mild or very mild	44	25.3	3.7
	145	23.1	2.9

no statistically significant differences could be discerned.

It is difficult to determine the validity of these measures, of course, but there is evidence that the criteria used to judge the three components are relatively independent. For example, the correlation between the evaluation of pain and that of cooperation was only 0.26. For further clarification, mean score values for the three questions were calculated (shown on Table 7) and there appear to be no discernable differences in the scores, except that the mothers uniformly saw their pain as more severe than was judged by the staff people. This finding is consistent with that of Freedman's[6] in an investigation of painless childbirth.

Since the scales did not discern differences between Negro and white responses or between the various personnel evaluations of these responses, it was decided to determine if they would discern any other meaningful differences. It has been felt that age and parity (number of births by a mother) would be factors in pain response, with the older and higher parity mothers exhibiting less pain. A subsample of 145 mothers was selected and the records researched to find the parity of these mothers. As is shown in Table 8, this evaluation brings out the expected differences by parity and age and therefore appears to have discriminatory value.

DISCUSSION

Since no differences can be demonstrated between the pain reaction patterns of Negro and white O.B. patients, the factors that determine pain expression would appear to be similar for the two groups. In other words, cultural differences between lower class Negro and white mothers do not appear to be significant determinants of the patients' pain response. It could be asserted that individual differences in pain response are determined by some other set of social, psychological and biological characteristics. Even though this study did not investigate intra-white cultural differences, it would appear that generalizations, as those offered by Zborowski, need further corroboration.

Further, all personnel tended to evaluate the patients' behavioral response to pain similarly. Since training of health personnel is focused on engendering consistency of observation regarding biological phenomena, it is not possible to assume that health personnel will also view behavioral phenomena in consistent ways. While it is clear that physicians and nurses should be able to reliably observe the physiologic phenomena relating to clinical situations, it is by no means clear that they must share frames of reference with regard to the behavioral phenomena. However, since the involved nursing personnel made observations of pain response very similar to the physicians', it appears that they do, in fact, share frames of reference with regard to the evaluation of at least this one type of behavioral response pattern.

SUMMARY

Differential response to the pain experience of Negro and white women in childbirth is investigated in this study, utilizing evaluations made by O.B. interns and residents and O.B. nurses and attendants of the cooperation, degree of pain, and response to pain of 365 women during normal, spontaneous obstetrical deliveries. Two hundred and seven white mothers and 158 Negro mothers were evaluated. The findings indicate that there is not difference between Negro and white patients of similar social class in the cooperation, pain response and estimated degree of pain as measured. Significant factors influencing the response appear to be age and parity. The older and higher parity patients appear to be more cooperative and stoical. Patients tended to see their pain as greater than did the medical staff. Further, close agreement was shown between the physicians and the para-medical personnel in evaluating the patients' response, which seems to indicate that physicians and nursing personnel share frames of reference with regard to evaluation of pain response.

[6] Lawrence Zelic Freedman, "Childbirth While Conscious: Perspectives and Communication," *Journal of Nervous and Mental Disease*, 137 (1963), p. 4.

SECTION FIVE

Laboratory manipulation of pain perception

Section five differs from Section three mainly by its attempt to seek cause-and-effect relationships rather than rely simply on correlational evidence, such as determining the underlying reasons for the association between pain tolerance and sex. Cause-and-effect relationships can best be obtained in the laboratory, where there are strict environmental controls except for what is permitted to vary. Cause and effect are usually inferred when the independent variable is manipulated to be present or absent. Often the extent to which it is present is also varied. Variation of the independent variable should produce a corresponding effect on the dependent variable.

There is no guarantee that the experimenter has chosen the correct variable to manipulate; nor can he be sure that alternative explanations are not possible, since he cannot be absolutely sure of control. However, there is a substantial amount of control possible, unlike in the clinic, where control becomes extremely difficult.

In pain research it is very desirable to combine research strategies so that both clinic and laboratory settings are used. For example, the Tursky and Sternbach study (Reading 18, Section four) was part of a laboratory series that was based on a hospital study by Zborowski (1969). Johnson's research (Reading 24) also used both the laboratory and the clinic setting. Unfortunately, this approach is usually given lip service but rarely practiced.

Beecher (Reading 5, Section two) has consistently argued that pain research is best carried out in the clinic. His argument is based on the ineffectiveness of morphine and placebos in the laboratory because of the absence of anxiety. It is probably valid to say that there is not as much anxiety in the laboratory setting as there is in the clinic. However, it is not impossible to create anxiety in the laboratory. Zimbardo, Cohen, Weisenberg, Dworkin, and Firestone (Reading 20) conducted a laboratory study using electric shock on naive subjects. On the basis of learning measures, a physiological measure of autonomic functioning, verbal reports, as well as observation, there was a little doubt that a substantial amount of anxiety was generated in naive subjects. Obviously, with trained subjects (Hardy, Wolff, and Goodell, 1952) there is a great deal less anxiety for a variety of reasons.

The readings in this section emphasize several of the major types of variables used in the laboratory as a means of influencing the reaction to pain: (1) choice and subject control, (2) rehearsal and preparation for the painful stimulation, (3) attention, and (4) modeling. Each of these procedures has important implications for understanding the basic reactions to pain, as well as for applying them to the clinical control of pain.

The success of these procedures does not necessarily mean that the pain sensation has disappeared. Clinically, also, success in treatment often occurs when the pain reaction is reduced from the intolerable to the tolerable level. In signal detection terms (see editor's comment for Section two), frequently what happens is that the sensation remains unaltered but is not judged as being as aversive. Feather, Chapman, and Fisher (1972), for example, applied a signal detection theory analysis to a laboratory study of the effects of placebos. They found no change in pain sensitivity but did find a difference in the willingness to report the sensation as painful.

The Craig and Weiss study (Reading 25) is probably an example of a similar effect. They used constant nonaversive shock. Each one of a group of subjects was paired with a model who rated the nonaversive shocks as increasingly painful. In contrast to a control group, the model-paired subjects began to give ratings of painful to levels of shocks usually judged as nonaversive.

In the real world this modeling process probably operates in a similar manner among social-cultural groups. Members learn that some sensations are to be tolerated, whereas others are not. Some are labeled as painful, whereas others are not.

In their other studies Craig and Weiss (1971) and Craig and Neidermayer (1974) have demonstrated other influences of models on pain tolerance in a laboratory situation. In the first study (1971) subjects rated the intensity of incremental shocks after a confederate model rated them. In one situation the model tolerated a great deal of shock before labeling it painful, whereas in a second situation he tolerated a great deal less before terming it painful. The high-tolerance group of subjects rated shock of a mean intensity of 8.65 ma. as painful. The low-tolerance group rated a mean intensity of 2.50 ma (approximately 70% less intense shock) as painful. Furthermore, Craig and Neidermayer (1974) were not able to demonstrate any heart rate or skin conductance differences between the high-tolerance and low-tolerance groups that would show that the subjects were not merely masking subjective discomfort.

The modeling process is a shorthand vicarious means of teaching a person the consequences of a behavior without necessitating trial-and-error experience. Bandura (1969) has called it the major mode of human learning. Of course, it is likely that both a modeling and trial-and-error combination are involved in teaching a person appropriate reactions to pain. Neufeld and Davidson (Reading 23) have demonstrated a similar effect of vicarious or cognitive rehearsal on pain tolerance. In the vicarious situation the subject watched another person experiencing the aversive stimulus, whereas in the cognitive situation the subject heard it described in detail. No differences were found between treatments. In the clinic modeling can be an extremely effective procedure for reducing fear, anxiety, and pain (Weisenberg and Epstein, 1973).

Preparation for aversive stimulation has been used effectively with surgical patients. (These studies will be discussed in greater detail in Section eight.) Neufeld and Davidson (Reading 23) suggest that rehearsal should be repeated over a period of time prior to the aversive event, such as several sessions separated by a week's time.

Johnson (Reading 24) presents evidence concerning the effectiveness of different types of preparations. She found that information fostering congruency between expectations and experience can reduce distress but not the perception of the sensation itself. Johnson has thus found that information regarding the sensations to be experienced is more effective in reducing stress than information regarding the procedures to be used. Reducing the incongruency between expectations and experience is one way of reducing anxiety based on fear of the unknown.

Allowing the subject to exert control over the onset of the aversive stimulation is another technique for reducing the aversiveness of noxious stimulation. Staub, Tursky, and Schwartz (Reading 21) have demonstrated how control can indeed affect the level of shock that subjects are willing to take. Zimbardo and others (Reading 20) have also demonstrated how choice and justification can be used to affect the reaction to pain.

In the clinic there is too often a fear of

allowing patients some degree of control over the situation. For example, Linn (1967) observed 27 dentists, their assistants, and 114 patients at two dental clinics to determine behaviors in the doctor-patient relationship that are necessary for the relationship to continue. The most important role for the patient was conformity, whereas the most important role for the dentist was authority to direct. Patients rarely directed or requested anything from the dentist. Yet, allowing the patient some degree of choice and control could probably have reduced the patient's distress and enhanced his ability to tolerate pain.

REFERENCES

Bandura, A. 1969. Principles of behavior modification, Holt, Rinehart and Winston, Inc., New York.

Craig, K. D., and Neidermayer, H. 1974. Autonomic correlates of pain thresholds influenced by social modeling, Journal of Personality and Social Psychology **29:**246-252.

Craig, K. D., and Weiss, S. M. 1971. Vicarious influences on pain-threshold determinations, Journal of Personality and Social Psychology **19:**53-59.

Feather, B. W., Chapman, C. R., and Fisher, B. A. 1972. The effect of a placebo on the perception of painful radiant heat stimuli, Psychosomatic Medicine **34:**290-294.

Hardy, J. D., Wolff, H. G., and Goodell, H. 1952. Pain sensations and reactions, Hafner Publishing Co., New York.

Linn, E. L. 1967. Role behaviors in two dental clinics: a trial of Nadel's criteria, Human Organization **26:** 141-148.

Weisenberg, M., and Epstein, D. 1973. Patient education as an alternative to general anesthesia, New York State Dental Journal **39:**610-613.

Zborowski, M. 1969. People in pain, Jossey-Bass, Inc., Publishers, San Francisco.

20

Control of pain motivation by cognitive dissonance

Philip G. Zimbardo, Arthur R. Cohen, Matisyohu Weisenberg, Leonard Dworkin, and Ira Firestone

Research on the "placebo problem" amply demonstrates that perception of pain may be influenced by psychological factors. One thorough survey *(1)* revealed that in nearly 100 independent studies of 29 different symptoms and sicknesses pain-reduction was achieved in an average of 27 percent of over 4500 cases of all types. In some studies the incidence of pain-reduction was as high as 75 percent, and in some a placebo was as effective as morphine.

While there is no clear understanding of the dynamics of a positive placebo reaction, the evidence suggests that experience of pain and other (aversive) motivational states may be influenced considerably by cognitive factors. Moreover, expectancies concerning future events (that is, that the "drug" will work and pain will be alleviated) can alter both psychological and physiological processes, thereby effecting changes in the way in which avoidance of pain motivates the individual.

This report describes one theoretical approach to the problem of control of motivational states by means of cognitive processes and an experimental study derived from this model which specifies several cognitive variables crucial in mediating pain-reduction.

Festinger's theory of cognitive dissonance *(2)* assumes a basic tendency toward consistency of cognitions about oneself and about the environment. When two or more relevant cognitive elements (or sets) are in a psychologically inconsistent relation, dissonance is created. For example, the cognition, "I believe cigarette smoking causes cancer," and the cognition, "I am voluntarily continuing to smoke cigarettes," are dissonant if the person does not want to get cancer. Dissonance can arise from one's awareness that he is behaving in ways which do not follow from his beliefs, opinions, values, or motives and can be defined as a tension state which motivates behavior; behavior which is followed by a reduction in dissonance is reinforced.

Our present concern is application of this theory to a situation in which a person is induced to commit himself voluntarily to a state of deprivation or to an aversive stimulus. If a person has knowledge of unpleasantness of the situation and of his freedom to choose to avoid it, his agreeing to endure more of the situation is dissonant. Although such a commitment obviously requires some coercive force, in order for dissonance to be aroused it is necessary for the person to maintain his perception of having choice to do otherwise (and thus of having responsibility for consequences of the decision). The greater the coercive force exerted (in the form of justification, reward, or punishment), the more consistent will be the "discrepant" behavioral commitment, and the less the dissonance. The magnitude of dissonance, therefore, will be a function of the propor-

From the Department of Psychology, University College, New York University, New York 10453.

tion of cognitions which are inconsistent with commitment and those which support the decision *(3)*. Attempts to reduce dissonance will be in the nature of redefining the situation by adding new cognitions or modifying existing ones. When it is difficult to deny the reality of one's behavioral commitment, a more likely dissonance-reducing behavior should be modification of one's cognitions about the drive state. For example, if one "feels" less thirsty or hungry, commitment to further deprivation of water or food would be less dissonant. The total process of dissonance-reduction may lead to an alteration of both the cognitive and noncognitive components of any motivational state and thus the drive itself may be functionally lowered. If so, then various consummatory and physiological behaviors correlated with that motive, as well as subjective and instrumental reactions to it, should decrease.

To test these derivations from dissonance theory, we employed an experimental paradigm in which 80 male undergraduate subjects were tested individually in a two-phase experiment. After their thresholds for painful shock had been determined and they had learned a practice list of words without shock, subjects had to learn a list of nine words by the serial-anticipation method while being given two unavoidable painful shocks per trial until they reached the criterion (two successive errorless trials). The list was composed of sets of semantically similar words *(4)* so that under conditions of shock-induced high drive it took more trials to memorize the list because generalization rather than discrimination was facilitated.

Three groups of subjects were not given a choice of continuing to a second part of the experiment, which was the same as the first except for a list of matched words. For one of these no-choice control groups shock was maintained at a high level in both parts of the experiment (Hi-Hi); for the second group it was lowered to a moderate level (Hi-Mod), while the third group received low shock throughout the study, and this group was used only as a specific control for effects of shock level on learning (Lo-Lo).

As subjects in the dissonance conditions were preparing to leave after the first part of the experiment (since they had been led to expect that the experiment was complete), they were asked to volunteer (explicitly given a choice) for the second part, a comparable experiment. Two levels of dissonance were created by giving half of these subjects (Lo-Dis) various justifications for engaging in discrepant behavior in terms of its importance to the experimenter, to science, the subject, the space program, and so forth. On the other hand, subjects in the Hi-Dis condition were given minimum justification before making their choice; in fact, verbal manipulation was designed specifically to deny a subject the possibility of generating justifications like those provided for the Lo-Dis subjects. This was done to increase the likelihood that cognitive reevaluations would be in terms of aversiveness of the shock and not in terms of extrinsic value of participation. There was not a differential attrition (self-selected dropout) rate in the two dissonance groups. In both parts of the experiment the following dependent measures were obtained: a subjective estimate of painfulness of a sample of the shock to be given, learning performance, and galvanic skin resistance to the shocks.

Control subjects (not given a choice) are treated comparably to subjects in standard laboratory studies of motivation, and their behavior should be primarily under control of physical intensity of the shock. Similarly, Lo-Dis subjects, having been provided with cognitions which are consistent with their choice, have little need for generating a psychological reinterpretation of shock-induced motive. For these subjects also there should be a close correspondence between stimulus intensity and reactivity. On the other hand, Hi-Dis subjects must engage in a psychological process (not necessarily conscious) of reevaluating painfulness of the shock. If they do so effectively, they reduce the dissonance occasioned by commitment to more shock. Thus, they should behave similarly to the Hi-Mod subjects for whom shock voltage has been physically reduced.

Assessment of experimental manipulations, by means of a questionnaire after the experiments, revealed that we had been successful in creating the impression that dissonance groups had considerable choice

Table 1. Mean perceived pain in relation to actual level of physical shock. An arbitrary scale of pain intensity was used to designate the perceived pain, and the numerical values were reported by the subjects. Scale values: 0, not painful; 20, slightly painful; 40, moderately painful; 60, very painful; 80, extremely painful; and 100, tremendously painful. The number of subjects in each group is shown in parentheses.

Mean shock (volts)	*Perceived pain (values on arbitrary scale)*		
	*Part 1 of expt.**	*Part 2 of expt.**	*Difference*
Lo-Dis group (20)			
38.0	49.4	47.6	−1.8
Hi-Dis group (20)			
49.5	46.0	36.8	−9.2
Hi-Mod control group (15)			
44.6	46.0		
22.0		19.8	−26.2
Hi-Hi control group (15)			
44.3	50.2	47.3	−2.9

*Part 1, precommitment, took place before the subject chose to continue the experiment; part 2, postcommitment, after the choice had been made.

in committing themselves to the second painful situation, while controls perceived that they had little choice ($p < .01$). Also, only the Lo-Dis group perceived that the importance of the "second experiment" was significantly greater than the first ($p < .05$). Therefore, the choice and justification conditions necessary for testing the dissonance theory hypothesis had been satisfied.

Table 1 presents data for subjective evaluation of painfulness of the sample shock in each part of the experiment. The Lo-Dis group, like the control group with high shock throughout, shows only a minor decrement due to adaptation. The control group, shifted from a high to a moderate level of shock, shows a corresponding shift in perception of pain and one that is quite veridical. Our attention centers upon the Hi-Dis group, which reports that the same high level of shock is less painful after commitment to more shock. The Hi-Mod group differs from all others by $p < .01$, while the Hi-Dis differs from the Hi-Hi and Lo-Dis groups by $p < .10$.

Thus we have the predicted trend of dis-

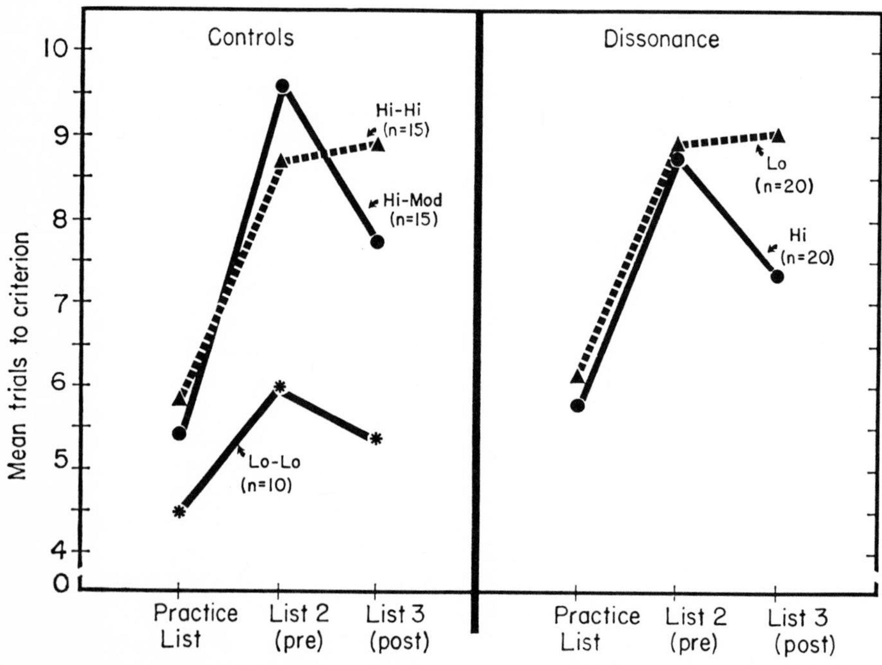

Fig. 1. Mean number of trials to reach criterion in a serial-anticipation learning task (the greater the number, the poorer the learning).

sonance influencing verbalization: many of the subjects said the shock "doesn't hurt so much." But did it really hurt less, or were they only role-playing? If there had in fact been a change in pain motive itself, then there should be a measurable effect upon learning behavior which is less amenable to conscious distortion and directly influenced by differences in strength of the shock stimulus which induces the pain motive.

Figure 1 reveals that for the three control groups the number of trials required to reach criterion is a function of the level of shock intensity; learning is poorer when shock level is higher and improves when shock level is reduced. These findings are reflected in kind by curves for dissonance groups which perform identically on the practice and premanipulation word lists. From this comparable base line, the groups diverge after commitment: the Lo-Dis group responds exactly like the Hi-Hi control, while the Hi-Dis group improves its performance in the same way as the Hi-Mod control group, in which shock is physically reduced by over 20 volts. These differences are statistically significant even when any initial differences in learning performance prior to commitment are covaried out (Hi-Dis versus Lo-Dis: $t = 2.38$, $p = .01$; control groups: $t = 2.03$, $p = .05$) *(5)*.

These average group effects are not due to a few extreme subjects since 70 percent of the Hi-Dis group and 60 percent of the Hi-Mod group improve, while for the Lo-Dis and Hi-Hi groups there is improvement by only 40 percent and 33 percent, respectively. This effect is revealed in statistically significant fashion on a number of different analyses of the learning performance. Thus we have been able to bring the learning performance of Hi-Dis subjects under a similar degree of control with verbal-cognitive manipulations, as has been possible with the Hi-Mod group by use of variations in shock intensity.

Next we turn to physiological data to determine whether changes noted above in cognitions and learning extend to the noncognitive component of pain. Figure 2 presents mean galvanic skin resistance (GSR) data for each of the four main groups, subtracting a subject's GSR to each of the first three shocks in list 2 from each of the first three shocks in list 3. These results clearly parallel those obtained at each of the other two levels of analysis. The control group given high shock throughout shows an increase in physiological responsiveness to shocks, while, as expected, lowering the shock for the Hi-Mod group produces a decrement in GSR. What is dramatic, however, is the fact that the Lo-Dis group again mirrors the Hi-Hi control, while the Hi-Dis group behaves physiologically as if shocks (of constant intensity) did not hurt as much after commitment as they had before ($F = 3.05$, $p < .05$; Hi-Dis versus Lo-Dis: $t = 2.00$, $p < .05$; control groups: $t = 2.24$, $p < .05$). These differences remain significant even after covarying changes in basal skin resistance.

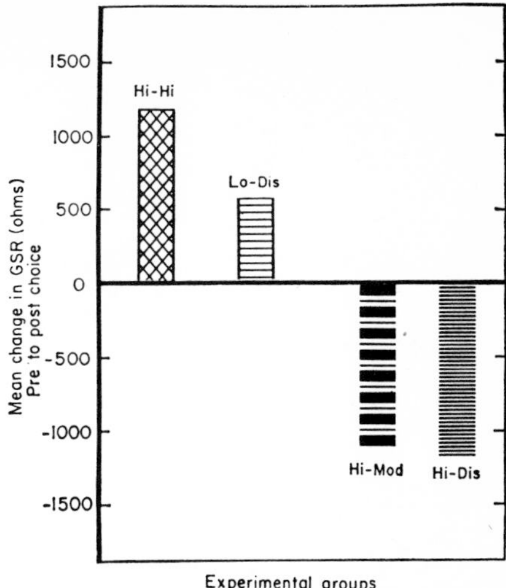

Fig. 2. Mean difference in galvanic skin response (GSR), expressed in ohms, from the first three shocks in word-list 2 (precommitment) to the first three shocks in word-list 3 (postcommitment). (Negative values indicate a reduction in GSR, while positive ones indicate an increase.)

Evidence has been presented which appears to validate the position derived from the theory of cognitive dissonance that voluntary commitment for minimal justification to a behavior which is discrepant with a motivational state can effectively limit the impact of that motive upon behavior. Recent studies in our laboratory and elsewhere *(6)* lead us to believe that this motivational control is demonstrable across a wide range of primary and socially acquired drives.

REFERENCES AND NOTES

1. H. Haas, H. Fink, G. Hartfelder, "Das Placeboproblem" which appeared in *Fortschr. Arzneimittelforsch.* **1,** 279 (1959); translation of selected parts appeared in *Psychopharmacol. Serv. Center Bull.* **8,** 1 (1963).
2. L. Festinger, *A Theory of Cognitive Dissonance* (Stanford Univ. Press, Stanford, Calif., 1957).
3. For a fuller discussion see J. Brehm and A. R. Cohen, *Explorations in Cognitive Dissonance* (Wiley, New York, 1962).
4. R. C. Carson, *J. Abnorm. Soc, Psychol.* **57,** 99 (1958).
5. Data analyzed by IBM program BMDO6V; general linear hypothesis with contrasts.
6. This research was financed by an NSF grant (GS-226) to New York University (P. Zimbardo, principal investigator) and represents part of a larger project initiated by A. R. Cohen before his recent death. A fuller report of this study is in preparation and will appear as a monograph published by Scott, Foresman and Company, Chicago.

21

Self-control and predictability
Their effects on reactions to aversive stimulation[1]

Ervin Staub,[2] Bernard Tursky, and Gary E. Schwartz

The ability to predict and control events in the environment is important for the comfort and safety of organisms. Consequently, control and predictability may come to be valued for their own sake, while lack of control, uncertainty, and unpredictability may become intrinsically aversive.

Both animals (Lockard, 1963; Perkins, Levis, & Seyman, 1963) and man (Badia, McBane, Suter, & Lewis, 1966; Lanzetta & Driscoll, 1966; Pervin, 1963) were found to prefer information about the onset of aversive stimuli, even when the information had no instrumental value. People preferred knowledge about what will happen, whether the outcome alternatives were shock versus no shock, reward versus no reward, or reward versus shock (Lanzetta & Driscoll, 1966). Furthermore, both predictability and control seem to reduce the impact of aversive stimuli on organisms. The ability to terminate electric shocks resulted in less disruption of eating behavior of rats (Mowrer & Vieck, 1948), as well as less ulceration (Weiss, 1968) than the same amount of uncontrollable shocks. The effects of aversive stimuli were diminished in several experiments by subjects' *belief* in their ability to terminate them (Bowers, 1968; Glass, Singer, & Friedman, 1969). Glass et al. found that an unpredictable loud noise disrupted subsequent problem-solving and task behavior more than a predictable one, but the differences disappeared when subjects believed that by pushing a button they could terminate the unpredictable noise. Predictability is usually a precondition for control, and unpredictability may have similar psychological effects to lack of control.

Reduction in the impact of stimuli was found even when there was no opportunity (perceived or real) to terminate or avoid aversive stimuli, only to regulate the manner of experiencing them (Staub, 1968). The ability to self-administer electric shocks rather than have them administered by the experimenter (Haggard, 1943) and instructions to the effect that the sequence of subtests of an intelligence test could be determined by subjects rather than predetermined by the experimenter (Stotland & Blumenthal, 1964) both resulted in less physiological arousal, as measured by galvanic skin response.

The present study aimed to extend the investigation of the "impact-reducing" effect of control and predictability by examining their effect on the subjective evaluation of aversive stimuli. Subjects were provided with control, in the sense of regulating the manner of experiencing aversive stimuli rather than terminating them; in many life situations this may be the only type of control possible. The effects of

From the Journal of Personality and Social Psychology **18:**157-162.

[1]This research was supported by National Institutes of Health Grant MH 04172(09) to Bernard Tursky, a Harvard Graduate Society grant to Ervin Staub, and United States Public Health Service Predoctoral Research Fellowship Grant MH 3613-02 to Gary E. Schwartz. The authors are grateful to Linda Onuska for her assistance.

[2]From the Department of Social Relations, Harvard University, William James Hall, Cambridge, Massachusetts 02138.

variation in control and in associated predictability on the perceived aversiveness of electric shocks, including a behavioral measure of endurance, and on physiological reactions to the shocks were explored. The first experiment was designed to determine whether simple control per se of the onset of electric shocks would influence reactions to the shocks. In the second experiment, control of the onset, the intensity, and the time of stimulation was given to the subjects. In both experiments, a yoked-control group was employed to assess the effects of the above variables; yoked subjects received an identical sequence of shocks. In addition, all subjects were given a second experience, also yoked, in order to study the effects of loss of control. It was predicted that subjects having control of the shocks would evaluate shocks as less unpleasant and would tolerate higher levels of stimulation than subjects having no control, and that the greater the difference in control and predictability, the greater the difference in tolerance. It was also expected that loss of control would decrease tolerance levels of self-control subjects.

EXPERIMENT I

Method

Subjects were seated in a lounge chair in a sound- and temperature-controlled experimental room. Verbal contact was maintained by means of a two-way intercom system, and the experimenter could observe the subject through a one-way mirror from the adjacent equipment room.

Electrical stimulation was delivered through an annular electrode (Tursky, Watson, & O'Connell, 1965) to the dorsal surface of the left forearm from a 60-Hertz controlled-current stimulator. Impedance of the electrode skin circuit was reduced to 5,000 ohms to insure uniformity of stimulus strength (Tursky & Watson, 1964). Duration of the shock, which was always 1 second, and other experimental events were controlled by Grason-Stadler solid-state programming equipment.

Heart rate was recorded on one channel of a Beckman Type R dynograph from a pair of standard electrocardiogram electrodes placed on the subject's left arm and right leg. Beat by beat rate information was obtained with a Lexington Instruments cardiotachometer. All experimental events were recorded on a second channel of the polygraph to insure accurate measurement of heart rate.

Subjects and procedure. Twenty paid subjects were divided into a self-control and a no-control group. Subjects were told that the experiment was designed to record physiological reactions to electric shock. Self-control subjects were given a switch which enabled them to administer the electric shocks to themselves. The experimenter increased the intensity of shocks in small steps (.2 milliamperes) from an imperceptible shock to the subjects' limit of endurance. The experimenter signaled the self-control subjects when a new level was set by turning on a light. Self-control subjects were told that they could deliver the shock to themselves at any time after the ready light went on. The switch and signal lights were not available to no-control subjects, who were administered the shocks by the experimenter. To insure that the no-control subjects received shocks in the identical temporal order as the self-control subjects, a brief tone was recorded on a continuously running audiotape at each shock. The tape record for a given self-control subject was used to operate the programming equipment to administer shocks to one no-control subject. This procedure ensured a temporally yoked no-control subject for each self-control subject. All subjects were instructed that shock intensity would increase in small steps and that they should report when they first felt the stimulus (sensation threshold), when it became uncomfortable, painful, and when they did not wish to go any higher (endurance). This last judgment represented a decision that subjects were unwilling to endure more shock. Subjects were told that they would be asked to make several "reports" of subjective intensity; after each report, they were told what intensity level they should report next.

After a short rest period, all subjects were given a second shock experience. In this session the control switch and light were taken away from the self-control subjects. Subjects were asked to make judgments about subjective experience and endurance as before. All shocks were delivered by means of the original audiotape recording, providing the same temporal sequence to each subject, as on the first administration.

Results

Differences between groups were evaluated by matched *t* tests, based on average differences in shocks received by yoked subjects, thus eliminating variability due to differences in the timing of shocks. No significant differences in average shock intensity were obtained on either the first or second administrations at any of the four levels of judgment, nor were any trends found that approached significance. Subjects in the self-control group tended to administer the shocks to themselves in rapid sequence (approximately 5 seconds between shocks). Cardiac responses to the shocks were not evaluated because of the overlap of responses from shock to shock.

Discussion

Because the subjects in the self-control group tended to administer the shocks to themselves as rapidly as possible, the timing of the shocks became predictable in the no-control group. Consequently, only the identity of the person who actually delivered the shocks, the subject or the experimenter, differentiated the two groups. The subjective level data indicate that under these conditions, variation in control over the onset of the stimulus did not, in itself, influence reactions to aversive stimulation.

EXPERIMENT II

Method

Subjects and procedure. Twenty paid male college students were divided into a self-control and a no-control group. As in Experiment I, self-control subjects were given a switch box that enabled them to deliver the shocks to themselves. However, in the present experiment, these subjects were given a second switch, which allowed them to control the increase in intensity of the shocks by one, two, or three increments (each increment was .2 milliamperes). In addition, self-control subjects received a light between shocks, varying in duration from 10 to 20 seconds. During this time they selected the increment of the next shock. Self-control subjects were instructed to deliver the shock any time after the light went off. The purpose of this light was to ensure variability in the timing of the shocks and thereby decrease predictability for no-control subjects. All subjects were asked to identify each of the four subjective levels of shock: sensation, uncomfortable, painful, and endurance. The temporal order of the shocks of self-control subjects was again recorded on an audiotape recorder, the tapes used to present the shocks for both administrations to the yoked–no-control subjects and for the second administration to the self-control subjects. In addition to temporal order, no-control subjects were also yoked to self-control subjects on the magnitude of shock increments. Thus, in addition to the basic self-control variable of delivering the shocks, self-control subjects in the present experiment controlled (and therefore could predict) the relative intensity of the next shock, as well as the time of shock presentation. This procedure insured that both the time of presentations and the size of shock increments were unpredictable in the no-control condition.

Table 1. Average shock intensity in milliamperes at four levels of judgment in the self-control and no-control groups, on the first and second administration of shocks

	Self-control (n = 10)		*No control (n = 10)*	
Judgment level	*First administration (self-control)*	*Second administration (no control)*	*First administration (no control)*	*Second administration (no control)*
Sensation threshold	.49	.43	.38	.32
Uncomfortable	3.78	2.16	2.29	2.29
Painful	4.86	4.15	4.02	4.24
Limit of endurance	6.54	6.19	5.15	5.67

RESULTS

Table 1 shows the mean levels of shock in each group, at each of the four levels of judgment, both on the first and the second administration. Differences between the two groups in the average amount of shock at each of the four levels of judgment were again evaluated by matched t tests, based on differences in shocks received by pairs of yoked subjects.

As predicted, both the evaluation of the aversiveness of the shocks and the willingness to endure it were affected by differences in control and predictability. Subjects in the self-control group reached significantly greater levels of shock before they reported it as uncomfortable than subjects in the no-control group ($t = 2.44$, $df = 9$, $p < .02$).[3] In addition, subjects in the self-control group endured somewhat stronger shocks than those in the no-control group ($t = 1.82$, $df = 9$, $p < .06$).

The effects of loss of control on reactions to shocks were also examined. Subjects who lost control evaluated significantly lower intensity shocks as uncomfortable under no control than they did under self-control ($t = 2.57$, $df = 9$, $p < .02$) and endured somewhat less shock ($t = 1.54$, $df = 9$, $p < .10$). Comparable changes in the no-control group, when the experimenter controlled both administrations of the shock, were negligible. Comparisons between changes from the first to the second administration of shock in the two groups showed that relative to subjects who did not have control, subjects who lost control came to perceive the shocks as uncomfortable at lower intensities ($t = 2.38$, $df = 18$, $p < .02$), and they came to endure somewhat less shock ($t = 1.81$, $df = 18$, $p < .05$).

Physiological reactions to the first administration of shocks were also evaluated. Heart rate was scored second by second for both the 5 seconds preceding and the 5 seconds following the offset of shocks. Analysis of variance of preshock scores showed that although self-control subjects tended to have higher average heart rates, neither the difference in average heart rate nor in the pattern of heart rate second by second was significant. To evaluate cardiac responses elecited by the shocks, average heart rates 5 seconds before and 5 seconds after stimulation were employed. An analysis of variance was performed with the factors, subjective judgment points (four levels), locus of control (two levels), preshocks to postshocks (two levels), and subjects (nine levels).[4] Overall, the average cardiac responses to the shocks at the four levels of judgment were acceleratory; heart rate after the shocks was significantly higher than before the shocks ($F = 62.50$, $df = 1/8$, $p < .001$). In addition, a marginally significant interaction was found between treatments, the four levels of judgment, and preshock and postshock values in heart rate ($F = 2.64$, $df = 3/24$, $p < .08$). These results are depicted in Figure 1. An examination of this figure shows that in the self-control group, the heart rate response to the shocks gradually increased from the sensation threshold to the endurance limit, from about 0 to almost 7 beats per minute. In contrast, in the no-control group, the increase in heart rate in response to the shock was already large at the sensation threshold, and the magnitude of the increase in heart rate was about the same at the other three judgment points.

Differences in cardiac response to electric shocks in the two groups at three discrete shock intensities, 1, 3, and 5 milliamperes, were also evaluated.[5] Comparison of average post- minus preshock heart rate in the two groups during the first adminis-

[3]The t tests of the difference between groups in average shock at subjective judgment points and at the limit of endurance, and of changes within groups following loss of control, are testing straightforward hypotheses described in the Introduction; related p values are therefore reported for one-tailed tests. p values related to physiological reactions to the shocks (see below) are all based on two-tailed tests.

[4]As in the above t tests, subjects were treated as matched yoked pairs, and the analysis of variance treated all factors, including locus of control, as repeated measures. Missing heart rate data restricted the analysis to nine pairs of subjects. Analyses were performed on an IBM 7094 using BIOMED 08V ANOVA programs.

[5]t tests rather than analyses of variance were employed because the number of remaining subjects decreased with increasing shock levels, thus causing problems with unequal ns in the repeated-measures design. Moreover, it was no longer possible to match subjects, since yoked subjects did not stop at the same point.

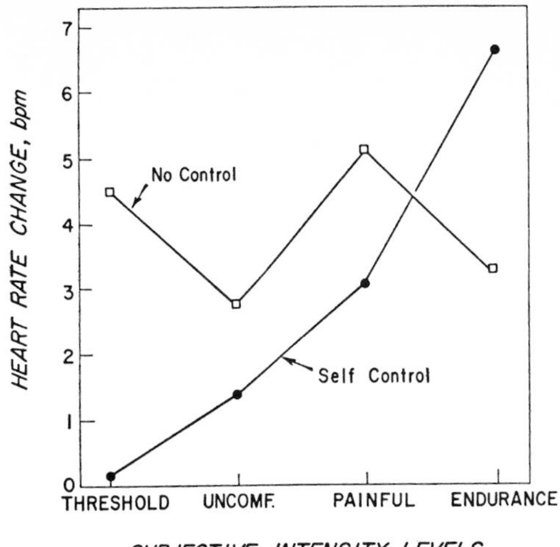

Fig. 1. Average heart rate responses (postshock minus preshock) of self-control and no-control subjects to shocks at each level of subjective intensity.

tration of shocks showed no difference at 1 and 3 milliamperes, but a significantly greater increase in heart rate was found in response to the shocks in the no-control group at 5 milliamperes ($t = 2.83$, $df = 12$, $p < .02$; seven subjects in each group reached the 5-milliampere intensity).

DISCUSSION

In Experiment II differences in control and predictability influenced reactions to aversive stimuli in the expected manner. Subjects in both treatment groups received identical sequences of shocks. However, subjects who could predict and had control over the administration of the shocks and the increase in their intensity evaluated significantly more intense shocks as uncomfortable and endured somewhat more intense shock than those who could not. With loss of control on the second administration of shocks in the self-control group, there was a decrease in the intensity of shocks that were evaluated as uncomfortable and in the intensity of shock endured.

Previous experiments discussed in the Introduction showed that control and predictability reduce tension and the disruption of behavior produced by aversive stimuli. The present findings show that perceived aversiveness as well as willingness to endure aversive stimulation are also influenced by predictability and control. Uncertainty or unpredictability may become intrinsically aversive (Berlyne, 1961), because it is likely to be associated with the inability to fend off aversive experiences. It is difficult to deal with the unpredictable. For this reason, uncertainty and lack of control may be intimately related. Lack of control represents a condition of helplessness; the ability to predict events may reduce the subjective experience of helplessness, even when control is not possible, and thereby reduce tension or anxiety.

Examination of heart rate reactions showed no difference between the self-control and no-control groups prior to the shocks. While some previous research showed heart rate deceleration in the last seconds before anticipated shocks (Obrist, 1968), in the self-control group, where the shocks were predictable, such deceleration may have been counteracted by cardiac acceleration, due to mental effort involved in the task (Tursky, Schwartz, & Crider, 1970), as well as to preparation for making an overt response (Elliott, 1969).

Comparison of cardiac responses at specific subjective intensities, where subjects presumably perceived the shocks as similar in intensity, demonstrated that subjects who could not control and predict the shocks tended to produce large heart rate responses at all levels of intensity, while self-control subjects made more differentiated responses. It is possible that control and predictability enables people to respond according to the significance of stimuli, while lack of control and predictability may enhance the potential importance of all stressful events, resulting in less differentiated reactions to them. Comparison of cardiac responses in the two groups at *given* physical intensities of shock, when subjects presumably perceived the shock as different in intensity, showed that reaction to a high-intensity shock (5 milliamperes) was significantly greater in the no-control than in the self-control group. Variation in control and predictability may influence expectations about aversive stimuli, such as probable intensity. Expectations created about a forthcoming stimulus have been found to influence physiological reactions to aversive stimuli (Cook & Harris, 1937; Epstein & Clarke, 1970).

The lack of significant differences in Experiment I suggests that the differences in Experiment II were not due to differential expectations created by self-control and no-control instructions, since these instructions were highly similar in the two experiments. The lack of differential effect of self-control and no control in Experiment I suggests, moreover, that a difference in who pushed the button was not, by itself, of great psychological significance. "Control" in this experiment did not mean the possibility of terminating or avoiding shocks, but rather the ability to influence the manner of experiencing them. Under such conditions the major importance of control may be that it increases predictability. Previous research findings (Glass et al., 1969) together with the present ones suggest the possibility that under some conditions, control and predictability may function interchangeably as safety signals that reduce threat and the impact of aversive stimuli; when the ability to terminate aversive stimuli is lacking, predictability may reduce impact, and when the ability to predict is lacking, perceived ability to terminate aversive stimuli may have a similar effect (Glass et al., 1969).

REFERENCES

Badia, P., McBane, B., Suter, S., & Lewis, P. Preference behavior in an immediate versus variably delayed shock situation with and without a warning signal. *Journal of Experimental Psychology,* 1966, **72,** 847-852.

Berlyne, D. E. *Conflict, arousal and curiosity.* New York: McGraw-Hill, 1961.

Bowers, K. S. Pain, anxiety, and perceived control. *Journal of Consulting and Clinical Psychology,* 1968, **32,** 596-602.

Cook, S. W., & Harris, R. E. The verbal conditioning of the galvanic skin reflex. *Journal of Experimental Psychology,* 1937, **21,** 202-210.

Elliott, R. Tonic heart rate: Experiments on the effects of collative variables lead to a hypothesis about its motivational significance. *Journal of Personality and Social Psychology,* 1969, **12,** 211-228.

Epstein, S., & Clarke, S. Heart rate and skin conductance during experimentally induced anxiety: Effects of anticipated intensity of noxious stimulation and experience, *Journal of Experimental Psychology,* 1970, **84,** 105-112.

Glass, D. C., Singer, J. E., & Friedman, L. N. Psychic cost of adaptation to an environmental stressor. *Journal of Personality and Social Psychology,* 1969, **12,** 200-210.

Haggard, E. Some conditions determining adjustment during and readjustment following experimentally induced stress. In S. Tomkins (Ed.), *Contemporary psychopathology.* Cambridge: Harvard University Press, 1943.

Lanzetta, J. T., & Driscoll, J. Preference for information about an uncertain but unavoidable outcome. *Journal of Personality and Social Psychology,* 1966, **3,** 96-102.

Lockard, J. S. Choice of a warning signal or no warning signal in an unavoidable shock situation. *Journal of Comparative and Physiological Psychology,* 1963, **56,** 526-530.

Mowrer, O. H., & Vieck, P. Experimental analogue of fear from a sense of helplessness. *Journal of Abnormal and Social Psychology,* 1948, **43,** 193.

Obrist, P. A. Heart rate and somatic-motor coupling during classical aversive conditioning in humans. *Journal of Experimental Psychology,* 1968, **77,** 180-193.

Perkins, C. C., Jr., Levis, D. F., & Seyman, R. Preference for signal-shock versus shock-signal. *Psychological Reports,* 1963, **13,** 735-738.

Pervin, L. A. The need to predict and control under conditions of threat. *Journal of Personality,* 1963, **31,** 570-587.

Staub, E. Reduction of a specific fear by information combined with exposure to a feared stimulus. *Procedings of the 76th Annual Convention of the American Psychological Association,* 1968, **3,** 525-527. (Summary)

Stotland, E., & Blumenthal, A. The reduction of anxiety as a result of the expectation of making a choice. *Canadian Journal of Psychology,* 1964, **18,** 139-145.

Tursky, B., & Watson, P. D. Controlled physical and subjective intensities of electric shock. *Psychophysiology,* 1964, **1,** 151-162.

Tursky, B., Watson, P. D., & O'Connell, D. N. A concentric shock electrode for pain stimulation. *Psychophysiology,* 1965, **1,** 296-298.

Tursky, B., Schwartz, G. E., & Crider, A. Differential patterns of heart rate and skin resistance during a digit-transformation task. *Journal of Experimental Psychology,* 1970, **83,** 451-457.

Weiss, J. M. Effects of coping responses on stress. *Journal of Comparative and Physiological Psychology,* 1968, **65,** 251-260.

22

Role of attentional focus in pain perception

Manipulation of response to noxious stimulation by instructions[1]

Bernard Blitz[2] and Albert J. Dinnerstein

It has long been recognized that the experience of pain is readily affected by motivational, perceptual, and cognitive processes. Recent experimental work has begun to explore the nature of this relationship of "higher order" processes to pain, with an interest both in theoretical formulation and in practical application to the management of clinical pain. One area of this research has been the role of instructions and suggestion in pain perception (Barber & Hahn, 1962; Blitz & Dinnerstein, 1968; Hilgard, Cooper, Lenox, Morgan, & Voevodsky, 1967; Wolff & Horland, 1967). This is the concern of the present study.

What are the processes whereby instructions and suggestion produce some degree of analgesia? It is the present authors' belief that attentional mechanisms serve a major function in producing analgesic effects. In a recent study of hypnotic analgesia, Hilgard et al. (1967) reported that one of their group of *S*s, who were asked to simulate hypnotic analgesia, achieved complete analgesia and did this by "focusing my eyes on a spot on my dress and concentrating on that, withholding attention from my arm [p. 509]." The degree of dissociation this *S* achieved so resembled that of the hypnotic state that her results were suspect and not included in the interpretation of the data. This observation, although it admittedly presents experimental difficulties, points to the potential role of attentional mechanisms in hypnotic and other forms of suggested analgesia.

One of the mechanisms which people frequently report using in their attempts to control pain is that of regulating their focus of attention. Ischlondsky (1949) stated that Pascal, who suffered from neuralgias, and Kant, who struggled with painful gout, relieved their pain by concentrating on challenging problems. This skill in self-distraction varies with individuals and can be affected by contextual variables. The studies of the masking of pain by concurrent stimulation might be viewed as contextual control of processes related to attention, although alternative mechanisms have been proposed to explain the analygesic outcomes (Benjamin, 1956; Duncker, 1937; Melzack, Weisz, & Sprague, 1963). It is also plausible that the analgesia shown by some schizophrenics and by practioners of oriental philosophies, such as Yoga, is achieved by a type of dissociation in which extreme concentration is attained. The effect of instructions may involve similar mechanisms to a lesser degree.

The present study is a demonstration of the potential effect of instructions in producing dissociation and analgesia in a pop-

From the Journal of Abnormal Psychology **77**:42-45.

[1]This research was supported by Grant MH 12097 from the National Institutes of Health and Grant RD 1372-P from the Vocational Rehabilitation Administration. The authors wish to express their indebtedness to M. Lowenthal, principal investigator of the latter grant, and to P. Klein for his assistance in collecting and analyzing the data.

[2]From the Department of Physical Medicine and Rehabilitation, New York Medical College, Flower and Fifth Avenue Hospitals, Fifth Avenue at 106th Street, New York, New York 10029.

ulation of normals. The *S*s, when placing their hands in freezing water, were instructed to dissociate their experience of coldness from that of pain and concentrate on the coldness. One group did this alone; another group was instructed to additionally attempt to interpret the cold as pleasant. (These latter instructions were similar to those used by Barber and Hahn (1962) in a study of hypnotic analgesia.)

METHOD

Subjects

There were 36 paid volunteers (18 male, 18 female) from a population of students and personnel at a metropolitan college.[3] Ages ranged from 17 to 50 yr. (mean, 23.8). Five *S*s were left-handed.

Apparatus

The noxious stimulus, cold, was presented by means of a tank containing an ice water mixture, slowly circulating. The temperature, measured before each trial was maintained at essentially .05° C. A warm water tank at 35° C. was used before each trial.

Procedure

The *S*s were randomly assigned to one of three groups, within the constraint that each group have an equal number of males and females (6 males and 6 females in each group).

The initial instructions were identical for all groups. They were as follows:

> First I would like you to place both your hands in this warm water tank. When I tell you to, I'd like you to place your right hand in the cold water up to this point (*E* demonstrated immersing his hand up to the finger-palm juncture) and report when you experience what you would call "pain." Then keep your hand in as long as you possibly can. If at any time your hand feels numb take it out.

After reaching maximum tolerance, *S* returned his hand to the warm water tank for a 2-min. period and then began the next trial. (The initial period in warm water was also 2 min.) There was a 4-min. maximum exposure set as the limit for each trial. The *S*s who did not report "quit point" by this time were stopped, and for that trial, quit point was recorded as 4 min. Also, numbness reported after pain threshold was treated as quit point. (This occurred with two *S*s.)

This initial trial was followed by two more identical trials for all three groups of *S*s. On the fourth and fifth trials the groups were treated differently. For one group, serving as controls, the instructions remained the same as those for the first three trials. For the second group, called Experimental 1 (E_1), the instructions were as follows:

> Now you have noticed that when you keep your hand in the ice water your experience has two components, cold and discomfort or pain. For the next trial, I'd like you to try to focus your attention and concentrate on the cold and try to ignore or focus away from the component of discomfort or pain. This is sort of a test of your powers of concentration. As before I'd like you to report when you experience what you would call "pain" and then keep your hand in as long as you possibly can.

The third group, Experimental 2 (E_2) was given the following instructions:

> Now for this trial I'd like you to try to imagine that it is a very hot day, as if you were in a very hot desert, and that the water is refreshing and pleasantly cool. That is, concentrate on the cool quality of the water and try to interpret it as pleasant. As before, I'd like you to report when you experience what you would call "pain" and then keep your hand in as long as you possibly can.

These instructions were read to the respective groups prior to the fourth and fifth trials while their hands were in the warm water tank for the 2-min. period waiting the next trial.

After the experimental trials, *S*s in the two experimental groups were informally questioned about the effect of the instructions on their experience of pain and their ability to follow the instructions.

RESULTS

The effect of the different instructions on pain threshold was determined by examining the mean threshold of the two trials prior to and subsequent to the instructions. The difference between these two means was computed for each *S*, and these difference scores for the three groups were compared. A large degree of varia-

[3]The original number of *S*s was 41; of these, 5 were dropped. Four *S*s (3 female, 1 male) reported numbness before pain threshold; and 1 *S* (female) reached the 4-min. limit before pain threshold, all of these in the preinstruction trials.

tion in response to the instructions in Group E_1 resulted in heterogeneity of variance, and consequently nonparametric techniques were used for this analysis.

For pain threshold, the median difference score, that is, elevation in pain threshold, for each group was as follows: Controls, .75 sec.; E_1, 14.50 sec.; E_2, 11.00 sec.

The difference scores for the three groups were tested for significance by the application of the Friedman two-way analysis of variance. The *S*s were matched on the basis of threshold scores on Trial 1. This analysis yielded a chi-square of 9.04 ($df = 2$, $p < .02$). Groups were then compared by the Wilcoxon matched-pairs signed-ranks test, and again *S*s were matched using Trial 1 thresholds. For this analysis, E_1 versus controls, $T = 11$ ($N = 12$, $p < .05$); E_2 versus controls, $T = 9.5$ ($N = 12$, $p < .02$); and E_1 versus E_2, $T = 20$ ($N = 11$, *ns*).

The effect of instructions on quit point was examined by an analysis equivalent to that for threshold. The median difference scores for quit point for each group were as follows: controls, 2.50 sec.; E_1 9.75 sec.; E_2 8.75 sec. The Friedman two-way analysis of variance yielded a chi-square of 4.17 ($df = 2$, *ns*).

The data were also examined for sex difference in response to the instructions. The median difference scores for pain threshold for males and females for the different groups were as follows: for the control, male = .75, female = 3.75; for E_1, male = 21.50, female = 10.00; for E_2, male = 23.50, female = 6.00. For quit point the median difference scores were as follows: control male = 3.00, female = 1.25; for E_1 male = 13.75, female = 9.75; for E_2 male = 16.75, female = 4.50. To test for sex differences, males and females were paired within each group according to pain threshold on Trial 1, and the difference (male minus female) of the pain threshold difference scores was obtained for each pair. These sex difference scores were then compared for the three groups by the Kruskal-Wallis analysis of variance. For this analysis, $H = 7.38$ ($df = 2$, $p < .05$). Comparisons of two groups at a time, by means of the Mann-Whitney *U* test, indicated that for controls versus E_1, $p < .03$; for controls versus E_2, $p < .02$; for E_1 versus E_2, *ns;* and for controls versus E_1 and E_2 combined $p < .01$. In all the comparisons, the male minus female scores were greater for the experimental groups than for the controls, indicating that the males showed a greater elevation in pain threshold in response to the instructions than did the females. The pain threshold scores prior to instructions for males and females were also compared. These were not significantly different. A similar absence of sex differences in response to cold pain has been reported by Voevodsky, Cooper, Morgan, and Hilgard, (1967).

Using the same procedure to analyze quit point scores, no significant differences were found.

DISCUSSION

As in the previous study by the present authors (Blitz & Dinnerstein, 1968), the results show an elevation in pain threshold in response to instructions. The present results demonstrate the analgesic effectiveness of attempts to redirect focus of attention, dissociate different aspects of the noxious stimulus complex, and reinterpret some of these aspects. These findings thus lend further support to the conceptualizations stressing the role of attentional and cognitive processes in pain perception.

The fact that the present instructions were not effective at quit point may be accounted for by the much greater attentional salience of pain at quit point levels of noxious stimulation. Consequently, greater ability is required to direct focus of attention away from pain at these levels.

The sex differences in response to the instructions were unexpected and are regarded as tentative. They might imply that males tend to have a greater ability than females in modulating attentional mechanisms when confronted with noxious stimulation This is consonant with the cultural stereotype of greater pain tolerance in males. However, because the results may reflect specific characteristics of the context of the present study, for example, *E* was a male, further work on this point is required before definitive conclusions can be drawn.

Also of interest are the special characteristics of the attentional mechanisms called for in Group E_1. The redirection of attention was not totally away from the noxious stimulus as is commonly the case in distraction. It was rather toward one aspect of the noxious stimulus complex and away from another. It represents a type of dissociation of stimulus qualities, separating one quality heavily loaded with emotional characteristics from others. Such restructuring of pain perception might be a useful technique in some types of clinical pain, where complete distraction cannot be achieved.

There was a wide range of individual difference in response to the instructions designed to produce dissociation. This difference may, as mentioned with respect to sex differences, reflect different degrees of skill in modulating focus of attention and may partially account for individual difference in pain tolerance encountered in everyday life. Training in such skills may thus be of some value for patients confronted with problems of chronic pain (Morgenstern, 1962).

A basic question which may be raised by the present results (as well as by those in the previous experiment by the present authors) is that with regard to response bias. Was the change in pain threshold a reflection of changes in perception, or might it simply reflect a change in the *S*s' reporting of pain in an attempt, for example, to please *E?* The present data cannot differentiate between these alternatives. However, the questioning of the *S*s at the end of the experiment strongly suggests that the effects were due to changes in perception. Most *S*s felt that on the instruction trials the pain was less intense, especially toward the beginning of the trial. Many reported that as the pain became more intense, they could no longer divert attention away from it. Further work is necessary, though, to clarify this question.

REFERENCES

Barber, T. X., & Hahn, K. W. Physiological and subjective responses to pain producing stimulation under hypnotically-suggested and waking-imagined "analgesia." *Journal of Abnormal and Social Psychology,* 1962, **65,** 411-418.

Benjamin, F. B. Effect of pain on simultaneous perception of nonpainful sensory stimulation. *Journal of Applied Physiology,* 1956, **8,** 630-634.

Blitz, B., & Dinnerstein, A. J. Effects of different types of instructions on pain parameters. *Journal of Abnormal Psychology,* 1968, **73,** 276-280.

Duncker, K. Some preliminary experiments on the mutual influence of pains. *Psychologische Forschung,* 1937, **21,** 311-326.

Hilgard, E. R., Cooper, L. M., Lenox, J., Morgan, A. H., & Voevodsky, J. The use of pain-state reports in the study of hypnotic analgesia to the pain of ice water. *Journal of Nervous and Mental Disease,* 1967, **144,** 506-513.

Ischlondsky, N. E. *Brain and behavior.* St. Louis: Mosby, 1949.

Melzack, R., Weisz, A. Z., & Sprague, L. T. Stratagems for controlling pain: Contributions of auditory stimulation and suggestion. *Experimental Neurology,* 1963, **8,** 239-247.

Morgenstern, F. S. The effects of sensory input and concentration on post-amputation phantom limb pain. *Journal of Neurology, Neurosurgery and Psychiatry,* 1964, **27,** 58-65.

Voevodsky, J., Cooper, L. M., Morgan, A. H., & Hilgard, E. R. The measurement of suprathreshold pain. *American Journal of Psychology,* 1967, **80,** 124-128.

Wolff, B. B., & Horland, A. A. Effect of suggestion upon experimental pain: A validation study. *Journal of Abnormal Psychology,* 1967, **72,** 402-407.

23

The effects of vicarious and cognitive rehearsal on pain tolerance

Richard W. J. Neufeld and Park O. Davidson

The importance of psychological factors involved in reaction to pain-inducing stimuli has been emphasized by several investigators [1]. They have presented evidence which demonstrates that such factors are responsible for the wide variety of responses to the same pain-inducing stimuli. Concurrently, manipulation of psychological factors has been shown to affect pain reaction [2-4].

It has been suggested that "cognitive style" relates to the way individual reactions to the same pain stimulus may differ. Petrie *et al.* [5], and Petrie [6] described two groups of individuals that they have classified on the basis of kinesthetic after effects. They were labelled "augmenters" and "reducers". The perceptions of augmenters were said to be less affected by prior perceptions than the perceptions of reducers. Petrie has contended that the responses to pain of augmenters are exaggerated while the responses of reducers are inhibited. Byrne [7] has described two types of individuals which he labels "repressors" and "sensitizers". Byrne states that those classified as repressors characteristically react to threat with denying, repressing and avoiding behaviors. Sensitizers, on the other hand are said to react with approaching and intellectualizing behaviors. It has been found that subjects classified as repressors tolerate pain less upon a second confrontation than upon the first, whereas the tolerance of sensitizers does not change from the first to the second confrontation [8].

Rehearsal of stress has been shown to be effective in reducing reactions to threat. Folkins *et al.* [9] investigated two components of systematic desensitization. These investigators designated relaxation and cognitive rehearsal as the two components. They found that cognitive rehearsal was more effective in reducing arousal to a stress film than the relaxation treatment of both cognitive rehearsal and relaxation together.

In investigating whether or not the effects of stress rehearsal on psychological stress extended to physical stress (pain), Bobey and Davidson [10] had subjects rehearse an experience involving radiant-heat pain. This detailed rehearsal was followed by actual application of the heat. It was found that the rehearsal was successful in lengthening the period of time subjects were willing to tolerate the heat.

A major function of rehearsing a stressful event could be that of reducing strangeness or uncertainty. There is evidence that uncertainty about an experience involving a noxious stimulus increases the aversiveness of the situation. In a study by Jones *et al.* [11], subjects were required to perform instrumental responses in order to receive information about electric shock. If the responses were performed, subjects were rewarded with information about the

Reprinted with permission from Neufeld, R. W. J., and Davidson, P. O. The effects of vicarious and cognitive rehearsal on pain tolerance, Journal of Psychosomatic Research **15**:329-335.
From the Dept of Psychology, University of Calgary, Calgary 44, Alberta, Canada. This study was supported in part by the Canadian National Research Council Grant. APA 213.

intensity and time of onset regarding the next shock. It was found that reducing uncertainty in this way was effective in establishing the instrumental responses. The authors of this study suggest that the removal of uncertainty decreases anxiety. Thus, responses which were followed by reduction in uncertainty would be reinforced.

Rehearsal of anticipated threat is often used in the clinic to reduce uncertainty about the upcoming event. Women awaiting childbirth often have the entire experience outlined to them beforehand.

London [13] and Folkins *et al.* [9] have emphasized that rehearsal must bear close resemblance to the actual experience if the person's preparation is to be effective. In addition, repeating the actual experience may affect reaction to it. However, systematic investigation of these factors has not been carried out.

The present study proposed to investigate whether or not pain tolerance was affected by the mode of rehearsing. In the present study, two modes were investigated. One involved observing another person experiencing an aversive stimulus. The other involved hearing the aversive experience described in detail.

A second factor considered was the relevance of the rehearsal. The "relevant" rehearsal had, as its subject matter, the specific pain to be experienced. The "irrelevant" rehearsal dealt with an aversive stimulus dissimilar to that which was subsequently experienced.

The effect of rehearsal when the aversive stimulus was repeated was also studied. It has been suggested that repetition of exposure may be an important factor to be considered in studying reaction to aversive stimuli [14].

The effect of alerting the subject to an impending threat, without actually rehearsing the threatening event, is not clear. It is possible that warning of a threat to come, with no further detail, is an effective technique for raising tolerance of the event. Janis [15], on the other hand, points to field observations that suggest an ambiguous warning increases stress. The present study compared subjects warned of pain to come with subjects unwarned. Neither group received information as the nature of the pain.

Davidson and Bobey [8] found that repressors differed from sensitizers in their reaction to repeated pain, with repressors showing a significant decrease in tolerance from trial one to trial two while sensitizers showed no significant change in tolerance. However, in their study, the pain stimulus was changed from the first to the second exposure. It is not clear how sensitizers would compare with repressors in reaction to repetition of the same pain stimulus. This study investigated the effects of repeating the same pain stimulus on the reaction of repressors as compared to that of sensitizers.

METHOD

Subjects

The subjects (*S*s) were 72 female volunteers from nursing classes at the Calgary General Hospital. 2 *S*s had to be replaced as their tolerance of pain stimulus exceeded that at which tissue damage has been found to occur [10]. Hence, the experimenter intervened and terminated the stimulus for these 2 *S*s. The 72 *S*s were divided into 6 groups with 12 *S*s per group. Four of these groups were used in a split-plot-factorial 22.2 design [16] to evaluate the following three interactions; mode of rehearsal [observation *(O)* vs. verbal description *(V)*]; relevance of rehearsal to the forthcoming pain [same pain *(S)* vs. different pain *(D)*]; repetition of exposure to the pain stimulus [first exposure *(1)* vs. second exposure *(2)*].

Two other groups were included in the study. One group was given no rehearsal but was informed that a pain stimulus was to be applied after 15 min. The second group of *S*s waited in the experimental room for the same length of time after which the stimulus was applied.

Apparatus

The radiant-heat apparatus was used to produce the experimental pain as this method has been shown to be reliable and convenient [17, 8, 10]. The radiant-heat apparatus resembled that used by Davidson and McDougall [12]. It was based on the Hardy-Wolff-Goodel model modified by Clark and Bindra [18]. A specially-constructed box contained a 250-watt i.r. lamp which delivered constant heat to a blackened portion of the *S*s forearm. The *S*'s arm was strapped to the box over a round hole 2 cm in diameter about 20 cm from the lamp. The heat was switched on by the experimenter *(E)* The switch which terminated the heat, was accessible to *S*. A Stoelting timer attached to the apparatus through a relay, recorded the duration of the heat.

Procedure

Prior to entering the room in which the experiment was conducted all *S*s completed the Repression-Sensitization scale [7].

*S*s were then administered the treatment appropriate to the group to which they were assigned. The specific treatments for the respective groups were as follows:

Observation-same (OS). The *S*s in this group were first given the following instructions:

> We want to find out how prior experience affects the way people react to a pain stimulus. A pain stimulus will be applied at the end of the session. A pain stimulus will first be applied to this person.

The model (a 23 yr old female) then sat in front of the heat apparatus and her right forearm was blackened. After the model's right arm was securely attached to the front of the box, the following instructions were read to her in the presence of *S:*

> The intensity of the heat will increase gradually until your arm begins to hurt. When it hurts a lot so you would like the stimulation stopped, press the switch near you with your free hand. This is not to see how much you can take, and as soon as you press the switch, the stimulation will be shut off.

A cardboard sheet had been placed in front of the hole before *S* entered the room so as to protect the model's arm. Before the *S* was fastened to the box, the cardboard was removed by the *E* sticking his finger through the hole in an inconspicuous manner while adjusting the position of the box. The model underwent the stimulation for 60 sec in a "serene" manner with no overt signs of stress. The timer was visible at all times to *E* only. The model watched *E*'s watch inconspicuously so as to know when 60 sec had elapsed. After pressing the switch that both terminated the heat and registered the duration of the stimulus on the timer, the model was unstrapped from the apparatus and left the room.

Observation-different (OD). The procedure for this group was identical to that for the *OS* groups except that after the *S* was told that a pain stimulus would be first applied to another person, the model received pain involving the pressure algometer [19]. The flat tip of the pressure algometer was placed just above the thumb nail of the left hand with the palm on the table. A constant pressure of 1 kg was applied for 60 seconds. The *E* simulated the appearance of moderate pressure being applied. The following instructions were given to the model in the presence of *S* prior to the simulated application of pressure.

> The pressure on your thumb will remain constant until it begins to hurt. Say "stop" when it hurts a lot so you would like the stimulation stopped. This is not to see how much you can take and as soon as you give the indication, the stimulation will be stopped.

Here also, the model underwent the stimulation in a "serene" manner with no overt signs of stress. After the pressure was terminated, the model left the room.

Verbal-description (VS). The *S*s in this group were given the following instructions:

> We want to find out how prior experience affects the way people react to a pain stimulus. A pain stimulus will be applied at the end of the session. The short tape you are now going to hear will give you practice in imagining scenes as well as a detailed pain-stimulus description. Please keep your eyes closed while listening to the tape.

The tape was adapted from Folkins *et al.* [9]. It involved instructions to imagine vivedly scenes which the *S* could choose herself. This "practice in imagining" was followed by instructions to imagine the experience involving the raidiant-heat apparatus. A detailed description of the heat apparatus, the procedure involved in the heat administration, and sensations associated with the radiant-heat stimulus were presented to *S*. The sensations described were those reported by three acquaintances of *E* to whom the radiant-heat had been applied before the tape had been made.

The three people had unanimously reported the following sequence of sensations: (a) a feeling of "warmth"; (b) a "pricking" sensation; (c) a "slight burning" feeling; and (d) a "burning feeling which hurt".

Verbal-description-different (VD). The procedure for this group duplicated that for the VS group except that after the "practice in imagining", the tape recording described the apparatus, procedure, and sensations involved in pressure pain as inflicted by the pressure algometer. The sensations described were those reported by the same three acquaintances of *E* who were used preparing the *VS* group.

Anticipation (A). The *S*s in this group were seated in the experimental room and given the following instructions:

> We want to find out how people react to a pain stimulus. A pain stimulus will be applied at the end of the session. There will now be a short interval – right after, the pain stimulus will be applied. The *E* then pretended to be busy with organizing papers for 15 min (the approximate time taken for the observational and verbal-description rehearsals).

Control (C). The *S*s in this group were unaware of the nature of the experiment at the time they entered the test room. They were told "We will be ready in 15 min". The *E* then pretended to be busy with organizing papers for 15 min (as in the *A* group's treatment, above). *S*s were told of the pain-tolerance and their consent obtained just prior to the test.

After being administered the assigned treatment, each *S* had both forearms blackened with washable black ink where the heat was to be applied. This was to reduce individual differences in conductance of the heat attributable to differential skin pigmentation. The heat was administered twice, once to each forearm after the arm was securely attached to the apparatus. Before the heat was switched on, the same instructions were read to *S*s as were to the model for the *OS* group. The *E* then switched on the heat and pain tolerance was recorded as the time in seconds between the onset of the heat and when the *S* pressed the switch terminating the heat [12].

Table 1. Analysis of variance summary

Source	*df*	*MS*	*F*
Mode *(A)*	1	30.4	
Relevance *(C)*	1	363.3	3.07
$A \times C$	1	348.6	2.94
*S*s within groups	44	118.2	
Exposure *(B)*	1	15.4	1.02
$A \times B$	1	18.2	1.21
$B \times C$	1	63.3	4.19*
$A \times B \times C$	1	1.0	
$B \times$ *S*s within groups	44	15.1	

*$p < 0.05$.

RESULTS

The summary of the SPF-22.2 [16] analysis of variance evaluating the three factors (mode of rehearsal, relevance of rehearsal and repetition of pain) is given in Table 1.

These results did not indicate a relationship between the manner in which the painful experience was rehearsed (observation of another's experience vs. having the experience described via a tape recording) and subsequent tolerance of the experience ($F < 1$). The main effects of rehearsal relevance to the ensuing experience only approached statistical significance ($F = 3.07$, $df = 1/44$, $p < 0.10$). Similarly, the interaction of relevance with mode of presentation only approached statistical significance ($F = 2.94$, $df = 1/44$, $p < 0.10$).

The interaction of relevance of rehearsal with first versus second exposures to the pain ($B \times C$) was statistically significant ($F = 4.19$, $df = 1/44$, $p < 0.05$). This interaction appeared reliable from one mode of rehearsal to the other as there was no interaction of $B \times C$ with A.

In examining simple main effects, it was found that the group which had the relevant rehearsal differed from the group which had the irrelevant rehearsal only on the second exposure to the pain ($F = 5.47$, $df = 1/44$, $p < 0.05$). Higher tolerance was found in the relevant rehearsal group. Also, difference in tolerance from exposure one to exposure two was found only for the group which had the irrelevant rehearsal. This group decreased in tolerance from the first to the second exposure ($F = 4.67$, $df = 1/44$, $p < 0.05$). The $B \times C$ interaction is presented in Fig. 1.

In order to evaluate the significance of

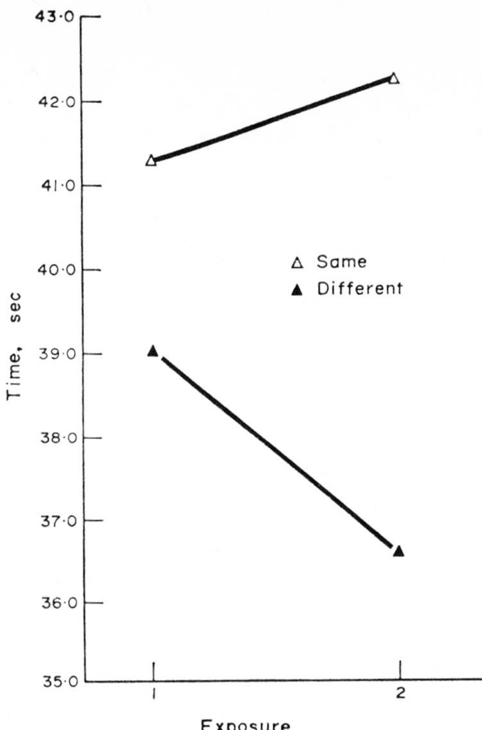

Fig. 1. Exposure by relevance interaction.

the change in tolerance over the two trials for both the relevant and irrelevant-rehearsal groups relative to a baseline change afforded by the control group, differences in mean change scores were tested. Neither the change for the relevant-rehearsal group nor the change for the irrelevant-rehearsal group was significantly different from the change over trials of the control group (t = 0.89 and t = −0.44 respectively, $df = 66$, $p > .05$).

Comparing the mean of group $A(\bar{\chi}=38.8)$ to the mean of group $C(\bar{\chi}=40.01)$ rendered a statiscally insignificant difference. Similarly, comparing the mean of group C with the combined mean of groups receiving rehearsal ($\bar{\chi}=39.68$) rendered a statistically insignificant difference.

The *S*s were classified according to whether they were above or below the *R-S* mean score of 41.54. Correlated *t*-tests were used to evaluate reaction to repeated pain for repressors as compared to sensitizers in the non-rehearsal groups (*C* and *A*). Only repressors in group *A* reacted significantly differently on the second exposure as compared to the first ($\bar{\chi}$ = 33.88 and 42.30, respectively); ($t = 2.53$, $df = 1/36$, $p < 0.01$). Changes for repressors in group *C* and changes for sensitizers in both groups *C* and *A* were statistically insignificant.

DISCUSSION

Preparation for a threatening experience through prior knowledge has been a much-used technique in everyday life. A student preparing for an examination often attempts to familiarize himself with the surroundings in which he will be writing. This reduces the strangeness of the situation when the time for the examination arrives. Young children in the primary grades are often introduced to the classroom, accompanied by their parents, before school officially begins. It is assumed that this type of prior experience will help allay anxiety when the child must attend classes on his own. One might contend that wedding rehearsals serve a similar purpose. In clinics, where patients must undergo procedures involving pain (such as most dental work), prior information is often used in an informal way. A nurse or fellow patient might describe what is to come.The common procedure of having long lineups for hypodermic injections allows the person at the end of the line to see what is to happen (many times).

Results from the current study indicate that vicarious rehearsal is no more effective than cognitive rehearsal in increasing pain tolerance. How relevant to the actual experience must the content be? From analysis of the data of this study, it appears that similarity of rehearsed to subsequently experienced pain affects tolerance of the pain. However, this was found only after the initial exposure to the direct pain. It was observed that the group which had the relevant rehearsal had greater tolerance than the group which had the irrelevant rehearsal. It is possible that the initial exposure made the *S*s in the irrelevant group aware that the preparation was irrelevant. Such awareness may increase anxiety and apprehension. Hence, the aversiveness of the painful situation could increase [11]. On the other hand, this would not be likely to occur with *S*s whose experience was in line with their rehearsal. The above possibility seems compatible with the observation that the irrelevant-rehearsal group's tolerance went down with the second exposure while the relevent rehearsal group's tolerance did not change.

While results from the present study did not support the frequent finding that rehearsal is preferable to no rehearsal in coping with stress and pain, these results did not indicate that—where rehearsal is used—appropriate or accurate rehearsal is preferable to inappropriate or inaccurate rehearsal. It would seem therefore that care should be taken assuring similarity between the rehearsal and the actual experience. Indications are that when a person's information about a forthcoming pain experience is contradicted by the actual experience, tolerance for the pain is reduced.

The effects on pain tolerance of warning a patient about future pain has needed clarification. Some physicians prefer not to give advance warning in some situations because anticipatory fears may develop. On the other hand "surprising" the patient with pain prevents him from mobilizing his defenses to cope with the pain. From the present results it appears as if anticipation neither significantly increases or decreases pain tolerance in comparison with no anticipation.

When subjects were given advance warning, however, personality factors seemed to affect subsequent pain tolerance. While repressors and sensitizers did not differ in this group on their first exposure to pain, repressors showed a reduction in tolerance on the second exposure while sensitizers did not change. These results confirm Davidson and Bobey's [8] findings, since the subjects in their experiment all anticipated the pain experience.

In the present study, *S*s rehearsing the pain were no more tolerant of it than those in the control group. Bobey and Davidson [10], on the other hand, found that rehearsal was effective in raising tolerance. However, they had their *S*s rehearse the pain twice. The rehearsals were separated by one day and the pain was experienced after the second rehearsal. From the present study, it does not appear that their findings are generalizable to a single rehearsal before pain. To the extent that such repetition of rehearsal is responsible for the difference in results between Bobey and Davidson's study and the present study, it would appear that the effective procedure is the more cumbersome one. If such repetition of rehearsal is an important factor (and this bears investigation) it would seem appropriate in clinical practice, to have the patient rehearse a day, wait a day, and then return for another rehearsal. It is possible that more details of the impending threat are perceived (and, consequently, uncertainty and strangeness is more effectively reduced) when rehearsal is experienced more than once. In addition, an intervening time period between rehearsal and the actual pain provide extended opportunity for the person to invoke strategies of coping with the impending harm [15]. Folkins *et al.* [9] found that rehearsal sessions separated by one week helped *S*s cope with psychological stress. However, Watkins and Davidson [19], who programmed rehearsal sessions only 8 hr apart, did not find this procedure effective in increasing tolerance of psychological stress.

A future experiment could examine the effects of giving *S*s multiple rehearsal as compared to *S*s receiving one rehearsal and *S*s receiving no rehearsal. The importance of a time interval between rehearsal and stressor should be investigated also.

SUMMARY

Several aspects of rehearsing an aversive experience were investigated in relation to subsequent tolerance of the experience. The aversive experience consisted of radiant-heat pain. Rehearsal by observing another person undergoing the experience was compared to rehearsal by hearing a detailed description of the experience. The content of rehearsal involving the same pain stimulus as that to be experienced (relevant) was compared to the content involving a different type of pain stimulus (irrelevant). The effect of rehearsal during the first vs. the second exposure to the pain stimulus was also investigated. Results showed no differences in effectiveness between vicarious and cognitive rehearsal, but after the first exposure to the pain, *S*s whose rehearsal was relevant had significantly higher pain tolerance than those whose rehearsal was irrelevant.

REFERENCES

1. Beecher H. K. The measurement of pain. *Pharmacol. Rev.* **9,** 154 (1957).
2. Kornetsky C. Effects of anxiety and morphine on the anticipation and perception of painful radiant thermal stimuli. *J. Compar. Physiol. Psychol.* **47,** 130 (1954).
3. Conn J. H. The inter-relationship between anxiety and pain. *J. Amer. Soc. Psychosom. Dent. Med.* **8,** 40 (1961).
4. Blitz B. and Dinnerstein A. Effects of different types of instructions on pain parameters. *J. Abnorm. Psychol.* **73,** 276 (1968).
5. Petrie A., Collins W. and Solomon P. Pain sensitivity, sensory deprivation, and susceptibility to satiation. *Science* **128,** 1431 (1958).
6. Petrie A. Some psychological aspects of pain and the relief of suffering. *Ann. N. Y. Acad. Sci.* **86,** 13 (1960).
7. Byrne D. The repression-sensitization scale: rationale, reliability, and validity. *J. Person.* **29,** 334 (1961).
8. Davidson P. O. and Bobey M. J. Repressor-sensitizer differences on repeated exposures to pain. *Percep. Motor Skills* **31,** 711 (1970).
9. Folkins C. H., Lawson K. D., Opton E. M. and Lazarus R. S. Desensitization and the experimental reduction of threat. *J. Abnorm. Psychol.* **73,** 100 (1968).
10. Bobey M. J. and Davidson P. O. Psychological factors affecting pain tolerance. *J. Psychosom. Res.* **14,** 371 (1970).
11. Jones, A., Bantler, P. M. and Petry, G. The reduction of uncertainty concerning future pain. *J. Abn. Psychol.* 1966, 71, 87-94.
12. Davidson P. O. and McDougall C. E. The generality of pain tolerance. *J. Psychosom. Res.* **13,** 83 (1969).
13. London P. *The Modes and Morals of Psychotherapy.* Holt, Rinehart & Winston, New York (1964).
14. Andrew J. M. Coping style, stress-relevant learning and recovery from surgery. Unpublished doctoral dissertation, University of California, Los Angeles (1968).
15. Janis I. L. Psychological effects of warnings. In *Man and Society in Disaster* (Edited by Baker G. W. and Chapman D. W.) pp. 55-92. Basic Books, New York (1962).
16. Kirk R. E. *Experimental design: procedures for the behavioural sciences.* Belmont, California: Brooks/Cole, 1968.
17. Hall K. R. L. Studies of cutaneous pain: a survey of research since 1940. *Br. J. Psychol.* **44,** (1953).
18. Clark J. W. and Bindra D. Individual differences in pain thresholds. *Can J. Psychol.* **10,** 69 274 (1956).
19. Merskey H. and Spear F. G. The reliability of the pressure algometer. *Br. J. Soc. Clin. Psychol.* **3,** 130 (1964).
20. Watkins R. E. and Davidson P. O. Stress reactions of psychiatric patients: An attempt at experimental reduction of threat. *Behav. Res. Ther.* **8,** 175 (1970).

24

Effects of accurate expectations about sensations on the sensory and distress components of pain[1]

Jean E. Johnson[2]

The effects of information on reactions to threatening stimuli have recently received a great deal of attention in the psychological literature. The role of information in emotional response has important implications for theory. In addition, there are practical implications. Preparatory information may reduce emotional response to procedures which are often an unavoidable part of health care, for example, diagnostic examinations, injections, dental procedures, and surgery. There is a great deal of information that could be transmitted about a threatening stimulus. Whether or not information can affect emotional response in a variety of threatening situations is no longer the issue. The type of information that reduces the emotional response and why it is effective are now our concern.

The classic experiment by Schachter and Singer (1962) demonstrated that information which described the sensations of emotional arousal combined with modeled behavior affected the emotional behavior that subjects displayed. As an extension of Schachter's (1964) model of emotion, Nisbett and Schachter (1966) reasoned that if subjects can be led to attribute their physiological arousal to a neutral source, they will be less apt to label their state as emotional than if the arousal is attributed to a threatening source. The attribution hypothesis has received support when subjects received electric shock (Nisbett & Schachter, 1966) and when they were threatened by shock (Ross, Rodin, & Zimbardo, 1969). In these attribution experiments, description of sensations frequently experienced when emotionally aroused and attribution to source of the arousal were confounded.

Accurate descriptions of sensations frequently experienced during confrontation with threatening stimuli may be the factor associated with reduced emotional response. Accurate descriptions of sensations allow the subject to form accurate expectations about the sensations he will experience. When accurate expectations of the sensations produced by threatening stimuli have been formed, the degree of incongruency between expectations and experience is reduced. The intensity of a response reflecting emotion during a threatening event may be a function of incongruency between expected and experienced sensations. The greater the incongruency the more intense the emotional response. The incongruency between expected and experienced sensations can change over the time a person is exposed to threatening stimuli. The change can be a result of reformulation of expectations, a change in

From the Journal of Personality and Social Psychology **27**:261-275.

[1]This research is based on a doctoral dissertation submitted to the University of Wisconsin. The author is indebted to her advisor, Howard Leventhal, for his help in all phases of this research. Support was provided by the National Institutes of Health, Division of Nursing, Research Grant NU 00302 to Howard Leventhal and Fellowship 5F04-NU-27185 to the author.

[2]From the Center for Health Research, 5557 Cass Avenue, Wayne State University, Detroit, Michigan 48202

the sensations, or both. If degree of incongruency changes, intensity of emotional response would also be expected to change over time.

The experiments reported here tested the incongruency hypothesis by exposing subjects to ischemic pain. Ischemic pain (pain caused by lack of blood supply) was used as the threatening stimulus for two reasons: *(a)* It has been demonstrated to be a satisfactory simulation of pain caused by pathology (Smith, Egbert, Markowitz, Mosteller, & Beecher, 1966) and therefore the potential for the laboratory research to be relevant to clinical situations is increased, and *(b)* the subject can be exposed to the stimulus for several minutes, thus allowing time for cognitive mechanisms to operate.

The pain experience was conceptualized as consisting of two components: sensory-discrimination component and reactive component (Beecher, 1959; Casey & Melzack, 1967; Melzack & Wall, 1965). The reactive component has emotional properties. Casey and Melzack (1967) suggest that the primary sensory output from a painful stimulus need not have a one-to-one relationship to responses indicating distress. The two components of the pain experience were measured separately in the experiments to be reported here. It was expected that accurate expectations about the physical sensations to be experienced during the painful stimulation would affect only the emotional component of the pain experience.

Expectations about sensations were manipulated by varying the relevance of preparatory information to physical sensations frequently experienced during the painful stimulation. To test the incogruency hypothesis it was necessary to vary expectations about the sensations caused by a painful stimulus without suggesting either the magnitude of those sensations or the degree of distress. To rule out alternative explanations based on other theoretical positions, the message could not differentially arouse fear (Janis, 1958, 1967), affect perception of being in danger (Lazarus, 1968), attribute cause of the sensations to alternative sources (Nisbett & Schachter, 1966), or affect feelings of helplessness (Mandler & Watson, 1966).

EXPERIMENT I

Method

Modified submaximum effort tourniquet technique.[3] The subject was seated with his forearm resting comfortably on a table. A standard adult-size blood-pressure cuff was applied to the upper arm and pressure pumped up to and left at 250 millimeters of mercury. The subject then squeezed a hand dynamometer 20 times. The 20-pound point was marked with a red line and subjects were instructed to squeeze just to the line. Each squeeze was timed to last 2 seconds, followed by a 2-second pause. The schedule was presented to the subject by tape-recorded signals consisting of "squeeze," "hold," "release." The experimenter observed the subject as he performed the exercises and corrected him if he deviated from the procedure.

The dial and bulb for inflation of the cuff were separated from the cuff by 10 feet of tubing. This allowed the experimenter to monitor the pressure in the cuff at a distance form the subject. During the time the cuff was inflated the experimenter was seated behind the subject with no physical barrier between them.

Subjects. Twenty male University of Wisconsin students served as subjects (10 per information condition). Names were randomly selected from students who filled out health survey questionnaires at summer registration; students were contacted by telephone and offered $2.50 to participate in a 1½ hour experiment relevant to health care. The subjects' ages ranged from 18 to 27 years with a mean age of 21.4 years. Subjects were studied individually by a female experimenter.

Procedure. The following introduction to the experiment was given to the subject:

> I want to tell you more about the experiment before you give your final consent to participate. In this experiment we are interested in learning about people's reaction to uncomfortable stimulation. We think the experiment will give informa-

[3] The procedure varied from that used by Smith et al. (1966). The arm was not exsanguinated by elevating it and applying Esmarch bandage. This was omitted because it was necessary to have subjects in a sitting position. Application of an Esmarch bandage and blood-pressure cuff while the seated subject's arm was extended above his head was an awkward procedure for both the subject and the experimenter.

> tion that will help patients who have pain from natural causes. I will put a tourniquet around your arm at a high pressure. This will cause you pain but no harm.
>
> We are not interested in how much pain you can take.[4] We want to know what the experience is like for you. You will be asked many questions about your experience. It takes about 1½ hours for the experiment, but most of that time you will be doing paper-and-pencil tasks. You will experience the discomfort for only a short part of the time. Are you willing to be in the experiment?

Each subject was questioned about his health that day, his general health, and about sports activities planned for the day. All students who gave a history of any chronic health problem, who were not presently feeling well, or who planned to participate in a competitive sport that day were not accepted as subjects. None of the students who met the criteria refused to be in the experiment.

The subjects' first task was to fill out a Mood Adjective Check List composed of 25 adjectives describing five moods (well-being, fear, anger, helplessness, and depression). The instructions asked for responses to indicate how they felt "right now" by placing 1, 2, 3, or 4 before each word. The numbers were labeled 1 = not at all, 2 = a little, 3 = somewhat, and 4 = very much. This Mood Adjective Check List provided a base-line measure before subjects were exposed to a message.

Subjects were asked to read one of the two messages. The experimenter told the subject that the folder on the table had more information about what to expect and that he should read it while she was getting equipment set up. This procedure allowed random assignment to information conditions and prevented the experimenter from knowing the subject's assignment. Both of the messages started with the statement: "Read the following information carefully. *You will be asked questions about it later.*" The relevant-information-condition subjects then read:

> You can expect to feel pressure and sensations such as tingling and aching, followed by numbness, very much like when your arm is "asleep." Your arm and hand will be temporarily very pale and blotched. This discoloration is typical when pressure is applied to the arm.

The irrelevant-information-condition subjects read:

> The sensations and discomfort you will experience are due to temporary ischemia of your arm (lack of blood in the arm). A tourniquet filled with air will cause high pressure on your arm. It is very unlikely that you have experienced discomfort of this kind before.

Subjects reported their judgment of the degree of sensation and distress they experienced while the cuff was inflated on two vertical scales, one labeled sensation and the other distress. The sensation scale was labeled 0, 25, 50, 75, and 100 at the appropriate points. The distress scale was labeled "slightly distressing" at the bottom, "moderately distressing" and "very distressing" at equally spaced intervals, and "just bearable" at the top. No numbers appeared on this scale. Subjects were shown the scales and told that sensation meant the physical intensity of what they would be feeling. The distress scale referred to the amount of distress the sensations caused. Subjects were asked to think of the degree of sensation they felt and how distressing that sensation was as two separate things. Zero on the sensation scale meant the way their arm felt then. One hundred meant the maximum amount they could imagine of the sensations they would experience. Tape-recorded directions told the subjects when to make their judgments. Each judgment was to be considered independent of previous ones and the sensation and distress ratings could also be independent. Subjects were again told that the experimenter was not interested in how much pain they could tolerate.

The subject was instructed about the use of the hand exerciser and a sample of the squeeze-pause sequence was presented by tape recording. The blood-pressure cuff was applied but not inflated. The second Mood Adjective Check List was administered.

The tasks the subject would be expected to do while the cuff was inflated were reviewed. The subject was asked to read again the information about what to expect. The cuff was inflated; the tape recording to pace the hand exercise began,

[4] The subject's expectations that traditional pain tolerance measures were to be used had to be corrected before he could be convinced that a new method of measuring pain perception was to be used.

followed by the requests for judgments of sensation and distress. The first judgment was made 2 minutes after the cuff was inflated and judgements were repeated every 30 seconds. The cuff was deflated and removed following a rating of distress at or above "very distressing." The maximum time the cuff was on was 18 minutes even if a rating had not reached "very distressing." If a rating as high as "very distressing" occurred before 5 minutes, the cuff remained on until 5 minutes had elapsed. The experimenter was seated behind the subject in a position which allowed her to observe unobtrusively the subject's marks on the scales.[5]

After the cuff was removed, the subject reported his feeling state on the third Mood Adjective Check List and then was given a long questionnaire asking about his reactions to and thoughts about the experience. This questionnaire provided checks on the manipulations and asked for information relevant to the cognitive processes in which the subject was engaged.

Subjects responded to a measure of tolerance for frustration and three personality scales. These data did not add to the understanding of the reactions to the pain experience and are not discussed further.

The experimenter explained the hypothesis to the subject and answered his questions. The potential relevance of the research to health care was also explained.

Results

Success of manipulations. The test of the hypothesis required that expectations about sensations differ for information conditions and that perception of the sensory experience not differ. The questionnaire included questions about the five sensations described in the relevant information and three other plausible sensations. The subjects were asked if they had been aware of, had expected, and remembered being told to expect each of the sensations. The data in Table 1 show that subjects in the relevant-information condition expected to experience significantly ($p < .02$)[6] more of the sensations they did in fact experience ($M = 5.2$) than those in the irrelevant-information condition ($M = 4.2$). The relevant-information subjects remembered being told what sensations to expect (3.5 on the average). The irrelevant-information subjects remembered that that they were not told the sensations. The different information conditions did not affect subjects' awareness of the five target sensations.

The ratings of intensity of sensations over the first 5 minutes the tourniquet was on did not differ for the information conditions (Figure 1 and Table 2). However, sensation ratings increased over time at a significant rate. The rate of acceleration was greater for the relevant-information than for the irrelevant-information condition, but the interaction with time was not significant. None of the comparisons between information conditions on sensation ratings (t tests) for each time of rating approached significance.

It was concluded that the manipulations were successful in that the information conditions differed significantly on number of sensations both expected and experi-

[5] One subject became pale as soon as the cuff was inflated and did not respond to the exercise instructions (he had read the irrelevant information). The cuff was removed and another subject was added to the sample.

[6] Two-tailed p is reported for all t tests.

Table 1. Experiment I: checks on manipulations

Information condition	*Mean number of sensations experienced and expected*	*Mean number of target sensations remembered being told*	*Mean number of target sensations aware of*
Relevant	5.2	3.5	4.9
Irrelevant	4.2	.6	4.6
t	2.61*	6.82**	.93

Note. $df = 18$.
*$p < .02$.
**$p < .001$.

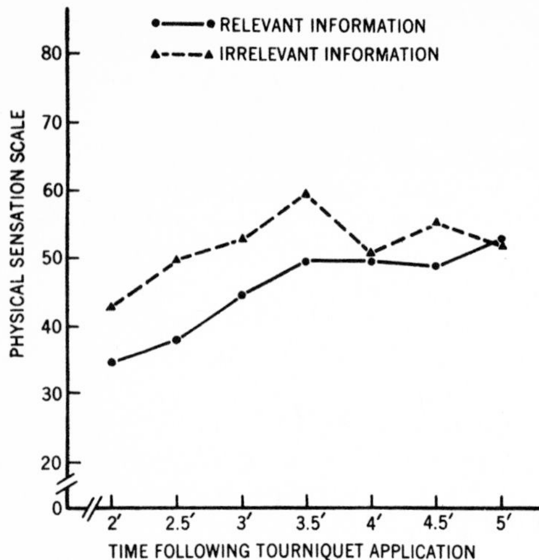

Fig. 1. Mean sensation ratings for information conditions over time for Experiment I.

Table 2. Experiment I: analysis of variance for sensation ratings

Source	*df*	*MS*	*F*
Between subjects			
Information (A)	1	1511.43	.83
Error	18	1830.21	
Within subjects			
Time (B)	6	620.25	4.45*
A × B	6	114.87	.83
Error	108	137.96	

*$p < .001$.

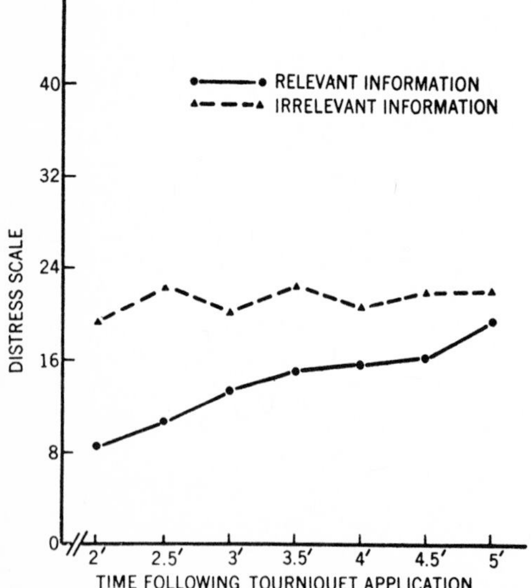

Fig. 2. Mean distress ratings for information conditions over time for Experiment I.

Table 3. Experiment I: analysis of variance for distress ratings

Source	*df*	*MS*	*F*
Between subjects			
Information (A)	1	1638.86	5.59*
Error	18	293.19	
Within subjects			
Time (B)	6	100.83	3.60**
A × B	6	47.75	1.70
Error	108	28.01	

* $p < .05$.
**$p < .01$.

enced while perceptions of the sensory experience did not differ significantly.

Distress ratings. The relevant-information condition resulted in significantly lower distress ratings than the irrelevant-information condition (Figure 2 and Table 3). The mean distress (14.4) over the first 5 minutes of the pain experience for the relevant-information condition was below the "moderately distressing" point on the scale (equal to a score of 16). The irrelevant-information-condition mean (21.8) was well above the moderately distressing point.

The distress ratings increased significantly over time (Table 3). There appeared to be a more rapid acceleration of distress in the relevant-information condition than in the irrelevant-information condition; however, the interaction between conditions and time of ratings was not significant. In addition, a trends analysis revealed no significant difference in linear trend in the information conditions. The lack of acceleration in mean distress ratings for the irrelevant-information condition was due primarily to two subjects. These subjects gave high distress ratings in the beginning (21 and 30) and low ratings after 5 minutes (2 for both subjects). The other eight subjects in the irrelevant-information condition tended to make increasingly higher distress ratings as time passed.

Time tourniquet tolerated. The mean time the tourniquet was on before a "very distressing" rating occurred was the same for both information conditions (M = 10 minutes for both groups). Thus, the difference in information did not significantly affect the subjects' motivation to tolerate the painful stimulus. This was not surprising since the experimenter had emphasized that she was not interested in "how much the subject could take."

Moods. The scores for the adjectives of the Mood Adjective Check Lists were summed to form scores for five moods (well-being, fear, anger, helplessness, and depression). Mood scores were analyzed with a repeated-measures analysis of variance. The between-subjects factor was information condition. The within-subject factor was the three repeated measures of mood. There were no significant differences for any of the five moods for the information factor. Neither did the information factor interact with time at a significant level for any of the moods. The only moods to change significantly over time were well-being ($F = 5.04$, $df = 2/36$, $p < .025$) and fear ($F = 7.33$, $df = 2/36$, $p < .01$). Tests between means at different times (Newman-Keuls) showed that neither well-being nor fear changed significantly from before to after the manipulation. Removal of the tourniquet was associated with an increase in a sense of well-being and a decrease in fear which probably reflected relief that the pain experience was over. The effect was strongest in the irrelevant-information condition.

Perception of being in danger. The measure of perception of being in danger was the subject's response to the request, "*While the cuff was inflated,* it might have occurred to you that your arm and hand were in danger of injury. Indicate for each of the sensations the degree that you thought your arm and hand might have been in danger of injury." The statement was followed by a list of eight sensations, each with a 7-point scale (1 labeled "not at all" and 7 "extreme") and a column to check if the sensation had not been experienced. Information did not systematically affect perception of the danger of the ischemic pain experience. None of the comparisons between the relevant- and irrelevant-information conditions for each of the sensations aproached significance. The t values ranged from .32 to .99.

Cognitive processes. There were no significant differences between the two information conditions on subject-reported search of past experience. All of the subjects in the relevant-information condition reported that they searched past experience to get an idea of what their arm would feel like; 8 of the 10 irrelevant-information subjects reported this activity.

Using the 7-point scale, subjects were asked to estimate the amount of attention paid to their arms between judgments in the beginning, middle, and end of the time the cuff was inflated. For the relevant-information subjects the amount of attention to the arm was nearly constant; the means were 5.2, 5.2, and 5.0. For the irrelevant-information subjects, attention to the arm was low in the beginning and increased with repeated measurement; the means were 3.7, 4.7, and 5.3. A repeated-measures analysis of variance produced an F ratio for the interaction between information conditions and time that approached significance ($F = 2.84$, $df = 2/35$, $p < .10$).

Discussion

The findings from Experiment I supported the hypothesis. The information relevant to forming accurate expectations about physical sensations was associated with less intense emotional response during painful stimulation. Accurate expectations about sensations did not prevent distress, but instead dampened the distress reaction in the beginning of the experience. After experiencing the painful stimulus for a few minutes, the effect of initial accurate expectations about sensations on distress diminished.

The effect of the messages on distress cannot be explained by the intervening process of different fear levels. The only variable affecting fear level was time. Subjects were less frightened after the painful experience than before. Neither of the messages significantly affected the level of reported fear. Similarly, the messages did not affect subjects' perceptions of danger. The sensations were perceived to be equally dangerous by subjects in both information conditions. Nor can the results be explained by differences in perceived helplessness. Perceived helplessness as reflected by the Mood Adjective Check Lists was not affected by the information manipulations.

The relevant-information manipulation was a composite of new information about sensations to expect and references to past experience (arm being "asleep"). The lack of a significant difference between information conditions on search of past experience suggests that such a search is not essential to forming accurate expectations about sensations.

The amount of attention paid to the sensations may be an important factor in the perception of the pain experience. The low distress ratings for the relevant-information condition could have been due to the information directing the subject's attention to his arm and the sensations. There was a trend for relevant-information subjects to attend to the sensations more than irrelevant-information subjects. On the other hand, Ross et al. (1969) have suggested that attending to the emotionally relevant source of arousal increases emotional response.

EXPERIMENT II

The effect of directing the subject's attention to his sensations on his perceptions of the pain experience was examined in Experiment II. The attention factor was manipulated orthogonally to the information factor in a 2 × 2 design. Attention to the sensations was manipulated by giving the subject a task which either directed his attention to or distracted him from the sensations. The distraction task also provided the means to test the effect on distress of interrupting ongoing behavior. Mandler and Watson (1966) hypothesized that distress is increased when ongoing behavior is interrupted. Interruption was accomplished by omitting the attention or distraction task for one of the intervals between the ratings of sensation and distress.

The content of the two information manipulations was more similar in Experiment II than in Experiment I. The messages were identical with one exception. The relevant information told subjects the sensations frequently experienced, and the irrelevant information explained the procedures to be carried out. Two experimenters were used; one delivered the information manipulations, and the other put the tourniquet on the subject. This allowed the messages to be delivered verbally to the subject and prevented the experimenter, who was present during the time the cuff was inflated, from knowing the subject's information condition.

Method

Subjects. Male subjects were selected by the same procedure used in Experiment I. Subjects who admitted, during the initial contact by telephone, to a health problem, were over 25 years old, or who had been in the armed services were not scheduled. It was discovered during Experiment I that men who had been in the armed services had often had their blood pressure measured by inexperienced people who left the cuff inflated for long periods of time. This causes sensations similar to the ischemic pain used in the experiment. The subjects who reported were again questioned about their health and sports activities. The sample consisted of 48 subjects.

The first experimenter assigned the subjects randomly to one of the four conditions. She placed a D or A after the subjects' names to inform the second experimenter about the assignment to attention or distraction conditions.

Procedure. Both experimenters were female. On the way to the experimental room, the first experimenter introduced the subject to the second experimenter. The introduction to the experiment varied from that used in Experiment I in two ways. The subject was told *(a)* that the second experimenter would put the tourniquet on him and *(b)* that every subject was to have the tourniquet on the same length of time (but they were not told how long the tourniquet would be on). The same Mood Adjective Check List that was used in Experiment I was administered.

To insure that would not vary, the information manipulations were read to subjects by the first experimenter. The relevant-information subjects heard the following relevant information.

> I want to tell you more about what you can expect to feel while the tourniquet is on. You can expect to feel pressure and sensations such as tingling and aching, followed by numbness. Your fingernails will probably turn blue. The tourniquet is a blood-pressure cuff, but the procedure we use is different from having your blood pressure measured. Our procedure causes lack of blood in the arm and it is unlikely that you have experienced a procedure of this kind before. The typical sensations you should expect to see and feel are pres-

sure, tingling, aching, numbness, and blueness of the fingernails.

The irrelevant-information subjects heard the following irrelevant information:

> I want to tell you more about what you can expect to happen while the tourniquet is on. You can expect that the cuff will be placed on your upper arm and then pumped up to 250 millimeters of mercury. The tourniquet is a blood-pressure cuff, but the procedure we use is different from having your blood pressure measured. Our procedure causes lack of blood in the arm and it is unlikely that you have experienced a procedure of this kind before. Typically the cuff is put in place and then pumped up to 250 millimeters of mercury so you should expect that to happen.

The directions for using the sensation and distress scales to record judgments and for the hand exercises were the same as in Experiment I. They were tape recorded by the second experimenter.

The first experimenter reviewed the tasks in the order the subject would be asked to do them, asked for questions, and then gave one of the following reviews of the manipulation, depending on the information condition to which the subject was assigned.

In the relevant-information condition:

> You have been given so many instructions you probably have forgotten what you can expect to feel. You can expect your arm and hand to tingle and ache, followed by numbness, and your fingernails will probably turn blue. Such things as tingling, aching, numbness, and blueness are typical for this procedure.

In the irrelevant-information condition:

> You have been given so many instructions you probably have forgotten what you can expect to happen. You can expect the cuff to be placed on your upper arm and then pumped up to 250 millimeters of mercury. This is the typical way that this procedure we use is carried out.

The subject was given the second Mood Adjective Check List to fill out and the first experimenter left the room.

The second experimenter entered the room, confirmed which was the subject's dominant hand, and placed the blood-pressure cuff on the upper arm of the non-dominant hand. She asked the subject if he had any questions. Then the subject was told the cuff was to be inflated, he would be directed to do the hand exercises, and then he would be asked to make his judgments about his experience.

The first ratings of sensations and distress were made 1 minute 25 seconds after the cuff was inflated. The ratings were repeated every 45 seconds. After the second set of ratings the distraction or attention task was introduced.

The distraction task consisted of a half sheet of paper with the word "multiplication" followed by three rows of three problems (3 digits × 1 digit).

The attention task was a half sheet of paper with the direction "Look at and think about your arm and hand. Which of these sensations do you have now?" The five sensations the relevant-information group was told to expect plus burning sensation and cramping were listed. Each sensation was followed with "Yes___ No___."

Following the second ratings, the task was placed in front of the subject as the experimenter said, "I would like for you to work these multiplication problems (check off this list)." When the next ratings were requested, the experimenter removed the paper from the subject's table.

The interruption of ongoing behavior manipulation consisted of withholding the distraction or attention task during the interval between the fourth and fifth ratings. The experimenter explained the withholding of the task by saying, "You don't have to work problems (check off a list) this time." The task was reinstated between the fifth and sixth ratings.

The cuff was deflated and removed following the sixth ratings. The subject was told that he was through with that part of the experiment and that he had only paper-and-pencil tasks left to do.

A questionnaire similar to the one used in Experiment I was filled out by the subject, after which he answered the third Mood Adjective Check List. Each subject was given a complete explanation of the experiment before being dismissed.

Results

Success of manipulations. For each of eight plausible sensations, the subject was asked if he had been aware of, expected, and remembered being told to expect the sensation. Relevant information resulted in subjects expecting more of the sensations they experienced than irrelevant-informa-

Table 4. Experiment II: checks on information manipulations

Condition	*Mean number of sensations experienced and expected*	*Mean number of target sensations remembered being told*	*Mean number of target sensations aware of*
Relevant information – attention	4.6[a]	3.8[b]	4.1[c]
Relevant information – distraction	5.2	3.8	4.4
Irrelevant information – attention	3.8	1.0	4.4
Irrelevant information – distraction	3.6	.7	4.2

Note. Analyzed with a two-way analysis of variance with information and attention as factors, $df = 1/44$ for all F ratios.
[a]For information, $F = 7.25$, $p < .025$; for attention – distraction, $F = .15$; for Information × Attention – Distraction, $F = .92$.
[b]For information, $F = 141.82$, $p < .001$; for attention – distraction, $F = .25$; for Information × Attention – Distraction, $F = 1.32$.
[c]For information, $F = .15$; for attention – distraction, $F = .15$; for Information × Attention – Distraction, $F = 1.32$.

Table 5. Experiment II: analysis of variance for sensation ratings

Source	*df*	*MS*	*F*
Between subjects			
Information (A)	1	1974.00	.84
Attention – distraction (B)	1	60.50	.03
A × B	1	4117.78	1.75
Error	44	2357.10	
Within subjects			
Time (C)	5	1594.04	17.78**
A × C	5	81.62	.91
B × C	5	138.45	1.54
A × B × C	5	202.56	2.26*
Error	220	89.65	

*$p < .05$.
**$p < .001$.

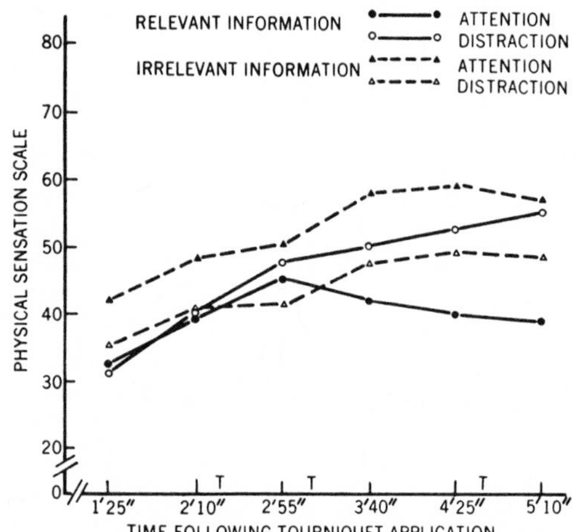

Fig. 3. Mean sensation ratings for conditions over time for Experiment II. (T indicates intervals during which subjects worked on a distraction or attention task.)

tion subjects (Table 4). Subjects in the relevant-information condition remembered that they were told to expect the five target sensations, while those in the irrelevant-information condition remembered that they were not told to expect the sensations. The subjects in all the conditions were aware of most of the five target sensations.

Sensation ratings were analyzed with a repeated-measures analysis of variance with information, attention-distraction, and time as factors. There were significant F ratios for time and the three-way interaction of Information × Attention – Distraction × Time (see Table 5). The three-way interaction was examined by a separate analysis of variance for each information condition with attention-distraction and time as factors. In the relevant-information condition, sensation ratings increased significantly over time ($F = 8.08$, $df = 5/110$, $p < .001$) and attention – distraction interacted with time ($F = 2.95$, $df = 5/110$, $p < .05$). In the relevant-information condition, attending to the arm and hand resulted in a trend for sensation ratings to level off after the third rating. Distraction was associated with an increase in ratings over time (see Figure 3). A trends analysis within the relevant-information condition revealed that the linear trends for attention and distraction differed at the .10 level (Linear Attention – Distraction × Time, $F = 4.14$, $df = 1/22$). In the irrelevant-information condition, the only significant F ratio

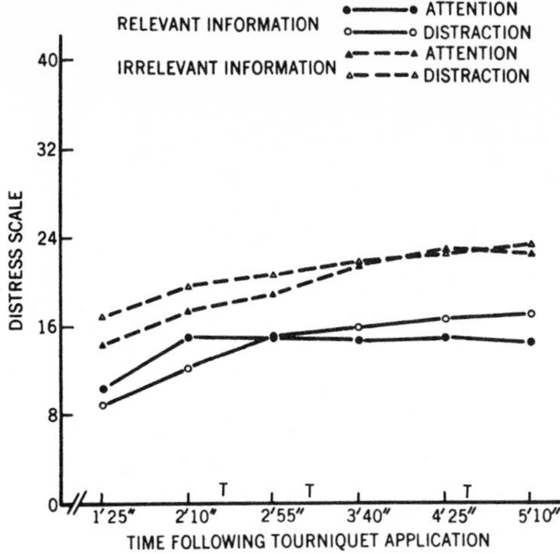

Fig. 4. Mean distress ratings for conditions over time for Experiment II. (T indicates intervals during which subjects worked on a distraction or attention task.)

was for time ($F = 11.28$, $df = 5/110$, $p < .001$).

The information manipulations were successful in establishing differences in expectations about sensations without affecting awareness of sensations. In the relevant-information condition, the perception of intensity of sensations during the last half of the time the cuff was inflated was affected by attending to the arm. But the differences in linear trend between attention and distraction were only of borderline significance.

Distress ratings. Distress ratings were analyzed with a repeated-measures analysis of variance with information, attention–distraction, and time as factors. The variables affecting distress ratings were information and time (Figure 4 and Table 6). As expected, irrelevant information resulted in higher distress ratings than relevant information. Distress increased with time.

If attention to sensations had affected the distress response, interactions with time would have occurred. None of the interactions was significant. As can be seen in Figure 4, attending to the arm when informed about the sensations to expect resulted in a slight decrease in distress ratings. On the other hand, attending in the absence of information about the sensations to expect resulted in distress ratings increasing with time. However, the

Table 6. Experiment II: analysis of variance for distress ratings

Source	*df*	*MS*	*F*
Between subjects			
Information (A)	1	2526.42	5.58*
Attention–distraction (B)	1	35.42	.08
A × B	1	21.67	.05
Error	44	452.61	
Within subjects			
Time (C)	5	322.68	16.68**
A × C	5	12.53	.65
B × C	5	7.01	.36
A × B × C	5	25.83	1.34
Error	220	19.35	

$^*p < .025$.
$^{**}p < .001$.

difference in linear trend between attention and distraction conditions within the relevant-information condition was not significant.

The expectation from the interruption of ongoing behavior theory (Mandler & Watson, 1966) was that withholding the distraction task would cause an increase in distress. As can be seen in Figure 4, the changes in distress ratings over the interval without a task were slight. A 2 × 2 analysis of variance of change scores between the fourth and fifth ratings with attention–distraction and information as factors produced no significant F ratios.

Moods. Repeated-measures analysis of variance (information, attention–distraction, and time as factors) of scores from the Mood Adjective Check Lists for three negative moods (fear, helplessness, and depression) produced only one significant F ratio for each mood. Each of the negative moods changed significantly with time (F ratios ranged from 35.41 to 40.65, $df = 2/88$, $p < .001$). There was a reduction in the negative moods after the tourniquet was removed. There was no significant changes for any of the three negative moods from before to after the information manipulations.

The only significant F ratio from analysis of the well-being scores was a three-way interaction (Information × Attention–Distraction × Time, $F = 4.05$, $df = 2/88$, $p < .025$). This interaction was primarily due to subjects in the irrelevant-information–distraction condition reporting a reduction in this positive mood after the tourniquet was removed in contrast to no significant changes (Newman-Keuls test) for the other conditions.

Perception of being in danger. A question about the subject's perception of being in danger appeared on the questionnaire. The question was "*While the cuff was inflated,* it might have occurred to you that your arm and hand were in danger of injury. Indicate the degree that you thought your arm and hand might have been in danger of injury." A 7-point scale followed the question (1 labeled "Did not think about being in danger," and 7 "Thought extensively about being in danger"). A two-way analysis of variance of these scores with information and attention–distraction as factors produced no significant F ratios. The overall mean was 1.9, which suggests that subjects did not perceive that they were in serious danger of injury.

Perceptions of the experimenters. Questions at the end of the questionnaire asked about perceptions of the experimenters. Subjects were asked to evaluate the competency of the experimenters and the degree of concern they showed for the subject as an individual. Two-way analysis of variance with information and attention–distraction as factors was used to analyze the responses to the questions. There were no significant differences in perception of competency of either experimenter attributable to the experimental conditions. Perceptions of concern of the first experimenter, who gave the subjects the information manipulation, did not differ by experimental conditions. Perceptions of concern of the second experimenter, who was present during the time the tourniquet was in place, produced an Information × Attention–Distraction interaction ($F = 5.81$, $df = 1/44$, $p < .025$). The order of the means from high to low was irrelevant information–attention (6.3), relevant information–distraction (5.7), and relevant information–distraction (5.2), and relevant information–attention (5.0). The responses were made on a 7-point scale with 1 labeled "Showed no concern" and 7 labeled "Showed extreme concern." These differences in perception of concern could not have systemically affected distress ratings. High distress ratings occurred in one of the conditions (irrelevant information–attention) with high concern, and low distress ratings in the other condition (relevant information–distraction) with high concern.

Discussion

The hypothesis that preparatory information which reduces the incongruency between expected and experienced sensations is associated with less intense emotional response during painful stimulation was supported by both Experiments I and II. The trend for the intensity of emotional response to increase over time suggests that expectations about physical sensations and experience may have become more incongruent as time passed. However, if expectations were reinstated, the increase in incongruency between expectation and experience could be stopped. This would result in lack of acceleration in distress response. In Experiment II, subjects who were asked to report the presence or absence of sensations could have had their expectations reinstated. Although the effect was very weak, distress ratings in the relevant–distraction condition tended not to accelerate after the attention task was introduced.

Attention to the sensations did not produce a main effect of distress or sensation ratings. In the relevant-information condition, attention to the arm resulted in lower sensation ratings than distraction. But this effect on sensations was not observed in the irrelevant-information condition. There was no significant overall effect for attention on distress ratings, nor was there a significant effect in either information condition.

The interruption of ongoing behavior theory received no support. Withholding the distraction task in Experiment II had no effect on distress ratings. This was a weak interruption manipulation and may not have provided an adequate test of Mandler and Watson's (1966) theory. However, perceived helplessness was not affected differentially by the information manipulations in either experiment. Thus, the perceived helplessness interpretation does not seem applicable to these data.

There were no indications that the manipulations affected the subjects' perceptions of the danger of the situation in either experiment. This lends no support to the interpretation that the differences in distress were due to differences in perceptions of danger (Lazarus, 1968). As could be expected from a laboratory-produced painful stimulation, subjects did not perceive that they were in much danger of injury. Even in this low-danger situation, distress was relatively high for the subjects who were not given information from which to form accurate expectations about the sensations.

The hypothesis from the emotional drive theory (Janis, 1958, 1967) that an optimum amount of fear before the threatening event results in low distress during the encounter with the event does not explain the findings in these experiments. The messages about what to expect did not differentially affect fear levels in either experiment.

Evidence to support the hypothesis that there is a functional relationship between degree of incongruency, between expected and experienced physical sensations and level of distress, was not especially strong. In both experiments, subjects in the relevant-information condition reported expecting significantly more of the sensations they experienced than those in the irrelevant-information condition, but the actual differences were not large. The subjects were asked to recall their expectations after the tourniquet was removed. Recall could have been distorted in the direction of experience.

EXPERIMENT III

Experiment III was designed to determine the effect of the different information on expectations about sensations before the painful experience. Anticipated levels of sensations and distress were also measured. The low distress observed in the relevant-information conditions in the first two experiments could have resulted from low levels of anticipated distress.

Method

*Subjects.*Subjects were selected, contacted, and screened by the same procedure used in Experiment II. The sample consisted of 24 male subjects who were randomly assigned to the two information conditions.

Procedure. The procedure of Experiment II was used up to the point of inflation of the tourniquet, with one exception. The experimenter who gave the information manipulation also placed the tourniquet on the subject's arm. After the tourniquet was in place, the experimenter told the subject that there were two paper-and-pencil tasks for him to perform before the tourniquet would be inflated.

Anticipated level of sensations and distress was assessed by asking subjects to demonstrate that they understood the sensation and distress scales by making hypothetical ratings. The instructions to each subject were:

> The sensation and distress scales are the main tool we provide subjects to help them describe their experience. Before I inflate the cuff, I would like for you to practice using the scales.
>
> Using an X, mark the sensation scale at the point you *think* the sensations will be at the time you are to make the first real judgment.
>
> Now place 2 X's on the sensation scale and the distress scale at the point you think the sensations and distress will be just before the tourniquet is removed.

The subject's second task was to report his expectations about the occurrence of specific sensations. He responded to questions about the likelihood of feeling each of nine sensations (the five target sensations plus four other plausible sensations) on a scale ranging from 0 to 100% chance.

The subject was informed that the tourniquet would not be inflated and it was removed. The experimenter explained the purpose of the research and paid the subject. Verbal and nonverbal behavior indicated that all but one subject had believed the tourniquet would be inflated. The nonbelieving subject's data was consistent with the data from other subjects and was included in the analysis.

Results

There was a trend for subjects in the relevant-information condition to report higher probability that they would experience the five target sensations and lower probability of experiencing infrequent sensations than those in the irrelevant-information condition. The difference between information conditions reached statistical

Table 7. Experiment III: accurate and inaccurate expectations about sensations to be experienced

Information condition	*Mean percentage chance of experiencing the 5 frequently reported sensations (accurate expectations)*	*Mean percentage chance of experiencing the 4 infrequently reported sensations (inaccurate expectations)*	*Mean accurate expectations minus inaccurate expectations*
Relevant	79.8	39.3	40.5
Irrelevant	72.6	48.3	24.3
t	1.02	1.60	2.14*

Note. $df = 22$.
$^{*}p < .05$.

Table 8. Experiment III: anticipated sensations and distress ratings

Information condition	*Sensation ratings*		*Distress ratings*	
	First	*Last*	*First*	*Last*
Relevant				
M	29.8	64.4	11.2	30.3
SD	9.20	22.13	7.28	7.96
Irrelevant				
M	40.4	75.2	14.7	29.8
SD	23.06	13.80	6.18	5.49
t	1.48	1.44	1.27	.18

Note. $df = 22$.

significance when expectations about frequently and infrequently experienced sensations were pooled (Table 7). Expectations about infrequently experienced sensations made the greatest contribution to this difference.

The level of sensations subjects anticipated at the beginning and the end of the experience did not differ significantly by information groups (Table 8). However, there was a trend for subjects in the relevant-information condition to anticipate the sensations to be lower than those in the irrelevant-information condition, thus replicating the same pattern as the actual sensation ratings in Experiment I and Experiment II. The first ratings in the irrelevant-information condition were more variable than those in the relevant-information condition. ($F_{max} = 6.28$, $df = 2/11$, $p < .01$). Information about sensations to expect may minimize the effects of individual differences.

The level of anticipated distress for the first or last ratings did not differ significantly by information conditions (Table 8). There was a trend for subjects in the relevant-information condition to anticipate that the distress would be lower in the beginning than those in the irrelevant-information condition; however, the last anticipated distress ratings were nearly the same for both information conditions.

This pattern of anticipated distress ratings was different from the actual distress ratings in Experiment I and Experiment II. In the first two experiments, distress ratings for the relevant-information group were consistently lower than for the irrelevant-information group.

GENERAL DISCUSSION

Experiment III demonstrated that information which resulted in accurate expectations about sensations experienced did not significantly lower the levels of anticipated distress. It is unlikely that the observed reduction in distress in the relevant-information condition in Experiments I and II was due to differences in anticipated levels of distress. Only when there was a combination of accurate expectations about sensations and experience with the sensations (Experiments I and II) did a reduction in distress ratings occur.

Information about sensations frequently experienced apparently structured subjects' expectations. Structured expectations increased subjects' confidence that they would not experience plausible but unlikely sensations, as well as increasing confidence that they would experience likely sensations (Experiment III). Attempts to measure the degree of incongruency between expectations and experience reflected significant differences in incongruency between information groups in each of the experiments. These consistent findings support the hypothesis that emotional response to a threatening event is affected by incongruency between expectations and experience. More refined methods of measuring or manipulating incongruency are required to test the nature of the functional relationship between incongruency and emotional response.

It was found (Experiment III) that expectations of sensations rarely experienced by subjects contributed to inaccurate expectations. In attribution experiments, subjects who are led to attribute physical sensations to a source relevant to emotional response are given descriptions of sensations rarely experienced by subjects during confrontation with the threatening stimulus (Nisbett & Schachter, 1966; Ross et al., 1969). The high emotional response observed in subjects in those conditions may be due to such descriptions of sensations contributing to inaccurate expectations about the sensory experience.

This research helps to make specific the characteristics of "appropriate" and "proper" information in Schachter's (1971) terms. An advantage the cognitive mechanism based on accurate expectations about sensory experience has over attribution processes is that it can accommodate situations where the threat is strong and the source of the threat is salient. Nisbett and Schachter (1966) demonstrated that the attribution hypothesis was supported only in a low-threat situation. These authors suggested that it is unlikely that attribution notions will apply to situations where threat level is high. The incongruency hypothesis has the potential for the theoretical notions to be useful in situations where people experience threatening events in real life. The potential for application in health care settings influenced the selection of the content of the irrelevant message in the experiments reported here. Health workers might assume that telling patients how a procedure was performed would reduce emotional response during the experience. The line of reasoning underlying the laboratory experiments has been used to design experiments conducted in the hospital (Johnson & Leventhal, 1973, in press; Johnson, Morrissey, & Leventhal, 1973, in press).

Patients scheduled for an endoscopic examination were subjects in the hospital experiments. The examination requires that a flexible tube 12 millimeters in diameter be passed into the stomach through the mouth. Information conditions were formed by playing tape-recorded messages to the patient before the examination. In both experiments the patients who heard a description of the sensations frequently experienced during the examination required less tranquilizer to enable them to tolerate the tube than patients who heard no taped message. Indications of emotional upset while the tube was in place were less for those patients who had heard a description of sensations as compared to those who heard a description of the endoscopic examination procedure. The theoretical notions about the role of incongruency between expectations and experience are guiding additional experiments in health-care settings.

The demonstration that the sensation and distress components of the pain experience can be rated separately and do not have a one-to-one relationship challenges the traditional methods of measuring pain by determining thresholds. The two thresholds that have received the most attention are the intensity of stimulation at which pain is reported and maximum tolerance. Attempts to determine the physiological and psychological loadings of each of the thresholds have not been very successful (Gelfand, 1964; Gelfand, Ullman, & Krasner, 1963; Wolff & Horland, 1967; Wolff, Krasnegor, & Farr, 1965). Direct separate measurement of the perception of the physiological and psychological components of the pain experience nullifies the issue of how the components of the pain experience are loaded in the traditional threshold measurements. The use of threshold measurements of pain in the laboratory has contributed to the problem of bridging the gap between laboratory study and the study of pain in the clinical setting. Treatment for relief of pain is usually begun before maximum tolerance levels are reached. In addition, analgesic drugs are selective as to the site of their primary action (Lim, 1967). For example, the appropriate drug for a patient reporting high painful sensations and low distress would be different from the drug appropriate for a patient with low sensations and high distress.

REFERENCES

Beecher, H. K. *Measurement of subjective responses: Quantitative effects of drugs.* New York: Oxford University Press, 1959.

Casey, K. L., & Melzack, R. Neural mechanisms of pain: A conceptual model. In E. Leong Way (Ed.), *New concepts in pain and its clinical management.* Philadelphia: Davis, 1967.

Gelfand, S. The relationship of experimental pain tolerance to pain threshold. *Canadian Journal of Psychology,* 1964, **14,** 36-42.

Gelfand, S., Ullman, L. P., & Krasner, L. The placebo response: An experimental approach. *Journal of Nervous and Mental Disease,* 1963, **136,** 379-387.

Janis, I. L. *Psychological stress.* New York: Wiley, 1958.

Janis, I. L. Effects of fear arousal on attitude change: Recent developments in theory and experimental research. In L. Berkowitz (Ed.), *Advances in experimental social psychology.* Vol. 3. New York: Academic Press, 1967.

Johnson, J. E., & Leventhal, H. The effects of accurate expectations and behavioral instructions on reactions during a noxious medical examination. *Journal of Personality and Social Psychology,* 1973, in press.

Johnson, J. E., Morrisey, J. F., & Leventhal, H. Psychological preparation for an endoscopic examination. *Gastrointestinal Endoscopy,* 1973, in press.

Lazarus, R. S. Emotions and adaptation: Conceptual and empirical relations. *Nebraska Symposium on Motivation,* 1968, **16,** 175-266.

Lim, R. K. S. Pharmacologic viewpoint of pain and analgesia. In E. Leong Way (Ed.), *New concepts in pain and its clinical management.* Philadelphia: Davis, 1967.

Mandler, G., & Watson, D. L. Anxiety and interruption of behavior. In C. D. Spielberger (Ed.), *Anxiety and behavior.* New York: Academic Press, 1966.

Melzack, R., & Wall, P. D. Pain mechanisms: A new theory. *Science,* 1965, **150,** 971-979.

Nisbett, R. E., & Schachter, S. Cognitive manipulation of pain. *Journal of Experimental Social Psychology,* 1966, **2,** 227-236.

Ross, L., Rodin, J., & Zimbardo, P. G. Toward an attribution therapy: The reduction of fear through induced cognitive-emotional misattribution. *Journal of Personality and Social Psychology,* 1969, **12,** 279-288.

Schachter, S. The interaction of cognitive and physiological determinants of emotional state. In L. Berkowitz (Ed.). *Advances in experimental social psychology.* Vol. 1. New York: Academic Press, 1964.

Schachter, S. *Emotion, obesity, and crime.* New York: Academic Press, 1971.

Schachter, S., & Singer, J. E. Cognitive, social, and physiological determinants of emotional state. *Psychological Review,* 1962, **69,** 379-399.

Smith, G. M., Egbert, L. D., Markowitz, R. A., Mosteller, F., & Beecher, H. K. An experimental pain method sensitive to morphine in man: The submaximum effort tourniquet technique. *Journal of Pharmacology and Experimental Therapeutics,* 1966, **154,** 324-332.

Wolff, B. B., & Horland, A. A. Effect of suggestion upon experimental pain: A validation study. *Journal of Abnormal Psychology,* 1967, **72,** 402-407.

Wolff, B. B., Krasnegor, N. A., & Farr, R. S. Effect of suggestion upon experimental pain response parameters. *Perceptual and Motor Skills,* 1965, **21,** 675-683.

25

Verbal reports of pain without noxious stimulation[1]

Kenneth D. Craig and Stephen M. Weiss[2]

In a recent investigation, Craig and Weiss (1971) noted that willingness to accept or reject electric shocks prior to expressions of pain was highly amenable to social control through the medium of having peers dissimulate less or more pain to essentially the identical noxious experience. When models reported incremental shock as increasingly more severe than the observing *S*s, *S*s reported low thresholds for pain, whereas when the model reported his discomfort to be less noxious, *S*s reported high thresholds for pain and voluntarily accepted high levels of shock. The effects appeared to be analogous to the analgesic control of pain that can be achieved through the use of placebos (Shapiro, 1960), hypnotic induction procedures (Barber & Hahn, 1962), and other similarly effective social techniques (Sternbach, 1968).

The effects noted by Craig and Weiss (1971) were sufficiently marked to suggest the possibility that vicarious influence processes could be utilized to elicit reports of pain even when individuals were subjected to stimulation which previously had not been reported as either painful or noxious. If reports of pain can be facilitated to non-aversive levels of stimulation, the findings would complement the earlier work where the emphasis has been on the inhibition of reports and experiences of distress to supraliminal levels of aversive stimulation (Meichenbaum, 1971).

METHOD

In an effort to maximize modeling effects *S* and the model ostensibly received identical shocks on each presentation, the model indicating his subjective reaction immediately after *S* responded by selecting one of five switches labeled along a scale of perceived aversiveness varying from "undetectable" to "pain."

Subjects

*S*s were 20 male volunteer students from the University of British Columbia, who did not have prior knowledge concerning conditions of the study. They were randomly assigned to one of two groups. The mean age was 18.9 yr., and the range was from 18 to 22 yr. The same paid male model and female *E* were used for all groups.

Apparatus

Electric shock was generated by a constant current stimulator and delivered to the volar surface of *S*'s right forearm through concentric electrodes. Gritty electrode paste was used to remove dead epidermis and to reduce the variability in *S*s' skin resistances. The technique eliminates progressive decrements in the subjective experience of the aversiveness of electric

Reprinted with permission of author and publisher: Craig, K. D., & Weiss, S. M. Verbal reports of pain without noxious stimulation. Perceptual and Motor Skills, 1972, **34,** 943-948.

From the University of British Columbia (K. D. Craig); and The John Hopkins University School of Medicine (S. M. Weiss).

[1]This investigation was supported by Research Grant APA-136 from the National Research Council of Canada. The assistance of Susan McBride and William Criddle is gratefully acknowledged.

[2]Now with the Peace Corps, Washington, D. C.

shock stimulation as contrasted with other shock electrodes (Tursky, Watson, & O'Connell, 1969). The electrode was positioned so that resistances on the electrode-skin circuit across the electrode were reduced to 5,000 ohms. The resistance was checked and returned to this level, if necessary, at the end of each shock series. There were no significant differences between groups in changes in resistance over trials.

To provide a constant nonaversive level of shock stimulation that level reported to be "slightly detectable" but not "painful" by 28 of the 30 *S*s in the earlier study was selected. This level of stimulation was 1.5 mamp. and was 60 Hz in frequency and sinusoidal in waveform. The 2 *S*s in the earlier study not reporting 1.5 mamp. as detectable did not report the shock to be at least "slightly detectable" until either 2.5 mamp. or 4 mamp. had been administered. Shock durations were .5 sec. Subjective intensities were rated by *S*s by depressing one of five microswitches which illuminated red jewel lights above printed labels reading from left to right: (5) "undetectable"; (4) "slightly detectable"; (3) "detectable"; (2) "questionably painful"; (1) "painful."

Procedure

The confederate arrived immediately after *S* and both were queried as to age, year at the university, and academic major, with the confederate posing in all instances to be a 21-yr.-old, second year, business student, changing to the study of English. *S* was seated to the right of the confederate with a wooden screen blocking each participant's view of the other excepting for their left hands as they selected a switch. Both were advised of *E*'s interest in, "how mild electricity influences your perception of when a shock becomes painful." The shocks were described as increasing in intensity, "from levels at which you cannot feel the shock through to the level at which you report pain," at which point no additional shock would be administered. Participation in the study was described as being completely voluntary and all *S*s were given the opportunity to withdraw then or at any other time. None withdrew. Electrodes were then attached and *S*s were requested to not move their arms. They were then advised:

> You will notice that each of your electrodes is connected to this box. This apparatus regulates the voltage, amperage, frequency, and other physical characteristics of the electric shock. On each trial I will press a switch and you will each receive the same shock at the same time. The initial shocks may be so slight as to be undetectable, some you may feel as a warm tickle, some may be stronger and somewhat painful. All I want you to do is to evaluate the intensity of the shock and indicate your response by means of these light switches.

The labels were then read and pointed out and they were advised that the recording equipment required *S* seated on the right to respond first. Five series of shocks were to be administered, ostensibly to study variations in the characteristics of the electricity.

After an opportunity to ask questions had been provided members of the control group were told that the foregoing instructions were intended only for other *S*s. *S* was told to respond as previously instructed, but the model was told to respond only if the shock was so painful that he wished to be disconnected for that particular series.

A minimum of 10 sec. was interposed between each shock administration. At the end of a series of shocks *E* simulated alterations in the shock by changing irrelevant dials on the shock stimulator. The confederate's electrode was not active. Questionnaires examining *S*s' experiences were administered after threshold determinations had been completed.

Confederates' instructions

The modeling group observed a confederate who endeavoured to reduce pain thresholds by selecting switches indicating that the shock was progressively more noxious to him than it was to *S*. *S*'s first switch selection was matched for the first shock followed by repeated selections of the next switch until *S* matched this selection. At that time the confederate remained there for one shock and advanced to the next switch. This procedure was continued until the pain switch was selected by *S*. If *S*s reversed to a switch indicating less experienced intensity the confederate remained on the previous switch for one shock presentation and then moved ahead. If *S*s skipped above the model, advancement would proceed with one switch per shock until the confederate again led *S*. The above rules then were to be followed.

If *S*s failed to follow the model, criteria were established for the discontinuance of a given trial. Twenty consecutive responses at the same switch or a total of 50 shocks without reaching the pain switch led to *E*'s arbitrarily terminating the trial.

The non-modeling group was paired with a model who did not respond to the shocks although ostensibly he also was receiving the identical shock. Since *S*s in this group conceivably could have continued to accept shocks without end, because there was neither physical nor social provocation for ending a series, each was yoked with *S* in the other group and received only as many shocks as did his reference partner.

An additional two groups of 10 *S*s were run randomly interspersed with *S*s in the above two groups. The additional groups received incremental shocks to provide a replication of the earlier findings and to evaluate the effects of having the model express verbal pain. Since the findings do not differ from those of Craig and Weiss (1971) and the effects of nonincremental and incremental shock cannot be contrasted because the rate of moving along the pain scale is a function of the size of the shock intensity increments these two groups were not considered in this paper.

RESULTS

The non-modeling group selected the pain switch but once out of the 50 opportunities, whereas the modeling group selected the pain switch on 37 of the 50 series administered to this group. The two groups differed significantly. A t test for independent groups on the frequency of selection of the pain switch was significant ($p < .001$). Although the non-modeling group did not select the pain switch with any degree of frequency their selections of the four remaining switches specifying lesser perceived aversiveness tended to be evenly distributed. Thus their mean frequencies of selecting switches 5, 4, 3, and 2 on each trial were 3.06, 3.70, 3.48 and 3.88 respectively. On the other hand, the modeling group tended to favor switches indicating that the shocks were of relatively strong intensity. The mean frequencies of selecting switches 5, 4, 3, and 2 were .68, 1.78, 3.12 and 8.18 respectively. Apparently, it was relatively easy to express the judgment that the shocks were progressively more noxious but difficult to describe them as painful.

On the five successive series of shocks the modeling group tended to require progressively fewer switches prior to selecting the pain switch. Thus the mean number of switch selections for each subsequent series was 23.6, 15.5, 10.8, 7.3 and 12.15. The decrease was statistically significant ($F = 6.21$, $df = 4/72$, $p < .01$).

The groups did not differ significantly on the frequencies of reversals or out of sequence switch selections on any specific trial or to any specific switch.

The questionnaire yielded the following findings. On no question did the two groups' ratings differ significantly. Both indicated that the severity of pain experienced on the last shock presentation was low to medium with the nonmodeling group assigning it a mean rating of 2.5 and the modeling group a mean rating of 3.6 on a 7-point scale with the polar extremes labelled "not painful" and "very painful." On the rating of the degree of difficulty involved in making the judgment as to whether the shock was painful or not both groups preferred the "very easy" end of the 7-point scale with the modeling and non-modeling groups providing means of 2.9 and 3.7 respectively. On a further question the model was rated as slightly less tolerant of the shock than *S*s. Finally, the groups tended to feel that the model had little influence on their ratings.

DISCUSSION

The findings confirmed expectations that reports of pain could be elicited to levels of shock usually perceived as nonaversive through exposure to a relatively intolerant model. In the previous study (Craig & Weiss, 1971) using an ascending series of incremental shocks, observing either intolerant or tolerant models led to mean verbal pain thresholds of 2.50 and 8.65 mamp., respectively. In the present study using nonincremental shock and a model who dissimulated less tolerance for the shock than *S*, reports of pain were being elicited at 1.5 mamp. In the previous study the group exposed to incremental shock and an intolerant model reached the verbal pain threshold after a mean of 5.0 shock presentations (2.5 mamp.), whereas, in the present study employing nonincremental shock and the modeling variable, the group required a mean of 13.8 shock presentations before reaching the pain criterion.

The tendency for the modeling group to require fewer shocks over time prior to selecting the pain switch suggested that in certain social contexts verbal expressions of pain are easier to express as time progresses. In natural social groups expressions of pain may have strong immediate social consequences because others frequently provide relief, sympathy, and attention. In the present study, selecting the pain switch may have had positive consequences for *S*s in that it led to the end of a trial and brought *S* closer to the end of the experiment.

Alternative explanations were available for the data. The first suggests that perceptual changes occurred in the actual aversiveness of the somesthetic experience. Studies of vicarious classical conditioning (Bandura & Rosenthal, 1966; Berger, 1962; Craig & Lowry, 1969) suggest that the model's report of greater aversiveness than that of *S* would instigate negative affect in *S* that would become conditioned to the shock. Subsequent presentations of the shock would in turn elicit and increase perceived aversiveness. An alternative response-bias explanation suggests that information specifying the appropriate role for *S* would lead to altered criteria for reporting the shock as being painful and that the subjective experience itself did not change. It may be, however, that conforming to a model's standards would deprive an observer of the opportunity to test more aversive experiences and that this in turn would lead to expectations that anything but very mild experiences would be painful (Schacter & Singer, 1962).

The effects of the modeling variables seem analogous to analgesic effects generated through the use of direct suggestion, hypnosis, and placebos. Social cues apparently function to alter the standards of those experiencing pain so that levels of pain normally leading to avoidance responses are accepted without expressions of undue discomfort. The earlier study provided a more direct analogue to studies of hypnosis and placebos since the intolerant model raised pain thresholds to the extent that *S*s were willing to undergo a mean of 8.65 mamp. of shock. Studies of hypnosis, placebo effects and direct suggestion have focused on the inhibition of the experience of pain and verbal reports. The present study attempted to facilitate these reports. If generalization effects occur *S*s exposed to intolerant models would be expected to report pain at relatively low levels of stimulation in other social contexts and to other forms of painful stimulation.

REFERENCES

Bandura, A., & Rosenthal., T. L. Vicarious classical conditioning as a function of arousal level. *Journal of Personality and Social Psychology,* 1966, 3, 54-62.

Barber, T. X., & Hahn, K. W. Physiological and subjective responses to pain-producing stimulation under hynotically-suggested and waking-imagined "analgesia." *Journal of Abnormal and Social Psychology,* 1962, 65, 411-418.

Berger, S. M. Conditioning through vicarious instigation. *Psychological Review,* 1962, 69, 450-466.

Craig, K. D., & Lowery, J. H. Heart-rate components of conditioned vicarious autonomic responses. *Journal of Personality and Social Psychology,* 1969, 11, 381-387.

Craig, K. D., & Weiss, S. M. Vicarious influences on pain threshold determinations. *Journal of Personality and Social Psychology,* 1971, 17, in press.

Meichenbaum, D. H. Examination of model characteristics in reducing avoidance behavior. *Journal of Personality and Social Psychology,* 1971, 17, 298-307.

Schacter, S., & Singer, J. E. Cognitive, social, and physiological determinants of emotional state. *Psychological Review,* 1962, 69, 379-399.

Shapiro, A. K. A contribution to a history of the placebo effect. *Behavioral Science,* 1960, 5, 109-135.

Sternbach, R. A. *Pain: a psychophysiological analysis.* New York: Academic Press, 1968.

Tursky, B., Watson, P.O., & O'Connell, D. N. A concentric shock electrode for pain stimulation. *Psychophysiology,* 1965, 1, 296-298.

SECTION SIX

Effects of hypnosis and acupuncture on pain

Section six deals with a revived interest in old and ancient techniques for the relief of pain: hypnosis and acupuncture. Chaves and Barber (Reading 27) describe reports dating back to the early 1800's, in which surgery was painlessly performed with the use of hypnosis. Acupuncture is an ancient Chinese approach to disease based on the restoration of an imbalance of bodily humors (Van Nghi, Fisch, and Kao, 1973). Current interest in acupuncture centers around its use for the relief of pain.

What is hypnosis? How does it work? What effects does it have on the individual? Barber (see Chaves and Barber, Reading 27) has argued that hypnosis does not place a person in a different state from that of the waking individual. Essentially, Barber has removed much of the glamour and magical notions associated with hypnosis by the use of carefully controlled laboratory research in which he has been able to demonstrate with awake simulators or with highly motivated subjects many of the same results claimed for hypnosis.

What Barber has stressed is that many of the claims of hypnosis are based on the individual's readiness to accept suggestions and not on a magical trance power that certain individuals possess to influence others. It would follow, therefore, that many of the procedures (such as deep relaxation) used to produce a "trance" are really not necessary. It would also follow that the variables affecting motivation and social influence would most probably affect hypnotic reactions. Much of what is done under hypnosis, such as distraction, could also be done with the waking individual. In fact, many good practitioners routinely use such procedures without labeling them hypnosis.

In terms of pain reduction specifically, Barber has argued that the spectacular results claimed for surgery under hypnosis are due to a heightened motivation, an increased readiness to accept suggestions from the physician, and the accompanying reduction in fear and anxiety. Hypnotic effectiveness in pain control depends mainly on a positive doctor-patient relationship. Then, too, most surgical pain is caused by the incision. There are very few pain receptors in the deeper tissues and organs. Local anesthetic, a frequent concomitant of hypnosis, is used to deaden the pain of the incision. The patient expresses little anxiety, and the surgery proceeds painlessly.

Although Barber's experiments have accomplished a great deal in changing hypnosis from the status of magic to science, many investigators disagree with his conclusions and regard hypnosis as something real—a state different from the waking one.

Hilgard (Reading 26) has also examined hypnosis in the laboratory under controlled conditions and would accept Barber's conclusion that there are no physiological changes produced simply as a result of hypnosis.

However, Hilgard's findings do not mean that physiological changes cannot occur with appropriate suggestions and conditions. For example, when subjects place their arms in cold water, there is a reduction in the perception of pain for those who are hypnotized but not for those who are awake. No difference between subjects is found in heart rate or blood pressure. However, when ischemic pain is used hypnotized subjects show both a reduced perception of pain and a lowered heart rate and blood pressure. Part of the lack of effect of hypnosis on the physiological measures for cold water might be a result of the specific pain stimulus used. Subjects may not be responding to pain but could be responding to the cold.

Hilgard has approached hypnosis on the basis of different levels of consciousness. There seem to be different systems of cognitive functioning, so that even though the pain stimulus is able to reach one level of consciousness, it is blocked from the more immediate level of awareness. That is, the person does perceive the pain stimulus at some lower level; however, he is capable of keeping it from coming to the level of awareness that makes it distressing.

From a Melzack and Wall point of view, both Barber and Hilgard stress the effects of hypnosis on the motivational-affective system of pain control (see Reading 1, Section one). Both view hypnosis as producing an increased readiness to respond to suggestion. Barber feels that there is no such thing as a trance state and that little is to be gained over the "waking" state by the use of hypnotic induction techniques. Hilgard, however, does feel that there is a state called hypnosis and that there the hypnotized individual's responses differ from those of the awake individual.

Clinically, both Hilgard and Barber have much to offer the practitioner in terms of their use of imagery, distraction, refocusing of attention, and so on, to relieve pain. However, on the basis of their personal experience, clinicians would probably disagree with both. Hilgard has argued that relaxation by itself does little to reduce the reactions to pain. However, Thompson (1975), a clinician, has seen great benefits in reducing pain reactions by merely relaxing her patients. Thompson has also produced a film showing the use of hypnosis for pain control during dermabrasion. Barber's argument is that surgery is done painlessly because there are few pain receptors in most organs and tissues other than in the skin. Dermabrasion, however, is performed directly on the skin, where most of the pain receptors are located.

One of the most imaginative and amazing clinicians to use hypnosis is Milton Erickson (Reading 28). He, too, has emphasized that hypnosis is used mainly as a means of securing and fixating the patient's attention and creating a receptive and responsive mental state in the patient to enable him to benefit from the unrealized potential he possesses. Erickson presents two amazing cases using a variation of his famous confusion technique. With the realization of what Erickson accomplished in the relief of intractable pain from cancer, one wonders why hypnosis is not more widely used in pain control.

Sarcedote (1970) has also presented several useful hypnotic techniques for the control of chronic pain. These techniques include such things as time distortion, hypnoplasty, and partial and total amnesia. These articles, among others, offer convincing evidence that the great potential in the clinical use of hypnosis for pain control has yet to be realized.

Acupuncture is another technique that has recently been flourishing in the United States. Melzack (Reading 29) describes some of the treatments in which it has been used along with modern medicine.

Three basic theoretical approaches have been formulated. The traditional Chinese approach describes acupuncture as working through a series of body meridians to correct an imbalance of bodily humors.

Kroger (1973) has argued that acupuncture is nothing more than hypnosis. He claims that he personally has carried out a great deal of surgery by using hypnosis and can demonstrate similar phenomena. Spiegel has also called acupuncture needle hypnosis (personal communication). He claims that his eye roll technique can determine if a patient would benefit equally from hypnosis or acupuncture and that both acupuncture and hypnosis operate on the same principles.

Melzack (Reading 29) presents an approach based on the gate control theory of pain that might account for its effectiveness. The explanation for its effectiveness, however, is still a mystery.

REFERENCES

Kroger, W. S. 1973. Acupunctural analgesia: its explanation by conditioning theory, autogenic training and hypnosis, American Journal of Psychiatry **130:** 855-860.

Sarcedote, P. 1970. Theory and practice of pain control in malignancy and other protracted or recurring painful illnesses, The International Journal of Clinical and Experimental Hypnosis **18:**160–180.

Thompson, K. F. 1975. Hypnosis in dental practice: clinical views. In Weisenberg, M., editor: The control of pain, Psychological Dimensions, Inc., New York.

Van Nghi, N., Fisch, G., and Kao, J. 1973. An introduction to classical acupuncture, American Journal of Chinese Medicine **1:**75-83.

26

A neodissociation interpretation of pain reduction in hypnosis[1]

Ernest R. Hilgard[2]

Pain reduction through hypnosis has baffled scientists ever since its successful use in major surgery in the early nineteenth century. The search for more satisfactory explanations might have continued except that the development of chloroform and ether brought an early end to the use of hypnosis for the purposes of general anesthesia. This was not actually quite the end, however, for hypnosis has been used for pain reduction to some extent ever since, and more recently there has been an upsurge of its use in obstetrics, in the relief of painful burns, in dental extractions, in terminal cancer, and (to a lesser extent) in a variety of surgical operations (e.g., Kroger, 1963; Schneck, 1963). While there are always some doubting Thomases, the evidence is overwhelming that some patients through hypnotic suggestion alone can endure normally painful experiences of stress without feeling any pain whatsoever.

The experiences of the clinic are duplicated in the laboratory. Laboratory pains can be produced in various ways: through cutting off the circulation of the blood in an arm, which is then exercised (ischemic test); through pressure on bone or tendon; through cold, heat, needle pricks, or electric shock. The widely scattered experiments with hypnosis can be summarized succinctly. When unselected subjects, with a minimum of prior exposure to hypnotic procedures, are studied under laboratory conditions, the suggestion of hypnotic anesthesia or analgesia results in a marked reduction in felt pain, honestly reported, and the amount by which quantitatively estimated pain is reduced is positively correlated with hypnotic susceptibility as measured on standardized scales (e.g., Hilgard, 1967, 1969, 1971). There is some ambiguity about the role of a formal prior hypnotic induction (Evans & Paul, 1970; Spanos, Barber, & Lang, in press), but the pain reduction through hypnotic suggestion is demonstrated by all of those who have tried it, including the most skeptical (e.g., Sutcliffe, 1961).

These facts pose difficult problems for a theory of cognitive control, but there are further facts that are even more puzzling. The first set of additional facts is that there are commonly no changes in the underlying physiological indicators of pain, even though the subject feels no pain. This circumstance led Sutcliffe to say that the subject was "deluded" into believing that he felt no pain. Sutcliffe made this assertion as an inference from the presence of physiological indicators normally associated with pain, but an inference to delusion goes beyond the evidence that he presented. Absence of pain is not a delusion if we accept the definition of pain as something that is felt as hurting, regardless of the physiological signs, which may be either present or absent. The evidence on

From the Psychological Review, **80**:396-411.

[1]The experimentation leading to this paper and its preparation have been aided by Research Grant MH-3859 from the National Institute of Mental Health. Acknowledgment is made to Hugh Macdonald for assisting the author in the conduct of the experiments described here and to Karl Pribram for assistance in summarizing current knowledge on the neurophysiology of pain.

[2]From the Department of Psychology, Stanford University, Stanford, California 94305.

the physiological consequences of pain reduction through hypnosis is incomplete and somewhat contradictory. Experiments from our laboratory have shown few signs of physiological changes associated with pain reduction in the cold pressor test, but in the experiments using ischemic pain the reduced pain is associated with both lowered heart rate and lowered blood pressure (Hilgard, 1969; Lenox, 1970). Experimenters have long noted the reduction in those components of the pain response under voluntary control, such as facial grimacing or overt restless movements (e.g., Sears, 1932).

A second set of facts has been hinted at in the literature for many years but has only recently been brought under careful laboratory investigation. As long ago as 1868, Durand de Gros, one of the magnetizers who had developed a theory of multiple layers of consciousness, believed that a person in hypnotic surgery suffered pain in one of his subegos, although his conscious ego remained ignorant of the suffering (Ellenberger, 1970, p. 146). Minor accounts have appeared since, one by William James, based on automatic writing (James, 1889). James demonstrated the subject's usual response to pain by pricking his normally sensitive arm twice. He then pricked the anesthetic arm several times, and the subject's hand, out of awareness, wrote that it was feeling added pin pricks. After removing the hypnosis, when James showed the subject what he had written, the subject could only explain the writing by assuming that his subconscious part had exaggerated the memory of the two earlier pin pricks into a belief that there had been more. I have found two similar cases reported since then, both involving consciously absent pain that is acknowledged as pain via automatic writing (Estabrooks, 1957, p. 98; Kaplan, 1960). There may be other accounts buried in case reports, but I have found no systematic or quantitative experiments other than those on which we are now engaged.

A REFERENCE EXPERIMENT FOR PAIN REDUCTION UNDER HYPNOSIS

An investigation now going on in our laboratory provides a useful reference experiment for a theory of hypnotic pain reduction. The purpose of such a reference experiment is to exhibit in clear form the problems that a satisfactory theory must encompass. The interpretation to be favored I am calling a neodissociation theory, because it derives from the classical dissociation theory of Janet (1889) but adds new dimensions. The exposition of a theory can often be carried out by relating it to a limited set of experimental or naturalistic observations. One can think of the swinging pendulum for Galileo, the moon and the tides for Newton, the salivating dog for Pavlov, the rat in the box for Skinner. If the theory fits the reference experiment, it then reaches out to encompass wider phenomena.

Because of a substantial amount of experience in our laboratory in reducing the pain of circulating ice water through hypnotic suggestion, we selected this arrangement for the experiment. We chose for the purposes of this reference experiment only subjects highly susceptible to hypnosis, representing the upper 1%-2% of hypnotic susceptibility as tested in an unselected student population. Each of the subjects was able to accept the suggestion of analgesia, so that essentially no pain was felt when the hand and forearm were inserted into the circulating ice water for a period of 45 seconds. In addition to this, there was another requirement: the subject had to demonstrate the ability to engage in automatic writing under hypnosis, either in the form of cursive writing with a soft pencil or of pressing keys according to an agreed-upon reporting system. In either case the hand out of awareness was shielded from sight in a covered box.

Under these circumstances the hand communicates something, but the subject is not aware of the hand, what it is doing, or that it is doing anything at all. For the quantitative part of the experiment, the subject uses a verbal pain scale in which 1 means no pain and higher numbers are assigned for increasing pain, going to 10 and beyond, with 10 defined as a reference point at which the subject would very much wish to remove his hand from the water, although he is able to endure pain beyond this. Under hypnosis, without analgesia but with the hand in automatic writing, the hand signals the pain level by pressing the keys—the left of two keys for the tens and the right key for the digits. In the normally painful condition the automatic writing yields the same numerical results for pain as the verbal reports do. Exactly the same instructions for conscious reporting and for automatic key pressing are used in sessions in which the hand in the water is analgesic. To avoid any subtle changes in the experimenter's voice associated with the conditions of experimentation, these instructions are given by electromagnetic tape over a loudspeaker, alike whenever pain reports are to be called for in words and through automatic key pressing.

Now what do we find? We initially tried this procedure with a young woman highly experienced in hypnosis. In the normal nonhypnotic state, she found the experience of the circulating ice water very painful and distressing. In the hypnotic analgesic state, she reported that she felt no pain and was totally unaware of her hand and arm in the ice water; she was calm throughout. All the while that she was insisting verbally that she felt no pain in hypnotic analgesia, the dissociated part of herself was reporting through automatic writing that *she felt the pain just as in the normal nonhypnotic state.* Subsequent experiments with her and with additional subjects have similarly reported no conscious pain but some pain reported in automatic writing, at a level usually below that of the full pain in the normal nonhypnotic condition. Some pain reduction is to be expected, even when the pain is felt, because of the quiescence of the hypnotic subject (Shor, 1962).

We are carrying on further experiments to see if there are depths of hypnotic involvement in which neither the verbal reports nor the automatic reports indicate an experience of pain. Too much must not be made of the precise technique of automatic reporting, because we have in some instances substituted automatic talking for automatic writing. By instructing the subject that when the hypnotist's hand is placed on his shoulder he will tell what is going on in the secondary consciousness, but will not know that he is talking, results similar to automatic writing are obtained. The subject describes the cold or pain that is felt by some part of himself, even though the ordinary waking consciousness is oblivious to pain.

Because this experiment provides in paradigmatic form the problems that a neodissociation theory must confront, I have proposed it as a reference experiment for such a theory. The essential relationships within it are diagrammed in Figure 1.

The left-hand box represents in simplified form the condition of the relevant cognitive systems when the hand is immersed in ice water in the normal state, a condition in which all channels are open. The normal response is of felt pain, and there is no barrier to reporting this as a communication to the experimenter or other witnesses. Associated with this report, there are visible signs of discomfort, as in grimacing or restless movements, and

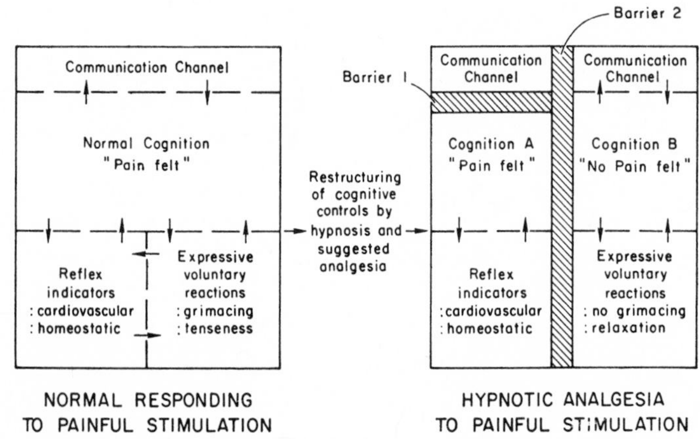

Fig. 1. Restructuring of cognitive controls in hypnotic analgesia. (For explanation, see text.)

instruments will report reflex changes in heart rate, blood pressure, and other physiological indicators. Some of these changes in bodily processes are reflected in the cognitive states, but the arrows go both ways because memories and anticipations also affect physiological indicators. The voluntary responses of grimacing, breath holding, and the like are noted separately from the reflex responses, but there is no communication barrier between them.

Now we move to the compartmentalized box on the right, with the changes in control structures that result because of the hypnotic interventions and the changes that follow the suggestion that the hand will feel no pain in the ice water. There has been a split between two cognitions, Cognition A and Cognition B, with some barriers around portions of them. Cognition A actually continues the normal consciousness of cold or pain, but because there is a barrier to communication (Barrier 1) this cognition remains hidden until exposed by automatic writing or automatic talking. It should be noted that this communication barrier is internal, so that the experience of Cognition A is not in the subject's awareness. In other words, the conscious part of himself is not withholding anything from social communication, for it has nothing to communicate.

Cognition B, reporting no pain, is bringing to light everything of which it is aware, so that, from the subject's point of view, he is making his private experience fully public. However, Cognition B is unaware that Cognition A continues to feel the cold or pain and is out of touch with its own reflex bodily state of stress, although it is aware of the relaxation of voluntary musculature. It is evident that Cognition B, although open in expressing what it feels, is a limited awareness.

Figure 1 is an incomplete diagram of what is happening in other respects. It deals only with the immediate control systems affecting the physiological responses to the stressful stimulation that normally causes pain and shows that one cognitive substructure (Cognition A) can still report the pain (but is normally concealed), while another one (Cognition B) now seems to be the ordinary dominant cognition because its communication channels are open, although it has limited access to what is going on and reports no pain.

This is the phenomenal situation, expressed as though it were static, but of course it is not static. How did the barriers get constructed, what is their nature, and how are they altered? Barrier 1, preventing communication of something known to Cognition A appears to be very much like familiar hypnotic amnesia, in which an intact memory is unavailable. It is not quite like amnesia, however, because in this case the felt pain never reaches the level of awareness in the subject himself until the barrier is broken; it is as though the felt pain is sealed in memory even while it is occurring. It is of interest that Barrier 1 can be broken (by the instructions for automatic writing or automatic talking), while Barrier 2 may continue to remain intact.

For some subjects, Barrier 2 is permeable in only one direction. For them, Cognition A, when it reports after Barrier 1 is weakened, asserts that it knows that Cognition B is reporting no pain; at the same time, Cognition B does not know about Cognition A. Thus far we have arrived at the basic problems for a dissociation theory: how to account for the split into the two Cognitions A and B, how to account for their interaction, and how to account for the nature of the barriers affecting awareness and communication, for their production and modification. The relationship to physiological indicators adds some additional problems.

The communication barrier between Cognition A and Cognition B brings to mind cases of fugues or alternating personality that turn up from time to time, either spontaneously or in connection with hypnosis experimentation. In one form of these alternations, there are two "personality integrations" – A and B, in which A knows B and B does not know A. An early case of this kind was published by Azam (1887) after many years of observation. His patient Félida in her normal personality, earning her living as a seamstress, was described as sullen and taciturn, with many headaches and neuralgias that would today be described as psychosomatic. After a crisis, however, she would awaken as a different person, gay, vivacious, and free of symptoms. This secondary "healthful" personality knew all about the symptoms of the primary personality, but the primary personality had no awareness of the secondary one except as she was told about it by others.[3] In Félida's case, we have an experiment of nature that shows a relationship between two cognitive control systems on a larger scale that have been reproduced in miniature in our laboratory experiment. Again I wish to point out that her dissociations were not produced by hypnosis, so that hypnotic procedures merely give us access to knowledge about cognitive functioning that need not be directly connected with hypnosis at all.

We now have before us the kinds of phenomena that gave rise to dissociation theory in the first place, and that I propose to consider in a more modern form of neodissociation theory. Before proposing the new interpretation, however, the classical theory and some of its alternatives may be examined.

CLASSICAL DISSOCIATION THEORY AND ITS CRITICS

The nature of the human mind has always been of interest to reflective men, who raise questions and formulate their answers according to contemporary beliefs expressed in theology, philosophy, science, or even as influenced by popular social movements. The doctrine of dissociation late in the nineteenth century and early in the twentieth rested upon the excitement created by discoveries showing hidden recesses of the mind, described as subconscious or unconscious phenomena, exhibited prominently in neurotic (especially hysterical) abnormalities, and paralleled in normal subjects through hypnosis. The trances of mediums (something of wide public interest at the same time), if interpreted naturalistically, led to similar conceptions.

The theories of mental organization that emerged can be concisely classified into two main groups, the theory of *dipsychism* and that of *polypsychism* (Ellenberger, 1970, pp. 145-147), implying either two "layers" of consciousness or more than two.

If there were two layers (dipsychism), the first was conceived as the normal waking consciousness, the second as usually hidden but occasionally revealing itself in dreams, abnormal symptoms, in hypnosis, and occasionally in unusual and unexpected creative acts. The two layers of personality (or consciousness) were assigned different qualities, depending on the authorities describing them. In what Ellenberger calls the "closed" form of the theory, the subconscious contains only tendencies and memories arising in the experience of the individual, but no longer available to the waking consciousness. According to Janet (1889), who was the first to use the expression "subconscious," the unavailable ideas have become "dissociated" or "disaggregated," so that they cannot be synthesized into waking awareness; Freud in his first concept of the unconscious believed that it consisted of "repressed" thoughts or wishes (Breuer & Freud, 1895; Freud, 1955). Hence, dissociation and repression described essentially the same facts of a closed subconscious layer.

In the "open" form of the theory, the subconscious layer is not only more extensive than the conscious layer, but it has access to some broader sets of experience that may never have been in the waking consciousness. Such a "subliminal self" was posited by Myers (1885, 1903) and was favorably supported by James (1902) in his *Varieties of Religious Experience*. The general position has found more recent expression in Jung's collective unconscious and in his belief in universal archetypes and mandala symbols in dreams (Jacobi, 1968). The issue is again of interest because of present-day romanticism about consciousness expansion and human potentiality. The iceberg analogy is often used, with consciousness merely the portion that is visible, with the larger (and more important) portion beneath the surface.

Another distinction differentiates various views of the subconscious in the "closed" and "open" form. In one position, common to Janet and Freud, the subconscious (or unconscious) portion is described as being fragmented, illogical, or as being impulse ridden (as in the seething cauldron picture of the unconscious associated with early psychoanalysis). The opposite view is that the subconscious

[3] An account, giving more details, can be found in Ellenberger (1970), p. 137f.

(whether closed or open) may be the source of morality, inspiration, or creativity. Oddly enough, the phenomenal observations are as contradictory as the theories explaining them.

The polypsychic theories accept the general notion of splits in the personality or ego but assert that the cleavages may result in more than two subordinate egos. Freud (1927) for example, moved from his earlier dipsychism[4] to a tripsychism in proposing the division into id, ego, and superego, and his later disciples have divided the ego into numerous apparatuses and substructures (Hartmann, 1958; Rapaport, 1967).

How independent were conscious and subconscious processes? This was always a matter of some dispute. Obviously they were not totally independent because there were usually some derivatives of the subconscious present to consciousness. The true nature of the unconscious thoughts might be disguised, as in dreams or hysterical symptoms. Morton Prince (1909) preferred the term "co-conscious" to avoid the connotation that the two consciousnesses were always isolated from each other.

The rapid fading of the dissociation concept has been discussed elsewhere (Hilgard, in press a, in press b). There were few attacks upon it. The main historical reasons for later neglect probably lay in the general disappearance of interest in hypnotic phenomena and the rise to prominence of psychoanalysis, whose followers seldom used the word at all.

After dissociation had all but disappeared from contemporary discussion, White and Shevach (1942) wrote a kind of epitaph for the concept, giving a clear and sympathetic account of Janet's use of the concept, reviewing experimental attempts to study it, giving some new data of their own, and reaching a clear conclusion: "Whatever the nature of the hypnotic state, it does not seem to be adequately characterized by dissociation [p. 327]." This conclusion has been favorably cited by recent writers (e.g., Sarbin & Coe, 1972).

If the evidence of White and Shevach is reviewed in detail, however, it is found to contradict only a rather extreme form of dissociation doctrine and not more qualified forms. Much of their evidence from hypnotic behavior lies in the direction of dissociated activities. They said, for example: "There is no doubt that hypnotic suggestion can bring about a separation of activities in a way that could not be duplicated by ordinary volition [White & Shevach, p. 326]." Their own experiment, while not yielding results that were very impressive statistically, still points in the direction of an exaggeration of dissociation through hypnosis. They chose for study a "dissociation" familiar outside hypnosis, the so-called Kohnstamm phenomenon that they called tensive perseveration. If a weight is sustained by an outstretched arm for a short time, when the weight is removed the arm tends to move upward. This will occur whether or not the person is attentive to some other task, such as reading aloud. What they found was that persons who became more deeply hypnotized tended to exaggerate the response beyond its normal amount when they were preoccupied at the same time with reading aloud. At various points in their discussion, they pointed out that a qualified form of dissociation theory might be appropriate, but they indicated no interest in following up this proposal and rested with the statement of their preference for suggestion as more useful than dissociation in explaining hypnotic behavior. The position was expanded in another place (White, 1941). Curiously enough, the preference for suggestion is a return to an earlier explanation that Janet (1889), Sidis (1898), and Prince (1909) had found too diffuse, which they had therefore replaced by the dissociation concept!

White and Shevach were attacking a strict form of dissociation theory. Their evidence was gathered carefully, and their discussion was temperate throughout. I believe, however, that with some modifications, a neodissociation theory can meet their objections to the classical doctrine.

ALTERNATIVES TO A DISSOCIATION THEORY

The decline of classical dissociation theory did not mean that the problems to which the theory addressed itself were

[4]For simplicity, I am considering the preconscious as part of the conscious control system because it consists largely of available memories.

neglected. The alternative theory that gained the widest support (and helped to divert interest from dissociation theory) was that of Freud. He and Jung and their associates made household words of unconscious processes, complexes, defenses, repression, and regression. Social psychologists with an objective social communication orientation have had their theories, too, of which Sarbin's role theory has been most directly related to the problems under discussion.

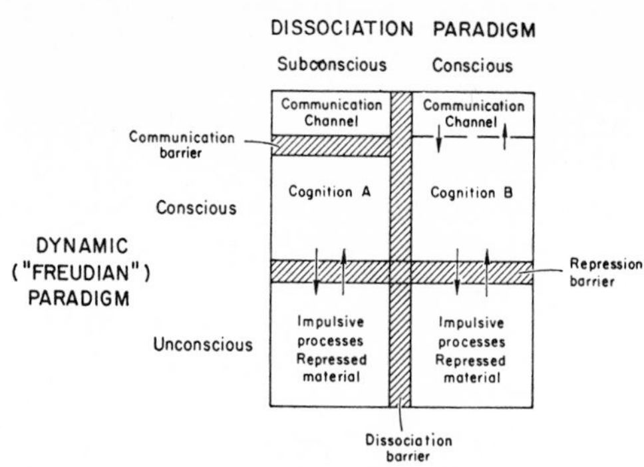

Fig. 2. Conceptual differences between dissociative and psychoanalytic interpretations. (The figure is simplified in order to indicate the differences between the dissociation barrier and the repression barrier.)

Psychoanalytic ego psychology

The later Freudians, in developing the psychoanalytic ego psychology, have modified the Freudian theory. In addition to the familiar id, ego, and superego, they speak of various ego substructures (in addition to defenses), including a wide range of "ego apparatuses" that serve the adjustment of the organization to the environment. They also favor a concept of partial and reversible regression called regression in the service of the ego, a concept that becomes central in the interpretation of hypnotic phenomena. In applying the ego theory to hypnosis, Gill and Brenman (1959) considered the regression in hypnotic induction to result in a fractionation of the ego. As the hypnotic state becomes stabilized, the ego is restructured at a slightly primitive (regressed) level, as evidenced by its uncritical thought processes. A regnant ego remains, but somewhat in the background, observing what goes on and introducing some control. It is evident that this conceptualization permits a discussion of the relationships of Figure 1 in these terms.

There are some conceptual differences between a regressive interpretation of hypnosis (the Gill and Brenman (1959) position) and the dissociative interpretation. The differences, schematic and oversimplified, are illustrated in Figure 2. For simplicity purposes, the cognitive controls in psychoanalytic theory are represented by a classification into a conscious and unconscious part of the cognitive apparatus. Then the conscious part represents chiefly the ego, with its reality orientation and conceptual thinking (secondary process thinking), while the unconscious part represents the id and whatever subsequent material has been repressed, characterized by impulsivity and irrationality (primary process thinking). Between them, there is some kind of barrier, across which some interchanges take place, as once-conscious material is repressed or once-unconscious material produces its derivatives in consciousness. This is an oversimplification of psychoanalytic thinking but is in essential agreement with its teaching. The subconscious and conscious splits that were characterized by my reference experiment are indicated as orthogonal to the psychoanalytic splits. Cognition A of Figure 1 (and the subconscious part of Félida), when they are manifested, represent essentially a psychoanalytic normal ego, in touch with reality, and with few intrusions of the reality distortions attributed to primary process. The fact that Cognition A is normally out of awareness does not fit the regressive concept of psychoanalysis, so that the dissociation barrier is indicated as at right angles to the repression barrier in Figure 2.

Cognition B of Figure 1, the conscious part in the midst of the hypnotic analgesia experiment, is the one showing reality distortion, and it is therefore partly regressed in Gill and Brenman's terms. However, I have not shown it as extending below the repression barrier, because there is no evidence that it has more access to the (Freudian) unconscious than Cognition A has. It would be stretching things to say that the wish to feel no pain is an unconscious striving, and the fact that no pain is felt might mean that there is a special unconscious influence upon consciousness. The desire to feel no pain was fully conscious, a wish encouraged by the hypnotist.

Note that my diagram does not deny the Freudian unconscious, but it makes it largely irrelevant to the major splits within cognitive structures that are found in hypnosis. It may be recalled that Gill and Brenman were able to carry out a normal psychoanalysis with the patient always in hypnosis within the analytic hour; dreams under hypnosis may serve as "projective techniques" similar to Thematic Apperception Test cards in the waking state, revealing hidden aspects of the personality. Figure 2 permits these interplays between unconscious and conscious (in the Freudian sense) within the dissociative splits.

The main point of my analysis is that the dissociations in hypnotic experiments belong primarily to the conscious cognitive controls and have little to do with the "deeper" unconscious. Psychoanalytic ego psychology allows for this, because within the ego there are "conflict-free" spheres not motivated by unconscious drives. Hence it is possible for psychoanalytic ego psychologists to agree with my interpretations, without abandoning their own vocabulary.

Gill and Brenman do, in fact, occasionally use the language of dissociation:

> We have already described the hypnotist's activities as directed toward a dissociation in which parts of the body develop an 'independent' functioning. It seems to us that the aspect of dissociation which is a decomposition is to be subsumed under deautomatization (and as we shall see later, function as an independent unit results from the establishment of a new automatization) [Gill & Brenman, 1959, p. 187-188].

To the extent that they are successful in explaining these processes of deautomatization and new automatizations, all at the ego level, they are presenting a theory that is indistinguishable from a neodissociation theory. The theory is, however, so intertwined with a metapsychology of five points of view (structural, dynamic, adaptive, genetic, and economic) that I am unable to apply it clearly to precise experimental findings.

Role theory

Role theory is pertinent to the cognitive splits found in experiments revealing dissociation because it is a social communication theory that assumes a person may enact several roles, public and private, either simultaneously or in succession. It therefore provides a set of labels that can be used alternatively to the dissociation label for such divisions as those between Cognition A and B. There are clearly many behaviors of the hypnotic subjects that can be characterized as role enactments, and there are some correlations between hypnotic susceptibility and dramatic abilities (e.g., Sarbin & Lim, 1963).

Sarbin and Coe (1972) were so impressed by the pervasiveness of role enactment that they took a limited view of the phenomena revealed in hypnosis. They believed that by conceptually removing the mystery from hypnosis, nothing remains that cannot be explained by quite familiar mechanisms. They had this to say about hypnotic analgesia:

> In another case a patient reported no pain after his hypnotherapist had burned his wrist as an experiment. The patient had to choose between disclosing that he felt the burn, thereby embarrassing and perhaps displeasing the therapist on whom he had become dependent, or not disclosing the private fact that he felt the burn and thus avoiding the risk of weakening the relationship. With the antecedent conditions of the verbal report made clearer the "secrets" metaphor helps to understand why the patient would not report: "You hurt me" [Sarbin & Coe, 1972, p. 136].

If a hypnotic subject is deliberately suppressing his report of felt pain to please the hypnotist (keeping the pain secret), then there is nothing to explain. This quotation, however, appears to be a misinterpretation of the facts of hypnotic analgesia, both as a subjective and social phenomenon. On both the phenomenal and social side, it is only necessary to call attention to the woman who having had one child with the help of hypnotic analgesia requests that she have hypnosis again for her next child (even though the original obstetrician is not around), or to one of our own subjects for whom the local anesthetic used by the dentist has not relieved pain sufficiently but now gains complete pain reduction in the dental chair through self-induced analgesia without any chemicals injected by the dentist. No hypnotist is around either to embarrass or to please.

If one concedes that the "private" experience of pain is so private that even the subject does not know he is feeling it, then dissociation and role theories converge. The role theorist uses a dimension of organismic involvement, which, at the extreme can cause psychic suicide, as in voodoo deaths. If depth of involvement were to be used to support role theory in the cases of genuine hypnotic analgesia, the impression created by the above quotation would be altered.

Psychoanalysis and role theory are not the only alternatives to dissociation theory, but they are the ones that have most prominently discussed the problems as they emerge in hypnosis.[5]

A NEODISSOCIATION INTERPRETATION

With this background, a new theory is appropriate if the evidence for dissociative splits can be comprehended better by the new theory than by earlier ones. It is particularly important, for the theory to be fruitful, that it should encourage quantitative testing, and hopefully, that it should recognize advances in psychophysiology. While the theory is at present speculative and incomplete, it is far enough along for its broad outlines to be formulated and for some specifics to be proposed in its favor.

Many of the arguments over classical dissociation theory and the efforts to provide experimental tests have assumed that if systems are dissociated there should be no interaction between them or at the very least that the interaction should be reduced by hypnotic dissociation. I propose, instead, that the problem of separation, both in awareness and in behavior, is an empirical one and may be a matter of both dimensionality and degree. That is, cognitive and behavioral systems that are separated in one dimension may be interacting in another, and the separation or interaction need not be sharp in order for some dissociative process to be demonstrated. Hence there may be partial dissociations, according to various criteria, and these may tell us about important aspects of cognitive functioning. For example, in experiments on dichotic listening to conversations, in which one message comes to one ear and a separate message to the other ear, the listener readily processes one message and ignores the other. Here one cognitive control system is dominant over another, and the two systems can be thought of as dissociated, because messages are surely reaching both ears. It is known, however, that while fully processing only one message, a subject may still report whether the other message is being delivered by a male or female voice, and, if interrupted, he can often tell you something of what was said to the nonattending ear (Norman, 1969). In other words, the dissociation is incomplete. Similar evidence can be found for the incompleteness of the dissociations in hypnotic experiments. In order not to become embroiled in arguments based on older interpretations, which are, in any case, somewhat muddled, I prefer to speak of the present standpoint as that of a *neodissociation* theory.

In experiments on task interference recently undertaken in our laboratory, it has been shown that there is some "cognitive cost" in maintaining hypnotic dissociation (Knox, Crutchfield, & Hilgard, 1973; Stevenson, 1972). If, for example, a subject is set the simple task of pressing two keys with the index and middle fingers of the right hand in the order 3 left-3 right, he soon picks up a rhythm and does this with very few errors. When, however, he does the same task in a procedure similar to automatic writing, through posthypnotic suggestion with the task out of awareness, he makes errors in perhaps 20% of the 3 left-3 right sequences, while maintaining approximately the same pace. Keeping the task out of awareness apparently uses some of his attentive ability and interferes with the performance. If there is added a simultaneous task, such as naming colors aloud from a panel of colors before him, with full awareness of what he is doing, this will, of course, interfere with conscious key pressing. If the key pressing is performed out of awareness, the errors

[5]Sarbin and Coe (1972) gave good expositions and critiques of several other theories pertinent to various aspects of hypnosis. I would add also Blum's (1961) speculative model. Sears (1936) developed a learning model bearing on dissociation, particularly as reflected in amnesia.

again rise, so that the performance with the two tasks dissociated is less efficient than when both tasks are conscious. This task interference, exaggerated when one of the tasks is performed automatically through hypnotic suggestion, is compatible with neodissociation theory. It is possibly analogous to the cost attributed by psychoanalytic theory to the act of continuing repression, in which creative activity may be lessened because of compulsive behavior that serves the purposes of repression.

A GENERAL FRAMEWORK

The earlier Figure 1 was an attempt to epitomize the end stage in an experimental demonstration of the dissociative aspects of pain control, but it was incomplete as a framework for a total theory. Such a framework is sketched in Figure 3.

The framework as proposed is a quite general one and not limited to hypnotic phenomena. There is, after all, only one nervous system, and it must serve all of behavior and awareness. What we want from hypnosis is to learn as much as we can about psychological processes, perhaps through the study of some neglected aspects of cognitive functioning. In its most general aspects, Figure 3 indicates that there are a number of control mechanisms, in a somewhat hierarchical arrangement, with a dominant system that may be called an executive ego, usually identified by the person as the self that plans and manages his affairs.

The basic assumption of neodissociation theory proposes that the unity which exists

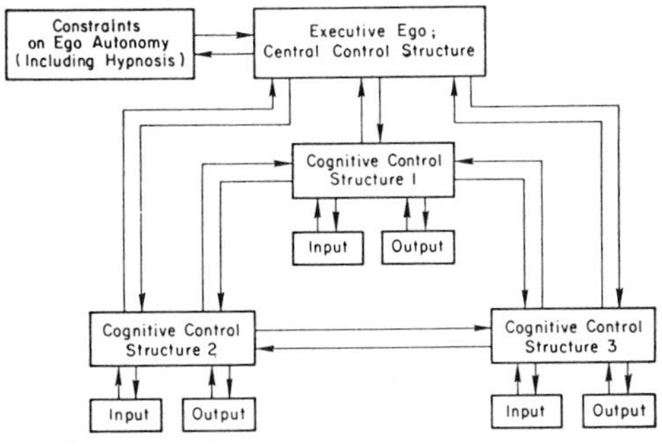

Fig. 3. Schematic conception of multiple cognitive control systems. (The assumption is that there are many substructures in hierarchical arrangement, of which only three are shown. Hypnotic interactions may alter the hierarchical positions.)

in personal cognitive functioning is somewhat precarious and unstable. An executive ego provides a basis for self-perception and for conceiving the self as an agent (Hilgard, 1949). Its integrity is provided largely through the continuity of the personal memories, not through any unusual self-consistency either in awareness or behavior. This executive ego has many constriants upon it, both through internal conflicts and insufficiencies, and through environmental pressures, physical and social, including hypnotic interactions. There are many subordinate control systems that represent fractions of total cognitive functioning, of which only three are shown, spaced as though one is superior to the other two. It is proposed that these substructures have at any one time a hierarchical arrangement, but their hierarchical positions can shift. For example in sleep, the cognitive control system that produces dreams is more prominent than it is in waking, though it is doubtless present at a lower level in waking also, as in daydreams and fantasy production generally. Once a system is activated, it may exert its controls autonomously, even though it is a subordinate system. When, for whatever reason, you start humming a haunting tune while working at something else higher in your hierarchy, the humming may have started spontaneously and continue unchecked. Daily life is full of many small dissociations, if we look for them.

Where hypnosis will enter into this framework is in *shifting the hierarchies of control*, so that what is normally voluntary may become involuntary, what is normally remembered may be forgotten, and (under some circumstances) what is normally unavailable to recall may be recalled. Furthermore, the dominance of the normal executive ego is reduced, though not obliterated. For example, if the hypnotic subject is given a suggestion that violates his self-conception, he is likely to be aroused from hypnosis, and the executive ego may be responsible for this arousal.

Each of the subordinate cognitive control structures is shown as related to a system of inputs and outputs, with feedback arrangements. As a control or monitoring system, the structure can seek or avoid inputs and enhance or inhibit outputs. While cognitive structures are not typically represented in quite this way, similar ideas have been suggested by many others, who may use quite different metaphors. Here are a few related concepts that refer to substructures of one sort or another that bear on the utilization of stored information, on the assimilation of new information, and on the transformation of information in the light of its context, so that the processing that goes on leads to outputs in the form of ideational activity or overt behavior:

1. Cognitive structures (Lewin, Tolman, Piaget).
2. Habit-family hierarchies (Hull, Berlyne).
3. Images, plans, and TOTE's (test-operate-test-exit) (Miller, Galanter, Pribram).
4. Subordinate ego structures (Gill and Brenman).
5. Role enactments (Sarbin).

The existence of substructures with some measure of autonomy is a prerequisite of neodissociation theory. Only if it is permissible to infer them can a plausible theory be developed based on modifying their interactions.

SPECIFIC APPLICATIONS TO THE PAIN EXPERIMENT

Although a theory should be embedded in a larger context, so that it is not narrowly ad hoc, its fertility can often best be shown by how well it meshes with concrete experimental data. I therefore wish to attempt a speculation regarding the awareness and control of pain, as earlier summarized in Figure 1.

It has become increasingly clear as the experiments have progressed that the pain perceived with Cognition A in Figure 1 is not ordinarily the full pain of the waking experience without suggested pain reduction. Writers on pain often point out that there is a difference between pain as a sensory experience and pain as an emotional-motivational experience, when it is described by such terms as distress, anguish, or suffering. When the hypnotized subject talks about these distinctions to the experimenter through automatic talking, the experimenter makes contact with a cognitive system that is hidden from the subject himself as well as from the experimenter. I shall refer to this usually secret communication system as the "hidden observer," for the reports contain a great deal of information not otherwise available.

The hidden observer came to my attention first from some experiments on hypnotic deafness.[6] A subject who was capable of shutting out all sounds, including pistol shots, still raised a finger when I asked him in a quiet voice to raise the finger (while he was still psychologically deaf) to let me know if some part of him was hearing me. He immediately requested that he have his hearing restored by the prearranged signal of my hand on his shoulder because he had felt the finger rise passively and wished to know what I had done to make it rise. Again able to hear, he replied to my question that he was totally unaware of any sounds prior to my restoring his hearing. A number of other demonstrations subsequently have shown that the words spoken by someone a subject cannot hear can be recovered from the hidden observer, and the number of fingers invisible behind a hallucinated opaque screen can be counted by him. Of course a skeptic may say that this proves that hypnosis is merely role playing, but the genuine surprises by the subjects when they hear the tapes of what they have reported out of awareness show quite convincingly that the split in awareness is genuine.

What the subjects commonly report through automatic talking, after they have experienced no pain in the ice water following suggested anesthesia, is that the sensory experience of the cold was actually as intense as ever, but the cold did not hurt: "So cold that it ordinarily would have been very painful, but it didn't bother me at all." This kind of report from the hidden observer is coherent with two behavioral facts: first, that the heart rate and blood pressure rise in the cold water, with changes corresponding to those of waking nonhypnosis, and second, that the subject appears altogether passive while experiencing the cold water under anesthetic conditions, showing none of the agi-

[6] I am grateful to James H. Stevenson and Gary Marshall for first calling some of these possibilities to my attention.

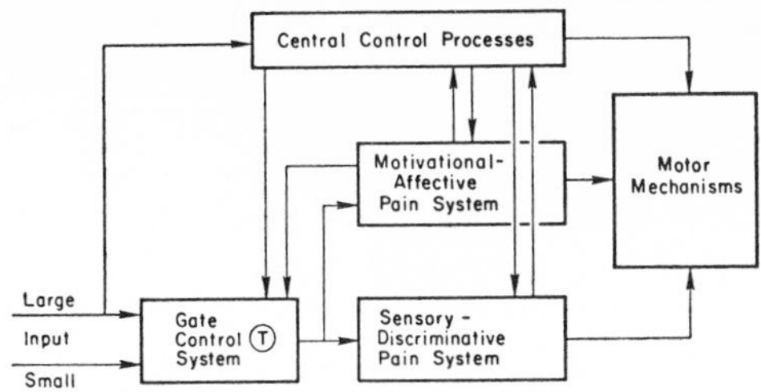

Fig. 4. Conceptual model of the sensory, motivational and central determinants of pain. (Reprinted with permission from an article by R. Melzack and K. L. Casey in *The Skin Senses,* D. Kenshalo (Ed.). Courtesy of Charles C Thomas, Springfield, Illinois.)

tation that the cold water normally produces.

Now for the proposed explanation. In this I shall rely heavily upon the gate theory of pain as proposed orginally by Melzack and Wall (1965), supplementing it with my own conjectures about hypnosis. Wall (1969), in a conference on psychophysiological mechanisms of hypnosis held in 1967, was the first to see the possibilities in this direction. He noted that the suggestions of the hypnotist might affect the modifiable afferent sensory pathways, that this action might suppress not only messages that trigger conscious sensation but also some segmental reflexes. At the same time (and here he unknowingly left room for my "hidden observer"), hypnosis would not be expected to modify the impulses in the more rigid pathway for pain or to modify signs of the activity of this pathway, such as evoked potentials in the cerebral cortex.

The essence of the conceptual model of pain, as developed by Melzack and Wall and in subsequent publications by them and their collaborators and others, is conveniently represented in Figure 4. Nearly all of its features have a bearing on the results of our reference experiment, because there are two pain systems anatomically distinct despite their occasional overlap, and a control over these systems by central processes permitting a place for hypnosis. My conjecture is that there are many other alternative physiological systems that have evolved to mediate cognitive processes of other kinds, having nothing to do with pain, such as the right and left hemispheres whose differences in function have lately received renewed attention. These alternative functional systems would allow conjectures about dissociation in relation to processes appropriate to them. However, the pain systems have been quite well worked out, so that an exposition in terms of them can serve as a heuristic model for other systems.

The following brief account of the pain control systems is based largely on Casey (1973). It is provided to give anatomical-physiological concreteness to the schematic representation in Figure 4.

A sensory-discriminative system begins with the large fibers (A alpha) entering the dorsal spinal column. Most of the fibers have long axons that travel up the white matter of the dorsal and dorsolateral spinal cord, making their first synapse in the dorsal column nucleus in the lower brainstem. From here the axons of the second-order neurons go to the ventral posterior lateral nucleus of the thalamus of the opposite side and in turn project to the parietal lobe somatosensory area of the cortex. This is a rapid-acting system that maintains information that is topographically organized for transmitting spatio-temporal information from innocuous stimulation. Lesions in it do not tend to reduce intractable pain (White & Sweet, 1969). Extensive lesions are necessary to produce deficits in this system, so that it appears to have considerable functional redundancy (Dobry & Casey, 1972a, 1972b).

A motivational-affective system for pain receives its input from the smaller fibers (C and A delta) entering the cord from the afferent roots. These make synapse with the short fibers of the dorsal horn cells (lamina 5 cells), and these cells form a gray-matter column running the length of the cord. From these cells the fibers cross the midline to the ventrolateral part of the spinal cord and make up the ascending ventrolateral spinothalamic tract. This ascending system has rich connections to the paramedial system in the core of the brain stem subserving aversive motivational and affective functions: the reticular formation, hypothalamus, medial and intralaminar thalamic structures, and (via the thalamic structures) the limbic forebrain structures. Because of the small fibers and many synapses, this is a relatively slow-acting system. Ventrolateral spinal tractotomy is a routine neurosurgical procedure performed for intractable pain, and Mark, Ervin, and Yakovlev (1963) have shown that medial thalamic lesions in man may in some instances relieve the distress of intractable pain without impairing motor or sensory functions.

The gate-control theory of Melzack and Wall attempts to account for some modification of the response to these systems by impulses from descending fibers. Some of this control comes from the intrasegmental interrelations between the two systems. There are, for instance, some relatively larger fibers (probably A delta, about 15% in cats and monkeys) that respond to pain; these make synapse in the dorsal horn. In addition, many collaterals are given off by A alpha fibers in their transit toward the midline – it is these collaterals that are believed to contribute to the gate-control system as shown in Figure 4. Basic to the theory is the idea that these larger collaterals antagonize the excitations produced by the smaller C (and A delta) pathways.

A suprasegmental central process is thought to control this relationship between the alpha collaterals and the smaller A delta and C fiber systems as shown in Figure 4. This is, of course, where hypnosis might come in. The proposal is that presynaptic inhibition (or enhancement) can occur through the interaction of the large and small afferent fibers at the level of the dorsal horn. Locally, this interaction is accomplished via short interneurons in the substantia gelatinosa. These in turn are said to be acted upon by efferent tracts that transmit impulses from the higher centers, as shown schematically in Figure 4.

The two afferent systems are well established both neuroanatomically and neurophysiologically, but the details of operation of the gate control system are still controversial. There can be little doubt, however, that a central control system exists. For instance, new evidence shows that electrical stimulation – and not ablation – of cells surrounding the cerebral aqueduct in the core of the brain stem abolish reactions to pain for the duration of the stimulation (Liebeskind, Guilbaud, Besson, & Oliveras, 1973). Furthermore, these periaqueductal cells have been shown to be exquisitely sensitive to morphine and are believed to be the biochemical receptors for this analgesic. These results provide new tools for the investigation of the physiology of the suprasegmental facets of the gate control of pain.

The parallels between this model of pain and our hypnotic findings are as follows: *(a)* The evidence clearly shows that central processes can modify the perception of pain that is produced by a normally painful source of stimulation. *(b)* The aspect of pain that is found more modifiable (by the testimony of the hidden observer as revealed in automatic talking and also from the lack of overt bodily response) is the suffering or anguish. This is coherent with the modifiable nature of the motivational-affective pain system. *(c)* The aspect of pain that is least modified (again according to the testimony of the hidden observer in automatic talking) is the information regarding the sensory aspects of stimulation, that is, the coldness of the water. This is again coherent with the uncensored information expected from the sensory-discriminative system.

These parallels provide provisional support for the neodissociational interpretation because of the differences in the information reported by the hypnotic reporting system and the automatic talking reporting system. The informational system is found to be more difficult to affect hypnotically as well as surgically.

The gate-theory interpretation of our findings leaves one possible area of disagreement and at least one source of ambiguity.

The possible disagreement lies in Wall's (1969) suggestion that if the gate is closed at the dorsal roots, the local reflexes should also be shut off. Our data suggest that the local reflexes, at least the vasomotor ones, persist, even though the pain is not felt. It may be, however, that in the cold pressor experiment, we are dealing with reflexes to cold rather than to pain, and the gate theory is specific to pain. Some support for Wall's conjecture is found in experiments from our laboratory with another kind of pain – ischemic pain produced by a tourniquet followed by exercise – in which there is no sensory stress corresponding to cold. In some of these experiments, suggested hypnotic analgesia has appeared to reduce both heart rate and blood pressure below the levels found in the normal nonhypnotic condition (Lenox, 1970). If these results are substantiated, they can be interpreted as evidence that local reflexes can be abolished by a gate control mechanism activated hypnotically, as suggested by Wall. Ischemic pain, by contrast with cold, may be mediated almost exclusively by the two pain mechanisms that interact at the dorsal horn level. Our subjects are able to distinguish between pain and discomfort in the normal response to ischemic (tourniquet) pain; this distinction is preferable, as a test of the pain-dissociation theory, to the distinction between cold and pain in the ice-water experiment. It is too early to say how the results will come out when analgesia in the ischemic pain experiment is studied with the aid of automatic talking.

The source of ambiguity in our results, in relation to the physiology of pain, rests in how hypnotic suggestions can work to cut off the perception of pain and cold entirely, despite some preservation of the bodily awareness, especially of the cold, as revealed by automatic talking. The problem of consciousness remains a baffling one, and the Melzack-Wall gate theory does not deal specifically with the nature of central control processes. While some speculations can be offered, such as the voluntary redirection of attention, or habituation and dehabituation of orienting responses, a fully satisfactory answer regarding hypnotic amnesia and other negations of normally conscious processes is not likely to be forthcoming in the near future.

I believe that the experimental results and the theory proposed fit sufficiently with psychophysiology to pursue further, not only in reference to pain but in reference to other dissociations found within hypnotic responsiveness. The experimental evidence here reported has all come from highly susceptible subjects, readily able to produce anesthesia, amnesia, automatic writing, and automatic talking. We have not had time to explore our somewhat novel findings over the range of individual differences in hypnotic susceptibility, and many parameters of what we have found remain to be investigated. One thing is abundantly clear: the powerful influences that hypnosis exerts over cognitive functioning make it a useful probe into these puzzling processes, quite apart from any interest in hypnosis per se.

REFERENCES

Azam, E. E. *Hypnotisme, double conscience et alteration de la personalité.* (Preface by J. M. Charcot). Paris: Bailliere, 1887.

Blum, G. S. *A model of the mind.* New York: Wiley, 1961.

Breuer, J., & Freud, S. Studies in hysteria. (Standard Edition) Vol. 2. London: Hogarth, 1955. (Originally published: Leipzig and Vienna: Deuticke, 1895.)

Casey, K. L. Pain: A current view of neural mechanisms. *American Scientist,* 1973, **61,** 194-200.

Dobry, P. J. K., & Casey, K. L. Coronal somatosensory unit responses in cats with dorsal column lesions. *Brain Research,* 1972, **44,** 399-416. (a)

Dobry, P. J. K., & Casey, K. L. Roughness discrimination in cats with dorsal column lesions. *Brain Research,* 1972, **44,** 385-397. (b)

Ellenberger, H. F. *The discovery of the unconscious.* New York: Basic Books, 1970.

Estabrooks, G. H. *Hypnotism* (Rev. ed.). New York: Dutton, 1957.

Evans, M. B., & Paul, G. L. (1970) Effects of hypnotically suggested analgesia on physiological and subjective responses to cold stress. *Journal of Consulting and Clinical Psychology,* 1970, **35,** 362-371.

Freud, S. *The interpretation of dreams.* New York: Basic Books, 1955. (Originally published: Leipzig and Vienna: Deuticke, 1900.)

Freud, S. *The ego and the id.* London: Hogarth, 1927. Originally published: Leipzig, Vienna, and Zurich: Internationaler Psychoanalytischer Verlag, 1923.

Gill, M. M., & Brenman, M. *Hypnosis and related states: Psychoanalytic studies in regression.* New York: International Universities Press, 1959.

Hartmann, H. *Ego psychology and the problem of adaptation.* New York: International Universities Press, 1958.

Hilgard, E. R. Human motives and the concept of the self. *American Psychologist,* 1949, **4,** 374-382.

Hilgard, E. R. A quantitative study of pain and its reduction through hypnotic suggestion. *Proceedings of the National Academy of Sciences,* 1967, **57,** 1581-1586.

Hilgard, E. R. Pain as a puzzle for psychology and physiology, *American Psychologist,* 1969, **24,** 103-113.

Hilgard, E. R. Pain: Its reduction and production under hypnosis. *Proceedings of the American Philosophical Society,* 1971, **115,** 470-476.

Hilgard, E. R. Dissociation revisited. In M. Henle, J. Jaynes, & J. Sullivan (Eds.), *Contributions to the history of psychology.* New York: Springer, 1973, in press. (a)

Hilgard, E. R. Toward a neo-dissociation theory: Multiple cognitive controls in human functioning. *Perspectives in Biology and Medicine,* 1973, in press. (b)

Jacobi, J. *The psychology of C. G. Jung.* (7th ed.). New Haven: Yale University Press, 1968.

James, W. Automatic writing. *Proceedings of the American Society for Psychical Research,* 1889, **1,** 548-564.

James, W. *Varieties of religious experience.* New York: Longmans, Green, 1902.

Janet, P. *L'Automatisme psychologique.* Paris: Alcan, 1889.

Kaplan, E. A. Hypnosis and pain. *A. M. A. Archives of General Psychiatry,* 1960, **2,** 567-568.

Knox, V. J., Crutchfield, L., & Hilgard, E. R. The nature of task interference in hypnotic dissociation. Paper presented at the Annual Meeting of Society for Clinical and Experimental Hypnosis, University of California at Irvine, November 1973.

Kroger, W. S. *Clinical and experimental hypnosis in medicine, dentistry, and psychology.* Philadelphia: Lippincott, 1963.

Lenox, J. R. Effect of hypnotic analgesia on verbal report and cardiovascular responses to ischemic pain. *Journal of Abnormal Psychology,* 1970, **75,** 199-206.

Liebeskind, J. C., Guilbaud, G., Besson, J. M., & Oliveras, J. L. Analgesia from electrical stimulation of the periaqueductal gray matter in the cat: Behavioral observations and inhibitory effects on spinal cord interneurons. *Brain Research,* 1973, **50,** 441-446.

Mark, V. H., Ervin, F. R., & Yakovlev, P. I. Stereotactic thalamotomy. *Archives of Neurology,* 1963, **8,** 528-538.

Melzack, R., & Casey, K. I. Sensory, motivational, and central control determinants of pain. In D. R. Kenshalo (Ed.), *The skin senses.* Springfield, Ill.: Charles C Thomas, 1968.

Melzack, R., & Wall, P. D. Pain mechanisms: A new theory. *Science* 1965, **150,** 971-979.

Myers, F. W. H. Automatic writing. *Proceedings of the Society for Psychical Research,* 1885, **3,** 1-63.

Myers, F. W. H. *Human personality and its survival of bodily death.* New York: Longmans, Green, 1903. 2 vols.

Norman, D. A. *Memory and attention: An introduction to human information processing.* New York: Wiley, 1969.

Prince, M. Experiments to determine co-conscious (subconscious) ideation. *Journal of Abnormal Psychology,* 1909, **3,** 33-45.

Rapaport, D. A historical survey of psychoanalytic ego psychology. In M. M. Gill (Ed.), *The collected papers of David Rapaport.* New York: Basic Books, 1967.

Sarbin, T. R., & Coe, W. C. *Hypnosis: A social psychological analysis of influence communication.* New York: Holt, Rinehart & Winston, 1972.

Sarbin, T. R., & Lim, D. T. Some evidence in support of the role taking hypothesis in hypnosis. *International Journal of Clinical and Experimental Hypnosis,* 1963, **11,** 98-103.

Sears, R. R. An experimental study of hypnotic anesthesia. *Journal of Experimental Psychology,* 1932, **15,** 1-22.

Sears, R. R. Functional abnormalities of memory with special reference to amnesia. *Psychological Bulletin,* 1936, **33,** 229-274.

Schneck, J. M. (Ed.) *Hypnosis in modern medicine.* (3rd ed.) Springfield, Ill.: *Charles C Thomas, 1963.*

Shor, R. E. Physiological effects of painful stimulation during hypnotic analgesia under conditions designed to minimize anxiety. *International Journal of Clinical and Experimental Hypnosis.* 1962, **10,** 183-202.

Sidis, B. *The psychology of suggestion.* New York: D. Appleton, 1898.

Spanos, N. P., Barber, T. X., & Lang, G. Cognition and self-control: Cognitive control of painful sensory input. In H. London & R. Nisbett (Eds.), *Cognitive alterations of feeling states.* Chicago: Aldine, in press.

Stevenson, J. H. The effect of hypnotic and posthypnotic dissociation on the performance of interfering tasks. Unpublished doctoral dissertation, Stanford University, 1972.

Sutcliffe, J. P. "Credulous" and "skeptical" views of hypnotic phenomena: Experiments in esthesia, hallucination, and delusion. *Journal of Abnormal and Social Psychology,* 1961, **62,** 189-200.

Wall, P. D. The physiology of controls on sensory pathways with special reference to pain. In L. Chertok (Ed.), *Psychophysiological mechanisms of hypnosis.* New York: Springer-Verlag, 1969.

White, J. C., & Sweet, W. H. *Pain and the neurosurgeon: A forty-year experience.* Springfield, Ill.: Charles C Thomas, 1969.

White, R. W. A preface to the theory of hypnotism. *Journal of Abnormal and Social Psychology,* 1941, **36,** 477-505.

White, R. W., & Shevach, B. J. Hypnosis and the concept of dissociation. *Journal of Abnormal and Social Psychology,* 1942, **36,** 309-328.

27

Hypnotism and surgical pain

John F. Chaves and Theodore X. Barber

In 1829, prior to the discovery of anesthetic drugs, a French surgeon, Dr. Cloquet, performed a remarkable operation on a 64-year-old woman who suffered from cancer of the right breast. After making an incision from the armpit to the inner side of the breast, he removed both the malignant tumor and also several enlarged glands in the armpit. What makes this operation remarkable is that, during the surgical procedure, the patient, who had not received any drugs, conversed quietly with the physician and showed no signs of experiencing pain. During the surgery, her respiration and pulse rate appeared stable and there were no noticeable changes in her facial expression. The ability of this patient to tolerate the painful procedures was attributed to the fact that she had been mesmerized immediately prior to the operation. Cloquet's case is one of the first reports of painless surgery with mesmerism or, as it was called later, hypnotism (Chertok, 1959; Kroger, 1957).

Cloquet was subjected to severe criticism when he reported his case to the French Academy of Medicine. Lisfranc, an eminent surgeon of that day, declared that Cloquet was either an imposter or a dupe. Larrey, the former Surgeon-in-Chief of the Grande Armee, claimed that Cloquet had been taken in by trickery. In spite of these criticisms, reports of painless surgery under mesmerism or hypnotism began to appear with some regularity and, in fact, still continue to appear.

Although Cloquet's case clearly indicates that at least some individuals can undergo surgery without manifesting signs of pain, it does not prove that mesmerism or "hypnotic trance" is the important factor in producing this effect. For instance, a very similar operation carried out about the same time, which did not involve mesmerism or hypnotism, has been described by Freemont-Smith (1950). The case involved a woman who had a breast removed for cancer. Since the operation was carried out in the early part of the nineteenth century, before drugs had been discovered that could produce anesthesia (absence of sensitivity) or analgesia (absence of sensitivity to pain), the patient underwent the surgery without medications. The operation took place in a large amphitheater before a group of eminent surgeons. Although the patient was not "hypnotized" and did not receive drugs, she tolerated the surgery ". . . without a word, and after being bandaged up, got up, made a curtsy, thanked the surgeon and walked out of the room."

Later in the nineteenth century, there were other cases of ostensibly painless surgery. For instance, some years later, Tuckey (1889) described the following case:

> There are few cases of this kind more remarkable than one related by Mr. Woodhouse Braine, the well-known chloroformist. Having to administer ether to an hysterical girl who was about to be operated on for the removal of two sebaceous tumors from the scalp he found that the ether bottle was empty, and that the inhaling bag was free from even the odor of any anesthetic. While a fresh supply was being obtained, he thought to familiarize the patient with the process by putting the inhaling bag over her mouth and nose, and telling her to breathe quietly and deeply. After a few inspirations she cried, "Oh, I feel it; I am going

Reprinted with permission from T. X. Barber, N. P. Spanos, and J. F. Chaves. Hypnosis, Imagination, and Human Potentialities, Chapter 8, Pergamon Press, 1974.

> off," and a moment after, her eyes turned up, and she became unconscious. As she was found to be perfectly insensible, and the ether had not yet come, Mr. Braine proposed that the surgeon should proceed with the operation. One tumor was removed without the least disturbing her, and then, in order to test her condition, a bystander said that she was coming to. Upon this she began to show signs of waking, so the bag was once more applied, with the remark, "She'll soon be off again," when she immediately lost sensation and the operation was successfully and painlessly completed [pp. 725-726].

Unfortunately, all of the early reports of painless surgery are quite anecdotal. Although the patients tolerated the surgery, it was not definitely established that they experienced no pain at all. It does appear likely that pain was markedly reduced, but it remains unclear what factors may have been responsible for the pain reduction.

The foregoing considerations lead to two major questions:

1. To what extent can pain be attentuated by suggestions given with or without a hypnotic induction procedure?
2. What factors are responsible for the reduction of pain?

We shall attempt to answer these questions. However, before we proceed, we need to look briefly at the complexity of pain and at methods that are used to measure it.

THE COMPLEXITY OF PAIN

The term *pain* refers to a variety of sensations—for example, pricking, throbbing, burning, and sharp sensations—that are described as unpleasant. Pain as an unpleasant sensation can vary, quantitatively, from very slight to very intense. However, pain as a sensation is usually closely intermingled with anxiety, fear, worry, anger, and other types of emotions. The total experience of pain thus usually involves a complex blending of unpleasant sensations with emotions.

It appears that when a patient becomes very anxious or fearful while he receives pain-producing stimulations, he tends to report that the pain is more intense. On the other hand, when a patient remains relaxed and does not become anxious about the pain-producing stimulation, he tends to report that the pain is less intense (Barber, 1959; Beecher, 1946, 1956).

Furthermore, it appears that some procedures that are said to reduce pain actually reduce anxiety, fear, worry, and other emotions that are usually intermingled with pain. For instance, the pain relief that follows the administration of morphine and other opiates may be closely related to the reduction in anxiety or fear. Although the patient who has received an opiate may still experience pain sensations, the reduction in anxiety, fear, or other emotions apparently leads him to report that pain is reduced (Barber, 1959, 1970; Beecher, 1959; Cattell, 1943; Hill, Kornetsky, Flanary, & Wilker, 1952a, 1952b; Kornetsky, 1954). Moreover, a surgical procedure—prefrontal lobotomy—that is said to relieve intractable pain, also appears to alter the patient's pain experience primarily by reducing anxiety or fear. Lobotomized patients typically report that they feel pain, but it does not bother them anymore.

MEASUREMENT OF PAIN

Since pain as a sensation is closely interblended with and affected by anxiety, fear, and worry or concern, it is a difficult phenomenon to measure. Clinicians and researchers concerned with the effectiveness of hypnotism or suggestions in relieving pain have used at least three indices to assess pain: verbal reports, physiological measures, and overt behavioral signs. Let us briefly examine these indices.

The patient's verbal report is generally the most informative measure concerning pain (Hilgard, 1969b). Patients can be asked to describe not only the magnitude of their pain but also its quality. Verbal reports can be readily obtained and require no special equipment. Although verbal reports are very useful, under certain conditions (such as when there is strong motivation to deny pain) they may be difficult to interpret. A strong motivation to deny pain may be present when the physician and other medical personnel have invested much time and effort in attempts to alleviate the patient's suffering (Mandy, Mandy, Farkas, & Scher, 1952). This possibility should be considered in evaluating suggested analgesia (suggested removal of pain), because verbal reports are typically used to evaluate pain and the patient may be motivated to deny that pain was experienced.

Investigators at times rely on physiological measures as indicants of pain. These physiological measures, which are commonly altered in normal individuals during painful stimulations, include, for example, blood pressure, heart rate, respiration, skin resistance or conductance, and forehead muscle tension. It should be noted, however, that alterations in these physiological measures during pain-producing stimulation are often closely related to anxiety, fear, anger, and other emotions (Barber & Coules, 1959; Doupe, Miller, & Keller, 1939; Hardy, Wolff, & Goodell, 1952; Levine, 1930; Sattler, 1943). Each of these physiological measures can also be altered by nonpainful stimuli and are especially affected by events that produce anxiety, fear, or emotional arousal. Although physiological measures are useful as indicants of pain when they are used in conjunction with the patient's verbal reports, they are insufficient by themselves to draw conclusions about the quality or degree of the patient's pain.

Investigators also commonly infer the presence of pain when the patient shows overt behavioral signs such as flinching, grimacing, moaning, or withdrawal from the stimulus. However, some patients who report pain can voluntarily inhibit these overt behavioral signs. Consequently, when the signs are absent, we cannot conclude with certainty that the patient is not experiencing pain. Also, patients at times flinch or grimace in *anticipation* of a painful stimulus. Consequently, the presence of the behavioral signs does not necessarily indicate that the patient is experiencing pain.

Taken separately, none of the three indices of pain has proven completely satisfactory. A major difficulty, as implied above, is that the indices are not always closely correlated. Since pain is comprised of a complex intermingling of "sensations" with "emotions," it is difficult to measure and evaluate its reduction by hypnotism and suggestions. Despite these difficulties, we believe that we can clarify some of the effects of hypnotism and suggestions on surgical pain. Let us begin our discussion by looking closely at the severity of the pain sensations that are due to surgical incisions.

SENSATIONS OF PAIN DURING SURGERY

When patients undergo major or even minor surgery, it is usually assumed that it would be impossible for them to tolerate the operation if drugs or special techniques were not used to reduce pain. Moreover, it is commonly assumed that, other things being equal, pain increases when the surgeon cuts into deeper and deeper body tissues and organs. Cutting the skin is thought to be less painful than incising the underlying muscles or the internal organs such as the stomach, liver, or kidney. The available evidence indicates that all of the foregoing assumptions are incorrect. Let us examine these assumptions.

Although surgical procedures give rise to anxiety, fear, worry, and other emotions, they usually give rise to fewer and less intense pain sensations than is commonly believed. Although the skin is very sensitive, the muscles, bone, and most of the internal organs of the body are relatively insensitive. More precisely, the skin is sensitive to a knife cut, but the skilled surgeon cuts through the skin smoothly and quickly and the underlying tissues and internal organs are generally insensitive *to incision*. Lewis (1942) has carefully documented the fact that the muscles, bone, internal organs, and most other parts of the body (with the exception of the skin) are insensitive *to cutting* (although they are generally sensitive to other stimuli such as pulling, traction, or stretching). For instance, he noted the following: The subcutaneous tissue gives rise to little pain when it is cut. Slight pain is elicited when muscles are cut. Compact bone can be bored without pain. The articular surfaces of joints are insensitive. The brain is quite insensitive. The lungs and visceral pleura are insensitive to puncture. The surface of the heart is insensitive. Surgeons have often painlessly removed pieces of the esophageal wall for histological examination. The abdominal viscera in man have been known for over a century to be insensitive to a knife cut. Cutting the great omentum is accomplished painlessly. Solid organs such as the spleen, liver, and kidney can be cut without the patient being aware of it. The stomach may be cut without pain. Lower portions of the alimentary canal, including the jejunum, ileum, and colon, are also insensitive to cutting. The uterus and internal portions of the vagina are also insensitive, although the mouth of the urethra is sensitive. In brief, although "pain receptors" may be found widely throughout the body, and although many tissues and organs of the body give rise to sensations of pain when they are stretched or pulled or when pressure is applied, most tissues and organs of the body (with the notable exception of the skin) give rise to little or no pain sensations when they are cut by the surgeon's scalpel.[1]

In the early 1900's, Lennander (1901, 1902, 1904, 1906a, 1906b) and Mitchell (1907) published a series of case reports indicating that major surgical operations could be accomplished painlessly with the use of only local anesthetics to remove sensitivity from the skin. Lennander performed a large number of abdominal operations using only local anesthetics, such as cocaine, to dull the pain of the initial skin incision. In the vast majority of cases, the remainder of the abdominal operation was accomplished painlessly, even though additional pain-relieving drugs were not used. Lennander consistently reported that the internal organs are insensitive to incision.

Mitchell (1907) also reported an extensive series of major operations performed with local anesthetics that were used to produce insensitivity of the skin. These operations included amputation of limbs, removal of thyroid glands, removal of female breast, removal of the appendix, cutting into and draining the gall bladder, suturing a hernia, excising glands in the neck and groin, and cutting the bladder. In addition, Mitchell noted that very extensive dissection of the neck was possible with the use of only local anesthetics.

Mitchell (1907) also confirmed Lennander's findings regarding the insensitivity of the internal organs. For instance, he wrote as follows:

> The skin being thoroughly anesthetized and the incision being made, there is little sensation in the subcutaneous tissues and muscles as long as the blood vessels, large nerve trunks and connective tissue bundles are avoided. . . . The same insensibility to pain in bone has been noted in several cases of amputation, in the removal of osteophytes and wiring of fractures. In every instance after thorough cocainization of the periosteum, the actual manipulations of the bone have been unaccompanied by pain. The patients have stated that they could feel and hear the sawing, but it was as if a board were being sawn while resting upon some part of the body [p. 200].

Taken together, these findings indicate that the pain associated with major surgery is not as great as is commonly supposed. Although many tissues and organs of the body give rise to pain when they are stretched, pulled, or when there is a deficiency in their supply of blood, most tissues and organs of the body (with the notable exception of the skin) give rise to little or no pain when they are cut by the surgeon. Of course, anxiety and fear of being cut play a major role in surgery. Nowadays, surgery is usually carried out with a general anesthesia primarily because of the anxiety and fear that is aroused and because it is difficult to carry out an operation when the patient is tense, when his muscles are not relaxed, and when he does not remain perfectly still. However, if the patient can tolerate the pain associated with the initial incision through the skin, and if he can remain relaxed and still, many major surgical procedures can be accomplished with little additional pain. Moreover, it is clear that the amount of pain that accompanies surgery is not related in any simple way to the extent of the surgical intervention – superficial surgery that involves the sensitive skin can be accompanied by much more pain than cutting compact bone, the cerebral cortex, the liver, and many other rather insensitive organs.

The findings summarized above imply that, in evaluating the effectiveness of any procedure in reducing surgical pain, it is important to have a base-line measure of pain. Thus, in order to determine the degree of pain reduction that is produced by hypnotism and suggestions, it is necessary to compare the results with those obtained with a control group. The control group should undergo the same surgery without drugs and without a hypnotic induction procedure or suggestions of analgesia. No study has utilized a control group comprised of the same kinds of patients undergoing the same kind of surgery. Of course, there are serious ethical and professional objections to using these kinds of controls in a surgical situation. Nevertheless, when controls are lacking, it is impossible to draw definitive conclusions about the degree of pain reduction produced by suggestions, hypnotism, or any other procedures that aim to alleviate pain. It simply cannot be assumed that all surgical procedures are painful.

With the above considerations in mind, we can begin to understand the effects of hypnotism and suggestions on surgical pain. We shall now discuss the following three points in turn:

1. Drugs for the relief of pain are usually used together with hypnotism and suggestions; in these cases, it is not clear to what extent hypnotism and suggestions reduce the pain.
2. The effects of hypnotism during surgery are commonly exaggerated.
3. There are data indicating that suggestions for pain relief given alone are as effective as the same suggestions given together with hypnotic induction procedures in producing a tolerance for pain during surgery.

USE OF PAIN-RELIEVING DRUGS TOGETHER WITH HYPNOTISM AND SUGGESTIONS

In most of the recent surgical cases, the effects of hypnotic induction procedures and suggestions for pain relief were confounded with the use of anesthetic or analgesic drugs. Let us look at a few illustrative cases.

The first case, presented by Werbel (1967), involved the removal of a tumor from the neck of a 69-year-old female patient. Although Werbel attributed the apparent painlessness of the operation to hypnotism, he also stated that "several cubic centimeters of procaine" (Novocain) were injected into the area where the skin was cut. Since the area of the skin incision was numbed by the local anesthetic, it appears possible that the operation might have been equally tolerable if hypnotism had not been used.[2]

In another illustrative case (Crasilneck, McCranie, & Jenkins, 1956), a temporal lobectomy was performed on a 14-year-old girl suffering from epilepsy. The patient was exposed to a hypnotic induction procedure and to suggestions of analgesia. The authors stated that "the scalp line of incision was injected with a 2% solution of procaine." The patient complained of pain when the dura mater was separated from the bone and she required additional local anesthesia. At another point in surgery, "as a blood vessel in the hippocampal region was being coagulated, the patient suddenly awoke from the hypnotic trance." Prior to the completion of the surgery, the patient was given 100 mg. of thiopental sodium intravenously. During most of the surgical procedures—when cutting through the bone of the scalp and into brain tissue—the patient appeared comfortable and did not seem to experience pain. Although the hypnotic induction procedure and the suggestions of analgesia were probably helpful in relaxing this patient and in reducing anxiety and fear, it is questionable whether they produced a marked reduction in pain sensitivity. It should be noted that (a) the patient showed pain, as would be normally expected, when the dura mater was separated from the bone and when a blood vessel was coagulated, (b) the scalp, which is sensitive to incision, was dulled by the use of Novocain, and (c) since compact bone and the brain are generally insensitive to incision, the patient naturally experienced little or no pain when these areas were cut. In brief, this case and also other similar cases (Finer, 1966; Schwarcz, 1965; Werbel, 1965) seem very amazing only when one wrongly assumes that insensitive body tissues such as compact bone and brain tissue are sensitive to cutting and when one fails to note that a local anesthetic was used to dull sensitive areas such as the skin.

In other recent studies, the effects of hypnotic induction procedures and suggestions for pain relief were confounded with the use of a wide variety of drugs including sedatives and local anesthetics. For instance, Marmer (1956, 1957, 1959) used hypnotism together with suggestions aimed at reducing pain in a large number of surgical cases, but these factors were always combined with many drugs that produce relaxation or pain relief. A typical operation reported by Marmer (1956) involved cutting the wall of the chest (thoracotomy) and then cutting out a considerable portion of a lung. (The lung is insensitive to incision.) The patient, a 25-year-old female, was exposed to a hypnotic induction procedure the night before surgery and again just before surgery. In addition to the hypnotic induction procedure and the suggestions for relief of pain, a wide variety of drugs were administered that were designed to produce sedation and to anesthetize the skin. The skin was dulled by infiltrating it with Novocain (25 cc. of 1% procaine hydrochloride). A wide variety of other drugs were also used including Nembutal, Benadryl, Demerol, scopolamine. Surital, and succinylcholine.[3] Although the hypnotic induction procedure and the suggestions for pain relief were probably effective in reducing anxiety and fear, it is not clear whether they had a direct effect on pain. The apparent lack of pain in this case might have been due to the wide variety of drugs that were used.

Before closing this section, let us look briefly at three additional illustrative cases presented by Betcher (1960). The first case involved an operation for the repair of a hernia. The patient, a 56-year-old male, was exposed to a hypnotic induction procedure the night before surgery and also immediately before surgery. However, the surgery itself was performed under spinal anesthesia. The second case involved a 12-year-old boy who underwent surgical correction of bilateral clubfoot. In this case, hypnotism and suggestions for pain reduction were combined with nitrous oxide and ether. In the third case, a 10-year-old girl underwent plastic surgery to remove scars on the neck. The operation was started after the girl had been exposed to a hypnotic induction procedure and to suggestions of anesthesia for the operative area. However, the patient "began to whimper softly at the incision of the scalpel" and, consequently, she was given drugs that produced "total chemical anesthesia."

In brief, hypnotism and suggestions are rarely used *alone* in present-day surgery. With few exceptions, hypnotism and suggestions are combined with pain-relieving drugs. Although the hypnotic induction procedure and the suggestions for pain relief often seem to be effective in reducing anxiety, fear, and tensions, the drugs seem to play an important role in relieving pain.

EXAGGERATION OF THE EFFECTS OF HYPNOTISM

If we look back at the early reports of painless surgery under mesmerism or hypnotism, we find that, although the procedures apparently reduced anxiety and fear, the extent to which they reduced pain as a sensation may have been exaggerated. For example, in a classic report, Esdaile (1850) stated that he had performed over 300 major operations and numerous minor surgical procedures during a six-year period while he was working in India. His report is frequently cited as demonstrating painless surgery utilizing mesmerism or hypnotism. However, a careful reading of Esdaile's cases indicates that, although anxiety, fear, and other emotions were apparently reduced to a marked degree, the surgery may not have been as painless as has been supposed.

Esdaile's procedures were studied by a commission appointed by the Bengal government (Braid, 1847). Esdaile first selected ten patients to be observed by the commission. However, three of the ten had to be excluded because they could not be mesmerized, even after attempts extending up to 11 days. One of the patients had one side of a double hydrocele (a circumscribed collection of fluid) tapped painlessly while in the "mesmeric state"; however, the same patient had the other side tapped painlessly while awake, so no conclusion could be drawn in this case regarding the efficacy of mesmerism in reducing pain. The remaining six patients underwent major surgery, including amputation and the removal of scrotal tumors, and all six denied experiencing pain. However, three of the six were described in the commission's report as showing ". . . convulsive movements of the upper limbs, writhing of the body, distortion of the features giving the face a hideous expression of suppressed agony." Two of the remaining patients showed physiological signs, including erratic pulse rates, suggesting the presence of pain. On the basis of the commission's report, it certainly seems possible that Esdaile's surgery was not as painless as has been supposed.

Soon after Esdaile completed his work in India, there was a rapid decline of interest in "mesmeric surgery" due to the discovery of the anesthetic properties of ether, nitrous oxide, and chloroform. Its staunchest advocates remained loyal, however, pointing out the dangers associated with gaseous anesthetics and noting with satisfaction that not a single death during surgery could be attributed to mesmerism!

About 50 years later, toward the end of the nineteenth century, there was a revival of interest in mesmerism or hypnotism, as it was called by that time. Bramwell (1903) reported that he could "sometimes induce anesthesia by suggestion and . . . occasionally performed surgical operations during hypnosis." Most of the cases reported by Bramwell involved minor dental or surgical procedures. A more critical evaluation of the use of hypnotism in surgery was made by Moll (1889), who noted that ". . . a complete analgesia is extremely rare in hypnosis, although authors, copying from one another assert that it is common" (p. 105). Moll also gave his own examples; for instance: ". . . I once hypnotized a patient in order to open a boil painlessly. I did not succeed in inducing analgesia, but the patient was almost unable to move, so that I could perform the little operation without difficulty" (p. 330). Moll went on to note that "The value of hypnotism for inducing analgesia is not very great. . . . The cases in which hypnotism can be used to make an operation painless are very rare; the care with which every such case is registered by the daily press shows this."

Beginning around 1930 and extending up to the present, interest in the reduction of pain by hypnotism or by suggestions has increased markedly. Numerous clinical reports, several books (Coppolino, 1965; Marmer, 1959; Werbel, 1965), and a symposium concerning "hypnotic analgesia" (Lassner, 1964) have been published. In most of the cases that have been reported, it appears that anxiety, fear, and worry or concern were reduced, but it is questionable whether there was a marked reduction in pain as a sensation. Let us look at a few examples.

Anderson (1957) performed an abdominal exploration on a 71-year-old male. Since the patient's general condition was poor, contraindicating general anesthesia, it was decided to use hypnotism. The patient underwent intensive hypnotic training sessions for two weeks prior to surgery. The training sessions included rehearsal of the operative procedure. It appears likely that this factor—rehearsing every step of the operation—may be sufficient to reduce anxiety and fear during the operation. During the surgery, the patient "partially broke trance" and, consequently, 5 cc. of 2% Pentothal was administered. A common duct stone was then removed. The report did not state how the patient "broke trance" but he presumably showed signs of pain. Physiological measures, such as changes in heart rate, blood pressure, or respiration, were not reported. Also, no mention was made of a verbal report from the patient regarding any pain he might have experienced. Thus, it is impossible to conclude from this report to what extent the sensory experience of pain was reduced. Furthermore, if we assume that pain was significantly reduced, we do not know whether to attribute the reduction to familiarity with the operative procedures obtained during the rehearsals, to the hypnotic induction procedure, to suggestions for pain reduction, to the Pentothal administered during surgery, or to some other variables.

Cooper and Powles (1945) reported using hypnotism to produce analgesia in six minor surgical procedures. Two cases involved infections in the tips of a finger, two involved abscesses in the palms, and two involved abscesses in the armpit. One of these cases was regarded as unsuccessful because of apprehension on the part of the patient. One of the six cases was described in detail since it was regarded as a good example of the successful use of hypnotism. The patient was an 18-year-old soldier who required incision of two abscesses in the armpit. The patient was premedicated with 1½ gr. Nembutal. Subsequently, he was told he would go to sleep because of the sleeping capsule. Suggestions for relaxation, fatigue, and sleep were continued for ten minutes. Additional suggestions were given for anesthesia of the armpit, arm, and shoulder. During the incision, ". . . there was considerable grimacing and some movement of the contralateral shoulder. . . ." Physiological measures were not reported and the patient's verbal report about his experience was not given. Although Cooper and Powles presented this as an exceptionally successful case demonstrating "satisfactory anesthesia," it is not clear to what extent pain as a sensation was reduced. Other investigators (e.g., Finer & Nylen, 1961; Schwarcz, 1965; Taugher, 1958) also implied that pain was obliterated by hypnotism even though the patients' verbal reports were not presented and either overt behavioral indices or physiological measures suggested that the patients may have experienced pain.

EFFECTS OF SUGGESTIONS OF ANALGESIA GIVEN WITHOUT A HYPNOTIC INDUCTION PROCEDURE

In a large number of studies, suggestions aimed at removing pain sensitivity were given together with the hypnotic induction procedure. Apparently, it was assumed that the surgery could not be carried out if the suggestions for pain relief or analgesia had been given alone, without a hypnotic induction procedure. This assumption is questionable. For instance, Esdaile (1850, pp. 214-215) reported that a few of his surgical patients who had received explicit or implicit suggestions for analgesia, but who could *not* be placed in "mesmeric trance," were able to tolerate major surgery in the same way as patients who had been placed in "mesmeric trance." Let us look at representative recent studies that indicate that suggestions for pain relief or analgesia given without a hypnotic induction procedure may be sufficient for some patients to tolerate surgical procedures.

During World War II, Sampimon and Woodruff (1946) were working under primitive conditions in a prisoner of war hospital near Singapore. Since the supply of anesthetic and analgesic drugs was practically depleted, hypnotism was used for surgery. Two patients could not be "hypnotized"; since the minor surgical procedures (incision for exploration of an abscess cavity and extraction of a tooth) had to be performed without drugs, they proceeded to operate after giving "the mere suggestion of anesthesia." To their surprise, they found that both patients were able to undergo the procedures without complaints and without noticeable signs of pain. Sampimon and Woodruff wrote: "As a result of these two cases two other patients were anesthetized by suggestions only, without any attempt to induce true hypnosis, and both had teeth removed painlessly."

Lozanov (1967) presented a more recent case of surgery in which suggestions of anesthesia were given without a hypnotic induction procedure. The patient was a 50-year-old man who required surgical repair of a hernia in the groin. Since he was ". . . convinced of the anaesthetizing power of suggestion," he offered to undergo surgery without drugs and without hypnotism. Before the surgery, he was given preparatory practice that involved breathing exercises. The patient did not appear to experience pain during the initial surgical incision – 12 cm. in the right groin – or when the muscle tissue was cut. Lozanov reported that "Pain appeared when the process of separation reached the testis. It became necessary to suspend the operation for one minute during which time the patient was subject to additional suggestions." Pain also appeared later "during the broaching of ligamentum inguinale and the periosteum of tuberculum pubicum." At that point, 12 cc. of 0.5% Novocain was injected and the remainder of the operation was performed apparently without pain. Lozanov noted that pain was apparently present during two minutes of the 50-minute operation.

In brief, there is evidence to indicate that suggestions for pain relief given *without* "hypnosis" may at times be as effective as suggestions for pain relief given *with* "hypnosis" in producing a tolerance for pain during surgery.

RECAPITULATION

It appears that with the exception of the skin, which is very sensitive, most tissues and organs of the body are rather insensitive to *surgical incisions*. Consequently, if a person is able to tolerate the pain that is associated with initial skin incision, he might then be able to undergo the rest of the surgery into tissues and organs that lie below the skin without experiencing much severe pain.

With the above facts in mind, reports of surgery performed with the use of hypnotism and suggestions are not as amazing as they first appear. Furthermore, they become even less amazing when we realize that (a) the effectiveness of hypnotism in reducing surgical pain has been exaggerated, (b) in the great majority of cases, *analgesic or anesthetic drugs* were used along with the hypnotism and the suggestions, and (c) although some patients were able to tolerate the surgery, they very commonly showed behavioral or physiological signs of pain, especially when those tissues were cut—for example, the skin or the area near the testis—which are normally quite sensitive.

The studies summarized in this chapter, together with other studies (e.g., Finer, 1966; Hoffman, 1959; Kroger, 1957; Kroger & DeLee, 1957; Mason, 1955; Reis, 1966; Wallace & Coppolino, 1960), indicate that, with at least a small proportion of patients, suggestions aimed at reducing pain given with or without hypnotic induction procedures are sufficient for the patients to tolerate the surgery, to minimize anxiety, fear, and other emotions, and probably to reduce (but not necessarily obliterate) the sensory experience of pain. This conclusion is in line with the results of recent experimental studies pertaining to the reduction of pain, to which we now turn.

EXPERIMENTAL STUDIES ON PAIN REDUCTION

Over the last 40 years, a number of investigators have attempted to clarify the phenomenon of suggested analgesia by bringing it into the laboratory. In these experiments, a wide range of procedures have been used to produce pain, including pressure from a sharp point, electric shock, radiant heat, immersion of a limb in ice cold water, occlusion of the blood supply to a limb, and application of a heavy weight to the bony part of a finger (cf. Barber, 1970). Obviously, the pain produced by these stimuli may differ in quality and may give rise to less anxiety and fear than the pain of surgery. However, it appears possible that some kinds of pain produced in the laboratory—for instance, the pain produced by occlusion of the blood supply to a limb or by application of a heavy weight to the bony part of a finger—may be as intense as the pain that is found during some surgical procedures.

Although the pain produced in the laboratory generally gives rise to less anxiety and fear than the pain produced by the surgeon's scalpel, it is nevertheless possible to draw some conclusions from the laboratory studies that are relevant to understanding how some patients are able to tolerate surgery without receiving drugs. Let us briefly state these generalizations before going on to examine the supporting data.

1. Implicit or explicit suggestions for pain relief or analgesia are effective in reducing reported pain regardless of whether or not a hypnotic induction procedure has been administered.
2. Reported pain is reduced when the subjects are distracted during the pain-producing stimulation.
3. Subjects report less pain when they are asked to imagine situations—e.g., to imagine a limb as a piece of rubber—which, if they actually occurred, would be imcompatible with the experience of pain.
4. Subjects who are not anxious report less pain than those who are anxious and fearful.

Let us examine some of the data that support these generalizations.

Suggestions for anesthesia or for relief of pain

Hilgard and his associates (Hilgard, 1967; Hilgard, Cooper, Lenox, Morgan, & Voevodsky, 1967; Morgan, Lezard, Prytulak, & Hilgard, 1970) confirmed earlier observations indicating that hypnotic subjects who have received suggestions of anesthesia report less pain than control subjects who have not received suggestions of anesthesia. However, several recent studies (Barber, 1969a; Evans & Paul, 1970; Spanos, Barber, & Lang, 1969), which will be discussed next, showed that, if nonhypnotic subjects are also exposed to suggestions of anesthesia, they show as much reduction in pain as hypnotic subjects who are exposed to the same suggestions of anesthesia.

Barber (1969a) gave identical suggestions of anesthesia ("Your hand is numb and insensitive . . .") to two groups of subjects—a group that had been exposed to a standardized hypnotic induction procedure and a group that had not been exposed to an induction. The pain stimulus was a heavy weight applied to the bony part of a finger for one minute. As compared to a no-suggestions condition (control group), the suggestions of anesthesia were effective in reducing reported pain in both the hypnotic and the nonhypnotic subjects. Moreover, the magnitude of the pain reduction was about the same in both the hypnotic and the nonhypnotic groups.

Spanos, Barber, and Lang (1969) confirmed the above results. These investigators also gave suggestions of anesthesia ("Your hand is numb and insensitive . . .") to subjects who had, and also to those who had not, been exposed to a standardized hypnotic induction procedure. The pain stimulus was again a heavy weight applied to the bony part of a finger. Again, as compared to control groups that did not receive any suggestions, the suggestions of anesthesia were effective in producing an equal reduction in reported pain in the hypnotic subjects and the nonhypnotic subjects. Most of the hypnotic and nonhypnotic subjects who received the suggestions of anesthesia showed a small reduction in reported pain and about one-fourth of these subjects showed a moderate reduction (3 or more points on a 10-point scale).

Evans and Paul (1970) cross-validated the above results in an experiment in which pain was produced by immersion of the hand in ice water at 0 to 2°C. Suggestions of anesthesia ("Your hand has no feeling at all . . .") were given to subjects who had been exposed to a hypnotic induction procedure and also to subjects who had not been exposed to an induction. Other subjects, assigned to control groups, were not given suggestions of anesthesia. The hypnotic and nonhypnotic subjects who received suggestions of anesthesia reported less pain than the control groups. Also, the hypnotic induction procedure was irrelevant in reducing pain; the two groups of subjects who received suggestions of anesthesia—hypnotic subjects and nonhypnotic subjects—reported the same degree of pain reduction.

Clinical studies also indicate that implicit suggestions for pain relief, given without hypnotic induction procedures, are effective in reducing pain in a substantial proportion of patients. For instance, pain was reduced when placebos were given with the implication that pain relief should be expected. Beecher (1955) and his associates (Lasagna, Mosteller, von Felsinger, & Beecher, 1954) found that satisfactory relief of pain, defined as "50 percent or more relief of pain at 45 and 90 minutes after administration of the agent," could be achieved with placebos in 35% of their postsurgical patients. These findings were confirmed in similar studies by Houde and Wallenstein (1953) and Keats (1956). Furthermore, Laszlo and Spencer (1953) found that "over 50% of patients who had received analgesics for a long period of time could be adequately controlled by placebo medication."

The data summarized above, and other data reviewed elsewhere (Barber, 1959, 1963, 1970), support the notion that explicit and implicit suggestions for pain relief tend to reduce anxiety, fear, and also the degree of reported pain in experimental subjects and in clinical patients.

The role of distraction

When attempts are made to produce "hypnotic analgesia," the patients are at times given instructions designed to focus their attention on something other than the painful stimulus. The available data suggest that a wide variety of distractions are effective in reducing pain (Barber, 1969a; Barber & Cooper, 1972; Barber & Hahn, 1962; Gammon & Starr, 1941; Gammon, Starr, & Bronk, 1936; Kanfer & Goldfoot, 1966; Notermans, 1966, 1967).

In one of these experiments (Barber, 1969a), student nurses were exposed to pain-producing stimulation (a heavy weight applied to a finger) while they listened to a tape recording that presented the interesting erotic escapades of an unnamed Hollywood actor. They were asked to guess the identity of the actor and to remember as many of the details of his escapades as possible. Immediately prior to the pain stimulation, some of the subjects had been exposed to a standardized hypnotic induction procedure and others had not. The distraction of listening to the interesting tape recording produced a significant reduction in reported pain. It is particularly interesting to note that the magnitude of the pain reduction was the same in both the hypnotic and nonhypnotic subjects. Similarly, in another recent study (Barber & Cooper, 1972), two distractions—listening to an interesting tape recorded story and adding numbers aloud—were both effective in reducing the degree of reported pain. An earlier study (Kanfer & Goldfoot, 1966) also showed that pain was reduced by three distractors (verbalizing the sensations aloud, self-pacing with a clock, and observing a series of slides).

Other kinds of distractions also appear to be effective in reducing the degree of reported pain. For instance, Notermans (1966) found that pain was apparently reduced when the subjects were engaged in the distracting task of inflating a manometer cuff and also when they were distracted by another noxious stimulus applied to another part of the body.

In brief, the available studies suggest that distraction can attenuate pain. Moreover, the distraction can either take the form of external stimulation or instructing the subjects to direct their attention to something besides the pain-producing stimulus.

Cognitive strategies

It also appears that certain kinds of "cognitive strategies" are useful in reducing pain. These strategies involve imagining situations which, if real, would result in the reduction or elimination of pain. For example, when a pain-producing stimulus is applied to a finger, the subject might try to think of pleasant events or might try to think and imagine that the finger is numb and insensitive (Spanos, Barber, & Lang, 1969).

Barber and Hahn (1962) showed that one kind of cognitive strategy—thinking of previously-experienced pleasant events—significantly reduced reported pain caused by the immersion of a hand in ice cold water (at 2°C.). Two physiological correlates of pain—irregular pattern of respiration and forehead muscle tension—were also diminished. The nonhypnotic subjects who thought of pleasant events during the painful stimulation showed the same degree of reduction in pain experience as "good" hypnotic subjects who had been exposed to a hypnotic induction procedure and to suggestions of anesthesia.

Chaves and Barber (in press) compared the degree of pain reduction that could be achieved by using two different cognitive strategies—imagining that a finger is insensitive and imagining pleasant events. In addition, other subjects were led to expect a reduction in pain but were not provided with any cognitive strategies. The subjects who were simply led to expect a reduction in pain, in fact, did report less pain than uninstructed control subjects. However, even greater pain reductions were shown by subjects who were asked to use the cognitive strategies for reducing pain—that is, who were instructed to imagine that the finger was insensitive or to imagine pleasant events.

In summary, a number of procedures are effective in reducing experimentally-produced pain including direct suggestions of anesthesia, distraction, leading subjects to expect a reduction in pain, as well as providing subjects with cognitive strategies for pain reduction.

Reduction of anxiety and fear

As stated in the beginning of this chapter, in the surgical situation and to a lesser degree in the laboratory, the experience of pain is usually closely intermingled with fear, anxiety, worry, and other emotions. There is evidence indicating that relief of postoperative pain due to the administration of morphine as well as placebos may be more closely related to the alleviation of fear or anxiety rather than to a marked alteration in the pain sensations (Barber, 1959; Beecher, 1959; Cattell, 1943). Even neurosurgical procedures designed to alleviate intractable pain, such as prefrontal lobotomy, seem to reduce anxiety and fear without markedly altering the pain sensations.

The reduction in anxiety and fear seems to dramatically reduce the overall pain experience. Many investigators appear to agree with Ostenasek's (1948) conclusion that ". . . when the fear of pain is abolished, the perception of pain is not intolerable."

Implications

In brief, it appears that a wide variety of procedures are capable of reducing pain. The variables mentioned above may also play an important role in producing the apparent reduction in pain that has been associated with hypnotism. To illustrate this contention, let us look briefly at the effects of distraction. The hypothesis that distraction plays an important role in reducing pain in "hypnotized" subjects was proffered many years ago by Liebeault (1885). He contended that, when suggestions are effective in reducing pain in hypnotic subjects, the mediating process involves a focusing of attention on thoughts or ideas other than those concerning pain. More recently, a similar conclusion was reached by August (1961) after a large-scale investigation of 1000 patients during childbirth. August concluded that hypnotic induction procedures and suggestions are effective in reducing pain during childbirth to the extent that they "direct attention away from pain responses to pleasant ideas" (p. 62).

Of course, distraction is not the only factor and may not be the most important factor in reducing pain in hypnotic situations. Hypnotic subjects are explicitly or implicitly led to believe that they are undergoing a procedure that will attenuate pain and attempts are made to reduce anxiety and fear. Furthermore, they are given various types of suggestions and instructions and some of these suggestions may give rise to "cognitive strategies" that are effective in attenuating pain. Also, a close interpersonal relationship may exist between the patient and the hypnotist. This relationship could affect the kinds of pain reports that are obtained from the patients (Barber, 1970, pp. 239-240; Egbert, Battit, Turndorf, & Beecher, 1963; Egbert, Battit, Welch, & Bartlett, 1964).[4]

Suggestions for further research

Although we have pointed to a number of variables that appear to play an important role in pain, a number of questions remain unanswered. One of the most striking questions pertains to individual differences. Some individuals seem to be able to adopt a detached attitude toward pain, treating it in the same way as other sensations and not being especially bothered by it. On the other hand, other individuals are hyperreactive to pain and are extremely disturbed by relatively minor pain-producing stimulation. A major research problem in this area is to identify the variables that produce these differences. If these variables could be specified, we might successfully train a large proportion of individuals to tolerate painful stimuli. . . .

Some success has already been achieved. Experimental data indicate that pain can be reduced by minimizing subjects' anxiety, by leading subjects to expect that they have the ability to control pain, by asking subjects to imagine situations that are incompatible with the experience of pain, by distracting the subjects, and by administering suggestions for pain reduction. Clearly, much additional work is needed to utilize these variables effectively in controlling pain. For example, what kinds of procedures are most effective in producing distraction? How can the effective variables be implemented in teaching tolerance of pain? . . .

SUMMARY

One of the most striking phenomena associated with hypnotism is its use in controlling the pain of surgery. This chapter has attempted to place this dramatic phenomenon in perspective by emphasizing that most tissues and organs of the body, with the notable exception of the skin, are rather insensitive to the surgeon's scalpel. Many individuals can tolerate the pain of surgery if local anesthetics such as Novocain are used to dull the skin for the initial incision. In addition, experimental and clinical data indicate that pain is reduced when the patients have low levels of anxiety and fear, when they have positive attitudes, motivations, and expectancies about the situation, when they are distracted, when they are given suggestions for analgesia or for pain reduction, and when they utilize a variety of "cognitive strategies" for pain reduction, such as thinking and imagining that the stimulated body part is a piece of rubber or is numb and insensitive. When some or many of these factors are present—in hypnotic situations, in nonhypnotic situations such as those described by Lozanov (1967) and others (Freemont-Smith, 1950; Sampimon & Woodruff, 1946; Tuckey, 1889, pp. 725-726), and also in acupuncture situations—some individuals are able to tolerate surgical pain.[5]

NOTES

[1]Although *most* tissues and organs of the human body are rather insensitive when they are cut, the surgeon's incision does produce pain when it cuts the skin and other external tissues such as the conjunctiva, the mucous membranes of the mouth and nasopharynx, the upper surface of the larynx, and the stratified mucous membranes of the genitalia. Also, it appears that a small number of deeper tissues, such as the deep fascia, the periosteum, the tendons, and the rectum, hurt when they are cut (Lewis, 1942).

[2]Other present-day investigators also use hypnotism together with local anesthetics during surgery. For instance, Van Dyke (1965) presented a case of a 9-year-old boy who was operated on for a bony cyst in the jaw which was delaying the descent of a permanent canine tooth. Prior to the surgery, the boy was given two training sessions in hypnosis. Immediately before the operation, he was exposed to a hypnotic induction procedure and to suggestions aimed at relieving pain. Although no preoperative medication was used, an unspecified amount of Novocain was administered immediately before surgery, making it difficult to determine to what extent the relief of pain was due to the hypnotic induction procedure, to the suggestions for pain relief, or to the use of Novocain. Similarly, Van Dyke presented another case involving surgical incision of the female vulvar orifice (episiotomy) in which the effects of hypnotism and suggestions in alleviating pain were confounded with the effects of 5 cc. of Novocain.

[3]In addition to the use of Novocain, the following drugs were administered to the patient: 0.10 gm. pentobarbital (Nembutal), 50 mg. diphenhydramine hydrochloride (Benadryl), 100 mg. meperidine hydrochloride (Demerol), 0.40 mg. scopolamine, and 50 mg. thiamylal sodium (Surital). Also, during dissection of the lung, 100 mg. of a 0.1% solution of succinylcholine was administered.

[4]Our analysis suggests that there are a host of variables that are effective in reducing pain. If these variables have broad relevance, we should also be able to see their effects in faith healing, in exorcism, in acupuncture, and in other situations in which pain is ostensibly reduced without the use of drugs. . . . We look at one of these techniques—the use of acupuncture in surgery—to see whether the variables that we have outlined in this chapter are helpful in understanding this technique for alleviating surgical pain.

[5]In this chapter, we have focused on *surgical pain.* The effects of hypnotism and suggestions on other kinds of pain—e.g., labor pain, postsurgical pain, and pain associated with cancer—are discussed by Barber (1970). . . .

• • •

Mitchell extract is from Mitchell, J. F. Local anesthesia in general surgery. *Journal of the American Medical Association,* 1907, **48,** 198-201.

Moll extract is from Moll, Albert. *The Study of Hypnosis.* New York: Julian Press, 1958.

REFERENCES

Anderson, M. N. Hypnosis in anesthesia. *Journal of the Medical Association of Alabama,* 1957, **27,** 121-125.

August, R. V. *Hypnosis in Obstetrics.* New York: McGraw-Hill, 1961.

Barber, T. X. Toward a theory of pain: Relief of chronic pain by prefrontal leucotomy, opiates, placebos, and hypnosis. *Psychological Bulletin,* 1959, **56,** 430-460.

Barber, T. X. The effect of "hypnosis" on pain: A critical review of experimental and clinical findings. *Psychosomatic Medicine,* 1963, **25,** 303-333. [Reprinted in T. X. Barber et al. (Eds.) *Biofeedback and Self-Control: An Aldine Reader.* Chicago: Aldine-Atherton, 1971, Pp. 724-754.]

Barber, T. X. Effects of hypnotic induction, suggestions of anesthesia, and distraction on subjective and physiological responses to pain. Paper presented at the annual meeting of the Eastern Psychological Association, Philadelphia, April 10, 1969.

Barber, T. X. *LSD, Marihuana, Yoga, and Hypnosis.* Chicago: Aldine, 1970.

Barber, T. X., and Cooper, B. J. Effects on pain of experimentally-induced and spontaneous distraction. *Psychological Reports,* 1972, **31,** 647-651.

Barber, T. X., and Coules, J. Electrical skin conductance and galvanic skin response during "hypnosis." *International Journal of Clinical and Experimental Hypnosis,* 1959, **7,** 79-92.

Barber, T. X., and Hahn, K. W., Jr. Physiological and subjective responses to pain producing stimulation under hypnotically-suggested and waking-imagined "analgesia." *Journal of Abnormal and Social Psychology,* 1962, **65,** 411-418.

Barber, T. X., Spanos, N. P., and Chaves, J. F. *Hypnosis, Imagination, and Human Potentialities.* New York: Pergamon, 1974.

Beecher, H. K. Pain in men wounded in battle. *Annals of Surgery,* 1946, **123,** 96-105.

Beecher, H. K. The powerful placebo. *Journal of the American Medical Association,* 1955, **159,** 1602-1606.

Beecher, H. K. Relationship of significance of wound to pain experienced. *Journal of the American Medical Association,* 1956, **161,** 1609-1613.

Beecher, H. K. *Measurement of Subjective Responses.* New York: Oxford University Press, 1959.

Betcher, A. M. Hypnosis as an adjunct in anesthesiology. *New York State Journal of Medicine,* 1960, **60,** 816-822.

Braid, J. Facts and observations as to the relative value of mesmeric and hypnotic coma, and ethereal narcotism, for the mitigation or entire prevention of pain during surgical operations. *Medical Times,* 1847, **15,** 381-382.

Bramwell, J. M. *Hypnotism.* New York: Julian Press, 1956. (Original date of publication: 1903.)

Cattell, M. The action and use of analgesics. *Research Publications Association for Research in Nervous and Mental Disease,* 1943, **23,** 365-372.

Chaves, J. F., and Barber, T. X. Needles and knives: Behind the mystery of acupuncture and Chinese meridians. *Human Behavior,* September 1973, **2,** No. 9, 19-24.

Chaves, J. F., and Barber, T. X. Cognitive strategies, experimenter modeling, and expectation in the attenuation of pain. *Journal of Abnormal Psychology,* in press.

Chertok, L. *Psychosomatic Methods in Painless Childbirth.* New York: Pergamon, 1959.

Cooper, S. R., and Powles, W. E. The psychosomatic approach in practice. *McGill Medical Journal,* 1945, **14,** 415-438.

Coppolino, C. A. *Practice of Hypnosis in Anesthesiology.* New York: Grune & Stratton, 1965.

Crasilneck, H. B., and McCranie, E. J., and Jenkins, M. T. Special indications for hypnosis as a method of anesthesia. *Journal of the American Medical Association,* 1956, **162,** 1606-1608.

Doupe, J., Miller, W. R., and Keller, W. K. Vasomotor reactions in the hypnotic state. *Journal of Neurology and Psychiatry,* 1939, **2,** 97-106.

Egbert, L. D., Battit, G. E., Turndorf, H., and Beecher, H. K. The value of the preoperative visit by an anesthetist. *Journal of the American Medical Association,* 1963, **185,** 553-555.

Egbert, L. D., Battit, G. E., Welch, C. E., and Bartlett, M. K. Reduction of postoperative pain by encouragement and instruction of patients. *New England Journal of Medicine,* 1964, **270,** 825-827.

Esdaile, J. *Hypnosis in Medicine and Surgery.* New York: Julian Press, 1957. (Original date of publication: 1850.)

Evans, M. B., and Paul, G. L. Effects of hypnotically suggested analgesia on physiological and subjective responses to cold stress. *Journal of Consulting and Clinical Psychology,* 1970, **35,** 362-371. [Reprinted in J. Stoyva et al. (Ed.) *Biofeedback and Self-Control: 1971.* Chicago: Aldine-Atherton, 1972. Pp. 380-389.]

Finer, B. L. Experience with hypnosis in clinical anesthesiology. *Särtryck ur Opuscula Medica,* 1966, **4,** 1-11.

Finer, B. L., and Nylen, B. O. Cardiac arrest in the treatment of burns, and report on hypnosis as a substitute for anesthesia. *Plastic and Reconstructive Surgery,* 1961, **27,** 49-55.

Freemont-Smith, F. Discussion of Beecher's paper on perception of pain. *Problems of Consciousness, First Conference.* New York: Josiah Macy, Jr. Foundation, 1950.

Gammon, G. D., and Starr, I. Studies on the relief of pain by counterirritation. *Journal of Clinical Investigation,* 1941, **20,** 13-20.

Gammon, G. D., Starr, I., and Bronk, D. W. The effect of counterirritation upon pain produced by cutaneous injury. *American Journal of Physiology,* 1936, **116,** 56.

Hardy, J. D., Wolff, H. G., and Goodell, H. *Pain Sensations and Reactions.* Baltimore: Williams & Wilkins, 1952.

Hilgard, E. R. A quantitative study of pain and its reduction through hypnotic suggestion. *Proceedings of the National Academy of Science,* 1967, **57,** 1581-1586.

Hilgard, E. R. Pain as a puzzle for psychology and physiology. *American Psychologist,* 1969, **24,** 103-113.

Hilgard, E. R., Cooper, L. M., Lenox, J., Morgan, A. H., and Voevodsky, J. The use of pain-state reports in the study of hypnotic analgesia to the pain of ice water. *Journal of Nervous and Mental Disease,* 1967, **144,** 506-513.

Hill, H. E., Kornetsky, C. H., Flanary, H. G., and Wikler, A. Effects of anxiety and morphine on discrimination of intensities of painful stimuli. *Journal of Clinical Investigation,* 1952, **31,** 473-480. (a)

Hill, H. E., Kornetsky, C. H., Flanary, H. G., and Wikler, A. Studies on anxiety associated with anticipation of pain. 1. Effects of morphine. *Archives of Neurology and Psychiatry,* 1952, **67,** 612-619. (b)

Hoffman, E. Hypnosis in general surgery. *American Surgeon,* 1959, **25,** 163-169.

Houde, R. W., and Wallenstein, S. L. A method for evaluating analgesics in patients with chronic pain. *Drug Addiction and Narcotics, Bulletin,* 1953, Appendix F, 660-682.

Kanfer, F. H., and Goldfoot, D. A. Self-control and tolerance of noxious stimulation. *Psychological Reports,* 1966, **18,** 79-85.

Keats, A. S. Postoperative pain: Research and treatment. *Journal of Chronic Diseases,* 1956, **4,** 72-80.

Kornetsky, C. Effects of anxiety and morphine in the anticipation and perception of painful radiant heat stimuli. *Journal of Comparative and Physiological Psychology,* 1954, **47,** 130-132.

Kroger, W. S. Introduction and supplemental reports. In J. Esdaile, *Hypnosis in Medicine and Surgery.* New York: Julian Press, 1957.

Kroger, W. S., and DeLee, S. T. Use of hypnoanaesthesia for cesarean section and hysterectomy. *Journal of the American Medical Association,* 1957, **163,** 442-444.

Lasagna, L., Mosteller, F., von Felsinger, J. M., and Beecher, H. K. A study of the placebo response. *American Journal of Medicine,* 1954, **16,** 770-779.

Lassner, J. (Ed.) *Hypnosis in Anesthesiology.* Berlin: Springer-Verlag, 1964.

Laszlo, D., and Spencer, H. Medical problems in the management of cancer. *Medical Clinics of North America,* 1953, **37,** 869-880.

Lennander, K. G. Ueber die Sensibilität der Bauchhöhle und über lokale und allgemeine Anästhesie bei Bruch-und Bauchoperationen. *Centralblatt für Chirurgie,* 1901, **8,** 209-223.

Lennander, K. G. Beobachtungen über die Sensibilität in der Bauchhöhle. *Mitteilungen aus den Grenzgebieten der Medizin und Chirurgie,* 1902, **10,** 38–104.

Lennander, K. G. Weitere Beobachtungen über Sensibilität in Organ und Gewebe und über lokale Anästhesis. *Deutsche Zeitschrift für Chirurgie,* 1904, **73,** 297-350.

Lennander, K. G. Ueber Hofrat Nothnagels zweite Hypothese der Darmkolikschmerzen. *Mitteilungen aus den Grenzgebieten der Medizin und Chirurgie,* 1906, **16,** 19-23. (a)

Lennander, K. G. Ueber lokale Anästhesie und über Sensibilität in Organ und Gewebe, weitere Beobachtungen. *Mitteilungen aus den Grenzgebieten der Medizin und Chirurgie,* 1906, **15,** 465-494. (b)

Levine, M. Psychogalvanic reaction to painful stimuli in hypnotic and hysterical anesthesia. *Bulletin of the Johns Hopkins Hospital,* 1930, **46,** 331-339.

Lewis, T. *Pain.* New York: Macmillan, 1942.

Liebeault, A. A. Anesthesia per suggestion. *Journal Magnestisme,* 1885, 64-67.

Lozanov, G. Anesthetization through suggestion in a state of wakefulness. *Proceedings of the 7th European Conference on Psychosomatic Research,* Rome, 1967, 399-402.

Mandy, A. J., Mandy, T. E., Farkas, R., and Scher, E. Is natural childbirth natural? *Psychosomatic Medicine,* 1952, **14,** 431-438.

Marmer, M. J. The role of hypnosis in anesthesiology. *Journal of the American Medical Association,* 1956, **162,** 441-443.

Marmer, M. J. Hypnoanalgesia: The use of hypnosis in conjunction with chemical anesthesia. *Anesthesia and Analgesia,* 1957, **36,** 27-32.

Marmer, M. J. *Hypnosis in Anesthesiology.* Springfield, Ill.: C. C Thomas, 1959.

Mason, A. A. Surgery under hypnosis. *Anesthesia,* 1955, **10,** 295-299.

Mitchell, J. F. Local anesthesia in general surgery. *Journal of the American Medical Association,* 1907, **48,** 198-201.

Moll, A. *The Study of Hypnosis.* New York: Julian Press, 1958. (Original date of publication: 1889.)

Morgan, A. H., Lezard, F., Prytulak, S., and Hilgard, E. R. Augmenters, reducers, and their reaction to cold pressor pain in waking and suggested hypnotic analgesia. *Journal of Personality and Social Psychology,* 1970, **16,** 5-11.

Notermans, S. L. H. Measurement of the pain threshold determined by electrical stimulation and its clinical application. Part I. Method and factors possibly influencing the pain threshold. *Neurology,* 1966, **16,** 1071-1086.

Notermans, S. L. H. Measurement of the pain threshold determined by electrical stimulation and its clinical application. Part II. Clinical application in neurological and neurosurgical patients. *Neurology,* 1967, **17,** 58-73.

Ostenasek, F. J. Prefrontal lobotomy for the relief of intractable pain. *Bulletin of the Johns Hopkins Hospital,* 1948, **83,** 229-236.

Reis, M. Subjective reactions of a patient having surgery without chemical anesthesia. *American Journal of Clinical Hypnosis,* 1966, **9,** 122-124.

Sampimon, R. L. H., and Woodruff, M. F. A. Some observations concerning the use of hypnosis as a substitute for anesthesia. *Medical Journal of Australia,* 1946, **1,** 393-395.

Sattler, D. G. Absence of local sign in visceral reactions to painful stimulation. *Research Publications Association for Research in Nervous and Mental Disease,* 1943, **23,** 143-153.

Schwarcz, B. E. Hypnoanalgesia and hypnoanesthesia in urology. *Surgical Clinics of North America,* 1965, **45,** 7547-7555.

Spanos, N. P., Barber, T. X., and Lang, G. Effects of hypnotic induction, suggestions of analgesia, and demands for honesty on subjective reports of pain. Department of Sociology, Boston University, 1969.

Taugher, V. J. Hypno-anesthesia. *Wisconsin Medical Journal,* 1958, **57,** 95-96.

Tuckey, C. L. Psychotherapeutics; or treatment by hypnotism. *Woods Medical and Surgical Monographs,* 1889, **3,** 721-795.

Van Dyke, P. B. Hypnosis in surgery. *Journal of Abdominal Surgery,* 1965, **7,** 1-5, 26-29.

Wallace, G., and Coppolino, C. A. Hypnosis in anesthesiology. *New York Journal of Medicine,* 1960, **60,** 3258-3273.

Werbel, E. W. *One Surgeon's Experience with Hypnosis.* New York: Pageant Press, 1965.

Werbel, E. W. Hypnosis in serious surgical problems. *American Journal of Clinical Hypnosis,* 1967, **10,** 44-47.

28

The interspersal hypnotic technique for symptom correction and pain control

Milton H. Erickson, M.D.[1]

Innumerable times this authors has been asked to commit to print in detail the hypnotic technique he has employed to alleviate intolerable pain or to correct various other problems. The verbal replies made to these many requests have never seemed to be adequate since they were invariably prefaced by the earnest assertion that the technique in itself serves no other purpose than that of securing and fixating the patient's attention, creating in him a receptive and responsive mental state, and thereby enabling him to benefit from unrealized or only partially realized potentials for behavior of various types. With this achieved by the hypnotic technique, there is then the opportunity to proffer suggestions and instructions serving to aid and to direct the patient in achieving the desired goal or goals. In other words, the hypnotic technique serves only to induce a favorable setting in which to instruct the patient in a more advantageous use of his own potentials of behavior.

Since the hypnotic technique is primarily a means to an end while therapy derives from the guidance of the patient's behavioral capacities, it follows that, within limits, the same hypnotic technique can be utilized for patients with widely diverse problems. To illustrate, two instances will be cited in which the same technique was employed, once for a patient with a distressing neurotic problem and once for a patient suffering from intolerable pain from terminal malignant disease. The technique is one that the author has employed on the illiterate subject and upon the college graduate, in experimental situations and for clinical purposes. Often it has been used to secure, to fixate, and to hold a difficult patient's attention and to distract him from creating difficulties that would impede therapy. It is a technique employing ideas that are clear, comprehensible, but which by their patent irrelevance to the patient-physician relationship and situation distract the patient. Thereby the patient is prevented from intruding unhelpfully into a situation which he cannot understand and for which he is seeking help. At the same time, a readiness to understand and to respond is created within the patient. Thus a favorable setting is evolved for the elicitation of needful and helpful behavioral potentialities not previously used, or not fully used or perhaps misused by the patient.

The first instance to be cited will be given without any account of the hypnotic technique employed. Instead, there will be given the helpful instructions, suggestions, and guiding ideas which enabled the patient to achieve his therapeutic goal and which were interspersed among the ideas constituting the hypnotic technique. These therapeutic ideas will not be cited as repetitiously as they were verbalized to the patient for the reason that they are more easily comprehended in cold print than when uttered as a part of a stream of utterances. Yet, these few repeated suggestions in the hypnotic situation served to meet the patient's needs adequately.

Reprinted with permission of the American Society of Clinical Hypnosis from the American Journal of Clinical Hypnosis **8:**198-209. Copyright 1966.

[1]32 West Cypress Street, Phoenix, Arizona 85003.

The patient was a 62-year-old retired farmer with only an eighth grade education, but decidedly intelligent and well-read. He actually possessed a delightful, charming out-going personality, but he was most unhappy, filled with resentment, bitterness, hostility, suspicion and despair. Approximately two years previously for some unknown or forgotten reason (regarded by the author as unimportant and as having no bearing upon the problem of therapy) he had developed a urinary frequency that was most distressing to him. Approximately every half hour he felt a compelling urge to urinate, an urge that was painful, that he could not control and which would result in a wetting of his trousers if he did not yield to it. This urge was constantly present day and night. It interfered with his sleep, his eating, his social adjustments and compelled him to keep within close reach of a lavatory and to carry a briefcase containing several pairs of trousers for use when he was "caught short." He explained that he had brought into the office a briefcase containing three pairs of trousers and he stated that he had visited a lavatory before leaving for the author's office, another on the way and that he had visited the office lavatory before entering the office and that he expected to interrupt the interview with the author by at least one other such visit.

He related that he had consulted more than 100 physicians and well-known clinics. He had been cystoscoped more than 40 times, had had innumerable x-ray pictures taken and countless tests, some of which were electroencephalograms and electrocardiograms. Always he was assured that his bladder was normal; many times he was offered the suggestion to return after a month or two for further study; and "too many times" he was told that "it's all in your head"; that he had no problem at all, that he "should get busy doing something instead of being retired, and to stop pestering doctors and being an old crock." All of this had made him feel like committing suicide.

He had described his problem to a number of writers of syndicated medical columns in newspapers, several of whom offered him in his stamped self-addressed envelope a pontifical platitudinous dissertation upon his problem stressing it as one of obscure organic origin. In all of his searching, not once had it been suggested that he seek psychiatric aid.

On his own initiative, after reading two of the misleading, misinforming and essentially fraudulent books on "do-it-yourself hypnosis", he did seek the aid of stage hypnotists, in all, three in number. Each offered him the usual blandishments, reassurances, and promises common to that type of shady medical practice and each failed completely in repeated attempts at inducing an hypnotic trance. Each charged an exorbitant fee (as judged by a standard medical fee, and especially in relation to the lack of benefit received).

As a result of all this mistreatment, the medical no better than that of the charlatans and actually less forgivable, he had become bitter, disillusioned, resentful and openly hostile, and he was seriously considering suicide. A gas station attendant suggested that he see a psychiatrist and recommended the author on the basis of a Sunday newspaper article. This accounted for his visit to the author.

Having completed his narrative, he leaned back in his chair, folded his arms and challengingly said, "Now psychiatrize and hypnotize me and cure this _____ bladder of mine."

During the narration of the patient's story, the author had listened with every appearance of rapt attention except for a minor idling with his hands, thereby shifting the position of objects on his desk. This idling included a turning of the face of the desk clock away from the patient. As he listened to the patient's bitter account of his experiences, the author was busy speculating upon possible therapeutic approaches to a patient so obviously unhappy, so resentful toward medical care and physicians, and so challenging in attitude. He certainly did not appear to be likely to be receptive and responsive to anything the author might do or say. As the author puzzled over this problem there came to mind the problem of pain control for a patient suffering greatly in a terminal state of malignant disease. That patient had constituted a comparable instance where a hypnotherapeutic approach had been most difficult, and yet, success had been achieved. Both patients had in common the experience of growing plants for a livelihood, both were hostile and resentful, and both were contemptuous of hypnosis. Hence, when the patient issued his challenge of "psychiatrize and hypnotize me," the author, with no further ado, launched into the same technique employed with that other patient to achieve a hypnotherapeutic state in which helpful suggestions, instructions, and directions could be offered with reasonable expectation that they would be accepted and acted upon responsively in accord with the patient's actual needs and behavioral potentials.

The only differences for the two patients was that the interwoven therapeutic material for the one patient pertained to bladder function and duration of time. For the other patient, the interwoven therapeutic instructions pertained to body comfort, to sleep, to appetite, to the enjoyment of the family, to an absence of any need for medication and to the continued enjoyment of time without concern about the morrow.

The actual verbal therapy offered, interspersed as it was in the ideation of the technique itself, was as follows, with the interspersing denoted by dots. "You know, we could think of your bladder needing emptying every 15 minutes instead of every half hour . . . . Not difficult to think that . . . . A watch can run slow . . . . or fast . . . . be wrong even a minute . . . . even two, five minutes . . . . or think of bladder every half hour . . . . like you've been doing . . . . maybe it was 35, 40 minutes sometimes . . . . like to make it an hour . . . . what's the difference . . . . 35, 36 minutes, 41, 42, 45 minutes . . . . not much difference . . . . not important difference . . . . 45, 46, 47 minutes . . . . all the same . . . . lots of times you maybe had to wait a second or two . . . . felt like an hour or two . . . . you made it . . . . you can again . . . . 47 minutes, 50 minutes, what's the difference . . . . stop to think, no great difference, nothing important . . . . just like 50 minutes, 60 minutes, just minutes . . . . anybody that can wait half an hour can wait an hour . . . . I know it . . . . you are learning . . . . not bad to learn . . . . in fact, good . . . . come to think of it, you have had to wait when somebody got there ahead of you . . . . you made it too . . . . can again . . . . and again . . . . all you want to . . . . hour and 5 minutes . . . . hour and 5½ minutes . . . . what's the difference . . . . or even 6½ minutes . . . . make it 10½ hours and 10½ minutes . . . . one minute, 2 minutes, one hour, 2 hours, what's the difference . . . . you got half a century or better of practice in waiting behind you . . . . you can use all that . . . . why not use it . . . . you can do it . . . . probably surprise you a lot . . . . won't even think of it . . . . why not surprise yourself at home . . . . good idea . . . . nothing better than a surprise . . . . an unexpected surprise . . . . how long can you hold out . . . . that's the surprise . . . . longer than you even thought . . . . lots longer . . . . might as well begin . . . . nice feeling to begin . . . . to keep on. . . . Say, why don't you just forget what I've been talking about and just keep it in the back of your mind. Good place for it—can't lose it. Never mind the tomato plant—just what was important about your bladder,—pretty good, feel fine, nice surprise—say, why don't you start feeling rested, refreshed right now, wider awake than you were earlier this morning (this last statement is, to the patient, an indirect emphatic definitive instruction to arouse from his trance). Then, (as a dismissal but not recognizable as such consciously by the patient) why don't you take a nice leisurely walk home, thinking about nothing (an amnesia instruction for both the trance and his problem, and also a confusion measure to obscure the fact that he had already spent 1½ hours in the office)? I'll be able to see you at 10:00 a.m. a week from today (furthering his conscious illusion, resulting from his amnesia, that nothing yet had been done except to give him an appointment)."

A week later he appeared and launched into an excited account of arriving home and turning on the television with an immediate firm intention of delaying urination as long as possible. He watched a two-hour movie and drank two glasses of water during the commercials. He decided to extend the time another hour and suddenly discovered that he had so much bladder distension that he had to visit the lavatory. He looked at his watch and discovered that he had waited four hours. The patient leaned back in his chair, beaming happily at the author, obviously expecting praise. Almost immediately he leaned forward with a startled look and declared in amazement, "It all comes back to me now. I never give it a thought till just now. I plumb forgot the whole thing. Say, you must have hypnotized me. You were doing a lot of talking about growing a tomato plant and I was trying to get the point of it and the next thing I knew I was walking home. Come to think of it I must of been in your office over an hour and it took an hour to walk home. It wan't no four hours I held back, it was over six hours at least. Come to think of it, that ain't all. That was a week ago that happened. Now I recollect I ain't had a bit of trouble all week – slept fine – no getting up. Funny how a man can get up in the morning, his mind all set on keeping an appointment to tell something, and forget a whole week has went by. Say, when I told you to psychiatrize and hypnotize me, you sure took it serious. I'm right grateful to you. How much do I owe you?"

Essentially, the case was completed and the remainder of the hour was spent in social small talk with a view of detecting any possible doubts or uncertainties in the patient. There were none, nor, in the months that have passed, have there occurred any.

The above case report allows the reader to understand in part how, during a technique of suggestions for trance induction and trance maintenance, hypnotherapeutic suggestions can be interspersed for a specific goal. In the author's experience, such an interspersing of therapeutic suggestions among the suggestions for trance maintenance may often render the therapeutic suggestions much more effective. The patient hears them, understands them, but before he can take issue with them or question them in any way, his attention is captured by the trance maintenance suggestions. And these in turn are but a continuance of the trance induction suggestions. Thus, there is given to the therapeutic suggestion an aura of significance and effectiveness deriving from the already effective induction and maintenance suggestions. Then again the same therapeutic suggestions can be repeated in this interspersed fashion, perhaps repeated many times, until the therapist feels confident that the patient has absorbed the therapeutic suggestions adequately. Then the therapist can progress to another aspect of therapy using the same interspersal technique.

The above report does not indicate the number of repetitions for each of the therapeutic suggestions for the reason that the number must vary with each set of ideas and understandings conveyed and with each patient and each therapeutic problem. Additionally such interspersal of suggestions for amnesia and posthypnotic suggestions among the suggestions for trance maintenance can be done most effectively. To illustrate from everyday life: A double task assignment is usually more effective than the separate assignment of the same two tasks. For example, a mother may say, "Johnny, as you put away your bicycle just step over and close the garage door." This has the sound of a single task, one aspect of which favors the execution of another aspect, and thus there is the effect of making the task seem easier. To ask that the bicycle be put away and then to ask that the garage door be closed has every sound of being two separate, not to be combined, tasks. To the separate tasks, a refusal can be given easily to one or the other task or to both. But a refusal when the tasks are combined into a single task means what? That he will not put away the bicycle? That he will not step over to the garage? That he will not close the garage door?

The very extent of the effort needed to identify what one is refusing in itself is a deterrent to refusal. Nor can a refusal of the "whole thing" be offered comfortably. Hence Johnny may perform the combined task unwillingly but may prefer to do so rather than to analyze the situation. To the single tasks he can easily say "later" to each. But to the combined task, he cannot say, "Later" since, if he puts away the bicycle "later", he must "immediately" step over to the garage and "immediately" close the door. This is specious reasoning, but it is the "emotional reasoning" that is common in daily life, and daily living is not an exercise in logic. As a common practice the author says to a patient, "As you sit down in the chair, just go into a trance." The patient is surely going to sit down in the chair. But going into a trance is made contingent upon sitting down, hence, a trance state develops from what the patient was most certainly going to do. By combining psychotherapeutic, amnestic and posthypnotic suggestions with those suggestions used first to induce a trance and then to maintain that trance constitutes an effective measure in securing desired results. Contingency values are decidedly effective. As a further illustration, more than once a patient who has developed a trance upon simply sitting down has said to the author, "I didn't intend to go into a trance today." In reply the author has stated, "Then perhaps you would like to awaken from the trance and hence, *as you understand that* you can go back into a trance when you need to, *you will awaken.* Thus the "awakening" is made contingent upon "understanding," thereby insuring further trances through association by contingency.

With this explanation of rationale, the problem of the second patient will be presented after a few preliminary statements. These are that the author was reared on a farm, enjoyed and still enjoys growing plants, and has read with interest about the processes of seed germination and plant growth. The first patient was a retired farmer. The second, who will be called "Joe" for convenience, was a florist. He began his career as a boy by peddling flowers, saving his pennies, buying more flowers to peddle, etc. Soon he was able to buy a small parcel of land on which to grow more flowers with loving care while he enjoyed their beauty which he wanted to share with others, and in turn, to get more land and to grow more flowers, etc. Eventually he became the leading florist in a large city. Joe literally loved every aspect of his business, was intensely devoted to it but he was also a good husband, a good father, a good friend and a highly respected and valued member of the community.

Then one fateful September a surgeon removed a growth from the side of Joe's face, being careful not to disfigure Joe's face too much. The pathologist reported the growth to be a malignancy. Radical therapy was then instituted but it was promptly recognized as "too late."

Joe was informed that he had about a month left to live. Joe's reaction was, to say the least, unhappy and distressed. In addition he was experiencing much pain, in fact, extremely severe pain.

At the end of the second week in October, a relative of Joe's urgently requested the author to employ hypnosis on Joe for pain relief since narcotics were proving of little value. In view of the prognosis that had been given for Joe, the author agreed reluctantly to see him, stipulating that all medication be discontinued at 4:00 a.m. of the day of the author's arrival. To this the physicians in charge of Joe at the hospital courteously agreed.

Shortly before the author was introduced to Joe, he was informed that Joe disliked even the mention of the word hypnosis. Also, one of Joe's children, a resident in psychiatry at a well-known clinic, did not believe in hypnosis and had apparently been confirmed in this disbelief by the psychiatric staff of the clinic, none of whom is known to have had any first hand knowledge of hypnosis. This resident would be present and the inference was that Joe knew of that disbelief.

The author was introduced to Joe who acknowledged the introduction in a most courteous and friendly fashion. It is doubtful if Joe really knew why the author was there. Upon inspecting Joe, it was noted that much of the side of his face and neck was missing because of surgery, ulceration, maceration and necrosis. A tracheotomy had been performed on Joe and he could not talk. He communicated by pencil and paper, many pads of which were ready at hand. The information was given that every 4 hours Joe had been receiving narcotics (1/4 grain of morphine or 100 milligrams of Demerol) and heavy sedation with barbiturates. He slept little. Special nurses were constantly at hand. Yet Joe was constantly hopping out of bed, writing innumerable notes, some pertaining to his business, some to his family, but many of them were expressive of complaints and demands for additional help. Severe pain distressed him continuously and he could not understand why the doctors could not handle their business as efficiently and as competently as he did his floral business. His situation enraged him because it constituted failure in his eyes. Success worked for and fully merited had always been a governing principle in his life. When things went wrong with his business, he made certain to correct them. Why did not the doctors do the same? The doctors had medicine for pain so why was he allowed to suffer such intolerable pain?

After the introduction, Joe wrote, "What you want?" This constituted an excellent opening and the author began his technique of trance induction and pain relief. This will not be given in its entirety since a large percentage of the statements made were repeated, not necessarily in succession but frequently by referring back to a previous remark and then repeating a paragraph or two. Another preliminary statement needed is that the author was most dubious about achieving any kind of success with Joe since, in addition to his physical condition, there were definite evidences of toxic reactions to excessive medication. Despite the author's unfavorable view of possibilities, there was one thing of which he could be confident. He could keep his doubts to himself and he could let Joe know by manner, tone of voice, by everything said that the author was genuinely interested in him, was genuinely desirous of helping him. If even that little could be communicated to Joe, it should be of some comfort, however small, to Joe and to the family members and to the nurses within listening distance in the side room.

The author began: "Joe, I would like to talk to you. I know you are a florist, that you grow flowers, and I grew up on a farm in Wisconsin and I liked growing flowers. I still do. So I would like to have you take a seat in that easy chair as I talk to you. I'm going to say a lot of things to you but it won't be about flowers because you know more than I do about flowers. *That isn't what you want.* (The reader will note that italics will be used to denote interspersed hypnotic suggestions which may be syllables, words, phrases or sentences uttered with a slightly different intonation.) Now as I talk and I can do so *comfortably,* I wish that you will *listen to me comfortably* as I talk about a tomato plant. That is an odd thing to talk about. It makes one *curious. Why talk about a tomato plant?* One puts a tomato seed in the ground. One can *feel hope* that it will grow into a tomato plant that *will bring satisfaction* by the fruit it has. The seed soaks up water, *not very much difficulty* in doing that because of the rains that *bring peace and comfort* and the joy of growing to flowers and tomatoes. That little seed, Joe, slowly swells, sends out a little rootlet with cilia on it. Now you may not know what cilia are, but cilia are *things that work* to help the tomato seed grow, to push up above the ground as a sprouting plant, and *you can listen to me Joe* so I will keep on talking and *you can keep on listening, wondering, just wondering what you can really learn,* and here is your pencil and your pad but speaking of the tomato plant, it grows so slowly. *You cannot see* it grow, *you cannot hear* it grow, but grow it does—the first little leaflike things on the stalk, the fine little hairs on the stem, those hairs are on the leaves too like the cilia on the roots, they must make the tomato plant *feel very good, very comfortable* if you can think of a plant as feeling and then, *you can't see* it growing, *you can't feel* it growing but another leaf appears on that little tomato stalk and then another. Maybe, and this is talking like a child, maybe the tomato plant does *feel comfortable and peaceful* as it grows. Each day it grows and grows and grows, *it's so comfortable Joe* to watch a plant grow and *not see* its growth *not feel* it but just know that *all is getting better* for that little tomato plant that is adding yet another leaf and still another and a branch and it is *growing comfortably* in all directions. (Much of the above by this time had been repeated many times, sometimes just phrases, sometime sentences. Care was taken to vary the wording and also to repeat the hypnotic suggestions. Quite some time after the author had begun, Joe's wife came tiptoeing into the room carrying a sheet of paper on which was written the question, "When are you going to start the hypnosis?" The author failed to cooperate with her by looking at the paper and it was necessary for her to thrust the sheet of paper in front of the author and therefore in front of Joe. The author was continuing his description of the tomato plant uninterruptedly and Joe's wife, as she looked at Joe, saw that he was not seeing her, did not know that she was there, that he was in a somnambulistic trance. She withdrew at once.) And soon the tomato plant will have a bud form somewhere, on one branch or another, but it makes no difference because all the branches, the whole tomato plant will soon have those nice little buds – I wonder if the tomato plant can, *Joe, feel really feel a kind of comfort.* You know, Joe, a plant is a wonderful thing, and *it is so nice, so pleasing* just to be able to think about a plant as if it were a man. Would such a plant *have nice feelings, a sense of comfort* as the tiny little tomatoes begin to form, so tiny, yet so *full of promise to give you the desire to eat* a luscious tomato, sun-ripened, it's so *nice to have food in one's stomach,* that wonderful feeling a child, a thirsty child, has and can *want a drink, Joe* is that the way the tomato plant feels when the rain falls and washes everything so that *all feels well* (pause). *You know, Joe,* a tomato plant just flourishes each day *just a day at a time.* I like to think the tomato plant can *know the fullness of comfort each day. You know, Joe, just one day at a time* for the tomato plant. That's the way for all tomato plants. (Joe suddenly came out of the trance, appeared disoriented, hopped upon the bed, waved his arms and his behavior was highly suggestive of the sudden surges of toxicity one sees in patients who have reacted unfavorably to barbiturates. Joe did not seem to hear or see the author until he hopped off the bed and had walked toward the author. A firm grip was taken on Joe's arm and then immediately loosened. The nurse was summoned. She mopped perspiration from his forehead, changed his surgical dressings, and gave him, by tube, some ice water. Joe then let the author lead him back to his chair. After a pretense by the author of being curious about Joe's forearm, Joe seized his pencil and paper and wrote, "Talk, talk.") "Oh yes, Joe, I grew up on a farm, I think a tomato seed is a wonderful thing, *think, Joe, think* in that little seed there does *sleep so restfully, so comfortably* a beautiful plant yet to be grown that will bear such interesting leaves and branches. The leaves, the branches look so beautiful, that beautiful rich color, *you can really feel happy* looking at a tomato seed, thinking about the wonderful plant it contains *asleep, resting, comfortable, Joe.* I'm soon going to leave for lunch and I'll be back and I will talk some more."

The above is a summary to indicate the ease with which hypnotherapeutic suggestions can be included in the trance induction and trance maintenance suggestions which are important additionally as a vehicle for the transmission of therapy. Of particular significance is Joe's own request that the author "talk." Despite his toxic state, spasmodically evident, Joe was definitely accessible. Moreover he learned rapidly despite the absurdly amateurish rhapsody the author offered about a tomato seed and plant. Joe had no real interest in pointless endless remarks about a tomato plant. Joe wanted freedom from pain, he wanted comfort, rest, sleep. This was what was uppermost in Joe's mind, foremost in his emotional desires, and he would have a compelling need to try to find something of value to him in the author's babbling. That desired value was there, so spoken that Joe could literally receive it without realizing it. Joe's arousal from the trance was only some minutes after the author had said so seemingly innocuously, "want a drink, Joe." Nor was the re-induction of the trance difficult, achieved by two brief phrases, "think Joe think" and "sleep so restfully, so comfortably" imbedded in a rather meaningless sequence of ideas. But what Joe wanted and needed was in that otherwise meaningless narration, and he promptly accepted it.

During the lunch time, Joe was first restful and then slowly became restless, another toxic episode occurred, as reported by the nurse. By the time the author returned Joe was waiting impatiently for him. Joe wanted to communicate by writing notes. Some were illegible because of his extreme impatience in writing. He would irritatedly rewrite them. A relative helped the author to read these notes. They concerned things about Joe, his past history, his business, his family and "last week terrible," "yesterday was terrible." There were no complaints, no demands, but there were some requests for information about the author.

After a fashion a satisfying conversation was had with him as was judged by an increasing loss of his restlessness. When it was suggested that he cease walking around and sit in the chair used earlier, he did so readily and looked expectantly at the author.

"You know, Joe, I could talk to you some more about the tomato plant and if I did you would probably go to sleep, in fact, *a good sound sleep."* (This opening statement has every earmark of being no more than a casual commonplace utterance. If the patient responds hypnotically, as Joe promptly did, all is well. If the patient does not respond, all you have said was just a commonplace remark, not at all noteworthy. Had Joe not gone into a trance immediately, there could have been a variation such as: "But instead, let's talk about the tomato flower. You have seen movies of flowers *slowly, slowly* opening, giving one *a sense of peace, a sense of comfort* as you watch the unfolding. So beautiful, *so restful* to watch. One can *feel such infinite comfort* watching such a movie.")

It does not seem to the author that more needs to be said about the technique of trance induction and maintenance and the interspersal of therapeutic suggestions. Another illustration will be given later in this paper.

Joe's response that afternoon was excellent despite several intervening episodes of toxic behavior and several periods where the author deliberately interrupted his work to judge more adequately the degree and amount of Joe's learning.

Upon departure that evening, the author was cordially shaken by hand by Joe, whose toxic state was much lessened. Joe had no complaints, he did not seem to have distressing pain, and he seemed to be pleased and happy.

Relatives were concerned about posthypnotic suggestions but they were reassured that such had been given. This had been done most gently in describing so much in detail and repetition the growth of the tomato plant and then, with careful emphasis, *"You know Joe," "Know the fullness of comfort each day,"* and *"You know, Joe, just one day at a time."*

About a month later around the middle of November, the author was requested to see Joe again. Upon arriving at Joe's home, he was told a rather regrettable but not actually unhappy story. Joe had continued his excellent response after the author's departure on that first occasion, but hospital gossip had spread the story of Joe's hypnosis and interns, residents, and staff men came in to take advantage of Joe's capacity to be a good subject. They made all the errors possible for uninformed amateurs with superstitious misconceptions of hypnosis. Their behavior infuriated Joe who knew that the author had done none of the offensive things they were doing. This was a fortunate realization since it permitted Joe to keep all the benefits acquired from the author without letting his hostilities toward hypnosis interfere. After several days of annoyance, Joe left the hospital and went home, keeping one nurse in constant attendance, but her duties were relatively few.

During that month at home he had actually gained weight and strength. Rarely did a surge of pain occur and when it did it could be controlled either with aspirin or with 25 milligrams of Demerol. Joe was very happy to be with his family and there was considerable fruitful activity about which the author is not fully informed.

Joe's greeting to the author on the second visit was one of obvious pleasure. However, the author noted that Joe was keeping a wary eye on him, hence, great care was taken to be completely casual and to avoid any hand movement that could be remotely misconstrued as an "hypnotic pass" such as the hospital staff had employed.

Framed pictures painted by a highly talented member of his family were proudly displayed. There was much casual conversation about Joe's improvement and his weight gain and the author was repeatedly hard pushed to find simple replies to conceal pertinent suggestions. Joe did volunteer to sit down and let the author talk to him. Although the author was wholly casual in manner, the situation was thought to be most difficult to handle without arousing Joe's suspicions. Perhaps this was an unfounded concern but the author wished to be most careful. Finally the measure was employed of reminiscing about "our visit last October." Joe did not realize how easily this visit could be pleasantly vivified for him by such a simple statement as, "I talked about a tomato plant then and it almost seems as if I could be *talking about a tomato plant right now. It is so enjoyable to talk about a seed, a plant.*" Thus there was, clinically speaking, a re-creation of all of the favorable aspects of that original interview.

Joe was most insistent on supervising the author's luncheon that day, which was a steak barbecued under Joe's watchful eye in the back yard beside the swimming pool. It was a happy gathering of four people thoroughly enjoying being together, Joe being obviously most happy.

After luncheon, Joe proudly displayed the innumerable plants, many of them rare that he had personally planted in the large back yard. Joe's wife furnished the Latin and common names for the plants and Joe was particularly pleased when the author recognized and commented on some rare plant. Nor was this a pretense of interest, since the author is still interested in growing plants. Joe regarded this interest in common to be a bond of friendship.

During the afternoon, Joe sat down voluntarily, his very manner making evident that the author was free to do whatever he wished. A long monologue by the author ensued in which were included psychotherapeutic suggestions of continued ease, comfort, freedom from pain, enjoyment of family, good appetite, and a continuing pleased interest in all surroundings. All of these and other similar suggestions were interspersed unnoticeably among the author's many remarks. These covered a multitude of topics to preclude Joe from analyzing or recognizing the interspersing of suggestions. Also, for adequate disguise, the author needed a variety of topics. Whether or not such care was needed in view of the good rapport is a debatable question, but the author preferred to take no risks.

Medically, the malignancy was continuing to progress, but despite this fact, Joe was in much much better physical condition than he had been a month previously. When the author took his departure, Joe invited him to return again.

Joe knew that the author was going on a lecture trip in late November and early December. Quite unexpected by the author, a long distance telephone call was received just before the author's departure on this trip. The call was from Joe's wife who stated, "Joe is on the extension line and wants to say 'hello' to you, so listen." Two brief puffs of air were heard. Joe had held the telephone mouthpiece over his tracheotomy tube and had exhaled forcibly twice to simulate "hello." His wife stated that both she and Joe extended their best wishes for the trip and a casual conversation of friends ensued with Joe's wife reading Joe's written notes.

A Christmas greeting card was received from Joe and his family. In a separate letter Joe's wife said that "the hypnosis is doing well, but Joe's condition is failing." Early in January Joe was weak but comfortable. Finally, in his wife's words, "Joe died quietly January 21."

The author is well aware that the prediction of the duration of life for any patient suffering from a fatal illness is most questionable. Joe's physical condition in October did not promise very much. The symptom amelioration, abatement and actual abolishment effected by hypnosis, and the freedom of Joe's body from potent medications, conducive only of unawareness, unquestionably increased his span of life while at the same time permitting an actual brief physical betterment in general. This was attested clearly by his improved condition at home and his gain in weight. That Joe lived until the latter part of January despite the extensiveness of his malignant disease undoubtedly attests to the vigor with which Joe undertook to live the remainder of his life as enjoyably as possible, a vigor expressive of the manner in which he had lived his life and built his business.

To clarify still further this matter of the technique of the interspersal of therapeutic suggestions among trance induction and trance maintenance suggestions, it might be well to report the author's original experimental work done while he was on the Research Service of the Worcester State Hospital in Worcester, Massachusetts in the early 1930's.

The Research Service was concerned with the study of the numerous problems of schizophrenia and the possibilities of solving some of them. To the author, the psychological manifestations were of paramount interest. For example, just what did a stream of disconnected rapidly uttered incoherencies mean? Certainly, in some manner, such a stream of utterances must be most meaningful to the patient in some way. Competent secretaries from time to time had recorded verbatim various examples of such disturbed utterances for the author's perusal and study. The author himself managed to record adequately similar such productions by patients who spoke slowly. Careful study of these verbal productions, it was thought, might lead to various speculative ideas that, in turn, might prove of value in understanding something about schizophrenia.

The question arose of whether or not much of the verbigeration might be a disguise for concealed meanings, fragmented and dispersed among the total utterances. This led to the question of how could the author himself produce a series of incoherencies in which he could conceal in a fragmented form a meaningful message. Or could he use the incoherencies of a patient and intersperse among them in a somewhat orderly fashion a fragmented meaningful communication that would be difficult to recognize? This speculation gave rise to many hours of intense labor spent fitting into a patient's verbatim, apparently meaningless, utterances a meaningful message that could not be detected by the author's colleagues when no clue of any sort was given to them. Previous efforts at producing original incoherencies by the author disclosed a definite and recognizable personal pattern indicating that the author was not sufficiently disturbed mentally to produce a bonafide stream of incoherent verbigerations.

When a meaning was interspersed in a patient's productions successfully, the author discovered that his past hypnotic experimentation with hypnotic techniques greatly influenced the kind of a message which he was likely to intersperse in a patient's verbigerations. Out of this labor came the following experimental and therapeutic work.

One of the more recently hired secretaries objected strongly to being hypnotized. She suffered regularly upon the onset of menstruation from severe migrainous headaches lasting 3 to 4 or even more hours. She had been examined repeatedly by the medical service with no helpful findings. She usually retired to the lounge and "slept off the headache," a process usually taking 3 or more hours. On one such occasion, she had been purposely rather insistently forced to take dictation by the author instead of being allowed to retire to the lounge. Rather resentfully she began her task but within 15 minutes she interrupted the author to explain that her headache was gone. She attributed this to her anger at being forced to take dictation. Later, on another such occasion, she volunteered to take certain dictation which all of the secretaries tried to avoid because of the difficulties it presented. Her headache grew worse and she decided that the happy instance with the author was merely a fortuitous happenstance. Subsequently she had another severe headache. She was again insistently requested by the author to take some dictation. The previous happy result occurred within ten minutes. Upon the occurrence of another headache, she volunteered to take dictation from the author. Again it served to relieve her headache. She then experimentally tested the benefits of dictation from other physicians. For some unknown reason, her headaches only worsened. She returned from one of these useless attempts to the author and asked him to dictate. She was told he had nothing on hand to dictate but that he could redictate previously dictated material. Her headache was relieved within 8 minutes. Later her request for dictation for headache relief was met by some routine dictation. It failed to have any effect.

She came again, not too hopefully since she thought she had "worn-out the dictation remedy." Again she was given dictation with a relief of her distress in about 9 minutes. She was so elated that she kept a copy of the transcript so that she could ask others to dictate "that successful dictation" to relieve her headaches. Unfortunately, nobody seemed to have the "right voice" as did the author. Always, a posthypnotic suggestion was casually given that there would be no falling asleep while transcribing.

She did not suspect, nor did anybody else, what had really been done. The author had made comprehensive notes of the incoherent verbigeration of a psychotic patient. He had also had various secretaries make verbatim records of patient's incoherent utterances. He had then systematically interspersed therapeutic suggestions among the incoherencies with that secretary in mind. When this was found to be successful, the incoherent utterances of another patient were utilized in a similar fashion. This was also a successful effort. As a control measure, routine dictation and the dictation of "undoctored incoherencies" were tried. These had no effect upon her headaches. Nor did the use by others of "doctored" material have an effect since it had to be read aloud with some degree of expressive awareness to be effective.

The question now arises, why did these two patients and those patients used experimentally respond therapeutically? This answer can be given simply as follows: They knew very well why they were seeking therapy; they were desirous of benefitting; they came in a receptive state ready to respond at the first opportunity, except for the first experimental patient. But she was eager to be freed from her headache, and wished the time being spent taking dictation could be time spent getting over her headache. Essentially, then, all of the patients were in a frame of mind to receive therapy. How many times does a patient need to state his complaint? Only that number of times requisite for the therapist to understand. For all of these patients, only one statement of the complaint was necessary and they then knew that the therapist understood. Their intense desire for therapy was not only a conscious but an unconscious desire also, as judged clinically, but more importantly, as evidenced by the results obtained.

One should also give recognition to the readiness with which one's unconscious mind picks up clues and information. For example, one may dislike someone at first sight and not become consciously aware of the obvious and apparent reasons for such dislike for weeks, months, even a year or more. Yet finally the reasons for the dislike become apparent to the conscious mind. A common example is the ready hostility frequently shown by a normal heterosexual person toward a homosexual person without any conscious realization of why.

Respectful awareness of the capacity of the patient's unconscious mind to perceive meaningfulness of the therapist's own unconscious behavior is a governing principle in psychotherapy. There should also be a ready and full respect for the patient's unconscious mind to perceive fully the intentionally obscured meaningful therapeutic instructions offered them. The clinical and experimental material cited above is based upon the author's awareness that the patient's unconscious mind is listening and understanding much better than is possible for his conscious mind.

It was intended to publish this experimental work, of which only the author was aware. But sober thought and awareness of the insecure status of hypnosis in general, coupled with that secretary's strong objection to being hypnotized – she did not mind losing her headaches by "taking dictation" from the author – all suggested the inadvisability of publication.

A second secretary, employed by the hospital when this experimental work was nearing completion, always suffered from disabling dysmenorrhea. The "headache secretary" suggested to this girl that she take dictation from the author as a possible relief measure. Most willingly the author obliged, using "doctored" patient verbigeration. It was effective.

Concerned about what might happen to hypnotic research if his superiors were to learn of what was taking place, the author carefully failed with this second secretary and then again succeeded. She volunteered to be an hypnotic subject and hypnosis, not "dictation" was then used to meet her personal needs. She also served repeatedly as a subject for various frankly acknowledged and "approved" hypnotic experiments and the author kept his counsel in certain other experimental studies.

Now that hypnosis has come to be an acceptable scientific modality of investigative and therapeutic endeavor and there has developed a much greater awareness of semantics, this material, so long relegated to the shelf of unpublished work, can safely be published.

29

How acupuncture can block pain

Ronald Melzack

The practice of acupuncture provides a unique and remarkable approach to the control of pain. During the past decade, acupuncture has been used increasingly in China to induce a profound analgesia (insensitivity to pain) in particular parts of the body so that major surgical interventions can be performed on the totally awake patient. Reports of these operations and of successful similar operations carried out elsewhere have captured the imagination of scientist and layman alike. Acupuncture may represent, also, a way to control a variety of terrible pain syndromes, such as the neuralgias and 'phantom limb' pain.

One of the most fascinating aspects of acupuncture analgesia is the distribution of acupuncture sites for insertion of needles for different operations. For a thyroid operation done in one hospital, for example, one of the special needles was inserted in each forearm at a point about 20 cm above the wrist and at a depth of a little more than 2 cm. A similar operation was carried out in another hospital with acupuncture needles in the neck and the backs of the wrists. An operation for the removal of the stomach, which was observed in Canton by the American physician E. G. Dimond, was carried out with four acupuncture needles inserted into the pinna of each ear. Dr Dimond reported:

'The patient was a slender 50-year-old man with a non-healing ulcer of the lesser curvature of the stomach. The procedure was to be a gastrectomy (removal of the stomach). This patient had not had medication at bedtime the previous night. He was given meperidine hydrochloride (an analgesic drug). Acupuncture anaesthesia was introduced by placing four stainless-steel needles in the pinna of each ear at carefully identified points. . . . The needles were connected to a phasic direct current battery source, delivering 6 volts at 150 cycles per minute. The patient remained awake, alert, and chatted throughout the procedure. A subtotal gastric resection was done by skilful surgeons, scrubbed, gowned, and disciplined thoroughly in modern or Western surgical practice. This patient required no additional anaesthesia but did note some sensation associated with visceral traction.'

It is clear that acupuncture analgesia involves fairly intense, continuous stimulation of tissues by the acupuncture needles. Sometimes electrical current is passed between two needles. At other times, the needles are continually twirled by hand, which would stimulate the tissues in which they are embedded. If the desired result is not produced, herbs may be placed on the acupuncture sites and burned. This would, of course, stimulate the tissues still more. The input produced by stimulation appears to be a critical factor. The injection of novocaine (a local anaesthetic) into the acupuncture points, which prevents them from projecting information to the nervous system, also blocks their ability to induce acupuncture analgesia at a distant site. The onset of analgesia, moreover, may not be instantaneous but sometimes develops slowly. Twenty minutes' stimulation was necessary to produce analgesia in one case. Furthermore, analgesia may outlast

Reprinted from Impact of Science on Society **23**:1, 1973, by permission of Unesco. From the Department of Psychology, McGill University, Box 6070, Montreal 101, Quebec (Canada).

A report on acupuncture in major surgery

A major operation, described by the British physician P. E. Brown, was carried out with a single acupuncture needle:

'My first introduction to this method of anaesthesia was during a visit to the Cheng Hwa Hospital in Shanghai. I was taken into the theatre to see a man in his mid-thirties, who was undergoing a right upper lobectomy (partial lung removal). . . . He was fully conscious and able to speak to me. There was only one acupuncture point, situated over the right biceps muscle. A needle, 5 cm long, was inserted and manually rotated by the anaesthetist. She was rapidly rotating the needle for ten to fifteen seconds, at intervals of half a minute. Every five minutes she checked the pulse rate and blood pressure, and her chart revealed a steady regular pulse of 80 per minute, and blood pressure varying from 150 to 130 mm Hg systolic and from 85 to 80 diastolic. . . . The patient remained extraordinarily calm. The anaesthetist occasionally spoke to him in a quiet voice, and he responded immediately. I was allowed to sit with him, and ask him questions about the amount of pain or discomfort he might be feeling, but he insisted there was no pain; in fact he seemed to enjoy the segments of orange with which I fed him. He was able to chew and swallow with no difficulty. His colour was good throughout, and he seldom showed any evidence of stress except when there was any traction on the trachea.

'From the surgical point of view, I noticed the extreme care taken by the surgeon and the very slow speed at which he operated. A further interesting feature was the very slight blood loss, which, I was told later by the surgeon, is a major advantage of acupuncture anaesthesia.

'The patient had been active during the week before the operation, and the only preoperative drug was . . . pethidine hydrochloride (an analgesic drug), intramuscularly. I examined him twelve hours after the operation, and he was sitting up in bed. He seemed quite comfortable, and the blood pressure and pulse were normal. I was told that the analgesic effect of acupuncture lasted for several hours after operation, and that postoperative sedation was seldom needed. The manual stimulation of the needle was given up when the wound was being sutured.'

the duration of stimulation by several hours.

ACUPUNCTURE ANALGESIA: MAJOR CHARACTERISTICS

We still have only fragmentary information about acupuncture analgesia. There are many unanswered questions. We do not know, for example, what percentage of patients report effective analgesia. The technique is not used routinely for all patients. Which patients are selected, and why are the others rejected? There is also evidence that the patients who choose acupuncture analgesia have complete faith in the effectiveness of the technique. It is important to know, then, whether this confidence in the method is necessary for effective analgesia to occur. Many of the patients who undergo acupuncture analgesia also get small doses of conventional analgesic drugs, which may have tranquillizing or euphoric effects. These, too, may interact with the effects produced by the acupuncture needles, but their role has yet to be determined.

Three major features of acupuncture analgesia appear to be so unusual that they immediately evoke scepticism in the physician who has been trained in Western medical practice and has learned a particular theory of pain. The traditional pain theory taught in medical schools, which is known as specificity theory, states that specific pain receptors in the body tissues project pain signals directly through a pain-transmission system to a pain centre in the brain. This concept of a direct transmission line resembles a simple telephone switchboard: a signal is dialled at one end and a bell rings at the other. The theory assumes that the amount of pain which is felt is proportional to the intensity of stimulation, and that the location of the pain is determined precisely by the location of the damaging stimulus.

Acupuncture analgesia, considered in the framework of specificity theory, is totally incomprehensible for three reasons: (a) a moderately intense stimulus, which cannot possibly block nerve impulses by any known pharmacological mechanism, nevertheless produces analgesia; (b) insertion of acupuncture needles at a given site produces an effect at a distant part of the body which has no known direct anatomical relationship; and (c) pain is relieved for hours after stimulation has stopped. At first glance, these three properties seem to defy all current knowledge. But, in fact, this turns out not to be the case. Each property is amply recorded in the medical literature.

Control of pain by intense stimulation of the body

It is well known that intense stimulation at the surface of the body sometimes produces relief of pain for variable periods of time. This type of pain relief, generally labelled as 'counter-irritation', is one of the oldest methods used for the control of pain. It includes such methods of folk medicine as application of mustard plasters, ice packs, or hot-water bottles to parts of the body.

Some of these methods are still frequently used, although there has not been until recently any theoretical or physiological explanation for their effectiveness. Suggestion and distraction of attention are the usual mechanisms invoked, but neither seems capable of explaining the power of the methods or the long duration of the relief they can afford.

There is, in fact, considerable evidence to show that brief, mildly painful stimulation is capable of bringing about substantial relief of more severe pathological pain for durations that long outlast the period of stimulation. Vigorous massage of the sensory nerve which innervates the lower head and jaw may permanently abolish the pain of *tic douloureux,* which is characterized by painful, convulsive spasms of the face and mouth. Similarly, injection of hypertonic saline (a strong solution of salt and water) into the tissues of the back may produce a sharp brief pain followed by prolonged relief of phantom limb pain. Saline injections into the stump may have the same effect.

There is also experimental evidence that one pain may produce a marked rise in threshold (the lowest stimulus level at which pain is reported) to other types of pain. Application of painful cold to the shin of either leg brings about a 30 per cent rise in threshold to pain produced by electrical stimulation of the teeth. The raised threshold may persist for two hours or more. Similarly, paraplegics who suffer pain have a higher threshold to experimentally evoked pain than paraplegics who are pain-free.

Interactions between distant body sites

It has long been known that patients with cardiac disease frequently develop pain – which is commonly called referred pain – in the shoulder and chest. Pressure on the trigger areas often produces intense pain that may last for hours. Surprisingly, similar examination of a group of subjects who do not have heart disease reveals an almost identical distribution of trigger areas. The application of pressure produces marked discomfort, which sometimes lasts for several minutes, and even increases in intensity for a few seconds after removal of the stimulus. There are many similar patterns of referred pain that relate other structures of the body.

The patterns of referred pain are so consistent from person to person that physicians often diagnose the diseased structure on the basis of the pain pattern. It is not surprising therefore that, within each area of referred pain, there are often one or more small trigger zones that are situated in more or less the same place in most people. Pressure on these trigger zones evokes pain in the referred area and, usually, pain in the related diseased visceral structure. Even more remarkable is the fact that injection of anaesthetic drugs like novocaine in the trigger zones removes the referred pain, and, very often, the pain of the diseased viscera. The frequency of painful attacks may decrease significantly after a single such injection. Sometimes the pain may disappear permanently.

Referred pain may also be relieved, astonishingly, by intense stimulation applied to trigger areas. Some physicians use intense stimulation to abolish referred pain in particular muscle groups. Dry needling of the trigger area – simply moving a needle in and out of the area without injecting any substance – is sometimes effective. Intense cold applied to the area may also be effective. This effect was presumed at first to be because of local analgesia produced by the cold, but it is more likely that it is the intense input itself that relieves the pain.

Interaction between distant body sites is sometimes also revealed by lesions of the central nervous system. Patients who have undergone operations on the spinal cord, mostly for the relief of cancer pain, report that pin pricks applied to analgesic parts of the body (such as the leg) evoke pain at some distant site (such as the chest or back) on the same or opposite side of the body. In some patients, the pain is referred to the site of an earlier injury.

Prolonged time-courses of pain phenomena

Many pain phenomena are characterized by unusual temporal properties. A brief intense stimulus may produce prolonged pain. In contrast, pains that have persisted for months or years may be abolished by temporary anaesthetic block of the input or even a brief stimulation to increase input. There are many such examples.

Teeth that have been drilled and filled without local anesthetic may be the site of referred pain when the nasal sinuses are stimulated as long as seventy days later. A single anaesthetic block of the appropriate nerve from the jaw abolishes the phenomenon. This effect cannot be attributed to a chronic local irritation after the dental manipulation: the anaesthetic block could not have affected the teeth themselves. The effect points, instead, to prolonged changes in central neural activity which may be initiated by a brief, painful input and stopped permanently by a single anaesthetic block.

There are many clinical observations which lead to the same conclusion. Momentary pressure on trigger areas in cardiac patients produces severe pain for several hours, and a single anaesthetic block of the areas may abolish recurrent cardiac pain for days, weeks, or longer.

How can a single, brief input produce such long effects, and how can a temporary block of input stop it? There is still no satisfactory explanation of these prolonged effects, which are among the most puzzling features of pain. It is clear, however, that the time-courses of events in the central nervous system do not always bear a simple one-to-one relationship to the duration of stimulation. Pain may long outlast the period of stimulation. Similarly, pain relief may long outlast the duration of an ameliorative procedure.

THREE THEORIES TO EXPLAIN THE ACUPUNCTURE ANALGESIA

The fact that the three major properties of acupuncture analgesia, taken individually, fit into an established body of medical observations does not explain how analgesia is brought about. It is still necessary to provide a theoretical framework to account for all the phenomena.

There are currently three theories to explain acupuncture analgesia: (a) the traditional Chinese explanation that acupuncture brings about harmony between the opposing forces of Yin and Yang; (b) the psychological explanation that the effects are due to hypnosis; and (c) a neural explanation in terms of the known functions of the central nervous system. Each theory will now be examined for its adequacy.

The traditional Chinese explanation

This explanation is that the two major universal forces are represented biological-

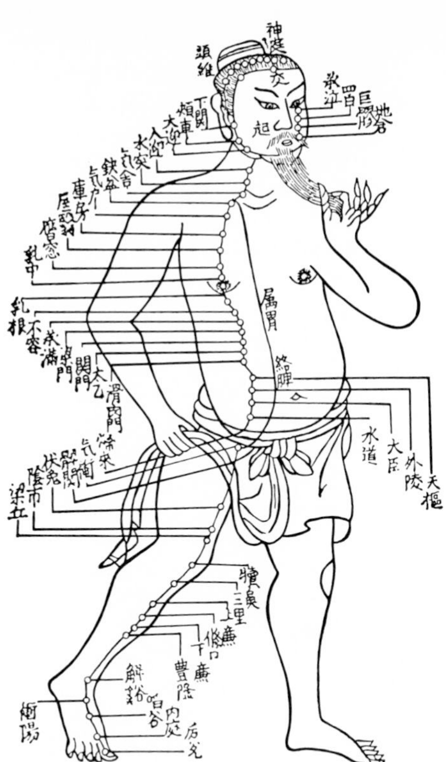

Fig. 1. A typical acupuncture chart, showing the sites for insertion of needles along several body meridians. After two or more needles are inserted, electrical current is usually passed through the needles for about twenty minutes. The resulting analgesia can permit major surgery. (Courtesy of *Abbottempo*, Vol. X, No. 1.)

ly in the body in the form of the spirit (Yin) and the blood (Yang). Each is carried along a series of separate channels called meridians. Acupuncture points lie on the meridians or at their intersections. Traditionally, there were 365 acupuncture sites along 12 meridians, but these numbers have changed in recent years. The theory maintains that when Yin and Yang fall into disharmony, disease and pain occur. The insertion of acupuncture needles at specific sites is assumed to permit them somehow to come into harmony again (see Fig. 1).

The choice of acupuncture sites is determined by the meridians, each of which controls specific internal or external body structures. Although the history of the evolution of these ideas is uncertain, it is clear that the acupuncture sites have been determined, to some extent at least, on the basis of empirical observation. That is, acupuncture needles inserted at particular points have presumably produced certain desired results.

The Yin-Yang theory is apparently still popular among the 'barefoot doctors' who practice folk medicine in the rural areas of China, although there is no evidence whatever for the tubules said to underlie the meridians. Physicians in large city hospitals in China, however, are currently searching for neurological explanations of acupuncture analgesia.

Interestingly, it has been claimed that the resistance to electrical current flow is different at acupuncture sites than at other skin areas. The evidence so far is scanty and merely suggestive. If this claim can be established as fact, however, it may be related to the two sets of observations. First, the acupuncture points may show some correspondence to the sites at which peripheral sensory and motor nerves emerge from muscles and other deep tissues and come to lie just below the surface of the skin. Second, some of these sites may, in turn, be related to the distribution of 'motor' points at the body surface which produce localized muscular contractions when they are electrically stimulated. Both of these possible correlations would certainly ensure maximal input to the central nervous system when needles are inserted under the skin and electrically stimulated, twirled, or heated by 'moxibustion' of herbs.

The explanation in terms of hypnosis

This is unsatisfactory for several reasons. First, hypnosis in the conventional sense involves prolonged training on the part of the patient. Professional medical hypnotists report that induction of a trance state sufficiently deep for surgical procedures usually requires from four to eight hours of initial training, with additional training for utilization of the trance in specific situations. This training is normally carried out over periods of days or weeks. This is in marked contrast to acupuncture analgesia, in which prior acquaintance with the procedure appears not to be essential. Furthermore, the induction of the trance state usually involves a set of specific procedures, but there is no evidence that these are employed in acupuncture analgesia.

Second, sufficient anaesthesia for major surgery can be achieved by highly competent, professional hypnotists in only about 20 per cent of people. Yet the available evidence suggests that a much higher proportion of patients in China (reported to be as high as 90 per cent) undergo surgery with the acupuncture procedure.

Third, subjects who achieve a deep hypnotic state rarely speak spontaneously or carry out normal movements unless they have received prolonged additional training. But patients who undergo acupuncture analgesia, without any apparent training, talk spontaneously, show interest in the operation (and sometimes examine the excised organ or tissue), eat oranges, and may even look after a baby just delivered by Caesarean surgery—and while suturing is still taking place.

Fourth, acupuncture analgesia is reported to be possible in animals, which cannot be hypnotized in the usual sense. Sudden immobilization of an animal in unfamiliar surroundings may sometimes greatly diminish the response to noxious stimulation. The effect varies from one animal species to another. It is less common in higher mammals than in birds or insects. Reports of surgery with acupuncture analgesia in the cat, dog, or horse suggest some mechanism other than 'animal hypnotism'.

These arguments against hypnosis as an explanation do not deny, of course, that psychological factors may play an important role in acupuncture analgesia. Their mechanism of action, however, is far more subtle than that implied by the concept of hypnosis.

The neural explanation

This is based on knowledge of the functions of the central nervous system. The 'gate control' theory of pain, now increasingly accepted by physicians, suggests that the transmission of pain signals from the body to the spinal cord and brain is not a fixed, immutable process but a dynamic one capable of modulation and plasticity. The theory holds that a gate-like mechanism exists in the pain signalling system. The gate may be opened or closed by variable amounts so that, in certain conditions, signals from injured tissues may be

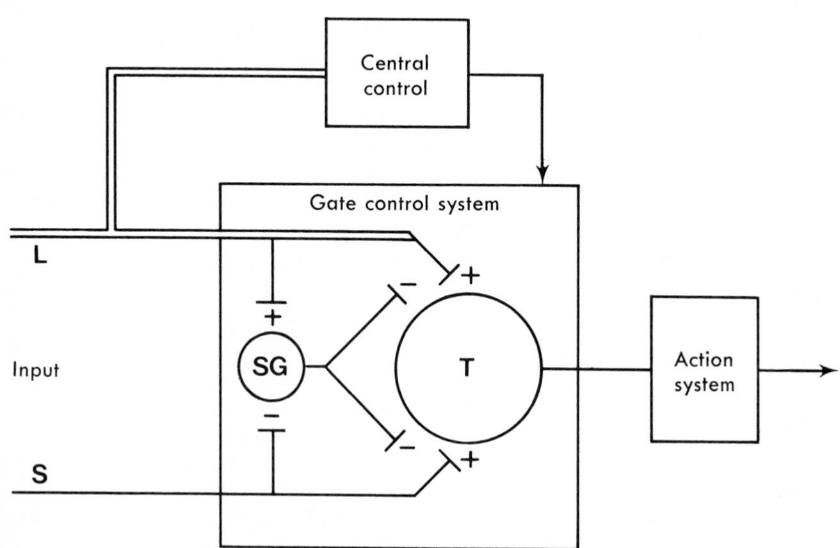

Fig. 2. Schematic diagram of the gate control theory of pain mechanisms. L, the large diameter fibres; S, the small diameter fibres. The fibres project to SG, the substantia gelatinosa, and T, the first central transmission cells. The inhibitory effect exerted by SG on the afferent fibre terminals is increased by activity in L fibres and decreased by activity in S fibres. Central control processes project to the gate control system. They include fibres from the brainstem which have a predominantly inhibitory effect, as well as fibres from the cortex. The T cells project to the entry cells of the action system. + stands for excitation; − for inhibition. (After Melzack and Wall.)

blocked and therefore fail to arrive at the brain. The gate control theory, which Professor Wall and I proposed in 1965 as a general theory of pain, suggests that the modulation of pain signals can occur in three ways (see Fig. 2).

THE MODULATIONS OF PAIN SIGNALS

First, there is evidence that the large fibres in sensory nerves that project from the body to the central nervous system tend to 'close the gate' and thereby diminish the level of perceived pain. Gentle electrical stimulation of the skin and underlying tissues would usually activate more large fibres than small fibres, tending to close the gate and block the pain signals that result from surgical trauma. This mechanism is plausible when the acupuncture needles are near the site of surgery. Indeed, in some cases of Caesarean surgery, the needles are inserted on each side of the line of incision. It seems less likely, however, when the needles are at distant sites, which is usually the case.

Second, it is known that portions of the brainstem (the lower part of the brain) exert a powerful inhibitory influence on transmission through the pain signalling system. This may be carried out by descending fibres that act on the gate control system in the spinal cord or by fibres that project to other transmission areas in the brain. This modulating system in the brainstem provides an explanation for the observations that analgesia of a body area may be produced by stimulation of distant sites. Certain brainstem areas are known to receive inputs from widespread regions of the body. When these areas are electrically stimulated, moreover, a profound analgesia is produced in a large part of the body.

Studies on the rat indicate that stimulation of these brainstem areas may produce analgesia in a quarter or half of the body, so that the rats fail to respond to painful pin prick, cold, pinching, or electrical shock. This brainstem modulating system can be activated by stimulation of widespread areas of the body surface. The system can block inputs from areas as large as a quarter or half of the body. The duration of the analgesia observed in these experiments, moreover, often outlasts the period of stimulation. This indicates that the stimulation evokes neural activities persisting for prolonged periods of time. All of these properties, taken together, appear to provide a satisfactory explanation of acupuncture analgesia.

Third, pain signals can be blocked by means of fibres that descend from the areas of the brain (predominantly the cortex) which are involved in the memory of cultural experiences, expectation, suggestion, and anxiety—those psychological processes known as higher central nervous system activities.

ANXIETY, FEAR, SHOCK AND PAIN

It is well known that these psychological processes can have a profound effect on pain. Anxiety and fear, for example, are known to enhance greatly the perception of pain. A given intensity of shock or heat is perceived as far more painful when a person is anxious than when he is not. The importance of anxiety is underscored by the observation that morphine effectively reduces pain only when the pain is accompanied by high levels of anxiety. It has little effect on pain in the non-anxious person.

Procedures that diminish the level of anxiety generally also decrease the level of perceived pain. It is well known that placebos, usually pharmacologically inert substances such as sugar or salt, produce marked relief of post-surgical pain in a third of patients if they believe that they are receiving an analgesic such as morphine. The more explicit the suggestion that a procedure will eliminate pain, the greater the likelihood that it will do so.

Relaxation, strong suggestion, faith in the physician and his techniques, and distraction have all been demonstrated to diminish both anxiety and pain. It is thus possible that the suggestion that acupuncture is effective (highly explicit in the Chinese hospital environment) may play a role. The knowledge that the procedure has worked in others would alleviate anxiety and fear, and thereby diminish the level of perceived pain.

We have seen that three mechanisms for the modulation of pain signals may all play a role in acupuncture analgesia. There is insufficient evidence at present to indicate the extent to which each contributes.

SECTION SEVEN

Surgical intervention to relieve pain

Nowhere is the complexity of the pain response better emphasized than in the surgical attempt to relieve pain. All notions of a simple wiring system in the nervous system to account for pain must be discounted. Almost every possible type of nervous connection from the periphery to the sensory cortex has been surgically cut without successfully permanently abolishing pain (see Reading 1, Section one). No matter what technique is used, the percentage of failures is significant.

Noordenbos (1972) has reviewed many of the causes of failures. Cordotomies have been relatively successful for patients with intractable pain caused by a malignancy when the patient is not expected to survive long. However, with an increase in survival time (beyond 18 months), there is an increase in the return of pain sensation. Despite the lack of regeneration of nervous tissue, it seems likely that other tissues take over the pain function. Noordenbos has (1972) pointed out that the spinal cord, especially the anterolateral quadrant, is a multisynaptic, multifiber system. Surgery must be done over a large area to produce longer-lasting pain relief. However, the larger the area cut, the more other functions, such as bladder control and strength in walking, tend to be lost. Noordenbos would limit surgery for pain to patients with fatal malignant diseases.

Schürmann (Reading 30) differentiates surgery on the basis of several major zones of the body. The first of these surgeries is in the region of the peripheral first neuron. It is described as being effective for facial neuralgias, herpes zoster, and pain from deep-lying organs. Facial pains, however, are currently being treated mostly with medication (Melzack, 1973). One problem is that cutting a mixed nerve produces both sensory and motor loss.

The second zone involves operations in the area of the second neuron in the spinal cord, where sensory and motor functions can be separated. These operations are cordotomies and tractotomies. Of the surgeries for pain, cordotomies seem to be the most successful, especially at the upper thoracic and upper cervical levels. The surgery usually requires removal of at least one quarter of the spinal cord. Unilateral sectioning is helpful only unilaterally. Pain from the pelvic area, abdomen, rectum, and genitalia involve both sides and require bilateral surgery. As previously noted, the more tissue that is removed, the more likely it is that pain relief will last longer, but the more chance there is for an increase in loss of other functions.

The percutaneous cordotomy is usually performed between C1 and C2; a surgical needle is inserted, frequent radiographs are taken, and electrical stimulation is used to see if the right area has been reached (Tasker and Organ, 1973).

Another zone of the body that has been used for the surgical control of pain is in the higher centers. These operations include thalamotomies and leucotomies. On the basis of observations made on 4,500 humans, Cooper (1965) has concluded that thalamic surgery should be limited to those patients with a central disorder of communication. The relative long-term success is only about 30%, and mortality from this surgery can be unacceptably high.

Frontal lobotomy or leucotomy abolishes the aversive feelings associated with pain. That is, the patient feels the pain, but it does not bother him. The major problem associated with this type of surgery is the change in personality—the patient can become an emotional vegetable. Roberts and Vilinskas (1973) have used a freezing technique whereby it is possible to determine the region to be cut and limit the lesion prior to the occurrence of irreversible tissue damage. They have reported successful pain relief without severe personality change. However, even so, they have recommended only limited use of this procedure.

Another zone of the body that has been cut is the autonomic nervous system. Schurmann believes that this surgery (sympathectomy) has proved disappointing and should no longer be performed.

Hackett (Reading 31) cautions against the free use of the scalpel to produce pain relief. He feels that there are many patients for whom surgery should not be undertaken and from whom physicians should accept the idea that there is no relief for their pain. These patients are characterized by three major problems: (1) the pain persists despite all medical and surgical intervention; (2) the persistence suggests the possibility of an emotional rather than a physical cause; and (3) the pain discomforts the doctor as much as the patient. Included in this group are many patients with low back pain, atypical facial neuralgias, and certain headache syndromes.

Hackett makes an important distinction between chronic and acute pain. The patient with chronic pain may lose all of the outward behavioral signs of someone in active pain. Autonomic reactions also tend to return to normal. Chronic pain may have been initiated by a relatively acute pain. However, once activated it can become self-sustaining. Hackett suggests a careful evaluation of the patient before embarking on a course of surgical procedures. Once more, the emphasis is on a multidisciplinary team to evaluate the patient.

REFERENCES

Cooper, I. S. 1965. Clinical and physiologic implications of thalamic surgery for disorders of sensory communication. I. Thalamic surgery for intractable pain, Journal of the Neurological Sciences **2:**493-519.

Melzack, R. 1973. The puzzle of pain, Basic Books, Inc., Publishers, New York.

Noordenbos, W. 1972. Causes of failure of surgical treatment. In Janzen, R., and others, editors: Pain: basic principles, pharmacology, therapy, Georg Thieme, Verlag, Stuttgart, Germany, pp. 220-222.

Roberts, M., and Vilinskas, J. 1973. Control of pain associated with malignant disease by freezing, cryoleucotomy, Connecticut Medicine **37:**184-186.

Tasker, R. R., and Organ, L. W. 1973. Percutaneous cordotomy, Confinia Neurologica **35:**110-117.

30

Surgical treatment

Fundamental principles of the surgical treatment of pain

K. Schürmann

The task of this paper is to point out the possibilities of surgical intervention in cases of "intractable" pain—i.e. for pain which can no longer be controlled by conservative therapeutic measures. In such cases the surgeon must also bear in mind that any operation on the peripheral or central nervous system causes a permanent lesion of nervous elements.

It is impossible to deal in detail with the diverse aetiology of intractable pain and with the very variable indications and choice of operation site which sometimes depend on this aetiology. This will be dealt with in the subsequent papers.

Broadly operations at three levels in the system of pain transmission must be differentiated:

1) In the region of the peripheral first neurone (resection in the area of the receptor apparatus of the peripheral afferent nerves and ganglia; and resection of the afferent spinal nerve roots, such as radicotomy or posterior rhizotomy);
2) in the region of the second neurone in the spinal cord (at the level of the thoracic medulla, the cervical medulla, the medulla oblongata and the midbrain; these are the chordotomies and tractotomies of the spinothalamic tract);
3) in the region of the third neurone or in the central synaptic junctions of the thalamus (stereotactic thalamotomies, cortectomies and divisions of the medullary fibres between the thalamus and the cortex).

Operations may also involve the autonomic nervous system (sympathectomies and resection of the sympathetic trunk) (Fig. 1).

OPERATIONS IN THE AREA OF THE PERIPHERAL FIRST NEURONE

These are resections in the area of the receptor apparatus; in the area of the peripheral afferent nerves and ganglia; in the area of the afferent spinal nerve roots, like radicotomy or posterior rhizotomy.

Operations on the peripheral neurone are still very common and effective, so for local "neuroma pain" of an amputation stump, for example resection of the focus of irritation itself should be considered first. As this involves total loss of the peripheral part of a mixed (motor and sensory) nerve, this is uncomplicated and the simplest kind of operation. But in order to prevent regeneration of the neuroma, which would of course always form again as long as the force of regeneration of the integument of the central nerve stump remains intact, it is necessary to devitalise it. In addition it is advisable to block the route of the axon cylinders which grow out of the nerve integuments.

Therefore after neuroma resection it will be necessary to: 1) destroy the whole nerve section centrally from the site of resection with an endoneural injection of alcohol or endoneural electrical destruction with a needle electrode and 2) close

Permission granted from Janzen and others, editors: Pain, Georg Thieme Publishers, Stuttgart/Churchill Livingstone, London, 1972.

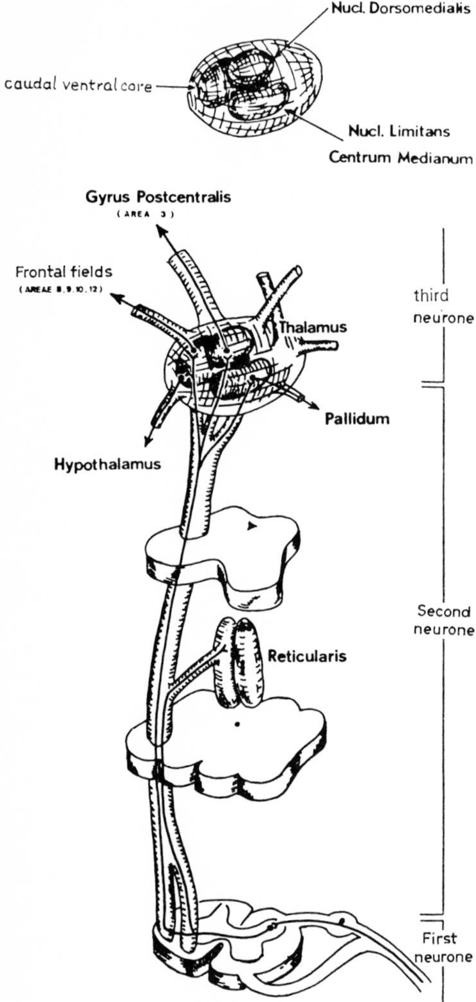

Fig. 1. Diagram of the pathway of pain impulses from the periphery through the spinothalamic tract to the thalamus, and from there the division to the cortical fields and to the hypothalamus.

First neurone – from the periphery of the body or the internal organs via the spinal ganglion (no synapse) to the posterior horn cell mechanism of the spinal cord (synapse).

Second neurone – from the posterior horn cell mechanism crossing over to the opposite side and extending upwards in the spino-thalamic tract through the cervical medulla oblongata and midbrain to the thalamus where the second neurone ends (synapse). A few of the fibres of the second neuron stop short in the substantia reticularis, from which the cerebrum is stimulated.

Third neurone – leading from the various cell bodies of the thalamus to various cortical fields of the cerebrum and to the hypothalamus (see text).

off the nerve integuments over the nerve stump.

The nerve stump should be treated in this way immediately after amputation as a preventive measure against the development of neuroma pain: unfortunately however, it does not guarantee protection.

In spite of everything pain frequently recurs after neuroma resection, and experience – especially since the last war – has shown that relapses are more common the longer the original state of pain lasted, i.e. the longer the operation was delayed. When it is no longer possible to cope with a recurrence of neuroma pain by resection of the neuroma – i.e. when simple removal of the focus of irritation is no longer sufficient – it means that an increase in the irritability of the dorsal horn cell mechanism of the spinal cord (substantia gelatinosa) has occurred with spontaneous discharging of impulses.

Now this primary synaptic junction must be separated from the centre. Section of the posterior root would no longer be adequate; chordotomy of the spinothalamic tract has now become imperative (see under: operations in the area of the second neurone in the spinal cord).

"Phantom pain" on the other hand can never be cured by neuroma resection; it need not even be tried. All the other operations that are to be discussed have also failed in practice – apart from transient improvements. What is the reason for this? The answer lies with the psychologists and psychiatrists. Physiologically phantom pain cannot be demonstrated; it is linked up somehow with the personality and probably represents some deviational reaction to psychic experience which cannot be dealt with surgically. That many operations have failed are in my opinion a clear proof of this.

Further examples of the possibility of operating on the peripheral neurone are seen in certain forms of facial neuralgia, such as neuralgia of the glossopharyngeal nerve, the intermedius nerve (sensory root of the seventh nerve) and the sphenopalatine nerve (ganglion sphenopalatinum, Sluder neuralgia). These can be treated by cutting through the pertinent nerves in the posterior cranial fossa or in the pterygopalatine fossa (ganglion sphenopalatinum).

In the same way some forms of trigeminal neuralgia may be successfully tackled by exheresis of the peripheral branch-

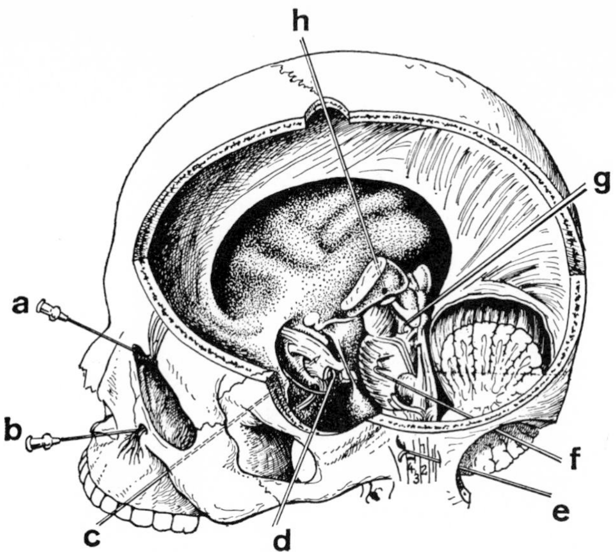

Fig. 2. *Various operations for trigeminal neuralgia* (from Riechert, Zbl. Neurochir. 18, 74 [1958]). a = Injection or exheresis of the first branch (N. supraorbitalis), b = Injection or exheresis of the second branch (N. infraorbitalis), c = *Electrical destruction* of the Gasserian ganglion (Partial and controlled by continual checking of sensitivity according to own modification), d = *Retroganglion root resection* subtemporally (Frazier), e = *Medullary tractotomy* or severing the spinal trigeminal root in the medulla oblongata (Sjöqvist), f = *Retroganglion* (parapontine) *root resection* through the subcerebellum (Dandy), g = Mesencephalic tractotomy (Dogliotti, Walker), h = Stereotactic thalamotomy.

Not all these operations have proved useful. The ones still most used and most reliable are: 1) Partial and controlled electrical destruction of the Gasserian ganglion (own modification) = c, 2) Retroganglion root resection in the middle cranial fossa subtemporally (extradural according to own modification) = d.

es. For example the *symptomatic* neuralgia of the second trigeminal branch of the maxillary nerve following chronic inflammation of the maxillary sinus. Here exheresis is equivalent to removal of the focus of irritation, namely the inflamed damaged nerves. On the other hand circumstances are quite different in the case of *idiopathic* trigeminal neuralgia, or "tic douloureux". In my experience exheresis practically never produces permanent results, and is not worth doing. Real "tic douloureux" is only successfully treated by surgery on the Gasserian ganglion, the trigeminal root or the trigeminal nucleus (tractus spinalis nervi trigemini) in the medulla oblongata. It is not clear why this is so, although there are a number of more or less plausible hypotheses (Fig. 2).

Among the operations affecting the peripheral neurone of the pain conduction system section of the posterior root (Foerster 1911) posterior radicotomy or posterior rhizotomy finally occupies a special position.

The first neurone does not end in the spindle ganglion, but in the posterior horn cell apparatus of the spinal cord and it is most practical to sever it intradurally, that is to say proximally from the spinal ganglion but distally from the posterior horn cells.

This operation has proved especially valuable for the exceptionally painful condition of paraspastic contractions as a result of partial or subtotal lesions to the spinal cord, whether of traumatic or degenerative origin (multiple sclerosis). The principle of the operation lies in curbing the excessive irritability in the posterior and anterior horns of the spinal cord (Fig. 3).

Following a lesion to the thoracic or cervical cord, extrapyramidal inhibiting devices that act on the anterior horn cell mechanism of the spinal cord are abolished. There is an increase in the tone of

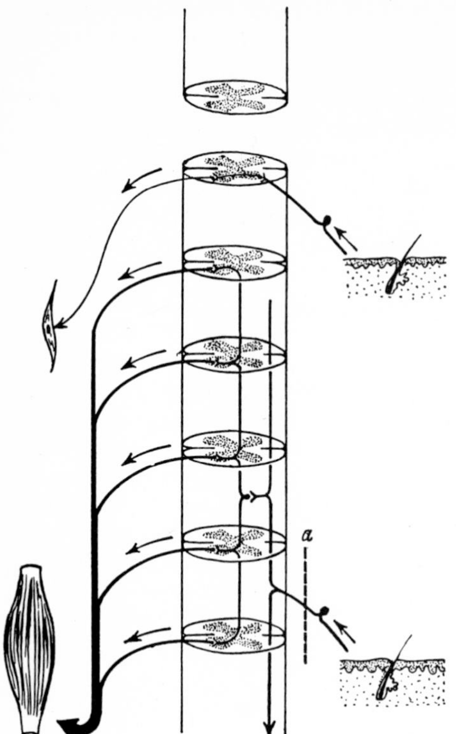

Fig. 3. The intramedullary synaptic neurones and reflex collaterals after Koelliker. Where there are lesions high up in the spinal cord these can transmit a stimulus arriving through a single posterior root to several anterior roots simultaneously and are therefore capable of causing a picture of exceptionally painful contractions (see text). a = resection of posterior root.

striated muscles. In addition all afferent influxes from the periphery are promoted pathologically, because they can be conducted in a central direction only partially or not at all. They are now in the main transmitted directly and without any inhibition via the spinal reflex arc to the anterior horn cell mechanism. Moreover this is still further strengthened by the intramedullary synaptic neurones, since they can transmit any stimulus entering through a single posterior nerve root simultaneously to several anterior nerve roots. The impulse is spread out over several segments. This means that the most minute irritation of the skin releases violent bending reflexes – i.e. reflexes of flight and defence. Eventually, even when just lying in bed, the least irritation to the skin from the sheet causes most violent and acutely painful bending contractions. Interrupting the afferent spinal reflex arc, that is, severing the numerous corresponding posterior nerve roots, ends the incessant flow of stimuli. 1) the pains and 2) the reactive contractions are eliminated.

Even today posterior radicotomy is justified for the treatment of intractable pain, so long as the correct operation technique is ensured with severance of a sufficient number of nerve roots at the necessary segment levels (Paillas p. 209).

Cutting through the posterior nerve root has also proved useful for neuralgia caused by Herpes Zoster and for chronic internal pain in different organs, although there is not quite the same certainty of success as in the case of pain due to contractions. Now and then one is obliged to supplement this operation with further surgical measures. This is because Herpes Zoster is caused by a neurotrophic virus whose point of attack is the peripheral nerve and the skin receptors and in particular the spinal ganglion. But it is not always restricted to these peripheral sites and may also lead to lesions of the posterior horn cell mechanism. In such cases simple posterior radicotomy is inadequate, and a more central site of attack is necessary – chordotomy of the spinothalamic tract. But often the cause of failure after radicotomy is not extension of the virus infection, but simply that surgery was not carried out extensively enough. Since the areas of sensitivity of the various roots overlap in up to two or three adjacent segments, radicotomy must be extended proximally and distally from the dermatome affected as far as these two or three neighbouring roots. Some authors are of the opinion that the surface pain in Zoster neuralgia is mainly attributable to a lesion of the skin receptors and their fibres and that resection of the dermatome can therefore relieve the pain, but this is not reliable (Poppen 1960, Verbiest personal communication 1964) (Fig. 4).

I have experience with only one case of dermatome resection for Herpes Zoster in the upper thoracic region. This was carried out on an 80-year-old woman who could not have tolerated a more major surgical operation. Before operation novocaine was injected subcutaneously to see whether or not the pain would disappear. As the pain disappeared for some four or five hours following the subcutaneous infiltration the skin segment was excised radically right into the adjacent healthy tissue: after this the patient was free from pain. This operation is, however, still too recent for it to be considered a complete success yet.

Posterior root resection may also be indicated for pain emanating from deep-lying

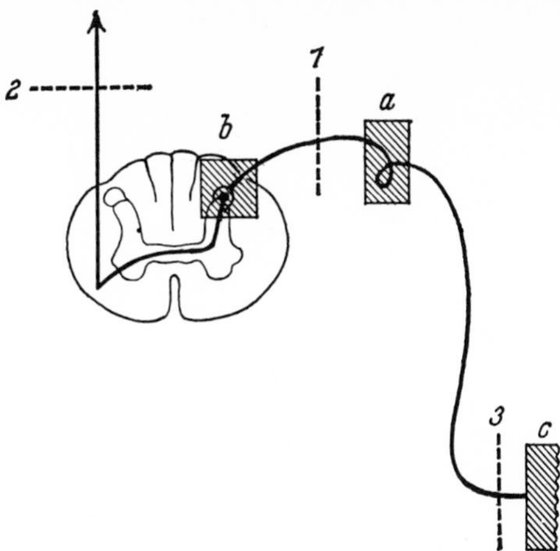

Fig. 4. Main points of attack of the neurotrophic virus in Herpes Zoster (shaded areas). a) spinal ganglion (Treatment: resection of posterior root = 1), b) posterior horn cell mechanism (Treatment: chordotomy of the spino-thalamic tract = 2), c) skin receptors (Treatment: possibly resection of the affected dermatome). The dotted lines indicate where the section should be made (see text).

parts of the body (visceral pain). However, it must be extended over a sufficient number of segments and in certain circumstances may also have to be combined with sympathectomy but not because the painful stimulus is conducted through the fibres of the sympathetic nerve. This view is wrong. There is no afferent pain conduction from the sympathetic nerve with a transfer in the sympathetic ganglion (Jung 1959). The real position is that enteroceptive pain fibres of the peripheral somatic nervous system simply use the pathways of the sympathetic trunk as guests (Fig. 5, Nr. 4), but are in fact normal posterior root fibres, whose neurones are situated in the spinal ganglion and end in the posterior horn cell mechanism of the spinal cord. Accordingly posterior radicotomy usually also meets with success in cases of visceral pain, provided it is carried out accurately and sufficiently extensively in the appropriate segments (e.g. gastric crises in cases

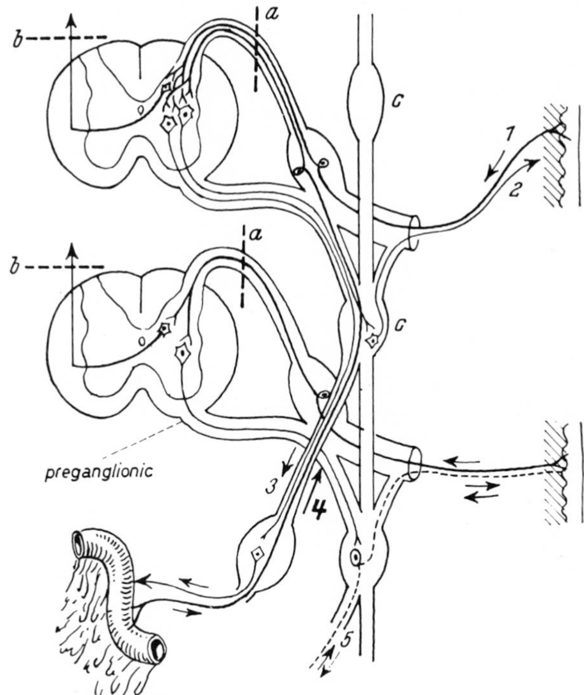

Fig. 5. Diagrammatic representation of the conduction of painful stimuli from internal organs (visceral pain). It should be noted that the enteroceptive pain fibres of the peripheral somatic nervous system (4) merely make use of the pathways of the sympathetic trunk as guests, but are in fact posterior root fibres, whose neurone lies in the spinal ganglion and ends in the posterior horn cell apparatus of the spinal cord (see text). Therefore there is good justification for posterior root resection (a) as well as chordotomy (b) of the spinothalamic tract for painful conditions from deep-lying organs (after Rein and Schneider 1956). a) posterior root resection, b) chordotomy of the spino-thalamic tract, c) sympathectomy (resection of sympathetic trunk).

of syphilis and pancreatic pain following chronic pancreatitis) (Fig. 5).

OPERATIONS IN THE AREA OF THE SECOND NEURONE IN THE SPINAL CORD

These are the intramedullary chordotomies or tractotomies of the spinothalamic tract at various segmentary levels of the thoracic or cervical cord, of the medulla oblongata or of the mesencephalon.

Undoubtedly the most effective operations for chronic pain involve surgery around the second neurone, chordotomies of the spinothalamic tract in the upper thoracic cord ($D_{2/3/4}$), high up in the cervical cord ($C_{1\text{-}2}$), in the medulla oblongata and in the mesencephalon. Of these, thoracic tractotomy is for various reasons superior to cervical and medullary tractotomies for relief of pain in the lower half of the body.

For painful conditions in the upper half of the trunk, i.e. in the thorax and its organs, the upper extremities and the shoulders, high cervical or medullary chordotomy is indicated. The higher the focus of pain is situated, the higher must be the site chosen for chordotomy and the deeper must be the cut into the cord. This is supported by the fact that the somatotopic construction of the anterolateral column has been elucidated neurophysiologically and neuroanatomically (Foerster 1932, Glees and Bailey 1951a and b, Hyndman and Van Epps 1939).

The second neurone of the spinal cord, belonging to the pain conduction system of the sacral segments, passes from segment to segment upwards to the surface of the posterior portion of the anterolateral column, close to the ligamentum denticulatum. The fibres of the lumbar segments that have just entered join rather further inside and ventrally; next, situated even further towards the centre of the cord section follow the thoracic and finally the cervical fibres, which are situated the furthest inside and the most ventrally (Fig. 6). This means not only that the level of a chordotomy is determined by the level of the focus of pain, but also that the cord must be cut into more deeply and more ventrally the higher the focus of irritation.

With thoracic chordotomy (Foerster 1913) at the level of the third or fourth segment, analgesia can seldom be achieved beyond D_8. Therefore it must be restricted to processes in the lower half of the body (Fig. 7).

With cervical chordotomy at the level of $C_{1\text{-}2}$, permanent analgesia very rarely extends higher than C_7 or D_1. This is why

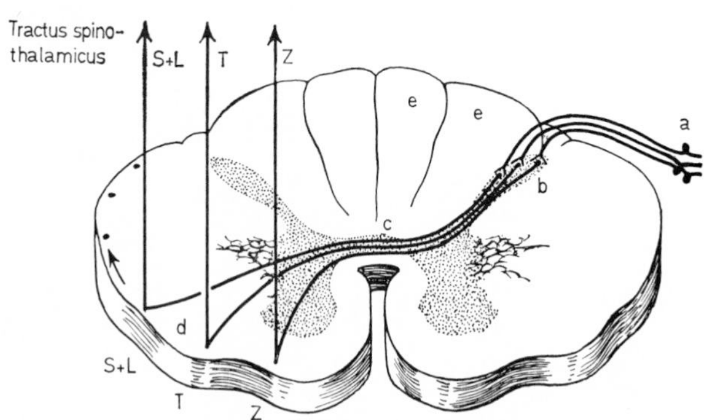

Fig. 6a. Diagram of the fibres crossing over to the other side of the *spino-thalamic system which conduct painful stimuli* in the entry segment of the spinal cord. (In contrast to this, tactile stimuli and the sensation of position are conducted towards the centre via the dorsal columns without crossing over. They do not cross over to the other side until high in the medial loop of the mesencephalon). Hence follows the essential fact for surgical purposes that the conduction pathways for *painful stimuli* (anterolateral column) and for *tactile stimuli* (posterior column) run separately through the spinal cord. a) Spinal ganglion, b) Substantia gelatinosa (synaptic posterior horn cell mechanism, where the first neurone ends and the second neurone starts), c) Crossing over of the second neurone in the anterior commisure of the spinal cord, d) Spino-thalamic tract in the anterolateral column of the spinal cord (somatotpically divided: S + L = sacral + lumbar, T = thoracic, Z = cervical), e) Posterior columns.

analgesia does not always extend to the radial and proximal extremities. In these cases either a medullary chordotomy is advisable straight away, or—preferred by many authors on account of the lower risks—cervical chordotomy combined with a supplementary posterior radicotomy should be performed (Fig. 7).

In my own experience medullary chordotomy at the level of the inferior olive is not in itself more risky than cervical chordotomy, but is perhaps technically rather more difficult, since at this level the spino-thalamic tract does not lie so near the surface and is slightly concealed medially from the (dorsal and ventral) spino-cerebellar tract.

Section as in the case of thoracic and cervical chordotomy would also damage this tract and bring about homolateral atactic disorders. Here, at the level between the superior accessory root and the inferior olive, the squared-off chordotome is simply pierced through both lateral tracts of the cerebellum and with gentle rotatory movements of the chordotomy stick around the puncture as the fulcrum point, the spino-thalamic tract in isolation is separated in the shape of the sector (Fig. 7).

But neither cervical nor medullary chordotomy should be carried out on both sides at once, since this considerably increases the dangers of oedema in the cord. Thoracic chordotomy can on the other hand be carried out bilaterally in a single session (it is then most practical to make the incisions into the cord at different segmental levels). High thoracic chordotomy on both sides is particularly recommended for visceral pain, since many painful stimuli emanating from internal organs are conducted via the pathways of the homolateral spino-thalamic tract and are not completely cut off by a unilateral chordotomy.

Mesencephalic tractotomy (Walker 1942b) has since been shown to offer no advantages. For relief of painful conditions it has proved inferior to chordotomies and in 50% of cases (Drake and McKenzie 1953) painful dysaesthesias have developed that were far worse than the original pain. Moreover in most patients side-effects were observed such as disturbances in the field of vision and in hearing (lowering of the threshold for hearing high sounds in the case of sections on one side, and even deafness in cases of sections on both sides (Fig. 7)).

The great advantage of chordotomies of the spino-thalamic tract is not only that their effectiveness has been proved over and over again but above all that they

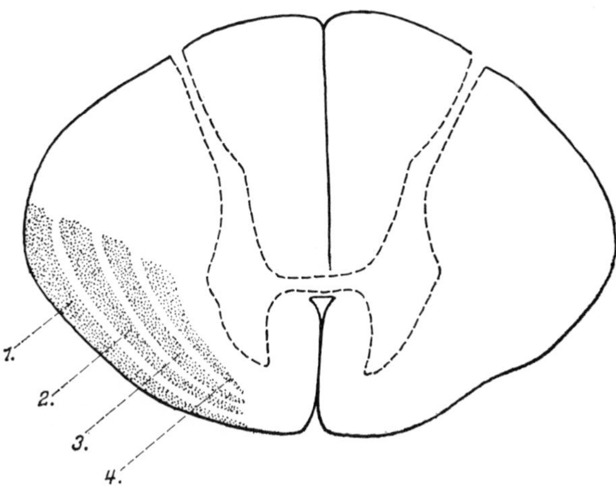

Fig. 6b. Diagrammatic representation of the *somatotopical construction of the spino-thalamic tract in the upper thoracic cord* (from Glees, P.: Acta neuroveg. 7:160, 1963). 1 = sacral fibres, 2 = lumbar fibres, 3 = thoracic fibres, 4 = cervical fibres. As regards chordotomy technique this means that the incision has to be made more deeply the higher the focus of pain is situated (see text).

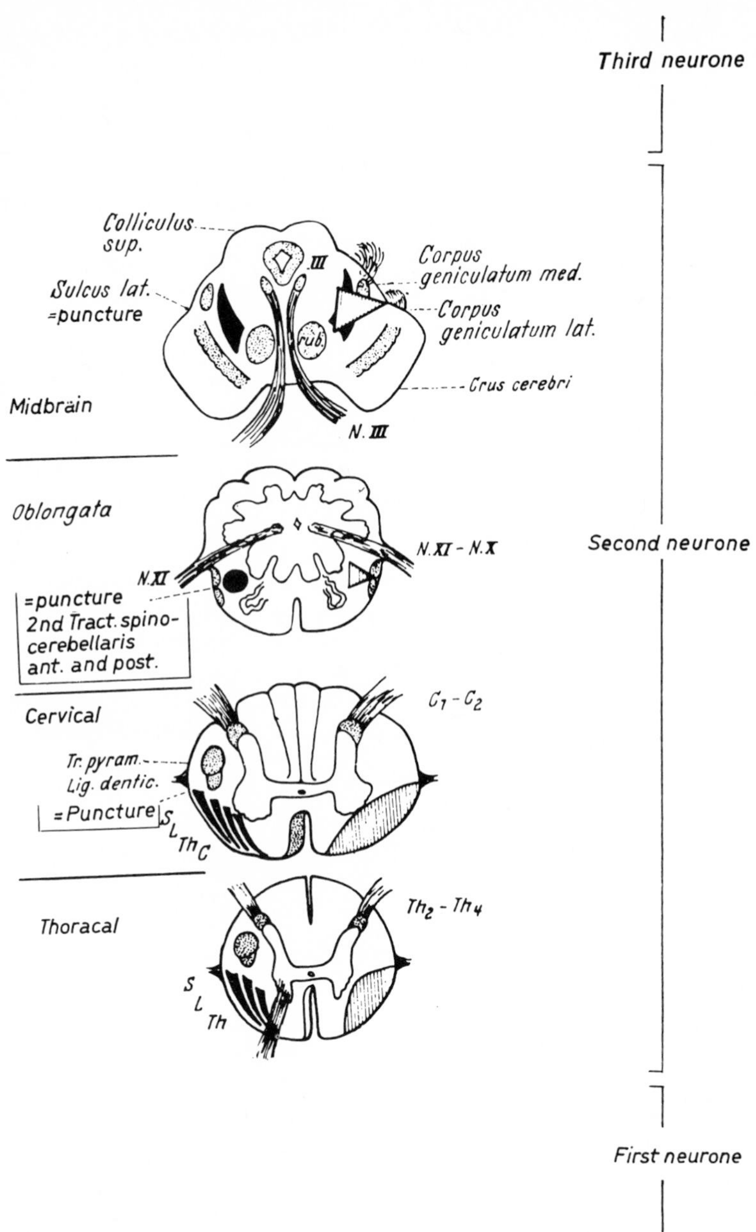

Fig. 7. Diagrammatic representation of *chordotomy of the spino-thalmic tract at different levels:* thoracic, cervical, medullary, mesencephalic (see text), (black areas on left = spino-thalamic tract), (shaded areas on right = sector for cutting).

leave behind only an isolated loss of sensations of pain and thermal changes, while leaving unaffected epicritic sensitivity, the sensations of touch and position which are mainly conducted via the posterior columns. In cases of extensive posterior radicotomy one unfortunately also has to put up with the loss of these important sensations. This may perhaps be of no great importance in the trunk, since the advantage of cutting off pain limited segmentally can outweigh the disadvantages – including those of chordotomy. But the loss of the positional sensation in the extremities is in certain circumstances hard to justify.

At this point it must again be stated that chordotomy of the spino-thalamic tract – especially when executed in the area of the upper thoracic cord and the upper cervical cord – is still one of the most successful operations for intractable pain in the trunk. This may be due to the fact that intractable pain is the result of an irritation or miscalculation in the first central nervous synapse, namely the substantia gelatinosa of the posterior horn cell mechanism of the spinal cord (neuronal pool), which this operation separates from centres situated higher up.

OPERATIONS IN THE AREA OF THE THIRD NEURONE OR THE CENTRAL SYNAPSES OF THE THALAMUS

These are the stereotactic thalamotomies: the cortectomies and separations of cord fibres between the thalamus and the cortex.

Although the so-called stereotactic pain thalamotomies may be counted among the less cumbersome operations, after initial successes an unexpectedly high quota of relapses (up to 50% or more) became apparent later including serious complications by damage to functionally important neighbouring structures and, not least, violent postoperative syndromes of thalamic pain which demanded active treatment. We ourselves have had no experience of this, but Reichert (1960) and Hassler (personal communication 1967) have warned against too much optimism. They emphasise that because of these complications and the high rate of relapse thalamotomy should be employed only when all other operative procedures have utterly failed. In Riechert's own words: "Stereotactic thalamotomy has only a qualitatively and quantitatively limited effect on painful conditions ("intractable pain")". Struppler (1968) also stresses the limited value of thalamotomy because of the high relapse rate and also because of the concomitant lesions. On the other hand the side-effects can now largely be avoided by more exact determination of the site of lesion by electrophysiological means. It is true that this drawback is thereby eliminated, but the high relapse rate still sets limits to the operation. For this reason Struppler (1968) sees the main indication for pain thalamotomy to be in cancer patients with a limited expectation of life, e.g. for patients with cancer in the region of the facial skeleton and the base of the skull.

Perhaps the partial failures of the thalamic synaptic system themselves should be considered as the cause of the so-called central pain syndrome. For example Hassler (1960) noted violent expressions of pain when the nucleus limitans, independent of the cortex, was stimulated, but when it was completely destroyed there was enduring relief from pain. Hassler therefore argued in favour of destroying both the nucleus ventralis *and* the nucleus limitans. Talairach, Tournoux and Bancaud (1960) too maintain that more extensive thalamotomies with more radical destruction of the caudal ventral nucleus and of the dorsomedian nucleus will probably make better results possible in the future (Fig. 1 and 2).

However, Hassler (personal communication) has admitted that successful relief of pain by means of thalamotomy presupposed on the one hand making a lesion that was sufficiently large, and that on the other hand much of the good effect could be attributed to cutting at the same time the terminal nuclei of the fronto-thalamic projection pathways situated rostrally in the thalamus. But this means that the good result of a more extensive pain-thalamotomy achieved in a few cases occurs not only by eliminating the terminal nuclei of the spino-thalamic tract, but also that such a radical operation affects the emotional experience of pain by damaging the terminals of the fronto-thalamic pathways, rather like a pre-thalamic section of the medullary fibres (comparable with selective "psychosurgical" leucotomy). But if this is so, the more extensive thalamotomy demanded would to some extent have a double action, one affecting the pain conduction system and the second – in the psychosurgical field – reducing the emotional tension of the actual individual experience of pain.

Here again the indication for such operative measures must be reserved for very particular cases, and be more closely circumscribed—just because of the inevitable psychic consequences.

Excision of cortical fields (cortectomies) and severing transfrontal medullary fibres (frontal lobotomies, or leucotomies) are not among the common operations for painful conditions. Cortectomy of the sensory cortical field (the postcentral gyrus or Area 3; according to David, Talairach and Hecaen 1947) affecting the area of the third neurone of the pain conduction system has been as completely disappointing as the more psychosurgical cortectomy of the frontomedial cortical fields of the midfissure (Gyrus cinguli; according to Le Beau, Bouvet and Rosier 1948). Frontal lobotomy has been variously employed as a last resort to attenuate the psychic and emotional experience of pain. But this operation is followed by not inconsiderable psychic changes and is therefore difficult to justify. Surgery to relieve pain and surgery for psychological reasons have their own realms of indications.

OPERATIONS IN THE AREA OF THE AUTONOMIC NERVOUS SYSTEM

These are the sympathectomies and resections of the sympathetic trunk. They have not achieved any outstanding significance for treating chronic and intractable pain since after long periods of observation their results have almost always proved disappointing. This may have been because conceptions of "sympathetic pain" were simply false. For it has since been demonstrated that there is no afferent conduction of pain from the sympathetic system with a synapse in the sympathetic ganglia (Jung 1959).

The position is rather that enteroceptive pain fibres of the peripheral somatic nervous system merely make use of the pathways of the sympathetic system as guests but are in fact normal posterior nerve root fibres, whose neurones lie in the spinal ganglion and end in the posterior horns of the spinal cord. For this reason posterior radicotomy for pain in deep-lying organs for example usually meets with success only if it is carried out accurately and sufficiently extensively in the right segments. Yet conversely extensive sympathetic denervation of the painful organ can sometimes be equally successful, since the sympathetic pathways contain a portion of the peripheral pain fibres of the spinal ganglion. But the intricate network of the sympathetic pathways with their multiple possibilities of diffusing stimuli and their great and proven power of regeneration make it clear that relapses soon occur, and that therefore specific segmental posterior rhizotomy offers greater effectiveness and durability (Fig. 5 and 8).

Sympathectomy may only be successful for causalgia in certain circumstances. The conditions in which stimuli are transmitted are obviously different, for there is a pathological referral from the excitation of sympathetic fibres to partially injured pain nerve fibres. The way Struppler (1968) expresses it is that there are in a way short-circuit formations between somatic

Table 1. Our personal experiences are based on the results of the following operations:

Operation	Number	Subtotal
Neurone resection	52	
Posterior radicotomy	36	
Thoracic chordotomy	58	
Cervical chordotomy	5	
Medullary chordotomy	6	
Combined cervical chordotomy and posterior radicotomy	3	
Combined medullary chordotomy and posterior radicotomy	2	
Frontal lobotomy (according to Busch)	3	
		165
Operations especially for trigeminal neuralgia:		
Peripheral exheresis (symptomatic neuralgia)	12	
Gasserian ganglion (destruction by alcohol, *prior* to 1955)	24	
Gasserian ganglion (electro-destruction from 1955-1969)	311	
Retroganglion resection (temporal) of trigeminal root	149	
Medullary tractotomy (according to Sjöqvist)	38	
		534
Pain sympathectomy (*prior* to 1958)	49*	
		49
Total:		748

*Most of the patient material for "pain sympathectomy" (40 cases) came from the Neurosurgical Clinic in Cologne (Prof. Tonnis). These were followed up by the author with Siess in 1962 to find out their effectiveness. The remaining nine cases were operated on by the author between 1955 and 1957. Because of the poor results as regards permanence (only three of the 15 cases of causalgia had been improved, and the others had no result) no more "pain sympathectomies" have been carried out by the author since 1958.

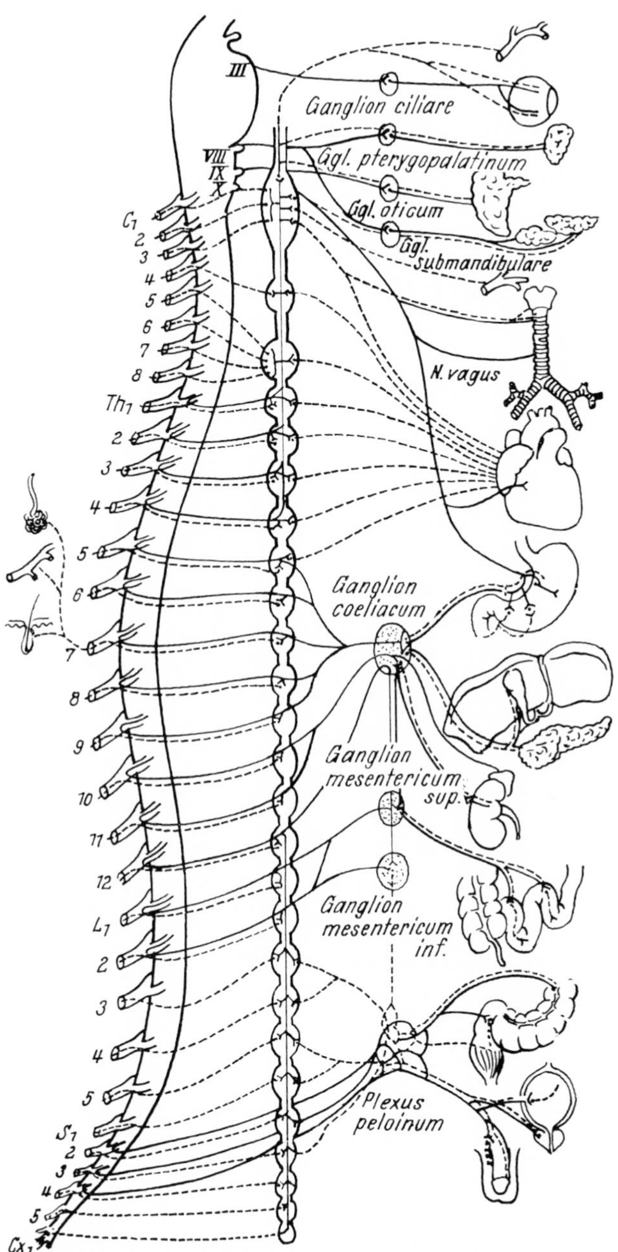

Fig. 8. Diagrammatic representation of the enteroceptive peripheral pain fibres of the somatic nervous system only passing via the *pathways of the sympathetic system* (but not belonging to it), which reach the spinal cord via the posterior roots and continue upward to the thalamus via the spino-thalamic tract (second neurone).

Therefore, in the case of visceral pain, resection of the posterior roots and chordotomy are effective and superior to sympathectomy because on account of the intricate network of the sympathetic pathways – which carry enteroceptive somatic pain fibres along only as guests – relapses practically always set in (see text).

and autonomic nerve fibres. This would be sufficient to explain why sympathetic denervation sometimes results in successful treatment for causalgia experimentally.

At any rate our own experience with 15 patients with causalgia from the last war who underwent sympathectomy between 1946 and 1949 was bad: only three produced lasting improvement over the next few years, while the other 12 cases reverted to their old state within a few months up to a maximum of a year or two (Table 1).

Sympathectomy should no longer be employed for other chronic painful conditions because it is known to be hopeless in producing permanent results.

AN ATTEMPT TO EVALUATE THE EFFECTIVENESS OF THE INDIVIDUAL OPERATIONS

It is hard to evaluate the effectiveness of individual operations and the decision to choose one or other surgical operation has always to hinge upon the individual patient and the underlying painful condition: this demands considerable personal experience. Some of the operations mentioned have become standardised and show a high success rate, whereas others—at first adopted enthusiastically—were later abandoned because of poor results.

The problem begins with deciding whether or not an operation is indicated, for we must bear in mind that every resection of a nerve pathway causes a permanent lesion which should be a positive gain for the patient. As for evaluation—this must also be reckoned with—even today we are very largely dependent on the subjective data provided by the sufferer. However reliable his or her remarks may seem to be as a source of information, they can sometimes provide the starting point for a chain of mistakes and wrong indications. Even though it has been demonstrated physiologically that pain is "measurable", yet as regards clinical practice there are so far no sufficiently exact methods for objectively demonstrating a chronic state of pain and suffering nor any exact technique for measuring the intensity of pain felt by the sufferer. Some of the disappointments in the surgery of pain may also be attributable to this inadequacy—with consequent wrong decisions by the physician. But some failures are in my opinion the consequence of defective surgical technique as a result of inadequate neurophysiological knowledge and a lack of experience. The failure of surgical treatment is discussed in more detail by Noordenbos (p. 220).

Although it is hard to evaluate the effectiveness of the various operations without including the individual case-history for judgment, it may be asserted at this point that *definite fields of indication* have become apparent for *particular operations*. It has been proved that the first two types of operations mentioned are the most effective and successful as regards a permanent result which is the aim in all cases. In this connection an important position is occupied by *operations on the Gasserian ganglion and the trigeminal root* for tic douloureux or idiopathic trigeminal neuralgia, *posterior rhizotomy* for the painful cramps of spastics, Herpes Zoster neuralgia and pain from deep-lying organs, *chordotomies and tractotomies of the spino-thalamic tract* for intractable pain in carcinoma and also from deep-lying organs, and in combination with rhizotomies for painful conditions of the upper half of the trunk. Today they are firmly entrenched in the surgical treatment of intractable pain. Mesencephalic tractotomy is inferior to tractotomies of the spino-thalamic tract at lower levels (medullary, cervical, thoracic). It is not yet possible to visualize completely the future of stereotactic thalamotomy. To begin with it should be reserved for the few patients in whom established operations have failed, as long as the deficiencies mentioned above—that gave rise to wrong indications or inadequate surgical removal—can safely be excluded.

In spite of all the problems involved in the operative treatment of pain, it may be noted with satisfaction that there are a number of very good and reliable surgical alternatives available for relieving the patient with chronic intractable pain. Nevertheless it must be admitted that many unsolved questions in the physiology and pathology of this phenomenon of "pain" still await clarification.

• • •

In the preparation of this article the

work of the following additional authors has been studied.

Adams and Munro (1944), Bernard (1851), Bernhard (1952), Crawford (1947), Crawford and Knighton (1953), Dandy (1925), Dejerine and Roussy (1906), Foerster (1908: 1927), Foerster and Kuttner (1909), Frazier (1918: 1925), Freeman and Watts (1942: 1946), Glees (1952: 1953a and b), Glees, Livingston and Soler (1951), Granit (1955), Grundfest and Campbell (1942), Hartel (1913), Hecaen et al (1949b), Hensel (1966), Hering (1879), Horrax (1946), Horrax and Price (1954), Jung (1954), Kahn and Rand (1952), Kirschner (1933: 1936: 1942), LeBeau and Gaches (1949), Leriche (1916: 1958), Mackenzie (1923), Monnier (1955: 1963), Noordenbos (1959, 1960), Riddoch (1938 and 1941), Schurmann (1956a and b: 1957: 1959: 1962: 1966), Schurmann and Butz (1968), Schurmann and Ulbricht (1966a and b), Sjoqvist (1937), Spiegl and Wycis (1953), Spiess (1966), Spiller and Frazier (1901), Taarnhøj (1952 and 1954), Talairach et al (1959), Talairach, Tournoux and Bancaud (1960), Walker (1942b), Weinberger and Grant (1943), White and Smithwick (1944), White and Sweet (1955).

REFERENCES

Adams, R. D., Munro, D. (1944) Surgical division of the spinothalamic tract in the medulla. Surg. Gynec. Obstet. **78,** 591

Bernard, C. (1851) Influence du grand sympathique sur la sensibilité et sur la calorification. C. R. Soc. Biol. (Paris) **3,** 163

Bernard, C. G. (1952) Pattern of organisation in the central nervous system. Res. Publ. Ass. Nerv. Ment. Dis. **XXX**

Crawford, A. S. (1947) Medullary tractotomy for relief of intractable pain in upper levels. Arch. Surg. (Chicago) **55,** 523

Crawford, A. S., Knighton, R. S. (1953) Further observations on medullary spinothalamic tractotomy. J. Neurosurg. **10,** 113

Dandy, W. E. (1925) Section of the sensory root of the trigeminal nerve at the pons: Preliminary report of the operative procedure. Bull. Johns Hopk. Hosp. **36,** 105

Dejerine, J., Roussy, G. (1906) Le syndrome thalamique. Rev. neurol. **14,** 521

Foerster, O. (1908) Über eine neue operative Methode der Behandlung spastischer Lahmungen mittels Resektion hinterer Rückenmarkswurzeln. Z. Orthop. Chir. **22,** 203

Foerster, O. (1927) Die Leitungsbahnen des Schmerzgefühls und die chirurgische Behandlung der Schmerzzustände. Urban & Schwarzenberg, Munich, p. 360

Foerster, O., Kuttner, H. (1909) Über operative Behandlung gastrischer Krisen durch Resektion der 7 bis 10 hinteren Dorsalwurzel. Beitr. Klin. Chir. **63,** 245

Freeman, W., Watts, J. W. (1942) Prefrontal lobotomy; the surgical relief of mental pain. Bull. N.Y. Acad. Med. **18,** 794

Freeman, W. Watts, J. W. (1946) Pain of organic disease relieved by prefrontal lobotomy. Lancet, **1,** 953

Glees, P. (1952) Der Verlauf und die Endigung des Tractus spinothalamicus und der medialen Scheife nach Beobachtungen beim Menschen und Affen. Verh. Anat. Ges. (Marburg) **50,** 48

Glees, P. (1953a) The central pain tract. Acta Neuroveg. (Wien) **7,** 160

Glees, P. (1953b) The interrelation of the thalamus and the sensorimotor cortex. Mschr. Psychiat. Neurol. **125,** 129

Glees, P., Livingston, R. B., Soler, J. (1951) Der intraspinale Verlauf und die Endigungen der sensorischen Wurzeln in den Nucleus gracilis und cuneatus. Arch. Psychiat. Z. Neurol. **187,** 190

Granit, R. (1955) Receptors and sensory perception. Yale University Press, New Haven, Conn.

Grundfest, H., Campbell, B. (1942) Origin, conduction and termination of impulses in dorsal spinocerebellar tract of cats. J. Neurophysiol. **5,** 275

Hartel, F. (1913) Die Leistungsanaesthesie und Injectionsbehandlung des Ganglion Gasseri und der Trigeminusstämme. Arch. Klin. Chir. **100,** 193

Heacaen, H., Talairach, J., David, M., Dell, M. B. (1949b) Coagulations limitées du thalamus dans les algies du syndrome thalamique; résultats thérapeutiques et physiologiques, Rev. neurol. **81,** 917.

Hensel, H. (1966) Allgemeine Sinnesphysiologie, Hautsinn, Geschmack, Geruch. Lehrbuch der Physiologie in zusammenhängenden Einzeldarstellungen. Springer, Berlin

Hering, E. (1879) Beiträge zur allgemeinen Nerven- und Muskelphysiologie. S.-B. Akad. Wiss. Wien, Math.-Nat. Kl. **7,** 237

Horrax, G., Price, W. T. (1954) High cervical chordotomy for the relief of intractable pain in the arm, shoulder and upper chest. Ann. Surg. **139,** 567

Jung, R. (1954) Die tätigkeit des Nervensystems. Handbuch d. inn. Medizin. Vol. I, Springer, Berlin

Kahn, E. A., Rand, R. W. (1952) On the anatomy of anterolateral cordotomy. J. Neurosurg. **9,** 611

Kirschner, N. (1933) Die Punktionstechnik und die Elektrokoagulation des Ganglion Gasseri; über "gezielte" Operationen. Arch. Klin. Chir. **176,** 581

Kirschner, M. (1936) Zur Behandlung der Trigeminusneuralgie. Erfahrungen an 250 Fällen. Arch. klin. Chir. **186,** 225

Kirschner, M. (1942) Die Behandlung der Trigeminusneuralgie (nach Erfahrungen an 1113 Kranken). Münch. Med. Wschr. **89,** 235

LeBeau, J., Gaches, J. (1949) Sur l'action de la topectomie dans les douleurs irreductibles à propos de deux cas de causalgie, Sem. Hôp. Paris, **25,** 2226

Leriche, R. (1916) De la causalgie envisagée comme une nevrite du sympathique et de son traitement par la denudation et l'excision des pleux nerveux periarteriels. Presse Med. **24,** 178

Leriche, R. (1958) Chirurgie des Schmerzes. Barth, Leipzig., p. 429

Mackenzie, J. (1923) Angina pectoris. Frowde, Hodder & Stroughton, London, p. 253

Monnier, M. (1955) Les résultats de la coagulation du thalamus chez l'homme (Nóyau ventro-posterieur). Acta Neurochir. (Wien) Suppl. III 291

Monnier, M. (1963) Physiologie und Pathophysiologie des vegetativen Nervensystems. Vol. II: Pathophysiologie. Hippokrates, Stuttgart, p. 960

Noordenbos, W. (1959) Pain: problems pertaining to the transmission of nerve impulses which give rise to pain. Elsevier, Amst.

Noordenbos, W. (1960) Einige theoretische Bemerkungen über den zentralen Schmerz. Acta Neurochir. **8,** 113

Riddoch, G. (1938) The clinical features of central pain. Three articles which make up the Lumleian Lectures for 1938 delivered before the Royal College of Physicians of London. Lancet **1,** 1093, 1150, 1205

Riddoch. G. (1941) Phantom limbs and body shape. Brain **64,** 197

Schürmann, K. (1956a) Die moderne Behandlung der "idiopathischen" Trigeminusneuralgie mit der subtemporalen extraduralen Wurzeldekompression. Therapiewoche **6,** 380

Schürmann, K. (1956b) Die "Rezidive" nach der Taarnhøj-Norlenschen Wurzeldekompression in der Behandlung der Trigeminusneuralgie, Zbl. Neurochir. **16,** 292

Schürmann, K. (1957) Die schweren spastischen Zustände. Handbuch der Neurochirurgie, Vol. VI, Springer, Berlin

Schürmann, K. (1959) Neurochirurgie im höheren Lebensalter. Zbl. Neurochir. **19,** 346

Schürmann, K. (1962) Neurochirurgische Therapie bei Schmerzzustanden. M. Kurse Arztl. Fortbild. **14,** 1

Schürmann, K. (1966) Schmerzbehandlung aus neurochirurgischer Sicht. Psychother. Psychosom. **14,** 459

Schürmann, K., Butz, M. (1968) Retroanglionare Trigeminuswurzelresektion durch temporale Schädeleröffnung oder kontrollierte partielee Elektroverödung des Ganglion Gasseri durch gezielte Punktion in der operativen Behandlung der idiopathischen Trigeminusneuralgie? (Bericht über 435 Fälle). Zbl. Neurochir. **29,** 139

Schürmann, K., Ulbricht, W. (1966a) Kopf und Gesichtsschmerz bei intrakraniellen Erkrankungen I. Fortschr. Med. **84,** 93

Schürmann, K., Ulbricht, W. (1966b) Differentialdiagnose des Kopfschmerzes. II Fortschr. Med. **84,** 148

Sjöqvist, O. (1937) Eine neue Operationsmethode bei Trigeminusneuralgie: Durchschneidung des Tractus spinalis trigemini. Zbl. Neurochir. **2,** 274

Spiegel, E. A., Wycis, H. T. (1953) Mesencephalotomy in treatment of intractable facial pain. Arch. Neurol. Psychiat. (Chic.) **69,** 1

Spiess, A. (1966) Operationsindikationen und Ergebnisse der Sympathikuschirurgie, Spätresultate von 371 Fällen. Inauguraldissertation, Mainz

Spiller, W. G., Frazier, C. H. (1901) The division of the sensory root of the trigeminus for relief of tic douloureux. An experimental, pathological and clinical study, with a preliminary report of one surgically successful case. Philad. Med. J. **8,** 1039

Taarnhøj, P. (1952) Decompression of the trigeminal root and the posterior part of the ganglion as treatment in trigeminal neuralgia. J. Neurosurg. **9,** 288

Taarnhøj, P. (1954) Decompression of the trigeminal root. J. Neurosurg. **2,** 499

Talairach, J., Tournoux, P., Bancaud, J., Djahanchahi, A. (1959) Exploration stéréotaxique du lobe pariétal dans trois cas de syndrome douloureux consécutif a des plaies des nerfs. Destruction thérapeutique des fibres thalamopariétales au niveau du pied de la couronne rayonnante. Acta Neurochir. (Wien) **5,** 130

Talairach, J., Tournoux, P., Bancaud, J. (1960) Chirurgie pariétale de la douleur. Acta Neurochir. (Wien) **8,** 153

Walker, A. E. (1942b) Mesencephalic tractotomy. A method for the relief of unilateral intractable pain. Arch. Surg. **44,** 953

Weinberger, L. N., Grant, F. C. (1943) Experiences with intramedullary tractotomy II. Immediate and late neurologic complications. Arch. Neurol. Psychiat. (Chic.) **49,** 665

White, J. C., Smithwick, R. H. (1944) The autonomic nervous systems, anatomy, physiology and surgical applications, Kimpton, London p. 469

White, J. C., Sweet, W. H. (1955) Pain. Its mechanisms and neurosurgical control. Thomas, Springfield, Ill. p. 736

31

The surgeon and the difficult pain problem

Thomas P. Hackett

The difficult pain patient is characterized by three problems: (1) his pain persists despite medical and surgical attempts to cure it; (2) the stubborn persistence of the pain often suggests the possibility of emotional rather than physical causes; and (3) the pain discomfits the doctor nearly as much as his patient. The most common examples of such pain are low back pain, reflex dystrophies, atypical facial neuralgia, cervical brachial neuralgia, visceral pain of the chest and abdomen of uncertain etiology, and headache and nerve compression syndromes. The pain problems under discussion in this presentation include all these syndromes except pains secondary to malignancies.

Before a rational approach to the management of the difficult pain case can be outlined, certain misconceptions about chronic pain must be considered. There are three basic misconceptions that commonly interfere with the evaluation of long-standing pain:

1. We traditionally examine chronic pain with the indices used for acute pain. Consequently, we are not convinced that the patient suffers unless he appears to be in pain. The chronic pain patient does not behave like a person in acute pain. More often than not, he learns to appear to be reasonably comfortable with his suffering. As a consequence of this adaptation, those in close contact with him may come to doubt that his pain exists.

2. Chronic pain raises the immediate question of narcotic addiction. Physicians assume that all patients with chronic pain, requiring control by a narcotic, are soon to become addicts. Often, the doctor's goal shifts from relieving his patient's pain to withdrawing him from drugs.

3. Too many physicians lose sight of the nature of chronic pain in their enthusiasm to cure it. Although a total cure is desirable, it is not usually possible. Compromises must be made, especially in selecting cases for various types of surgery, or we risk damaging the patient irremediably, often with scant benefit to him in the way of pain relief.

As a result of the first factor, the patient whose pain is under investigation often ends up by feeling that he is on trial, that his probity is being tested. If the doctor-patient relationship has not been firmly established, it can be severely undermined by any insinuation that the patient may be imagining or exaggerating his discomfort. Furthermore, should a psychiatrist unexpectedly appear to complete the evaluation, insult is added to injury. First, the patient's honesty is questioned, and next his sanity undergoes psychiatric scrutiny.

NATURE OF CHRONIC PAIN

The fundamental difference between acute pain and chronic pain is that the latter can be endured and the former cannot. When pain persists over days, weeks, and months, a highly subjective change appears to occur either in the original sensation or in the way the sufferer feels it. The pain somehow becomes bearable without seeming to change in any other specific way. The longer it lasts, the less it comes to resemble acute pain. For example, the fearful affect which so often accompanies acute pain is absent in the chronic pain

Reprinted with permission of Little, Brown and Co. from The International Psychiatry Clinics 4:179-188.

case. The chronic pain patient is concerned but not obviously frightened. The autonomic signs of distress are absent or sharply modified in chronic pain.

In short, aside from what the chronic pain patient tells you, there is little in his manner to alert the examiner to his discomfort. Acute and chronic pain are widely separated conditions, even though they occupy the same spectrum of sensation. For the purpose of analogy, if we consider acute pain to be the model for pain, chronic pain can be thought of as its shadow. A shadow can closely resemble the primary object, but by shifting the position of the light source, the shadow can become larger or smaller, wider or narrower, than the object in any one of innumerable distortions.

It is practical and probably correct to view the experience of pain as containing two components [1, 4], the original sensation and the reactive component. The original sensation is what is felt as pain, and the reactive component is the psychological response to it. Henry Beecher [2] in his thorough and brilliant work on pain, explains the lack of effect morphine has on experimental pain in humans by using this concept. Pain that is produced in the laboratory contains no threat to the subject because he knows its origin and can control its intensity. As a consequence, its reactive component is weak. Morphine acts against the reactive component of pain. Since the pain produced by disease or injury always contains a threat to health, it responds to morphine because in this type of pain one can easily see that the psychological factors (reactive component) are more important. Cobb [3] felt that chronic pain was always initiated by a relatively acute type of pain which acted as a trigger mechanism to set off what he termed "reverberating circuits" between the thalamus and frontal lobes; once activated, they could be self sustaining even when the original sensation was absent. This is a particularly attractive model for conceptualizing chronic pain because it links the sensation to the peripheral nervous system, but anchors it rightly in the central neuraxis. Chronic pain is largely a factor of the reactive component and is probably cerebrally determined.

The vocabulary of pain is largely derived from the acute painful conditions. Pain is described essentially in three dimensions: quality (dull or sharp), anatomical location, and duration. The patient in acute pain has little or no difficulty in depicting his discomfort along these lines. Yet, the chronic pain sufferer often balks at such a mechanical breakdown of his pain because he cannot fit it satisfactorily into any conventional descriptive pattern. One has only to ask a person with phantom limb pain to give a detailed description of his sensations in the stump over a week's time to learn that we need a new lexicon for chronic pain. Over many months of suffering, pain becomes a state of mind. To inform another person of it demands some capacity for introspection and objectification. As every weary house officer knows, the chronic pain patient is apt to confuse accuracy with repetitiveness and exactness with the compulsive recall of insignificant details of his pain. Taking a case history from such a patient is often an exasperating task. Since a sizable number of these patients are able to write and are interested in doing so, I generally ask all chronic pain cases to write a personal account of their trouble. This technique can save time.

Running parallel to the patient's trouble in describing pain is the listener's difficulty in empathizing with the sufferer. Unlss the doctor has been through a siege of chronic pain himself, he generally finds it hard to understand the effect pain has on the sufferer. He may find it especially difficult to explain why his patient does not seem to be suffering. The next step is for him to question the pain's authenticity and to turn to more objective methods to appraise it.

Methods of detection

By and large, there are three ways in which this so-called objective evidence is obtained. The first is to ask nurses and relatives whether or not the patient appears to have genuine pain, the second is to give the patient a trial of placebos; and the third is to request a psychiatric evaluation. I would like to consider each of these methods separately.

Observations of nurse and family. Although it is a laudable gesture to ask a nurse for her opinion about a patient's state of mind, the physician must remember that this opinion is only as reliable as the nurse. The same holds true for relatives. Only when the nursing staff is well known to the doctor, and only when they have been especially trained in chronic pain techniques, can their judgments be relied upon.

Placebo trial. The proper use of placebo trials in the evaluation of pain ought to be the subject of a series of lectures in the medical school curriculum. It is difficult to think of a comparable subject, with the exception of hypnosis, about which there is so much misinformation circulating in the presence of a considerable body of fact. The most important fact about the placebo reaction is that it exists. Beecher and his coworkers [2] have demonstrated that it accounts for much of morphine's effectiveness in postoperative pain. The next most important fact is that, in order to use the placebo as an instrument in the evaluation of pain, its administration must be carefully controlled. It must be given to the patient in a randomized fashion along with the usual narcotic under double-blind conditions for at least two to four days. Without this type of control, the placebo trial is useless. The time-worn custom of slipping in a few shots of saline for Demerol and calling this deception a placebo trial demonstrates only the ignorance of the perpetrator. It also underlines the chief hazard of the placebo trial: the patient must be tricked. If he discovers that placebos have been used (as he generally does), it is natural for him to feel on trial and wrongly accused. Consequently, to avoid this, it is advisable to tell the patient beforehand that over the next few days his pain medication will be changed a number of times and different agents will be used, all in an attempt to assess his pain more closely. He should be further informed that neither the nurse nor the doctor will know what he has been given dose by dose until after the test is through. Depending upon the patient's intelligence and interest, a more complete or less detailed explanation can be offered. The point is to avoid trickery. The best way to do this is to include the patient in the plot.

The results of controlled placebo trials are apt to be disappointing in the evaluation of chronic pain, and may raise several questions. For example, is the person's pain more likely to be legitimate because he is not a placebo reactor? Would you consider him more seriously for surgery? If you did, your decision would have less precedent in the literature than you might imagine. The main value of the placebo trial is identification of the positive placebo reactor, and programming therapy along the lines of suggestion and support. I have also used the placebo trial method to determine the baseline narcotic requirement for conditions that are apt to need these drugs permanently.

The important thing to remember is that no device or test exists to verify the presence of pain, much less the degree of suffering. As a consequence, we are well advised by Wilder Penfield, who counsels us to consider every patient complaining of pain to be in pain. The only exception to this rule of thumb is the malingerer, and he can generally be identified without great trouble.

Psychiatric evaluation. The service of a psychiatrist is essential to the evaluation of chronic pain. He should be brought into the case early and should be introduced as a regular member of the medical team. The physician in charge should inform the patient that every pain case is seen by a psychiatrist just as each is examined by a neurologist. This approach, in my experience, is rarely resisted by patients. It is only when the psychiatrist is called in at the end of a long, frustrating, and unprofitable hospitalization that the patient balks and protests.

The psychiatrist's contribution to the evaluation is ostensibly simple. He should determine whether the patient falls into any one of the following categories: hysteria, malingering, compensation neurosis, depression, or schizophrenia. The psychiatrist should rule out the possibility that a serious mental disease may be masquerading as pain rather than focus on the psychodynamics of pain. Depression is the most difficult of the five psychiatric conditions to evaluate, because it is present in a reactive form in practically all patients with chronic pain. As a consequence, it is sometimes impossible to determine whether pain or depresssion is the primary condition. When this is the case, it is advisable to treat the depression before resorting to surgery.

The pitfall that snares the psychiatric consultant in pain cases is the senseless issue of separating the functional from the organic. Short of doing so along the broad lines advocated in the above paragraph, I have little more to suggest than to avoid the whole question. In any illness, the functional and the organic are so inextricably woven that they comprise the warp and woof of disease. To try to separate one from the other or even to consider them as possibly separate is unsound and unnecessary.

Use of narcotics in treatment of pain

The problem of narcotic addiction in the patient with chronic pain needs to be looked at with an eye to revising some of our prejudices. As a profession, we tend to stint on issuing narcotics, even in cases where the need is evident. It is difficult to trace the source of this frugality, but perhaps a portion of it stems from the fear that we will be duped by patients who are secret addicts or that any liberality will evoke criticism from our colleagues. Whatever the reason, the fact remains that we are too quick to act on the basis of our suspicions when pain patients ask us for narcotics. Although it is true that patients in chronic pain run a greater danger of becoming addicted, if only because of propinquity, in my experience this hazard becomes realized in only a small percentage of cases. Only 8 in my series of over 200 cases with chronic pain who have been on narcotics at one time or another have become addicted, as this term is used by Wikler et al. [5]. In each of the 8, the drug tolerance, and the consequent need for increasing doses, were evident early in the course of management.

It is probable that those individuals who are likely to become addicted can be spotted long before trouble begins. In sharp contrast to the small group who readily become addicted, there is a larger group who can remain on a moderate dose of a narcotic for years at a time, without developing a troublesome tolerance.

My point in bringing drugs into this discussion is only to minimize their importance in the evaluation of pain. When a patient with chronic pain states that he can't go on taking medication all his life, it is wise to tell him that he may be required to do so. Just as a diabetic needs to take insulin and the heart patient digitalis, so the chronic pain patient may require his anodyne. Quite often, when a patient does make a complaint, his doctor is apt to agree with him simply because the anodyne is a narcotic. The same physician will readily give vasodilators for anginal pain and cafergot for migraine, but will stop short at ordering codeine for another type of pain even though the patient has shown no tendency to addiction. There seems to be a moral bias implicit in dispensing narcotics.

What of the patient who is already addicted when he is admitted for evaluation of his pain? When this is the case, our first effort should be directed at finding out how the addiction developed, whether the patient has a long history of addiction, and whether it is iatrogenic. He should then be denarcotized, if this is possible, or at least switched to methadon. The majority of patients with chronic pain problems are not addicted, even though they may consume large amounts of a narcotic.

PAIN WHICH SHOULD NOT BE CURED

Although most physicians would agree that not all pain can be cured, only a much smaller number would concur with the proposal that not all pains should be cured. All of us have had experience with pain that defied therapeutic attempts to relieve it. If we learned not to respond to chronic pain with the urgency we do to acute pain, the patient would be the better for it. The patient's shibboleth, "Something must be done for this pain," should never be joined in chorus by the physician. In point of fact, we must admit that there are types of pain we can do nothing about, just as there are some illnesses we are powerless to help. Simply hearing that a specific cure does not exist often prepares the way for a patient to regard his pain differently. I think it is our duty in these cases to change the psychological set from cure to compromise. We can usually help such pain even if we can't cure it. In assessing the degree of desperation expressed by a given patient when told that his pain can't be cured by surgery, it is well to remember that the incidence of suicide is no higher in patients with chronic pain than it is in the general population.

Case history

A well-known case at our hospital exemplifies the type of pain that should not be cured. The man was a mechanic who sustained damage to his brachial plexus as the result of a motorcycle accident which occurred on the way to his wedding. He married nonetheless and had two children. He also had as extensive a series of pain operations as any patient I have ever known. The arm was amputated shortly after the accident. Phantom pain was present as soon as he came out of the anesthesia. The stump was revised and three neurectomies were done without success. A rhizotomy followed, and then another. Cordotomy was next on the list, followed by mesencephalic tractotomy. There was no change in his pain. He was given long drug trials on the phenothiazines, MAO inhibitors, and antidepressants, respectively, all without success. Hypnosis was attempted, but he was unable to be put in trance even though three experienced hypnotists tried. Six ECT's did nothing but dull his memory and intensify his phantom pain. A half year of intensive inpatient psychotherapy was no more successful than surgery. Radiofrequency leucotomy was next employed; bilateral lesions in the frontal white matter neither altered his personality in any detectable way nor modified his pain. Thalamic electrodes were next used in the dorsomedial nucleus and in other thalamic nuclei. One of these electrodes penetrated the midbrain, putting the patient in coma for two weeks. When he awoke the pain was there unchanged and it remained so even after parts of his thalamus were ablated. When the patient died, of an unrelated infection, four years after his motorcycle accident, we could not help but speculate what his life might have been if surgery had stopped after the first unsuccessful neurectomy. If he had been told then that we would help him adjust to the pain without resorting to surgery, he would probably have become depressed and spoken of suicide. He might have been openly angry with his physician and threatened to go elsewhere for medical help. (The latter is the usual rationalization we use to justify doing the procedure ourselves rather than have it done at some unsavory place where unscrupulous and possibly unhygienic practitioners will do anything for personal gain.) These are common responses, displayed by most pain patients when an anticipated procedure is denied them. They can be dealt with effectively in psychotherapy.

SUMMARY

The foregoing discussion suggests a few broad principles of management in the case of long-standing pain. To begin with, unless the role of surgery is so evident that no one would argue its necessity for treatment, it should be underemphasized, if anything, and the surgeon himself should play no greater part in the evaluation than the other specialists. The patient should be prepared to have a psychiatrist interview him, and this examination ought to be incorporated into the workup of every chronic pain case. Assuming that these cases are hospitalized for the period of evaluation, the use of placebo trials should be conducted by the psychiatrist or someone who is trained in their use. As has been mentioned earlier, chronic pain should be assessed by physicians and not by untrained nurses or interested third parties. The question of addiction is another issue and should not complicate the evaluation of an individual's pain. If the patient is already addicted when he comes in for evaluation, the emphasis must be shifted to determining the sources of his addiction and potential for readdiction before the pain itself is attacked. Finally, it is important to keep in mind that a cure does not exist for every pain, some do not require a cure and in other cases the patients may manage to carry on despite their pain. Too often, it is the doctor who insists on a cure, and damages the patient unnecessarily in the process.

REFERENCES

1. Beecher, H. K. Pain, placebos and physicians. *Practitioner* 189:141, 1962.
2. Beecher, H. K. *Measurements of Subjective Responses: Quantitative Effects of Drugs.* New York: Oxford University Press, 1959.
3. Cobb, S. *Emotions and Clinical Medicine.* New York: Norton, 1950. P. 243.
4. Strong, G. A. *Psychol. Rev.* 2:329, 1895.
5. Wikler, A. *Opiate Addiction.* Springfield, Ill.: Thomas, 1953.

SECTION EIGHT

Pain control associated with selected diseases

Section eight is concerned mainly with behavioral correlates and intervention in pain associated with disease. The readings in this section demonstrate the variety of approaches to the pain of disease even when organic tissue damage is evident.

As seen in the preceding section, no simple procedure for producing relief from chronic pain is available. Even the effectiveness of pharmacological intervention for pain is enhanced by appropriate behavorial control. Beecher (1959), for example, has reported that the greater the pain and anxiety concerning an operation, the more effective placebo treatment was. Under conditions of severe pain accompanied by a great deal of anxiety (inferred by Beecher), 40% of his patients found relief with placebos, whereas 52% found relief following injection of morphine. Under conditions of reduced severity of pain with less inferred anxiety, the same dose of morphine brought relief to 89%; the placebo affected only 26%. Beecher places the average effectiveness of placebos at 35% of patients obtaining relief from clinical pathological pain. Placebo relief undoubtedly is produced not so much by removing the sensory component of pain but mainly by reducing the input from the motivational-affective component of pain (Feather, Chapman, and Fisher, 1972).

Reduction of the motivational-affective component of pain can be achieved through a variety of means. In his review Melzack (1973) has included desensitization techniques enabling the patient to gain control, hypnotic suggestion, progressive relaxation, control of body function through biofeedback, attention distraction, and relief from depression.

When the effectiveness of any of these techniques is evaluated, it is important that one use adequate controls–laboratory study or double-blind techniques. Clinicians are not always willing to arrange controlled conditions when treating a given individual. The treatment per se usually is confounded in many ways, such as by interpersonal factors, patient expectations, and simultaneous administration of several drugs. Furthermore, professional training does not always prepare a clinician to deal with data collection. Friedson (1970) has described what he calls the development of the clinical mind in physicians. Whereas scientists use both specific phenomena to arrive at general principles of knowledge and general principles to apply to specific situations, physicians are interested in dealing with individuals, not groups. Therefore, they place a greater reliance on firsthand, clinical experience than on general rules. Arguments based on experience carry greater weight than scientific data.

A physician with a clinical mind is described as having the following characteristics:

1. He puts an emphasis on action, not knowledge.
2. He believes that whatever he does makes a difference, that it is better than no action at all.
3. He is a pragmatist; he relies on results, not theory.

4. He trusts firsthand experience more than abstract principles.
5. He puts an emphasis on uncertainty rather than on lawfulness.

Audioanalgesia is an illustration of how lack of thorough experimental evaluation led many astray. Gardner and Licklider (1959) and Gardner, Licklider, and Weisz (1960) effectively used music and white noise to suppress pain during 5,000 dental operatons. They proposed that the music promotes relaxation while the noise directly suppresses pain. Many dentists quickly followed the lead and purchased expensive noise and stereo equipment. According to Melzack's description (1973), with some dentists and on some patients the results were dramatic. However, with other patients it did not work at all. Many dentists became quickly disillusioned. In a controlled laboratory study Melzack, Weisz, and Sprague (1963) were able to demonstrate that auditory stimulation did not abolish pain. What it did (when accompanied by strong suggestion) was divert attention away from pain. Therefore, in the hands of a dentist who could relate well to his patients, it was effective. For dentists who could not build up expectations of effectiveness, it did not work.

When one is dealing with the pain of disease, preconceived notions on the part of staff and patients can affect the treatment. Loan and Morrison (Reading 32) review the evidence regarding postoperative pain. According to their review, the factors related to severity of pain include a patient's age, sex, physical status, site of operation, and surgical management. As measured by the amount of anesthetic given, a small reduction in the severity of postoperative pain appears to occur with age. However, Loan and Morrison point out that a staff bias could account for this finding; their willingness to give anesthesia appeared to decrease as the patients' advanced in age. Similarly, women received anesthetic earlier than men. Public ward patients received an average of 3.2 does of analgesic, whereas a comparable group of private patients received an average of 13.4 doses. The site of the operation seemed to be important. Upper abdominal surgery produced severer pain than lower abdominal surgery. For lower abdominal surgery as many as 52% of the patients studied did not require any anesthetic following surgery.

Pilowsky and Bond (Reading 37) studied 21 women and 15 men suffering from malignant disease. They recorded the number of times the patient asked for pain relief and the number of times the staff offered it on their own. Female patients were more likely than male patients to be provided drugs to reduce pain on staff initiative when these patients were very concerned about their pain and illness. Older patients were not given powerful analgesics as frequently and were not treated by the nursing staff on the staff's own initiative. Thus, relief from pain was more related to the staff's definition of what was appropriate than to the degree of illness. Treatment was determined by the patients' social characteristics.

Preparation for surgery has been credited with reducing the severity of postoperative outcomes. Egbert, Battit, Welch, and Bartlett (1964) prepared one group of patients by a preoperative visit. The patients were told about the preparation for anesthesia, the time and approximate duration of the operation, and that they would wake up in the recovery room. They were also told they would feel pain, how severe it might be, and how long it would last. The patients were reassured that feeling pain was normal after abdominal surgery and that they would be able to cope with the effects of the surgery through relaxation procedures, the use of a trapeze, and instructions on how to turn their bodies. They were also told that they could ask for medication if they needed it.

In comparison with a control group, the specially instructed patients requested significantly less narcotic following surgery and were sent home an average of 2.7 days earlier.

What were the crucial ingredients that went into the patient preparation? Janis

(1958) has emphasized anxiety. There is an optimal relationship between the amount of suffering expected and the amount obtained that seems to be conducive to a feeling of mastery over a difficult situation and to speeding recovery. The optimal degree of worry or anxiety prior to the stressful event is best reached when the patient receives realistic information and is able to listen to and accept what is being told to him. The credibility of the practitioner is enhanced, and the patient is helped to prepare for the event.

In his study of surgical patients, Janis (1958) identified three basic groups of surgical patients. The *very apprehensive group* had feelings of vulnerability to bodily damage both before and after surgery. They found it difficult to develop inner defenses to help cope with the threat of surgery. They could not sleep without sedation and would shrink with fear at routine postoperative procedures. Many of these patients had a history of neurotic disorder.

The second category of patients was the *group with little fear.* They felt calm and invulnerable, denying or minimizing the danger prior to surgery. With the inescapable pain of major surgery, they lost their calm and tended to blame the staff for their suffering. Adequate warning before surgery would have helped them to cope with postsurgical pain and stress.

The *moderately fearful group* asked for and received realistic information about what would happen. After surgery they were able to reassure themselves about their fears and felt secure.

These results, further supported by a second study of 150 college students, indicate that high-stress tolerance is associated with moderate anticipatory stress. The moderately fearful group had been better informed prior to surgery and felt worried before surgery. Fewer patients in this group became angry, resentful, or emotionally upset following surgery. They had time to build up psychological defenses prior to surgery. Janis has described a different sequence of events when the "work of worrying" is absent. There is little anticipatory fear. Thus, there is no mental rehearsal of the impending danger. The result is a feeling of helplessness when the danger manifests itself, and this feeling of helplessness results in feelings of disappointment in protective authorities, intense fear, anger, and "victimization"—the sense of deprivation, loss, and suffering from a stressful experience.

Unfortunately, subsequent studies have not supported Janis's emphasis on fear and anxiety. Cohen and Lazarus (Reading 33) emphasize the importance of coping strategies in dealing with the stress of surgery. Unlike Janis, they feel that denial would be a beneficial strategy to use when the outcome is expected to be positive.

Wolfer and Davis (Reading 34) also fail to confirm the relationship between anxiety and postsurgical recovery. Undoubtedly, many things are occurring when patients are being realistically informed. In the study by Egbert and others (1964), although patients were told of the pain, they were also instructed in how to cope with any difficulties. What the critical ingredients for reducing postsurgical pain are still requires greater classification. A period of advanced notice (Johnson, Dabbs, and Leventhal, 1970) with prior information and coping techniques however, does seem to help. (Additional discussion can be found in Section five.)

The problem of chronic pain is a more difficult one for the clinician. Many of the outward signs of acute pain are lacking, and as Hackett (Reading 31) points out, the physician is often at a loss for dealing with the pain; as a result the physician ends up questioning the sanity of his patient. The inability to deal with chronic pain also encourages patients to seek relief elsewhere, often from quacks who at least provide a sympathetic ear while relieving the patient of his money. These quacks can teach practitioners that there is more to medicine than surgery or simply prescribing another pill. Gordon (1966) has summarized the issue well.

> Why do people go to quacks? Repeatedly we have said that they go "seeking that which they have not found elsewhere." Perhaps the incurable may not be seeking a cure for their disease at all although they profess to be. Perhaps they are seeking sympathy, understanding, kindness, friendliness, and an attitude of concern on the part of someone. Admittedly the quack can't cure the disease, but he has for a brief time patched and soothed the patient's fractured ego and led the family to believe they have left no stone unturned in seeking the cure. I often believe that at an exorbitant fee, the patient and the quack play a game of make-believe, with each knowing that it is make-believe. But at this stage, the patient may consciously or unconsciously believe that it is better to play games than to stare at a gaping void into which he is about to step. The quack has nothing to sell but himself, but he sells himself well. Could the ethical practitioner of medicine learn a lesson from this? Should he not visualize himself in the patient's place when he explains his diagnosis and proposed course of treatment? (1966, p. 46)

Even though there is no cure for many types of pain problems, it is still possible to let the patient realize that he can be taught how to deal with what he has. Everything will be done to help him obtain as much as he can from life, even with his pain problem.

Pain reactions can become reinforced independently of the original physiological sensation and tissue damage. This finding was demonstrated by Fordyce, Fowler, and DeLateur (Reading 35) in their treatment of a woman who had suffered from back pain for 18 years. She had undergone 4 major surgical operations without relief. She was taking 4 or 5 habit-forming drugs each day and could not remain active continuously for more than 20 minutes without reclining. Treatment essentially involved breaking the contingency between the cry of pain and relief while at the same time reinforcing increased physical activity. At the end of 30 days she was able to maintain continuous out-of-bed activity for at least 2 hours. After her discharge from the hospital, she was able, with continuous outpatient visits, to maintain her increased activity level, and her complaints of pain ultimately ceased. Undoubtedly, pain relief did not eliminate the sensation of pain. Instead the patient was taught to cope and function despite her pain.

Moldofsky and Chester (Reading 39) point to another type of patient who requires help in coping with life. They conducted a study of patients with rheumatoid arthritis and found two basic mood patterns associated with pain. One group showed a positive association of joint tenderness and moods of hostility and anxiety. A second group, however, showed a paradoxical reaction with an inverse relationship between intensity of joint tenderness and mood. This latter group did not manage as well on a long-term basis. They felt despair regarding a future with the amelioration of their pain. They apparently achieved self-worth by being cared for when sick or helpless. This group probably would benefit from psychological help to allow them to cope with life.

Coping strategies can help bring pain relief. Woodforde and Fielding (Reading 36) point out that contrary to expectations, the incidence of severe intractable pain from cancer is low. Pain is frequently a concomitant of depression based on a feeling of hopelessness caused by not being able to deal with the disease. Pain can become an assurance of obtaining help and not being abandoned.

Greene and Laskin (Reading 40) have used different behavioral strategies in helping patients cope with myofascial pain-dysfunction syndrome (MPD). MPD patients show a high rate of placebo responsivity. Stress reactor patients respond well to physical treatment combined with a cognitive program, whereas psychoneurotics respond favorably to an interpersonal type of counseling.

Spear (Reading 41) has shown that pain is a common complaint in psychiatric patients. Treating the underlying symptoms seems to relieve the pain. Depression is very strongly related to pain, and antidepressants can provide relief.

This section emphasizes the large behavioral component associated with disease processes. Pain relief, too, can be obtained by utilizing behavioral strategies to help patients cope with their situations. Success may be based on helping the patient tolerate his pain rather than on relieving it.

REFERENCES

Beecher, H. K. 1959. Measurement of subjective responses: quantitative effects of drugs, Oxford University Press, Inc., New York.

Egbert, L. D., Battit, G. E., Welch, C. E., and Bartlett, M. D. 1964. Reduction of postoperative pain by encouragement and instruction of patients, The New England Journal of Medicine **270:**825-827.

Feather, B. W., Chapman, C. R., and Fisher, S. B. 1972. The effect of a placebo on the perception of painful radiant heat stimuli, Psychosomatic Medicine **34:**290-294.

Freidson, E. 1970. Profession of medicine, Dodd, Mead & Co., New York.

Gardner, W. J., and Licklider, J. C. R. 1959. Auditory analgesia in dental operations, Journal of the American Dental Association. **59:**1144-1149.

Gardner, W. J., Licklider, J. C. R., and Weisz, A. Z. 1960. Suppression of pain by sound, Science **132:** 32-33.

Gordon, W. H. 1966. Why people go to quacks. In: Proceedings of the Third National Congress on Medical Quackery, American Medical Association, Chicago.

Janis, I. L. 1958. Psychological stress, John Wiley & Sons, Inc., New York.

Johnson, J. E., Dabbs, J. M., and Leventhal, H. 1970. Psychosocial factors in the welfare of surgical patients, Nursing Research **19:**18-29.

Melzack, R. 1973. The puzzle of pain, Basic Books, Inc., Publishers, New York.

Melzack, R., Weisz, A. Z., and Sprague, L. T. 1963. Strategies for controlling pain: contributions of auditory stimulation and suggestion, Experimental Neurology **8:**239-247.

32

The incidence and severity of postoperative pain

W. B. Loan and J. D. Morrison

A knowledge of the natural history of postoperative pain is of importance in at least two respects. It will help the clinician, who finds its treatment is at present unsatisfactory. There is a pressing need for greater efficiency in meeting this problem (Editorial, 1953; Leading articles, 1964; Simpson and Parkhouse, 1961). In the field of research, the extent of the relief of postoperative pain has been much used in clinical trials designed to assay the efficacy of analgesic agents (Lee, 1942; Denton and Beecher, 1949; Masson, 1962; Parkhouse, 1967). To be meaningful, the design of such trials must take into consideration the various factors influencing the degree and course of postoperative pain.

Although incidence and severity are obviously closely related, these two facets of pain after operation will be dealt with separately.

INCIDENCE OF POSTOPERATIVE PAIN

There have been very few well-documented reports on the incidence of significant pain in patients following operation. Such as there are have been derived from data of patient demand for analgesic drugs in the postoperative period.

Jaggard, Zager and Wilkins (1950) found that, of a consecutive series of over 1,000 patients who had had general surgical or urological operations, 36 per cent had no need for any analgesic drug in the entire postoperative period.

Reprinted with permission of John Sherratt and Son Ltd. from the British Journal of Anaesthesia **39:**695-698. Copyright 1967.
From the Department of Anaesthetics, The Queen's University of Belfast, Northern Ireland.

Papper, Brodie and Rovenstine (1952) reported that after laparotomy or thoracotomy, 23 per cent of patients did not require any analgesia, while this proportion increased to 49 per cent in patients who had had superficial operations. Keats, Beecher and Mosteller (1950) found that 21 per cent of 104 patients who had had abdominal surgery required either one only or no dose of opiate postoperatively.

In a much more detailed study of the incidence of pain following operation, Parkhouse, Lambrechts and Simpson (1961) analyzed the data from a series of almost 1,000 general surgical patients. They found that the proportion of patients requiring analgesia in the postoperative period correlated closely with the site of the operation, as follows: gastric and gall bladder surgery, 95 per cent; upper abdominal operations, 82 per cent; appendicectomy, 75 per cent; inguinal herniorrhaphy, 48 per cent; neck and superficial head operations, 55 per cent; minor chest wall and scrotal operations, 20 per cent. They were unable to demonstrate any differences between the sexes in these groups, but did find that the proportion of patients requiring pain relief was less in the over-50 age group.

Loan and Dundee (1967) in a series of 1,220 general surgical patients also found that in the immediate postoperative period the proportion of patients requiring relief of pain depended on the site of operation. Their incidence of patients requiring analgesics was as follows: thoracotomy, 74 per cent; upper abdominal operations, 63 per cent; lower abdominal operations (excluding gynaecological operations), 51 per cent; inguinal operations, 23 per cent;

body wall operations, 20 per cent; limb operations, 27 per cent; neck operations, 12 per cent.

SEVERITY OF POSTOPERATIVE PAIN

Bonica (1953) listed the various factors which may influence the severity of postoperative pain as the personality of the patient himself, his age, sex and physical status, site of operation, and surgical management. To these, Simpson and Parkhouse (1961) added conditioning, fatigue, fear, and nausea, along with discomfort from such things as abdominal distension, drainage tubes and dressings.

As with incidence, almost all reported data on degrees of severity of pain in the postoperative period have been related to the patients' needs for analgesics. It is, therefore, apparent that in this type of assessment severity and duration of pain are frequently inseparable. Where results are stated in terms of total analgesic requirement in the postoperative period both of these factors contribute to the result, albeit in unknown proportions.

Age

Keats, Beecher and Mosteller (1950) were unable to find any relationship between the age of the patient and the analgesic requirement. Pratt and Welch (1955) reported that the requirement for postoperative analgesia lessened with increasing years, but these authors also admitted to being rather more cautious in administering opiates to the older age groups. Parkhouse, Lambrechts and Simpson (1961) found a small but significant reduction in analgesic requirements in patients over 50 years of age as compared with those under 50.

Sex

It is not always easy to compare groups of postoperative patients with respect to sex distribution, because of the bias of the different types of operation. For example, it has been suggested that gynaecological patients may react quite differently to patients having other lower abdominal operations (Parkhouse, personal communication). Keats, Beecher and Mosteller (1950) found no difference in the postoperative analgesic requirements of patients of different sex groups. Parkhouse, Lambrechts and Simpson (1961) were also unable to demonstrate any statistical difference between the sexes in the total requirement for analgesics following operation, but stated that there was a tendency for female patients to receive the drugs earlier. Swerdlow, Murray and Daw (1963) reported that female patients obtained more prolonged pain relief from a single dose of analgesic drug than did comparable male patients.

Site of operation

Keats (1956) found that in respect to total postoperative analgesic requirements there were no statistically significant differences between comparable groups of patients who had been subjected to the operations of cholecystectomy, gastrectomy, pyelolithotomy, pneumonectomy, colectomy or hysterectomy. On the other hand, Parkhouse, Lambrechts and Simpson (1961) found a very high degree of correlation between the severity of the pain (again judged by total postoperative analgesic requirements) and the site of the operation. Most postgastrectomy patients required three or four injections of analgesic drug at all. They also showed that the lower abdominal surgery required one or two injections; after appendicectomy only one injection was required; 50 per cent of herniorrhaphy patients required no analgesic drug at all. They also showed that the interval between the end of the operation and the demand for analgesics was shortest in those groups which required the greatest amount of analgesia, i.e. there was a short interval in the case of upper abdominal operations, and a much longer average interval in the case of herniorrhaphies. Swerdlow, Starmer and Daw (1964) found that patients who had had upper abdominal operations required a greater amount of analgesia, and obtained less prolonged relief from any single dose, than did patients who had had lower abdominal operations.

One of the authors (Loan, 1967) attempted to obtain a direct correlation of the severity of pain with the site of the operation, not by reference to the patients' ultimate need for analgesics but by having the patients estimate the degree of pain in the immediate postoperative period before any analgesic had been administered. The results were recorded on a five-point scale (most severe pain = 4, no pain = 0). After upper abdominal operations the mean score was 3.45 pain units (SE 0.039) and after lower abdominal operations the mean score was 3.10 pain units (SE 0.036).

Environment

It has been shown that the experimental pain threshold is altered by such diverse factors as distraction, anxiety, fear, prejudice and suggestion (Hardy, Wolff and Goodell, 1940; Hill et al., 1952) and although there are no comparable documented findings in respect to postoperative pain severity it is not unreasonable to expect that similar factors, dependent to a large degree on his immediate environment and the general attitudes of those attending him, will affect the reaction component of the pain in the postoperative period and thus will exert considerable influence on the severity of the patient's total pain experience (Simpson and Parkhouse, 1961). Parkhouse, Lambrechts and Simpson (1961), however, found little difference in the incidence and severity of postoperative pain within the general surgical wards of one hospital, although one of the same authors (Parkhouse, 1967) did give data which seemed to indicate differences between similar surgical units in different hospitals. Keats (1956) has presented evidence of considerable differences in analgesic requirements in different wards within one hospital complex. Public ward patients received an average of 3.2 doses of analgesic drug postoperatively whilst a comparable group of private patients in single rooms received an average of 13.4 doses. These results probably reflect differences in the attitudes of the attendants of these two groups of patients as well as any differences attributable to variation in severity and incidence of pain.

Patient

Psychic factors affecting the patient's personality and emotional state apart from those directly connected with the patient's environment may also exert considerable influence on the severity of postoperative pain. Roe (1963) reported that the usual total requirement of "50-100" mg morphine in the entire postoperative period was reduced to an average requirement of 4 mg by pre-operative instruction of the patient in relaxation and what to expect postoperatively, coupled with constant postoperative encouragement and reassurance. Egbert et al. (1964) found that pre-operative encouragement and instruction in a group of 97 patients having intra-abdominal operations reduced the requirement for analgesia by 50 per cent in comparison to a similar control group who had had no such pre-operative conditioning.

The effects of heightened emotional states due to fear and excitement have not been investigated with respect to postoperative pain. In traumatic wound pain, however, Beecher (1956) showed that there was a significantly lower requirement for analgesics in a group of recently wounded soldiers compared to a matched group of men with similar wounds sustained under civilian conditions. He suggested that the difference was largely accounted for by the reaction of the patient to the differing significance of the injury, the recently wounded soldier frequently being euphoric about his escape from the battlefield. It is also commonly found that injuries sustained in states of heightened emotional activity often pass unnoticed by the recipient at the time of his injury (Beecher, 1959). Petrie (1960) states that the previous personality of the patient has an effect on his attitudes to pain, and Malmo (1954), claims that continuing psychological stress affects the ability of the patient to tolerate pain.

Premedication and anaesthesia

Especially where analgesic agents are used, premedication and anaesthetic drugs could be expected to exert considerable influence on the course of postoperative pain. Gravenstein and Beecher (1957), in a series of 54 patients, one half of whom was given as premedication 10 mg of morphine and the other half saline, found that the requirement for postoperative analgesia was quantitatively similar in both groups, but that the request for the initial postoperative administration was delayed in the group who had had the opiate premedication. Pratt and Welch (1955) found no difference in postoperative analgesic requirements in patients who had had either an opiate or a barbiturate as premedication. Parkhouse, Lambrechts and Simpson (1961) found that where anaesthetic agents with marked analgesic properties, such as trichloroethylene and diethyl ether, were used in gastric operations there was a significant tendency for less analgesia to be required in the postoperative period, and that the time interval to the first postoperative injection was increased. The postoperative "analgesia" which is believed to follow methoxyflurane anaesthesia, however, may merely reflect the slow recovery after this drug. Several authors have also commented on the reduction of the total requirement for postoperative analgesia, and an increase in the interval between operation and first analgesic administration, where opiates have been used during operation to supplement anaesthesia (Corssen, Domino and Sweet, 1964; Martin et al., 1967).

In a series of 55 matched pairs of patients, one in each pair was given 2 mg levorphanol at the time of induction of anaesthesia. It was then found that 82 per cent of the levorphanol group did not require any analgesic in the first 6 postoperative hours compared with only 11 per cent in the control group. The average total analgesic requirement in the first 24 hours after operation was 19.5 mg methadone (2.3 injections) in the levorphanol group, and 29.0 mg methadone (3.7 injections) in the control group (Dundee, Brown and Hamilton, personal communication).

• • •

It will be apparent from this brief review that many aspects of these complicated relationships remain unexplored, and that further detailed investigation must benefit both the clinician and the research worker.

ACKNOWLEDGEMENT

The work of both Dr. Morrison and Dr. Loan in the Department of Anaesthetics at the Queen's University of Belfast is supported by Medical Research Council grants.

REFERENCES

Beecher, H. K. (1956). Relationship of the significance of wound to the pain experienced. *J. Amer. med. Ass.*, **161**, 1609.

——— (1959). *Measurement of Subjective Responses*, ch. 9. New York: Oxford University Press.

Bonica, J. J. (1953). *The Management of Pain*, 1st ed. London: Henry Kimpton.

Corssen, G., Domino, E. F., and Sweet, R. B. (1964). Neuroleptanalgesia and anesthesia. *Curr. Res. Anesth.*, **43**,748.

Denton, J. E., and Beecher, H. K. (1949). New analgesics. I: Methods in the clinical evaluation of new analgesics. *J. Amer. med. Ass.*, **141**, 1051.

Editorial (1953). Reduction of postoperative pain. *Brit. med. J.*, **2**, 385.

Egbert, L. D., Battit, G. E., Welch, C. E., and Bartlett, M. K. (1964). Reduction of postoperative pain by encouragement and instruction of patients. *New Engl. J. Med.*, **270**, 825.

Gravenstein, J. S., and Beecher, H. K. (1957). The effect of preoperative medication with morphine on postoperative analgesia with morphine. *J. Pharmacol.*, **119**, 506.

——— Smith, G. M., Sphire, R. D., Isaacs, J. P., and Beecher, H. K. (1956). Dihydrocodeine: further development in measurement of analgesic power and appraisal of psychologic side effects of analgesic agents. *New Engl. J. Med.*, **254**, 877.

Hardy, J. D., Wolff, H. G., and Goodell, H. (1940). Studies on pain: a new method of measuring pain threshold; observations on spatial summation of pain. *J. clin. Invest.*, **19**, 649.

Hill, H. E., Kornetsky, C. H., Flanary, H. G., and Wikler, A. (1952). Effects of anxiety and morphine on discrimination of intensities of painful stimuli, *J. clin. Invest.*, **31**, 473.

Jaggard, R. S., Zager, L. L., and Wilkins, D. S. (1950). Clinical evaluation of analgesic drugs: a comparison of Nu-2206 and morphine sulphate administered to postoperative patients. *Arch. Surg. (Chicago)*, **61**, 1073.

Keats, A. S. (1956). Postoperative pain, research and treatment. *J. chron. Dis.*, **4**, 72.

——— Beecher, H. K., and Mosteller, F. C. (1950). Measurement of pathological pain in distinction to experimental pain. *J. appl. Physiol.*, **1**, 35.

Leading article (1964). Postoperative pain. *Lancet*, **1**, 751.

——— (1964). Relief of postoperative pain. *Lancet*, **2**, 188.

Lee, L. E. (1942). Studies of morphine, codeine and their derivatives. XVI: Clinical studies of morphine, methyldihydromorphinone (Metopon) and dihydrodesoxymorphine-D (Desmerphine). *J. Pharmacol. exp. Ther.*, **75**, 161.

Loan, W. B. (1967). A comparative study of some drugs used systemically in the relief of pain. M. D. Thesis. The Queen's University of Belfast.

——— Dundee, J. W. (1967). The clinical assessment of pain. *Practitioner*, **198**, 759.

Malmo, R. B. (1954). Higher functions of the nervous system. *Ann. Rev. Physiol.*, **16**, 371.

Martin, S. J., Murphy, J. D., Colliton, R. J., and Zeffiro, R. G. (1967). Clinical studies with Innovar. *Anesthesiology*, **28**, 458.

Masson, A. H. B. (1962). Clinical assessment of analgesic drugs. 2: Observer trial. *Anaesthesia*, **17**, 411.

Papper, E. Brodie, B. B., and Rovenstine, E. A. (1952). Postoperative pain: its use in the comparative evaluation of analgesics. *Surgery*, **32**, 107.

Parkhouse, J. (1967). Subjective assessment of analgesics. *Anaesthesia*, **22**, 37.

——— Lambrechts, W., and Simpson, B. R. J. (1961). The incidence of postoperative pain. *Brit. J. Anaesth.*, **33,** 345.

Petrie, A. (1960). Some psychological aspects of pain and the relief of suffering. *Ann. N. Y. Acad. Sci.*, **86,** 13.

Pratt, J. H., and Welch, J. S. (1955). Hyatrobal and methadone hydrochloride in preoperative preparation of patients. *J. Amer. med. Ass.*, **157,** 231.

Roe, B. B. (1963). Are postoperative narcotics necessary? *Arch. Surg. (Chicago)*, **87,** 912.

Simpson, B. R. J., and Parkhouse, J. (1961). The problem of postoperative pain. *Brit. J. Anaesth.*, **33,** 336.

Swerdlow, M., Murray, A., and Daw, R. H. (1963). A study of postoperative pain. *Acta anaesth. scand.*, **7,** 1.

——— Starmer, G., and Daw, R. H. (1964). A comparison of morphine and phenazocine in postoperative pain. *Brit. J. Anaesth.*, **36,** 782.

33

Active coping processes, coping dispositions, and recovery from surgery

Frances Cohen, MA, and Richard S. Lazarus, PhD

Clinical workers have long observed that surgical patients under roughly comparable medical conditions differ greatly in the course of postsurgical recovery. One of the psychological explanations of this variation is based on personality-related and hospital-induced differences in the modes of coping with stress (1-5). Questions about the role of coping have major theoretical as well as practical implications. From the practical standpoint, knowledge about the relevant coping processes, and the personality factors associated with them, could ultimately contribute greatly to improved patient care; for example, it may be possible to intervene selectively with suitable communications designed to facilitate coping.

From the theoretical standpoint, we must consider, among other things, the mechanisms by which coping styles and the course of recovery from surgery might be linked. One such link is via the relations between coping and stress or emotion. Some types of coping activities reduce or short-circuit stress reactions by modifying stress-induced threat appraisals (6) (see also, Lazarus, Averill, and Opton (7) for a recent review), and others presumably provide an opportunity for anticipatory coping, that is, for working out prior to an impending crisis the harms and threats to be faced (1, 8). It is assumed in such analyses that the course of postsurgical recovery would be related to the increase or decrease of psychological stress during this period.

Evidence suggesting a possible physiological link between stress and bodily illness has been reported (9-13). Another possibility, more psychological in nature, is that the course of recovery is not only a matter of physical healing and the return of strength and energy, but involves a complex of behavioral events which could be influenced by coping styles, for example, complaints of pain, use of tranquilizers, use of pain medication, willingness to get out of bed and move around, response to the suggestion that the patient is ready to leave the hospital shortly, etc. The various elements of the recovery process have not been carefully analyzed and they probably include physiological, behavioral, and social events operating in a complex chain of causation.

The present study focused mainly on the relationship between individual differences in coping and the course of recovery. No plans were made to intervene experimentally in the patients' situation, although there has been evidence that such inter-

Reprinted with permission of the Americian Psychosomatic Society, Inc., from Psychosomatic Medicine **35**:375-389. Copyright 1973.
From the Department of Psychology, University of California, Berkeley.
The research reported here was supported in part by a research grant (MH-2136) from the National Institute of Mental Health. Financial support for the senior author was provided by a predoctoral traineeship from the Rehabilitation Services Administration (Grant No. RH4), and to the junior author through a Miller Professorship at the University of California, Berkeley.
Part of this research was presented at the Western Psychological Association Convention, Los Angeles, California, April, 1970.

vention can facilitate recovery (2, 3), depending on the patient's original coping dispositions (4, 5). Rather, we wanted to assess further the role of individual differences in coping and their importance in affecting surgical recovery. In particular, two approaches to coping activity were compared—dispositional measures and measures of ongoing coping activity.

Among the coping styles most commonly assessed by personality researchers is the dimension of repression-sensitization (14, 15), and the closely related concepts of repression-isolation (e.g., Ref. 16), and avoidance-coping (17). The latter dimension was employed, for example, in Andrew's (4) and DeLong's (5) research with surgical patients. Although these diverse assessment approaches to theoretically similar concepts have not been linked empirically (18), and may, therefore, represent different psychological processes (19), all three appear to deal with a general type of coping activity, avoidance versus vigilance, which could have an important bearing on the way a patient manages stressful events prior to and following surgery.

The above measures of coping style are all basically *dispositional,* that is, prior to a stressful event they assess the disposition or tendency in the person to use one or another coping process. Whether or not an avoider will actually display avoidance behavior in a given stress situation depends on the generality of the disposition and the relevance of that stress situation to the coping disposition (20). However, one can also study coping more directly in the very stress situation which calls for it. That is, by observing the person who is faced with stressful demands, measures can be obtained of the *active coping processes* being employed. It is of great theoretical and practical interest simultaneously to examine the patterns of relationship between such dispositional measures and measures of active coping obtained on the spot, as well as their relationship to recovery from surgery (or any other adaptive outcome). The central focus of this study of patient coping and recovery from surgery is, therefore, centered on comparisons of dispositional and active coping measures in such recovery.

METHOD

Subjects

Sixty-one surgical patients (22 male, 39 female) between the ages of 21 and 60 ($\bar{X}$= 39.9, SD = 11.1) were studied.[1] They had entered the Kaiser Foundation Hospital in Hayward, California between November 5, 1968 and May 7, 1969 for elective operations for hernia (22), gall bladder (29), and thyroid (10) conditions. Patients who had previously had an operation of the same type were excluded from the sample.

In this sample, each of the 10 thyroid patients (age range 22-49, all female) had an admitting diagnosis of a nontoxic thyroid nodule. No cancer of the thyroid was present and final diagnoses included chronic thyroiditis, colloid adenoma with degeneration, involutionary nodule (4), thyroid adenoma, nodular colloid goiter, follicular adenoma, and parathyroid cyst. Admitting and final diagnoses for the hernia patients were similar with one exception. Diagnoses included 18 patients with left or right inguinal hernia, left inguinal hernia with lipoma of the spermatic cord, or right femoral hernia (age range 27-58, 15 male, 3 female), 2 with bilateral inguinal hernia (age range 34-49, 1 male, 1 female), and one (age 40, male) with an admitting diagnosis of left inguinal hernia and a final diagnosis of sliding left inguinal hernia (with incarceration of sigmoid colon).

Admitting diagnoses for the gall bladder patients, excluding the 2 eliminated because of serious complications (as explained below), included 6 with cholecystitis (age range 26-52, 1 male, 5 female), 20 with cholelithiasis, cholelithiasis with cholecystitis, or cholecystitis with calculi (age range 22-56, 2 male, 18 female), one (age 21, female) with cholelithiasis (probably choledocholithiasis with obstructive jaundice), and one with hiatal hernia (age 32, male). The latter patient was included in the gall bladder category upon the advice of the physician, since the severity of the surgical procedure and the postoperative course were most comparable to that of a gall bladder operation. Diagnoses changed following surgery for 6 of the patients, resulting in one patient with a final diagnosis

[1]Patients over 60 years old were excluded because of the greater chance of complications due to age.

of cholecystitis (age 27, female), 24 with cholelithiasis, cholelithiasis with cholecystitis, or cholecystitis with calculi (2 male, 22 female), one with chronic cholecystitis, cholelithiasis, obstructive jaundice, one with chronic cholecystitis, cholelithiasis, choledocholithiasis, cholecystoduodenal fistula (age 44, male), and one with hiatal hernia (with hiatal hernioplasty, vagotomy, Finney pyloroplasty, and gastrostomy performed).

Procedure

Each patient in the sample was approached individually by the senior author, and asked if he or she would participate in a program of research.[2] All those accepting were interviewed in the hospital the afternoon or early evening of the day before their operation, approximately 1-3 hrs. after being admitted. In the interview (which was tape-recorded, and usually lasted 10-15 min.), questions were asked about the patient's emotional state, what he knew about his operation, what other information he wanted to know, etc., questions based on the procedures developed by Janis (1).

Following the interview, Andrew's (4) version of the Goldstein coper-avoider Sentence Completion Test (SCT) was administered, some general background questions were asked concerning education and occupation, and two pencil and paper tests were given, namely, the Epstein and Fenz (21) modified Repression-sensitization scale (modified R-S), and the Holmes and Rahe (22) Schedule of Recent Experiences (SRE). In a few instances where the experimenter felt it was in the patient's best interest to terminate the interview session (e.g., due to an excessively long interview that was interfering with the duties of the medical staff), the SRE was not given. Occasionally the patient terminated the interview session himself by refusing to continue to fill out questionnaires.[3]

[2]Three subjects were lost by refusal. Two subjects were lost because their operations were cancelled for medical reasons. These subjects are not included in the totals listed above.

[3]Some patients rejected the SCT as being too personal, too difficult, too time-consuming, or as something they did not feel like answering. Although encouraged, patients were not forced to continue if they did not want to.

Thus, full questionnaire data were not obtained on every patient, and as a result, the N's vary slightly for different measures. While the patient was filling out the questionnaires, the interviewer took notes on the patient's behavior and general demeanor, and made two ratings, one on his use of avoidant and vigilant coping mechanisms, and another on anxiety, as explained later.

Control data were also obtained on a different sample of patients (N = 101) by examining the hospital records of the thyroid, gall bladder, and hernia operations performed by each of the four participating surgeons over the 6 months to 1 year prior to the start of the present research. These data were collected in order to test differences on several subsidiary variables, such as whether the surgeons as individuals contributed significantly to their patients' course of recovery. These control patients were not interviewed or tested; however, recovery measures were obtained for them as with the group that was interviewed and tested.

Recovery index

This index was devised using a modified version of the criteria employed by Andrew (4) in her study.[4] Four separate measures were obtained, namely, number of days in the hospital, number of pain medications, number of minor complications, and number of negative psychological reactions. They were also summed to give a fifth variable which is more or less

[4]The minor complications category was greatly revised, omitting variables which did not reflect medical complications or which had no psychological implications (for example, the number of intravenous feedings), and weighing certain complications somewhat differently from Andrew. Minor complications were totalled as follows: inability to void, requires catheterization (2 points); inability to move bowels, enema given (2); nausea (1); nausea requiring medication (2); nausea plus vomiting plus medication (2); slight headache (1); severe headache, persistent (2); discomfort requiring hot water bottle (1); discomfort requiring ice pack (1); rectal tube for gas (1); routine postoperative antibiotics (1); antibiotics given to combat fever and infection (3); medication to prevent constipation or for urine stimulation (1); antacids given (1); medication given to counteract tetany (calcium gluconate) in thyroid operations (3); medication for diarrhea and/or gut irritability (1); medication (Aminophylline) for bronchial spasms (2); cough medication given when there was no fever (1); and nurse's observations that patient looked pale, dizzy, weak, etc. (1).

equivalent to Andrew's recovery index. *Number of days in the hospital* requires no further explanatory comment. In the case of *pain medications,* analgesics and sedatives were both included. *Minor complications* included treatment for slight medical difficulties, such as fever and infection or bronchial spasms, and symptoms thought to be common manifestations of conversion reactions, such as nausea, inability to void, inability to move bowels, and headache (23). Anyone with serious complications, such as wound dehiscence (i.e. wound reopening), atelectasis (i.e. lung collapse), pneumonia, rehospitalization with high fever, and hypocalcemia (i.e. deficiency of calcium in the blood) after a thyroid operation, was excluded from the analysis, since the additional medical problem would interfere with a clear evaluation of the patient's recovery. The category of *negative psychological reactions* included such things as complaints by the patient and the number of tranquilizers given.

It should be pointed out that the three types of operations used are heterogeneous—that is, the medical characteristics and severity of each varies. (Each has a differing course of recovery, with gall bladder patients, for example, staying more days in the hospital, etc.) On the other hand, the three operative groups did not differ to any significant extent in the proportion of patients in each of the 3 avoidant-vigilant groups. Due to the heterogeneity in the course of recovery for each operation, however, standard scores were employed as follows to equate for these differences.

Each patient's five recovery indexes were separately transformed for each operation into a T-score distribution with a mean of 50 and a standard deviation of 10, thereby transforming the range of scores within each type of operation to a common scale. Thus, a recovery score falling at the mean for the gall bladder patients and one at the mean for hernia patients will each be given a score of 50, regardless of the fact that gall bladder patients as a group take longer to recover. This statistical procedure, designed precisely for this sort of situation, allows us to talk in general about the effect of psychological coping activity on recovery from surgery without the results being distorted by the type of medical condition and the divergent surgical procedures.

Process ratings

These refer to several on-the-spot assessments of how the patient was coping with and reacting to the surgical threat. There were three such assessments: a rating of mode of coping, anxiety as judged by the interviewer, and anxiety as rated by the patient.

Mode of coping. Avoidance and vigilance, as judged from the interview data, were treated as a dimension, and rated on a scale from 1 to 10, with high ratings (8-10) implying vigilant modes, low ratings implying avoidant modes (1-3), and a middle group (4-7) designed for patients emphasizing neither one nor the other. The rating was made by listening to tape recordings of the interviews, by the interviewer, as well as by an advanced clinical psychology graduate student,[5] so that reliability could be assessed. The correlation between the two sets of independent ratings was +0.878.

Avoidance and vigilance[6] were based on the following general characterizations:

Avoidance. The patient shows avoidance or denial of emotional or threatening aspects of the upcoming medical experience, as indicated by restriction of knowledge or awareness about the medical condition for which surgery was recommended, the nature of the surgery, and the postsurgical outlook, and by unwillingness to discuss thoughts about the operation.

Vigilance. The patient is overly alert to emotional or threatening aspects of the upcoming medical experience, as indicated by the seeking out of knowledge about the medical condition, the nature of the surgery, and the postsurgical outlook, and by the readiness to discuss thoughts about the operation.

An example from a response considered avoidant is, "All I know is that I have a hernia. . . . I just took it for granted . . . doesn't disturb me one bit. . . . have no

[5]Warren Gould, University of California, Berkeley.

[6]No distinction between the concepts of defense and coping was made (e.g., Ref. 24).

thoughts at all about it." An example from a vigilant response is, "[after a detailed description of the medical problem and the operation's procedure] . . . I have all the facts, my will is prepared. . . . it is major surgery . . . It's a body opening . . . you're put out, you could be put out too deep, your heart could quit, you can have shock. . . . I go not in lightly."[7]

The middle group were those who gave evidence of both avoidant and vigilant modes of coping.

The distribution of scores on this dimension of coping had a mean of 5.51, and a standard deviation of 2.22. Twenty-three percent of the patients (N = 14) were classed as avoiders, 16% as vigilant copers (N = 10), and 61% as falling in the middle group (N = 37). No strong differences were found among these coping groups with respect to the type of surgery they underwent, their sex, or social class as assessed by Warner's (25) revised scale for rating occupations.

Anxiety. The interviewer rated the amount of anxiety shown by the patient on a scale from 1-10, based on verbal and nonverbal cues such as jitteriness, nervous laughter, tremulousness, and rapid or impaired speech. It was impractical to obtain an independent set of ratings to check reliability, but these data are reported nonetheless. This distribution of anxiety ratings had a mean of 4.38 and a standard deviation of 2.23. On the basis of these scores, patients were divided into groups, with 51% (N = 31) classed as low anxiety, 13% (N = 8) as high anxiety, and 36% (N = 22) in the medium group.

In addition, a self-rating of anxiety was also obtained from each patient by having him respond to the following question as employed by Janis (1): "How worried or concerned about your operation are you? If I asked you to rate yourself on a 10-point scale, with 1 being not very worried or concerned at all and 10 being very worried or upset about your operation, where would you put yourself, from 1 to 10?" The resulting distribution of these self-ratings had a mean of 3.69, and a standard deviation of 2.76. Fifty-seven percent were classified as low anxiety (N = 35), 15% as high (N = 9) and 28% as medium (N = 17). The correlation between interviewer-rated anxiety and self-rated anxiety was +0.455 ($p < 0.01$).

Dispositional measures

These included a special form of the Goldstein Sentence-Completion Test of coping disposition (4), a modified version [by Epstein and Fenz (21)] of the Byrne scale of repression-sensitization, and the Schedule of Recent Experiences as developed by Holmes and Rahe (22).

SCT coping disposition scores. This test consists of a series of sentence-completion stems, the responses to which are scored for "avoidance" if the emotional content of the stem is not acknowledged by the person, or for "coping" (sensitizing or vigilant modes) if the person accepts the emotional content, elaborates it and relates it to himself. Some examples of the items are: "My greatest fear is . . .", and "Sexual intercourse would be better if. . . ." *S*'s

[7]Many detailed criteria were used in determining the process rating, and a clinical judgment was made for each patient based on his total interview responses. For example, knowledge of any of the following kinds of information put a person closer to the vigilant end of the dimension: a description of the medical problem (including etiology), the risks if surgery were not performed, the nature of the hospital experience, the operation's procedure, medical problems which could occur during the operation, the expected general course of postoperative recovery, possible postoperative complications, and the possibility of recurrence of the medical condition. Patients who stated they had sought information beyond what their doctor had told them were also placed toward the vigilant end.

Lack of knowledge about the medical condition put the person closer to the avoidance end, as did statements that he had no thoughts at all about his operation and had not discussed it with anyone, that he did not want to know anything about it, denial that an operation was anything to be concerned about, and unusually positive statements ("having an operation is like having a vacation").

Categorizing patients as "vigilant" implies either that they sought out information about their operation or that they were sensitized (in terms of noting and remembering) to information when it was discussed, or both. It was difficult to separate out these two processes; from the interview data it appeared they usually occurred together, and our assumption is that they are related aspects of a vigilant mode. Similarly, we were not able to determine if those classed in the avoider group were unwilling to recall information, or to discuss it, or if they simply did not know certain things. Since all the surgeons had given information preoperatively as usual, we have assumed that there was avoidant activity in these patients, either in recall or in discussion.

are divided into coping types depending on whether they display predominantly a "coping" or vigilant pattern of responses, an avoidant pattern, or fall in between the two extremes, thus being classed as "nonspecific defenders."

In scoring this test, the method reported in Andrew (4) was followed. Dividing points (upper and lower 25%) for the three types of coping were determined separately for males and females, following Goldstein's (17) recommendations, since in his data and ours there was a difference between the distributions by sex. With a possible scoring range from 0 to 80, cutoff points were as follows: for females, 24-39 for avoiders, 42-50 for nonspecific defenders, and 53-64 for copers; for males, 15-30 for avoiders, 33-45 for nonspecific defenders, and 47-51 for copers. A second judge independently scored the SCT's, yielding a reliability of +0.926.

Modified R-S coping disposition scores. Epstein and Fenz developed a modification of the Byrne scale in order to eliminate some of the overlap between repression-sensitization and anxiety (e.g. Refs. 26, 27). Byrne himself admits that the correlations between his MMPI-derived scale, the Taylor Scale of Manifest Anxiety, and the Edwards Social Desirability Scale are generally around +0.90 (15, 28). With the overlap with anxiety items eliminated, the Epstein and Fenz version should be more purely related to coping dispositions.

The R-S distributions for males and females were nearly identical, so separate cutoff points were not necessary as in the case of the SCT. The combined distribution had a mean of 13.21, and a standard deviation of 3.28. Selection of the upper and lower 25% required cutoff points as follows: 5-10 for repressors, 11-15 for middle group, and 16-20 for sensitizers. The possible range of scores is 0-30.

SRE-based life change units. This scale lists a number of life events which are either indicative of or require some change (positive or negative) in the ongoing life pattern of the individual. In our study this list was modified in a minor way to make it more personal and easy to understand. The subject indicated how many times in the preceding two-year period each of these life events had occurred. These events have been given life change unit (LCU) values by Holmes and Rahe (29), depending on how much social readjustment or coping was judged necessary to accommodate to each event. LCU values range from 11 (for the occurrence of minor violations of the law) to 100 (for the occurrence of the death of a spouse). Scoring was done by totaling the number of LCU's for each patient for the previous two years. This score was used in the analyses reported below. Patients were also divided into two groups, those who had LCU totals of 250 or more (N = 21), and those with totals of less than 250 (N = 31), according to the findings of Holmes and Rahe (30) concerning the likelihood of developing (or in a sense, disposition to develop) a stress-related illness.

RESULTS

In the analysis of relationships among most preoperative variables, all 61 patients were used (except for 55 in the case of the SCT). Only 59 could be used in the analysis of the course of recovery since 2 patients who had severe complications had to be eliminated. Moreover, of these only 53 completed the SCT and 52 the SRE. In the control group, 99 out of the total of 101 patient records were used, since 2 had to be eliminated for major postsurgical complications.

The control data were analyzed for any differences in the recovery indexes on several subsidiary variables (including male-female, surgeon, previous surgical experience). No significant differences were found, so these variables were ignored in the analysis of the data in the patient group that had been interviewed and tested.

Relationships between recovery variables

Table 1 shows the correlations found between each of the recovery variables for the interviewed patient group.

Course of recovery and process ratings

Simple one-way analyses of variance were separately performed with each of the four indexes of recovery, and the sum of these making a fifth. Below are the findings for each.

Avoidant vs. vigilant coping. The avoid-

Table 1. Correlations among the recovery variables

	Pain medi-cations	*Minor compli-cations*	*Negative psycho-logical reactions*	*Sum*
Days in hospital	0.465[b]	0.154	0.354[b]	0.543[b]
Pain med-ications		0.224	0.259[a]	0.820[b]
Minor com-plications			−0.133	0.662[b]
Negative psycho-logical reactions				0.345[b]

Note – $N = 59$.
[a]$p < 0.05$.
[b]$p < 0.01$.

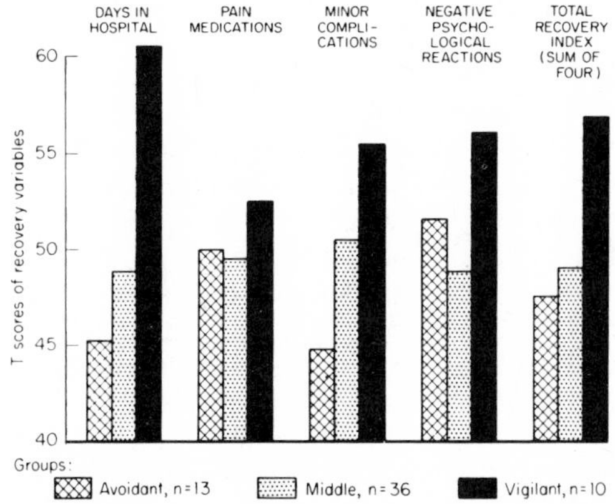

Fig. 1. Rate of recovery on 5 variables for groups differing in mode of active coping.

ant and middle groups of patients recovered somewhat faster from their operations than did vigilant patients. This trend could be observed in 4 recovery variables, but it was statistically significant only for days in the hospital ($F = 9.14$, $p < 0.01$), and minor complications ($F = 3.54$, $p < 0.05$). These relationships are diagramed in Figure 1.

Observer-rated anxiety. No significant relationships were found between anxiety, as rated by the interviewer, and any of the 5 recovery indexes.

Self-rated anxiety. These self-ratings were significantly related only to the incidence of negative postoperative psychological reactions ($F = 11.42$, $p < 0.001$), with patients high in self-reported anxiety showing more such reactions.

Course of recovery and dispositional measures

A simple one-way analysis of variance was employed to relate each of the coping dispositional measures to each of the indexes of recovery.

SCT coping disposition scores. Amount of pain medication was the only recovery index which showed a significant relationship with groups varying in the SCT measure of coping disposition ($F = 4.20$, $p < 0.05$). Patients classified as copers took significantly more pain medications than did the other two groups.

Modified R-S coping disposition scores. No significant differences were found between patient groups differentiated into repressors, sensitizers, or in-between, and any of the five recovery indexes.

SRE-based life change scores. Using a T-test analysis on each recovery index, no significant differences emerged between patients with high and low life change scores for the previous two years. Correlations between the total LCU score and each of the recovery indexes similarly showed no significant relationships.

Correlations among process ratings and dispositional measures

Table 2 reveals a few small, but significant, relationships. Two dispositional measures (SCT and modified R-S) showed a correlation of +0.369 ($p < 0.01$) with each

Table 2. Correlations of dispositional measures and process ratings

	Anxiety	*Self-rating of anxiety*	*SCT*	*Modified R-S*
Active coping process rating	0.283[b]	0.481[c]	0.082[a]	0.268[b]
Anxiety rating		0.455[c]	0.220[a]	0.247
Self-rating of anxiety			0.056[a]	0.216
SCT				0.369[a, c]

[a]$N = 55$.
[b]$p < 0.05$.
[c]$p < 0.01$.
$N = 61$ for other variables.

other. The modified R-S showed a low but significant correlation (i.e. $r = +0.268$, $p < 0.05$) with the process rating of coping, but the SCT did not show any significant relationship to this process rating. The correlations between the dispositional measures and the process ratings of anxiety showed no significant relationships.

Other findings

Low, insignificant correlations were found between age and social class, and the recovery variables. Years of schooling showed a significant relationship with two recovery variables, days in hospital ($r = +0.276$, $p < 0.05$) and number of negative psychological reactions ($r = +0.278$, $p < 0.05$).

A one-way analysis of variance showed no significant differences between coping groups on how anxious they were rated by the observer. Further, a discrepancy score was obtained by subtracting the self-rated anxiety score from the anxiety score given by the interviewer. A one-way analysis of variance showed there were no significant differences in this discrepancy among the three process-rated coping groups.

A one-way analysis of variance of LCU scores for the process-rated coping groups revealed no significant differences between groups on their total life-stress score.

It is quite possible that intervention of any sort, even an interview before surgery, may affect the recovery process by singling out the patient and thereby implicitly expressing concern for him. This possibility was examined by comparing the recovery pattern of a control group not so interviewed and the interviewed group. However, T-tests revealed no significant differences between the control ($N = 99$) and interviewed ($N = 59$) groups on any of the 5 recovery variables, showing that the interview itself did not affect the patients' recovery.

The correlation of $+0.481$ ($p < 0.01$) between the process rating of coping and the self-reported anxiety rating, reported in Table 2, suggests that the latter was confounded somewhat with the ratings of coping behavior. To eliminate this confounding, a one-way analysis of covariance was done on each of the 4 recovery variables (omitting the sum), thus partialing out the rating of self-reported anxiety. The results showed slightly reduced statistical significance, but remained essentially the same. Days in the hospital remained significantly related to process ratings of coping beyond the 0.01 level ($F = 6.45$), but the relationship between minor complications and coping was reduced to just below statistical significance at the 0.05 level ($F = 3.11$). Negative psychological reactions continued to show a trend in the same direction.

DISCUSSION

The main positive finding of this study was that inferences made just before surgery about whether patients coped with the threat by avoidance or vigilance were significantly related to various indexes of postsurgical recovery. Patients using vigilant modes of coping generally showed a slower course of recovery in 4 of the 5 recovery variables—number of days in the hospital, frequency of minor complications, negative psychological reactions, and a combined index created by summing the other four variables. Although this trend was found for 4 of the 5 indexes of recovery, it was strongest for number of days in the hospital and frequency of minor complications, reaching statistical significance in these instances. Patients using avoidant modes of coping generally did best in recovery, although their recovery measures were not significantly different from those of the middle group. Overall these findings should be considered suggestive, rather than definitive, considering the fact that many statistical analyses were performed, thereby increasing the possibility of obtaining significant relationships by chance. However, there do seem to be indications of a clear trend.

It is important to note that there are many factors of a medical and clinical nature which could have a bearing on both a patient's attitude toward his operation and his subsequent recovery from surgery. The procedure, discussed earlier, of obtaining separate standard score distributions for each type of operation adequately takes care of this heterogeneity across operations, but it does not control for heterogeneity within operative groups. For example, one type of gall bladder condition could be far more serious than another. And although in this study we did not try to investigate the influence of individual differences in medical condition, since we were oriented toward investigating more general factors—coping activity and recovery variables—it is possible that such influence could have occurred and could, in part, account for our results. For example, a patient who discovers he has a more severe condition could become more vigilant about his operation than the patient with a routine medical problem; in addition, since the disorder is more serious, he may take longer to recover postoperatively.

In effect, if seriousness of medical condition is a prime factor in affecting recovery and it also affects how much information the patient is told or seeks out, any relationship between the patient's knowledge of his medical problem and recovery would, in fact, be controlled by a third factor, namely the seriousness of the medical condition. It is, therefore of some interest to explore this possibility, in order to clarify the relationship we observed between psychological coping and recovery from surgery.

Due to the small number of subjects and the lack of a wide variety of clinical diagnoses for which the operations were performed, it was not possible to determine the extent of this relationship statistically. Scatter plots of the 2 recovery variables that showed significant results—days and minor complications—were made separately for each operative group. Diagnoses for each operation (e.g. gall bladder) were divided into least, middle, and most serious types, and the recovery variables were plotted for each type. In addition, scatter plots relating the seriousness of the medical condition and the avoidance-vigilance grouping were made. These plots revealed no relationship between seriousness of medical condition within each type of operation and either the recovery variables for that operation, or the avoidance-vigilance classification.

If, however, those patients with the 4 most serious medical conditions contained in the sample[8] are examined, there appears to be some indication that seriousness of medical condition may have some bearing on coping classification and possibly on recovery. Concerning mode of coping, 3 of these 4 patients were classified as vigilant, and 1 was classified in the middle group. On both the days and minor complications recovery variables, 2 (both vigilant) of the 4 patients had scores greater than one standard deviation above the mean, and the other 2 had scores close to the mean. These data are suggestive, but are not sufficient to explain the significant relationships found between coping activity and recovery. Further research using a larger sample and detailed clinical examinations and ratings of seriousness of medical condition might be desirable to determine the way individual medical factors could affect both recovery from surgery and mode of coping with its threats.

Contrary to anything we expected from past research, those who knew the most about their operation—the vigilant group—showed the most complicated recovery from surgery. One possible interpretation is that the vigilant copers are more demanding patients—who act in such a way that doctors keep them in the hospital longer, etc. However, this interpretation does not seem plausible, since this group did not show significantly higher use of pain medications. This variable was the one most under their control, because in this hospital patients must ask for pain medications to get them.

It is possible that the vigilant group was actually more anxious postoperatively, but then we might have expected increased use of pain medications (31), which was not found. The possibility that the vigilant group was more "stressed," and thus more vulnerable, was also not substantiated, since there were no differences among coping groups on the total SRE-based life stress scores. Thus, an explanation based simply on anxiety or stress does not especially fit our data.

Another possible interpretation can be offered if we view vigilant copers as individuals who were using a strategy of actively trying to master the world by seeking information and trying to learn everything about their operation. In the postoperative hospital context, however, with its incapacitation and pain, they can-

[8]Final diagnoses were 1) chronic cholecystitis, cholelithiasis, obstructive jaundice, 2) chronic cholecystitis, cholelithiasis, choledocholithiasis, cholecystoduodenal fistula, 3) hiatal hernia (hiatal hernioplasty, vagotomy, Finney pyloroplasty, and gastrostomy performed), and 4) sliding left inguinal hernia (with incarceration of sigmoid colon).

not "master" the situation actively as they would wish, but are forced to be dependent and passive. This could produce lowered self-esteem and an increased sense of vulnerability, which could conceivably impede the patient's recovery. This hypothesis is consistent with the findings that the vigilant group did not show increased use of pain medications, which their strategy of coping might lead them to reject as a solution. It is important to note, too, that vigilant patients not only had more detailed medical information but usually were also aware of possible negative complications. Perhaps knowledge of these threatening possibilities, obtained and remembered in their search for information, helped create their more complicated recovery, though we have no clear idea of the processes involved.

It is not appropriate to compare these findings with those of Andrew (4) and DeLong (5) since both these researchers used only a dispositional measure of coping. Moreover, even Andrew's and DeLong's findings were not entirely consistent with each other in the obtained pattern of relationship between coping disposition and recovery from surgery. Nonetheless, our findings are also not in accord with other studies that have suggested that the avoidant patient should show the poorest course of recovery, since this form of coping prevents the working through of the threat (1, 8, 32). However, it should be pointed out that Janis' work (1), which has never been replicated, dealt only with relationships between pre- and postoperative emotional reactions, and did not examine modes of coping separately or look at medical recovery variables, as we did.

The inconsistencies among studies do suggest, however, the possibility that given coping processes may be more useful for certain stressful situations than for others, or in particular periods of a prolonged crisis yet not in others. Thus, for example, many parents of children dying of leukemia profited from avoidant-denial defenses prior to the child's death (33) but suffered more afterwards (32). It is possible that surgery is one of those stressful occurrences that can be more effectively dealt with by avoidant-denial forms of coping than by vigilant ones, since although many threats exist in the surgical context, few actually materialize. This is consistent with Hackett and Weisman's (34) observations that patients can benefit more from denial if there is the possibility of a positive outcome (as in coronary infarction, for example, as opposed to terminal cancer). This possibility needs to be tested. In any case, our data do provide some support for the idea that individual differences in active coping may have an important bearing on the course of recovery from surgery.

A second major finding is that measures of dispositional coping, as distinguished from active coping processes, do not appear to be clearly or consistently associated with the course of recovery, or even strongly correlated with active coping processes, although one might have assumed they should be. It is becoming increasingly clear that behavior is determined by many factors, including situational ones to which the person must accommodate (35, 36), as well as factors within the individual. Research in this area has not yet determined how specific situational demands interact with coping dispositions.

There is another negative finding that bears comment, especially in the light of the great current interest in the relationship between life changes and susceptibility to illness. One might have anticipated from the research of Holmes and Rahe and their associates that patients with high life change scores should have fared worse in recovery from surgery than those with low life change scores. Our data did not bear out this expectation, although the approach used here (assessing recovery from surgery) is quite different from theirs (predicting the development of illness), making comparisons with their findings somewhat tenuous. Different factors may be operating in these two processes, or, as Spilken and Jacobs (37) have recently suggested, it may be that life stress (or perhaps the perception or judgment of life stress) increases treatment-seeking behavior, rather than illness. If so, a simple relationship to recovery would not be expected.

A final comment is also in order about the indexes of recovery. There is a sense in which it is arbitrary to say that the course of recovery is better or worse insofar as the patient goes home sooner, takes less pain medication, has fewer minor complications, and exhibits fewer complaints. Such allegations adopt a particular set of values, largely behavioral in sphere, generated in part by practical considerations within the hospital setting. However, nothing seems to be known about the determinants of each of these indexes, and the decision process related to discharging a patient, giving tranquilizers, etc. Nor do we have a calculus of the importance of these recovery variables in reflecting the patient's return to health. We have kept the indexes separate, as well as combining them in order to keep better track of the contribution of coping style to each.

From a practical point of view, clinical workers look toward the possibilities of using knowledge about individual differences in coping to understand the process of recovery from illness, as well as to develop methods of intervention to speed recovery, or make its course more favorable in other ways. Effective intervention will ultimately depend on what we can learn about the factors influencing recovery, especially those related to coping. This study also raises many questions concerning whether and when avoidance or vigilance as styles of coping are effective in helping people to adapt to inevitable life stresses. Research to date has not provided the answers, but has strongly suggested the fruitfulness of the questions.

SUMMARY

Surgical patients with similar medical problems often differ greatly in their course of postoperative recovery. This study investigated the relationship between mode of coping with preoperative stress—using both measures of ongoing coping activity and dispositional coping—and recovery from surgery.

Sixty-one preoperative surgical patients were interviewed and classified into avoidant, vigilant, or middle groups based on whether their interview responses showed avoidance of or vigilance toward information about their operations, or both kinds of behavior. Coping dispositions or traits referring to the same type of dimension were also measured using two different personality tests. Self-report and observer ratings of preoperative anxiety were made, and a measure of previous life stress was obtained. The five recovery measures included days in hospital, number of pain medications, minor medical complications, negative psychological reactions, and the sum of these four.

Results showed that the vigilant group—those who knew the most about their operation—had a more complicated recovery than did the other two groups on 4 of the 5 recovery measures, although only two (days in hospital, and minor complications) were statistically significant. The dispositional tests were not clearly or consistently associated with the course of recovery, nor correlated with the active coping processes. No significant relationships were found between observer ratings of preoperative anxiety, previous life stress, and any of the 5 recovery variables. Self-reported anxiety showed a significant relationship with only one recovery measure (negative psychological reactions).

Ways in which the mode of coping may have influenced recovery measures were discussed. These findings raise the possibility that knowledge of threatening aspects of surgery, if untempered by denial, could result in a more complicated postoperative recovery, and that an avoidant orientation may be an effective mode of coping in a medical situation where the likelihood of threats occurring is small.

• • •

The authors greatly appreciate the assistance of Norman T. Walter, M.D., Surgery Department, Kaiser Foundation Hospital, Hayward, California, who was instrumental in arranging for permission for this study to be done, and who willingly gave his time and expertise to advise and answer questions. We are also grateful to the administrator of Kaiser Hospital for approving this study, to the medical and nonmedical staff for their cooperation, and to Edward M. Opton, Ph.D., for his efforts during the preliminary stages of this study.

REFERENCES

1. Janis I: Psychological Stress. New York, Wiley, 1958
2. Egbert LD, Battit BE, Welch CE, Bartlett MK: Reduction of postoperative pain by encourage-

ment and instruction of patients. N Engl J Med 270:825–827, 1964
3. Healy KM: Does preoperative instruction make a difference? Am J Nurs 68:62–67, 1968
4. Andrew JM: Coping styles, stress-relevant learning and recovery from surgery. Unpublished doctoral dissertation, University of California, Los Angeles, 1967
5. DeLong DR: Individual differences in patterns of anxiety arousal, stress-relevant information and recovery from surgery. Unpublished doctoral dissertation, University of California, Los Angeles, 1970. (Referenced in Goldstein MJ: Individual differences in responses to stress. Paper given at conference entitled "Stress: Its Impact on Thought and Emotion," University of California Medical Center, San Francisco, June 2–3, 1972)
6. Lazarus RS: Psychological Stress and the Coping Process. New York, McGraw Hill, 1966
7. Lazarus RS, Averill JR, Opton EM: Towards a cognitive theory of emotion, Feelings and Emotions (Edited by MB Arnold), New York, Academic Press, 1970, pp 207–232
8. Goldstein MJ, Jones RB, Clemens TL, Flagg G, Alexander F: Coping style as a factor in psychophysiological response to a tension-arousing film. J Pers Soc Psychol 1:290–302, 1965
9. Rahe RH, Meyer M, Smith M, Kjaer G, Holmes TH: Social stress and illness onset. J. Psychosom Res 8:35–44, 1964
10. Rahe RH, McKean JD, Arthur RJ: A longitudinal study of life change and illness patterns. J Psychosom Res 10:355–366, 1967
11. Wyler AR, Masuda M, Holmes TH: Magnitude of life events and seriousness of illness. Psychosom Med 33:115–122, 1971
12. Jacobs MH, Spilken A, Norman M: Relationship of life change, maladaptive aggression, and upper respiratory infection in male college students. Psychosom Med 31:31–44, 1969
13. Querido A: Forecast and followup: an investigation into the clinical, social, and mental factors determining the results of hospital treatment. Br J Prev Soc Med 13:33–49, 1959
14. Byrne D: The Repression-sensitization scale: rationale, reliability, and validity. J Pers 29:334–349, 1961
15. Byrne D: Repression-sensitization as a dimension of personality, Progress in Experimental Personality Research, Vol 1 (Edited by BA Maher), New York, Academic Press, 1964, pp 170–220
16. Gardner RW, Holzman PS, Klein GS, Linton HB, Spence DP: Cognitive control: a study of individual consistencies in cognitive behavior. Psychol Issues 1:No. 4, 1959
17. Goldstein MJ: The relationship between coping and avoiding behavior and response to fear-arousing propaganda. J Abnorm Soc Psychol 58: 247–252, 1959
18. Levine M, Spivack G: The Rorschach Index of Repressive Style. Springfield, Ill. Charles C Thomas, 1964
19. Lazarus RS, Averill JR, Opton EM: The psychology of coping: issues of research and assessment. Paper given at conference entitled "Coping and Adaptation," Stanford University Department of Psychiatry, Stanford, California, March 20–22, 1969
20. Averill JR, Opton EM: Psychophysiological assessment: rationale and problems, Advances in Psychological Assessment. Vol 1 (Edited by P McReynolds), Palo Alto, Cal. Science and Behavior Books, 1968, pp. 265–288
21. Epstein S, Fenz WD: The detection of areas of emotional stress through variations in perceptual threshold and physiological arousal. J Exp Res Pers 2:191–199, 1967
22. Holmes TH, Rahe RH: Schedule of Recent Experiences. Seattle, University of Washington School of Medicine, 1967
23. Engel GL: Psychological Development in Health and Disease. Philadelphia, WB Saunders Company, 1962
24. Haan N: A tripartite model of ego functioning: Values and clinical research applications. J Nerv Ment Dis 148:14–30, 1969
25. Warner WL (with Meeker M, Feels K): Social Class in America. New York, Harper & Row, 1960
26. Golin S, Herron EW, Lakota R, Raineck L: Factor analytic study of the Manifest Anxiety, Extraversion, and Repression-sensitization scales. J Consult Psychol 31:564–569, 1967
27. Lefcourt HM: Repression-sensitization: a measure of the evaluation of emotional expression. J Consult Psychol 30:444–449, 1966
28. Schwartz M, Krupp N, Byrne D: Repression-sensitization and medical diagnosis. J Abnorm Psychol 78:286–291, 1971
29. Holmes TH, Rahe RH: The social readjustment rating scale. J Psychosom Res 11:213–218, 1967
30. Holmes TH, Rahe RH: Life crisis and disease onset: II. Qualitative and quantitative definition of the life crisis and its association with health change, Seattle, University of Washington School of Medicine, unpublished paper
31. Drew FL, Moriarty RW, Shapiro AP: An approach to the measurement of the pain and anxiety responses of surgical patients. Psychosom Med 30:826–836, 1968
32. Chodoff P, Friedman SB, Hamburg DA: Stress, defenses and coping behavior: observations in parents of children with malignant disease. Am J Psychiatry 120:743–749, 1964
33. Wolff CT, Friedman SB, Hofer MA, Mason JW: Relationship between psychological defenses and mean urinary 17-hydroxycorticosteroid excretion rates: I. A predictive study of parents of fatally ill children. Psychosom Med 26:576–591, 1964
34. Hackett TP, Weisman AD: Reactions to the imminence of death, The Threat of Impending Disaster. (Edited by GH Grosser, H Wechsler, M Greenblatt), Cambridge, Massachusetts, MIT Press, 1964, pp. 300–311
35. Wicker AW: Attitudes versus actions: the relationship of verbal and overt behavioral responses to attitude objects. J Soc Issues 25:41–78, 1969
36. Brigham JC: Racial stereotypes, attitudes, and evaluations of and behavioral intentions toward Negroes and whites. Sociometry 34:360–380, 1971.
37. Spilken AZ, Jacobs MA: Predictions of illness behavior from measures of life crisis, manifest distress, and maladaptive coping. Psychosom Med 33:251–264, 1971

34

Assessment of surgical patients' preoperative emotional condition and postoperative welfare

John A. Wolfer and Carol E. Davis

The present investigation was designed as a preliminary study for testing the effects of preoperative psychological preparation on postoperative recovery and adjustment of patients undergoing major elective surgery. A review of the literature and consideration of some of the major theoretical and methodological issues involved suggested a number of areas that needed further work before the original experiment could be done. These areas can be stated as five problems: 1) the definition and measurement of preoperative emotional state, particularly in terms of fear and anxiety, 2) how to define and measure postoperative recovery and adjustment, 3) the relationship among different measures and indicators of postoperative recovery, 4) the relative incidence or "base rate" of untoward preoperative and postoperative emotional and physiological states, and 5) the relationship between preoperative emotional state and postoperative recovery and adjustment.

Reprinted with permission from Nursing Research **19**: 402-414. Copyright September/October 1970, The Americal Journal of Nursing Company. Reproduced, with permission, from the Americal Journal of Nursing Company.

From Yale University School of Nursing, New Haven, Conn. (J. A. Wolfer), and the University of Utah College of Nursing (C. E. Davis).

The original project members were Mildred D. Quinn, dean, University of Utah, College of Nursing; Maxine Cope, associate professor of nursing, University of Utah, College of Nursing; and Verla B. Collins, director of nursing. Latter-day Saints Hospital, Salt Lake City, Utah. The project was supported by the nursing staff and patients at Latter-day Saints Hospital and by USPHS, Division of Nursing Grant NU 00246-01.

This study was undertaken to provide further information regarding these questions.

1. Preoperative emotional condition. The assessment of patients' preoperative emotional state has been primarily in terms of anticipatory "fear" and "anxiety," usually without any consistent operational distinction between fear and anxiety. Several different approaches have been taken. Most often these have been in the form of clinical judgments based on interviews with the patient (1, 2, 3, 4, 5). Surveys of the types of fears experienced have been done (6, 7). Self-reports have been made by patients using checklists, rating scales and inventories (8, 9, 10, 11). An important distinction in connection with self-report tests is one between measures of what has variously been called "chronic," "dispositional," or "trait" anxiety and measures of "transitory," "situational," or "state" anxiety. According to Spielberger trait anxiety refers to individual differences in anxiety proneness, that is, the disposition to appraise many situations as threatening and respond accordingly (12). This type of anxiety has been measured by such tests as the Cattell IPAT Anxiety Scale and the Taylor Manifest Anxiety Scale (13, 14). State anxiety, on the other hand, refers to subjective feelings of apprehension and fear in the presence or anticipation of a specific situation as registered on measures such as the Today form of the Zuckerman Affect Adjective Check List (AACL) or a simple rating scale of present affect (15). Some recent investigators have found that state or situationally specific measures of anxiety were better predictors of emotional responses to stress situations than were chronic or trait measures (16, 17). An attempt was made in the present investigation to include measures of preoperative fear and anxiety which represented several of the different approaches. These included observer ratings and self-reports on scales and inventories.

2. Postoperative recovery and welfare. The general need for reliable and valid criterion measures of patient welfare for determining the effectiveness of nursing procedures has been clearly recognized for some time (18, 19). A wide variety of measures and indices of postoperative condition have been used such as: smoothness of emergence from anesthesia, length of hospitalization, time to ambulation stage, amount of physical activity and independence, days of fever, skin condition, number of narcotics, analgesics and sedatives, vital signs, urinary retention, incidence of vomiting, recurrence of physical complications, number of complaints, pain and comfort ratings, and so on (20, 21, 22, 23, 24, 25). Usually, only one or two recovery indicators are included in surgery studies. An attempt was made in the present investigation to collect data on a large number of these measures in order to determine the extent to which the various aspects of the physical and psychological condition of the patient following surgery are interrelated. Are there, for example, some measures or indices that correlate high enough with most facets of the patient's condition to be taken as general measures of postoperative welfare? Are there some that are relatively independent of the others and seem to reflect separate aspects of postoperative recovery?

3. The base rate problem. One important consideration in selecting criterion measures is the rate of occurrence or most typical severity of undesirable patient conditions. This can be described as a "base rate" problem (26). If the task is to predict postoperative complications and degree of adjustment or to assess the effectiveness of special nursing procedures in terms of postoperative condition of the patient, it is necessary to have some idea of the relative incidence or severity of the undesirable state in a given clinical population. If, for example, only ten to fifteen per cent of patients having a certain type of surgery vomit postoperatively under usual conditions, a fairly large sample would be required to demonstrate the effectiveness of a nursing intervention that should, among other things, reduce the incidence of vomiting. The lower the base rate of the condition the more difficult it will be to relate it to other variables, such as the preoperative emotional state, and show differential effects of nursing and medical procedures, especially where large samples might be very difficult or impossible to obtain. Similarly, when the patient welfare measure produces scores on a continuum, such as with pain or comfort ratings, and most of the scores cluster around a mean or medium that falls close to the favorable end of the continuum, such as very low mean pain ratings, it would be much more difficult to demonstrate effectiveness of different procedures and find antecedents and correlates, especially with small samples. The same point holds for preoperative measures. If an undesirable state of affairs such as anticipatory fear and anxiety is comparatively rare, large clinical samples would be necessary in order to discover antecedents and correlates of the condition or test the effectiveness of nursing techniques designed to remedy the situation. Consequently, one of the objectives of the present investigation was to obtain initial normative data regarding base rates and the amount of variation for the variables under consideration.

4. Relationship between preoperative fear and postoperative recovery. Two general theoretical positions on the relationship between preoperative fear and anxiety and postoperative recovery can be found in the literature. One holds that there is an inverse linear relationship between the preoperative level of fear and postoperative recovery and adjustment. The greater the fear and apprehension, the poorer the recovery. This is the position held by many practitioners. Clinical studies based on this view attempt to reduce or minimize high levels of anxiety with some type of special preoperative psychological preparation and evaluate the procedure in terms of one or two criterion measures of postoperative recovery (27, 28). The other position calls for a curvilinear relationship between preoperative fear level and postoperative welfare and adjustment; both high and low levels of fear are associated with more difficult postoperative convalescence (29). But all of these studies have employed very small clinical samples and only a few measures of recovery. The present study examined the relationship between preoperative fear and postoperative recovery with larger samples and multiple recovery indicators.

Five separate but closely related studies were conducted as part of a larger project; two master's theses which involved small samples of patients undergoing gynecologic (GYN) and cardiovascular surgery and three larger studies of patients undergoing gynecologic surgery, male abdominal surgery, and both male and female patients undergoing cardiovascular surgery (30, 31). The present report is based on the two larger studies of patients undergoing gynecologic and male abdominal surgery.

METHOD

Clinical setting. The setting for the studies was Latter-day Saints Hospital, Salt Lake City, Utah. All the GYN patients were obtained from a single gynecology ward. This unit consisted of 37 beds; all but two of these beds were in semiprivate rooms. Seven full-time and three part-time registered nurses, eight full-time and two part-time licensed practical nurses, two full-time and two part-time female attendants, and two ward clerks made up the 24-hour nursing staff of the unit. Team nursing was employed on all three shifts with registered nurses acting as team leaders.

Four surgical wards were selected for obtaining the sample of male patients. The units contained private rooms, semiprivate rooms, and 4-bed wards. The staffing patterns were similar to the GYN floor.

GYN sample. The female sample consisted of 76 white female patients who underwent elective surgery under general anesthesia. The number and types of surgery were: 46 abdominal hysterectomies, 10 ovarian cystectomies, 7 tuboplasties, 2 wedge resections of the ovaries, 2 resections of pelvic endometriosis, 2 salpingectomies, and one uterine suspension. Preoperative data only were collected on five patients who had vaginal hysterectomies. All but three of the patients were admitted to the gynecology unit one day prior to scheduled surgery. One patient was admitted three days prior and two patients were admitted two days prior to scheduled surgery.

Male abdominal surgery sample. The male sample was composed of 70 white patients who underwent major abdominal surgery under a general anesthetic. They were selected on the basis of convenience and availability. The number and types of surgery were as follows: 21 gastric resections, 13 cholecystectomies, 10 colon resections, 7 exploratory laparotomies, 7 ureterolithotomies, 5 hiatal herniorrhaphies, 5 appendectomies, two excisions of bladder diverticuli, and one procedure for removal of sigmoid polyps. One patient expired on his second postoperative day, one was dropped from the study because he had a transthoracic surgical approach and another was dropped because of his very complicated postoperative course. Therefore, complete data were obtained on 67 patients.

Because of the nature of the surgery being performed and the need for preoperative diagnostic tests and x-rays, 22 of the patients were admitted from three to fourteen days (Mean = 6.3 days) prior to surgery.

Preoperative procedures. The preoperative measures were administered following dinner but before visiting hours. The nurse introduced herself and explained the general nature of the study, what would be required of the patient, and then asked if the patient was willing to participate. It was emphasized that the results were for research and that it was extremely important for the patients to give honest and frank responses. After the patient's consent was obtained, she or he was given the first of the test forms. The instructions for all the self-report tests were written on the forms. The nurse remained with the patients while they read the instructions to help answer any questions that came up and then left while the patient made his responses to the tests that took longer than ten minutes.

An attempt was made to select and develop measures of preoperative emotional state that would represent the following different approaches and formats for this type of assessment: a) direct self-ratings of present affective state, b) standardized inventories of predispositional or "chronic" anxiety, c) observers' ratings, and d) a more indirect approach via general attitude towards hospitalization and surgery. In a pilot study 27 hysterectomy patients were given a) the IPAT Anxiety Scale, b) the Affect Adjective Checklist, and c) Palmer's Patients' Perceptions Toward Surgery scale the night before surgery (32). None of these measures were significantly intercorrelated nor were they correlated with the number of analgesics and sedatives taken postoperatively. Furthermore, many of the patients questioned the psychiatric connotation of the IPAT and some found the longer tests somewhat tiresome. On the basis of these results other anxiety measures were selected and developed for the main study.

Attitude towards surgery and hospitalization. The first instrument administered was the "Hospital Reaction Questionnaire" which was developed to measure attitude toward surgery and hospitalization. An attitude scale was included in order to determine if patients' general attitude was related to preoperative fear and anxiety and postoperative recovery. The form given to the female sample consisted of 33 Likert-type items, five of which were from Palmer's Patients' Perception Toward Impending Surgery and eleven of which were taken from Giller's Attitude Toward Surgery Scale. The remaining items were composed by the project staff. The intent was to select and develop items which would reflect the degree to which patients were favorably or unfavorably predisposed towards surgery and its immediate consequences in the hospital. The response alternatives were: Strongly agree, agree, undecided, disagree, and strongly disagree. Each item was scored from 0 to 4 with a high score indicating a more favorable attitude. On the basis of the results from the female sample some items were slightly revised to make them clearer, more personal and less general in nature.

S-R Inventory of Anxiousness. The second preoperative test given was the S-R Inventory of Anxiousness (33). This new approach to assessing fear and anxiety requires the respondent to rate the strength of his response to 11 different situations (e.g., "You are crawling along a ledge high on a mountain side." "You are getting up to give a speech before a large group.") in terms of 14 different modes of response, mostly physiological (e.g., "heart beats faster," "perspire," "mouth gets dry," "experience nausea," etc.). Because the original situations were selected for a college-age population, five of them were changed to be more appropriate for adults (e.g., "You are going to a counseling session to seek help in a personal problem," was changed to "You are going to a psychiatrist to seek help in solving a personal problem."). In addition, a twelfth situation was added to the inventory, "You are waiting to be taken to the operating room for surgery," and scored separately. A high score on the inventory would be indicative of a person who tended to show strong physiological reactions to a variety of specific situations. One of the reasons for giving this inventory was the possibility of scoring only those situations where the stress was primarily one of threat of physical harm. It was reasoned that patients who show the strongest physiological reactions to the possibility of physical harm might also have more recovery difficulties postoperatively. Accordingly, "physical fear" subscores based on six of the situations describing the possibility of physical pain or discomfort were obtained.

On the basis of the results and the fact that the inventory was rather long and tedious for many of the patients, the S-R Inventory was given only to the GYN patients.

Moods and Feelings Inventory. The "Moods and Feelings Inventory" was developed by the authors as a short, self-report measure of fear and anxiety for hospitalized patients. It consisted of 20 adjectives describing both negative and positive affect. Ten of the words formed a fear-anxiety scale. They were: apprehensive, uneasy, concerned, tense, frightened, disturbed, anxious, worried, upset, and nervous. The other ten adjectives which were intermixed with the first ten were: relaxed, confident, angry, peaceful, indifferent, comfortable, optimistic, resigned, depressed, and calm. Each word appeared on a separate sheet along with a six-point rating scale which varied from "not at all" to "very much." This format provided for an expression of the degree to which each feeling was experienced in contrast to the usual adjective checklist which allows only for the presence or absence of a feeling. Separate sheets for each adjective and rating scale were used to encourage independent ratings since the rater was unable to see, immediately and continuously, how he had rated the other words as he turned from one sheet to the next. Each rating scale was scored from zero to five and the fear-anxiety ratings were summed for a total "fear-anxiety" (F-A) rating. The word "concerned" was eventually dropped from the scale because some patients noted they were "concerned" about their surgery but not necessarily frightened. Accordingly, the "concerned" rating had low intercorrelations with the other fear-anxiety items. As an internal check on the consistency of response, the ratings on relaxed, peaceful, comfortable, and calm were also summed and used as an index of "positive affect (PA)." The PA ratings were expected to correlate negatively with the F-A ratings. In addition the individual items could be scored and considered separately. The instrument was also administered on two consecutive days postoperatively as an indicator of the patient's emotional state following surgery.

Nurse ratings of emotional distress. In addition to the self-report measures that were given to the female sample, the research nurse and the evening team leader responsible for each patient made independent ratings of how emotionally distressed the patients seemed to be on the night before surgery. These ratings were made on a six-point scale and were based on the nurses' general impression of the patient without special intervention for the specific purpose of ascertaining the patient's emotional condition. These impressionistic ratings were included in the first study to see if they were related to the self-report measures and any of the postoperative recovery measures. Not surprisingly they did not correlate significantly with any of the other pre- and postoperative measures. The research nurse and the team leaders became increasingly aware and somewhat chagrined at the fact that without more systematic observation of and interaction with the patients, their emotional distress ratings were largely guesses and probably invalid. Consequently, these ratings were discontinued with the male sample.

The final preoperative measures taken were pain-threshold and pain-tolerance readings devised by the authors in an attempt to determine if pain threshold and tolerance were related to preoperative fear and postoperative recovery. It seemed reasonable to expect patients with high pain thresholds and tolerance to be less anxious preoperatively and perhaps more comfortable postoperatively. Separate threshold and tolerance readings were taken because several investigators have found that pain threshold and tolerance measures are somewhat different and independent aspects of pain (34, 35). The test consisted of wrapping a sphygmomanometer cuff around the calf of the extended left leg, with the comment, "Now I'm going to pump this up and I would like you to tell me when it first begins to be painful." The bulb of the cuff was squeezed to a specific height every three seconds until the patient indicated it was painful. After a 60-second rest, the test was repeated. The mean of five such readings was taken as the pain *threshold.* After a two-minute-rest interval, the patient was instructed, "Now I'll gradually make it stronger until you tell me you don't want to go any higher." The level at which the patient asked to stop was taken as the pain *tolerance* reading.

Postoperative recovery measures. Information regarding postoperative welfare consisted of two general types of data: 1) information routinely available regarding the patient's condition and course of recovery such as number of analgesics, h.s. sedations, elevated temperatures, wound complications, incidents of nausea and/or vomiting, etc. for the postoperative period. These are called "indicators" hereafter. 2) specially developed inventories and scales that were completed by the patients and the nurses—called "ratings."

The selection and construction of the postoperative recovery measures were governed by several important considerations. On the one hand an attempt was made to include as many aspects of the recovery process and patients' condition as possible; including indicators and criterion measures frequently used in other investigations. On the other hand, it was considered necessary to minimize the demands and inconvenience placed on the patient. The assessment process certainly should not interfere with the course of recovery or cause the patients additional discomfort. Furthermore, the data collection procedures should be as clinically practical as possible in order not to place an undue burden on the staff. The goal then was to collect information that was already available or could be obtained regarding the patient's condition with a minimum of interference and inconvenience. It was also intended that the self-report recovery scales and inventories have the potential for routine clinical assessment.

Recovery Room rating. The head nurse and the assistant head nurse of the Recovery Room were asked to rate the amount and vigor of physical activity ("delirium") the patients exhibited upon emergence from anesthesia (36, 37). The intention here was to observe any relationship between preoperative emotional state and the type of emergence from anesthesia. Following Smessaert, *et al.*, physical activity was rated on the basis of:

> Mode 1 – Those patients who make a tranquil and uneventful recovery. They exhibit little or no moaning, very little movement or turning, and are content to lie completely still without any demands on the nursing staff.
> Mode 2 – Those patients who show a moderate degree of restlessness. They exhibit moaning, sobbing, cries for the nurse, and much turning and movement on the stretcher.
> Mode 3 – Those patients who are markedly delirious and uncooperative, requiring special care and restraints. They exhibit flinging and thrashing of the body, no effort to cooperate or control movements, and are continuously trying to remove I.V. tubes, airway, O_2, and other apparatus (38).

Because 80 per cent of the GYN patients received a rating of Mode 1 and the ratings did not correlate significantly with any of the preoperative or postoperative measures, the ratings were discontinued in the male sample. Mode of recovery from anesthesia as measured here therefore did not turn out to be a useful and promising criterion measure.

Recovery Inventory. A "Recovery Inventory" was devised by the authors as a self-report measure for assessing patients' welfare primarily in terms of their *physical* condition. The items included sleep, appetite, strength and energy, stomach condition, bowel condition, urination, self-assistance, movement, and interest in surroundings. The patient rated each item on a six-point scale: very poor, poor, fair, good, very good, and excellent. The responses were scored from zero (very poor) to five (excellent). On the sleep, appetite, strength, and stomach items the patient also indicated his usual condition at home. This provided a combined rating for these items which reflected the patient's state relative to what it usually was outside of the hospital. The individual ratings were summed for a total Recovery Inventory score. The higher the score, the better the patient's general physical condition was judged to be.

Three other separately scored items completed the Recovery Inventory for the female sample. Two of these were six-point ratings of (a) the *amount* and (b) the *intensity* of pain experienced during the day. The amount item was to reflect the duration of pain while the intensity item was to indicate the severity of pain even if it occurred only once for a very short time. This difference was explained to the patient. The last item called for the patient to note whether there were any circumstances at home or in the hospital that were upsetting. The item was coded simply as the presence or absence of an "upsetting life situation" for the GYN sample. The male patients were also asked to rate on a six-point scale how upsetting or distressing the episode or circumstance was. This item was included as a check on the possibility that disturbing events not necessarily directly connected with the patient's hospitalization and condition might be associated with his recovery status, especially his psychological condition.

One further item was added to the Recovery Inventory for the male sample in order to provide a simple estimate of the amount of activity the patient engaged in during the day. This item required the patient to keep track of and record the number of times he got out of bed.

The research nurse explained how each

item in the Inventory was to be completed and remained in the room to answer any questions the patient had while making his rating.

Moods and Feelings Inventory. As an index of the patient's emotional condition, the Moods and Feelings Inventory was given again postoperatively in the same form as it occurred preoperatively. This provided self-ratings on the Fear Anxiety scale and the Positive Affect scale as well as ratings on the other individual adjectives (confident, angry, concerned, indifferent, optimistic, resigned, depressed).

The Recovery Inventory and the Moods and Feelings Inventory were administered on two consecutive days in order to determine if they would reflect the expected average improvement in the patient's physical and emotional condition. Although the rating scales are very simple and easy to complete in three or four minutes, most patients prefer not to be bothered the day of surgery. In fact, 24 per cent of the female sample and 28 per cent of the male sample did not feel up to taking the scales until their third and fourth postoperative days. "Test Day I" and "Test Day II" are used hereafter to refer to the first and second administration of the instruments regardless of the actual postoperative day. The patients took the two Inventories shortly before dinner and visiting hours.

Nurse and family member ratings. During the evening of the third postoperative day the head nurse or assistant head nurse rated the patient's general "Physical Progress" and "Emotional Progress" on six-point rating scales (very poor, poor, fair, good, very good, excellent). Physical progress was defined as the patient's improvement in terms of strength, appetite, independence, and physical appearance. Emotional progress referred to the patient's morale, mood, level of spirits, et cetera. A family member, usually the patient's husband or wife, was also asked to make the same ratings on the same evening. This was a preliminary attempt to ascertain a patient's condition from the point of view of someone who has known him for some time previous to the hospitalization. One question was the extent to which the family members' evaluations would correlate with the other recovery measures.

Number of complaints. The number of complaints made by the patient from postoperative day one to day four was recorded by ward personnel on a special sheet inserted into the chart. The complaint sheet was devised largely on the basis of information and recommendations from the nursing staff. Complaints were categorized according to type, such as pain, noise, food, temperature, nursing and medical care. One check in the appropriate complaint column was made for each complaint received by any of the nursing staff. If the same complaint was repeated, it was recorded accordingly. Complaints were recorded for all three shifts.

Postoperative interview. On the fourth or fifth postoperative day the patients were interviewed by the research nurse regarding their overall experience in the hospital primarily as it related to upsetting or disturbing experiences. The patients were also asked if taking the scales and inventories had in any way contributed to their discomfort or apprehension. None of the male patients and only two of the female patients indicated they were made any more uncomfortable by the data collection procedures.

Recovery indicators. The following information was collected systematically and treated as "indicators" of patient welfare: 1) number of analgesics, 2) number of sedatives, 3) number of anti-emetics, 4) number of days in the hospital, 5) number of elevated temperatures (100° and above), 6) incidence of nausea, 7) incidence of vomiting, 8) wound complications, 9) respiratory complications, 10) use of tranquilizers postoperatively, 11) number of days until catheter removed, and 12) number of repeated catheterizations. These variables were quantified by simply counting, where appropriate, or scoring the presence or absence of a condition as "1" or "0." One important question regarding these types of data is whether the frequency of occurrence and/or amount of variation within patient populations is high enough to suggest that the indicator would be an effective criterion measure for assessing nursing procedures.

As a check on the possible influence of biographical and situational factors on the pre- and postoperative measures, the fol-

Table 1. Means, standard deviations, and p levels for preoperative measures

Preoperative measures	*Female*			*Male*			
	N	*M*	*SD*	*N*	*M*	*SD*	*p*
Fear-anxiety self-rating	76	22.9	12.66	70	18.4	11.28	.05
Positive affect self-rating	76	10.6	5.55	70	11.6	5.06	NS
Hospital reaction (attitude)	76	63.3	8.34	70	66.0	11.05	NS
Pain threshold (mm. of mercury)	74	99.1	47.32	60	103.6	47.21	NS
Pain tolerance (mm. of mercury)	74	155.8	69.73	60	201.3	70.44	<.001

lowing information was also collected: age, number of children, number of previous major and minor surgeries, diagnosis, other extenuating diseases, the possibility of cancer, time in the hospital prior to surgery, length of time between leaving the ward and the beginning of surgery, total time in the operating room and total time in the recovery room.

RESULTS AND DISCUSSION

The results consist of four types of data: 1) descriptive characteristics of the pre- and postoperative variables and measures, 2) mean differences on measures which were repeated pre- and postoperatively, 3) correlations between the preoperative and the postoperative measures, and 4) intercorrelations of preoperative and postoperative measures.

Table 1 gives the means, standard deviations, and p levels for t test comparisons of the female and male means on the preoperative measures. The main purpose of these descriptive data is to provide some initial normative information regarding base rates and variability of the ratings and indicators. The sample size varies somewhat from variable to variable because complete information was not always available for all patients.

Preoperative emotional state. The preoperative F-A self-ratings showed wide variation with the lowest and highest possible scores (0-45) being obtained by some patients in both samples. The female mean of 22.9 is very close to the middle of the possible range and the male mean of 18.4 is slightly below the mid-point. The female patients reported significantly more fear than the male patients on the average. Dividing the ranges of F-A ratings into equal thirds with the top third indicating a "high" level of fear, the middle third a "moderate" level of fear, and the bottom third a "low" level of fear, the percentages for the two samples were as follows: GYN, High = 30 per cent, Moderate = 40 per cent, Low = 29 per cent; males, High = 15 per cent, Moderate = 39 per cent, Low = 46 per cent. The difference in reported fear and anxiety between the male and female patients may indicate that GYN surgery, especially hysterectomies, with its symbolic and practical significance for the female role may be appraised as very threatening for many women in comparison to the abdominal surgery faced by the male patients. Women also may be more willing to publicly admit fear than men. That a sex difference in willingness to admit fear does not entirely account for the higher F-A ratings in the female group is suggested by the fact that there was no significant difference in mean F-A ratings between male and female in another sample of 40 patients undergoing cardiovascular surgery.

Self-ratings of fear and anxiety most likely underestimate the number of patients who are considerably worried and upset about their forthcoming surgery because the ratings are subject to two possible response sets; "social desirability" in the form of an unwillingness to publicly admit fear, and "denial" of anxiety as a coping technique. To the extent that either or both of these response sets are operating, the percentages in the high fear category are conservative. A conservative estimate that 15 per cent to 30 per cent of the patients facing major surgery experience a relatively high degree of fear and anxiety preoperatively would suggest there are enough patients to warrant special consideration from the nursing and medical staff.

The mean Positive Affect self-ratings for both samples were very near the middle of the possible range and some patients in both groups obtained the lowest (0) and the highest (20) scores possible. There was no significant difference in these ratings between the male and female patients.

The mean score and standard deviation on the Hospital Reaction questionnaire fell in the third quartile of the possible range (0 to 104). Taken at face value this reflects a moderately favorable general attitude towards hospitalization and surgery on the part of most of the patients. There was no significant difference in these ratings between the male and female patients.

The pain threshold and pain tolerance readings showed extremely wide variation within both samples indicating large individual differences in reported sensitivity to and tolerance for pain. The difference in mean for pain threshold readings between the female and male patients was not significant but the male patients had a significantly higher mean score for pain tolerance.

Postoperative measures. Table 2 gives the means, standard deviations, and significance levels for differences in means between the female and male patients on the recovery ratings and indicators. Considerable variation was obtained on all the rating scales and inventories, indicating that these instruments are sensitive to individual differences. With the exception of the Recovery Inventory total scores, there were some patients who obtained the lowest and highest ratings possible on the scales. Table 3 presents the mean differences and significance levels for the ratings that were given pre- and postoperatively and for the ratings that were given on the two consecutive days postoperatively.

The male patients continued to have lower mean F-A self-ratings than the female patients postoperatively, although not quite significantly so on testing day I ($p < .10$). In both samples there was a highly reliable decrease in the F-A ratings from the night before surgery to the first and second testing days following surgery, as would be expected. This finding provides some support for the validity of the Fear-Anxiety self-ratings. There were exceptions to this general trend and these could be very important clinically if the shift in affect was picked up by the nurses. Male patients showed another significant decrease in F-A ratings from the first to the second testing day postoperatively while the mean rating of the female patients remained essentially the same. Hence the scale seemed to reflect an improved emotional condition for the males but not for the females from one day to the next, postoperatively. The male patients also showed a reliable increase in their mean Positive Affect ratings from testing day I to day II while there was no change for the females. At this point it is not clear why there was a significant change in these ratings only for the male patient.

The total scores on the Recovery Inventory showed wide dispersion which indicates considerable differences in the patients' self-ratings of their recovery in terms of sleep, appetite, strength and energy, stomach condition, voiding, self-help, movement, and interest. The scores were generally very low on day I as would be expected. The striking increases in the mean Recovery Inventory scores from testing day I to testing day II in both groups were significant at beyond the .001 level and show substantial improvement in the condition of the patients at this point in their convalescence. The female and male scores are not directly comparable because two items were added to the Inventory for the male sample. Since the top score possible on the Inventory was 35 for female patients and 45 for the male patients, considerable further improvement is possible. The means of 7.1 and 11.3 on day I indicates that most of the patients were checking "very poor" or "poor" on most of the items. The means of 20.0 and 27.1 on day II indicate they were typically checking "fair" or "good." Although there is a mean increase in ratings, obviously some patients do not show as much improvement in ratings as others. If the Recovery Inventory could be administered each day throughout the postoperative period, individual recovery ratings could then be evaluated in relation to the typical curve. Knowing that an individual patient's recovery curve deviates substantially from the general trend in a negative direction would be useful. It is possible that a patient's recovery rating across several postoperative days would be a more important

Table 2. Means, standard deviations, and *p* levels for postoperative measures

	Female			*Male*			
Postoperative measures	*N*	*M*	*SD*	*N*	*M*	*SD*	*p*
Ratings							
Fear-anxiety self-rating I	69	12.9	9.74	67	10.3	7.75	.10
Fear-anxiety self-rating II	67	13.2	11.71	67	8.6	7.62	<.01
Positive affect I	69	12.2	4.69	67	11.7	4.49	NS
Positive affect II	67	12.6	5.36	67	13.1	5.06	NS
Recovery inventory I	69	7.1	5.32	67	11.3	5.54	NS
Recovery inventory II	67	20.0	6.14	67	27.1	7.29	NS
Amount of pain rating I	69	2.6	.99	67	2.4	1.10	NS
Amount of pain rating II	67	2.2	1.22	67	1.9	.95	NS
Intensity pain rating I	69	2.4	1.08	67	2.2	1.15	NS
Intensity pain rating II	67	1.9	1.13	67	1.6	1.13	NS
Nurse physical rating	69	3.7	.83	67	3.5	1.03	NS
Nurse emotional rating	69	3.5	.96	67	3.7	.91	NS
Family physical rating	62	3.7	.91	57	3.4	1.07	NS
Family emotional rating	62	3.6	1.15	57	3.5	1.02	NS
Indicators							
Days in hospital	70	8.6	3.44	68	13.0	5.05	<.001
Number of analgesics	70	24.1	11.38	68	20.0	12.67	.05
Number of h.s. sedations	70	3.1	2.10	68	3.6	2.94	NS
Number of elevated temperatures	70	6.3	6.75	68	6.9	5.35	NS
Number of anti-emetics	70	.31	.94	69	.25	1.09	NS
Day catheter removed	69	1.3	1.05	68	.84	1.67	NS
Number of times catheterized	69	.59	2.60	64	.92	1.41	NS
Number of complaints	46	11.6	6.51	53	6.1	7.2	<.001
Number of times out of bed I	**	**	**	67	3.2	2.28	—
Number of times out of bed II	**	**	**	67	5.5	3.42	—
Wound complications*	70	.07	—	68	.1	—	NS
Respiratory complications*	71	.08	—	69	.39	—	NS
Nausea*	70	.60	—	**	**	—	—
Vomiting*	70	.21	—	**	**	—	—
Upsetting life situations*	72	.31	—	67	.34	—	NS

*Scored no = 0, yes = 1
**Data not collected

and meaningful criterion measure than either his absolute or relative position on any one day.

The mean amount and intensity of *pain* self-ratings on day I were about in the middle of the six-point scales. The mean decreases in pain ratings on both samples from day I to day II for both amount and intensity were significant (Table 3). The full scale (0-5) was represented in the obtained ratings. These distributions were skewed positively with most of the ratings falling in the bottom half of the scales. The reliable decreases in mean ratings from day I to day II along with their sensitivity to individual differences suggests self-ratings of pain are promising criterion measures of recovery. If the scales were administered a day or so earlier and continued throughout the postoperative period, a typical pain reduction curve could be obtained and individual daily pain ratings as well as patterns could be interpreted accordingly. As with the Recovery Inventory, a patient's profile of pain ratings across several days in relation to a typical curve might be more meaningful than the rating for any single day.

It is interesting to note that the mean ratings of the family members and nurses on the patient's emotional and physical condition were very similar in both samples. The most typical ratings were "good" and "very good." These rating distributions were negatively skewed with most of the ratings being in the upper half of the scale. Although the mean ratings of the family members and nurses were about the same, they did not correlate significantly in the female sample but did in the male sam-

Table 3. Mean differences and p levels for repeated pre- and postoperative measures

Measures	*Females*		*Males*	
	Mean diff	*p*	*Mean diff*	*p*
Preop. F-A vs. postop. F-A I	−10.70	.001	−8.10	.001
Preop. F-A vs. postop. F-A II	− 9.70	.001	−9.80	.001
Preop. PA vs. postop. PA I	1.60	.10	.13	NS
Preop. PA vs. postop. PA II	1.90	.05	1.50	NS
Postop. F-A I vs. II	.30	NS	−1.70	.05
Postop. PA I vs. II	.30	NS	1.37	.05
Recovery inventory I vs. II	12.90	.001	15.90	.001
Amount of pain I vs. II	− .40	.05	− .48	.001
Intensity of pain I vs. II	− .50	.02	− .61	.001

ple (physical, $r = .52$; emotional, $r = .39$). Since many family members expressed doubt about their ratings because they felt unqualified to evaluate the patient's progress, since it was difficult to obtain the ratings, and since they did not provide additional information about the patient's condition, these ratings have dubious potential.

Turning now to the recovery "indicators" listed in Table 2 it can be noted that most of the indicators had a high enough base rate and variance to qualify as potential criterion measures. Wound complications, respiratory complications, nausea, and vomiting were scored "0" or "1" to indicate their absence or presence for each patient. Hence the means for these variables are the proportions of patients who had these difficulties. Number of analgesics had the highest means and standard deviations. The lowest means and variances occurred with number of anti-emetics and number of times catheterized. Along with wound and respiratory complications, the base rates on these four variables are too low in the present samples to make them promising criterion measures for evaluating nursing procedures. Of course there are many situational variables such as diagnosis, anesthetic agent, specific type and duration of surgery, the patient's age and general physical condition, et cetera that can influence these indicators and should be taken into account or controlled whenever possible to make the indicators useful as valid criterion measures of nursing actions. Nevertheless, if the frequency of occurrence and/or variability of the indicator is very low to begin with, it has a low potential for differentiating between nursing procedures even if there is a very real difference, unless very large samples are used.

Since the procedure for determining the number of complaints patients made each day was not operational from the beginning of the study and required full cooperation from all the staff, smaller samples were obtained. Nevertheless, there was wide variation in total number of complaints in both samples. The significantly higher mean number of complaints in the female compared to the male sample could be due to any number of differences such as type and significance of surgery or amount and quality of care given in different units, but presumably not to differences in defining, monitoring, and recording of complaints, which was standardized across units. Female patients also spent significantly fewer days in the hospital but received more analgesics. The possibility of reliable sex differences with these indicators should be checked out in further studies which control for relevant intervening variables.

The patient's own count of the number of times he got out of bed each day (collected on the male sample only) showed good variation across patients and the increase in the mean from testing day I to day II was significant (Table 3).

That 31 per cent of the female patients and 34 per cent of the males reported Upsetting Life Situations of one kind or another points to the possibility that episodes and circumstances not directly related to or resulting from surgery and hospitalization could influence the patient's

Table 4. Intercorrelations of preoperative measures for female patients

	1	*2*	*3*	*4*	*5*	*6*	*7*
1. Fear-anxiety self-rating	1.00						
2. Positive affect self-rating	.77*	1.00					
3. S-R inventory of anxiousness	.33*	−.32*	1.00				
4. S-R surgery situation	.62*	−.58*		1.00			
5. Hospital reaction (attitude)	−.26				1.00		
6. Pain threshold		.32*		−.27		1.00	
7. Pain tolerance		.25				.78*	1.00

*$p < .01$

Table 5. Intercorrelations of preoperative measures for male patients

	1	*2*	*3*	*4*	*5*
1. Fear-anxiety self-rating	1.00				
2. Positive affect self-rating	−.71*	1.00			
3. Hospital reaction	−.44*	.43*	1.00		
4. Pain threshold	−.22	.28	.22	1.00	
5. Pain tolerance	−.24	.22	.24	.62*	1.00

$p < .01$

condition, especially the emotional state. In fact, the male patients' ratings of the significance to them of the upsetting events were correlated significantly with their individual ratings on the Moods and Feelings Inventory from .40 to .77. These results underscore the necessity of taking into account extra-hospital episodes and circumstances as at least partial determinants of the patient's postoperative conditions independent of the type and quality of care received in the hospital.

Intercorrelations of preoperative measures. Tables 4 and 5 contain the intercorrelations of the preoperative measures for the female and male patients respectively. Only correlations reaching the .05 level of confidence or better are listed.

The F-A self-ratings correlated in the expected direction with the other measures. Patients who rated themselves high on fear and anxiety the night before surgery tended to be low on Positive Affect, have higher scores on the S-R Inventory of Anxiousness (especially for the specific surgery situation in the female sample), have less favorable general attitudes towards hospitalization and surgery, and in the male sample have a slight tendency for lower pain threshold and tolerance readings. In the female sample the lower correlation between the F-A ratings and the total S-R Inventory of Anxiousness scores (.33) compared to the correlation between the F-A ratings and the specific S-R Situation score (.62), along with the absence of any correlation between the total S-R Inventory scores and the specific Surgery Situation score, provides further support for the point that measures of general trait anxiety are not always highly related to measures of fear for specific situations.

Although the Pain Threshold and Pain Tolerance readings were correlated with all of the other measures in the male sample and three of the others in the female sample, the correlations are so low that it can be concluded that patients' pain threshold and tolerance are not substantially related to their affective state preoperatively. The negative correlations between the PA and F-A ratings of −.77 in the female group and −.71 in the male group point to a fairly high degree of internal consistency of responses to the Moods and Feelings Inventory.

Relationships between preoperative emotional state and postoperative recovery. Pearson correlations were calculated between all the preoperative and postoperative measures including subscales and individual items on the postoperative measures and all quantifiable descriptors of patients' convalescences.

The most striking feature of these results was the almost complete absence of any significant and substantial (.50 and above) correlations between the pre- and postoperative measures. Where the comparatively few significant correlations did occur they were in the range of .23 to .46 with the large majority of these being under .35. The significant correlations were therefore by and large too low to be of any value for predicting patients' postoperative recovery from their preoperative emotional states. With very few exceptions patients' self-ratings of fear and anxiety, positive affect, attitude toward hospitalization and surgery, and pain threshold and tolerance the evening before surgery were not related to the many different aspects of their physical and emotional recovery following surgery.

Janis found a curvilinear relationship between preoperative anticipatory fear and postoperative emotional adjustment (39). Both high and low fear patients had more difficulty adjusting postoperatively than did moderate fear patients. As a provisional test of Janis' findings and hypotheses, scattergrams for the preoperative F-A ratings and the following postoperative measures were examined: total F-A and Positive Affect ratings, separate ratings for the individual ratings of apprehension, anger, and depression, and total number of complaints. Careful scrutiny revealed no sign of curvilinear relationships between preoperative F-A ratings and other ratings of postoperative emotional state. There was no evidence of low fear patients being more angry, depressed, lower on PA, or complaining more than either high or moderate fear patients. Where there was an indication of a relationship, it was linear. The correlations between pre- and postoperative F-A ratings were .41 ($p < .01$) for the females and .28 ($p < .01$) for the males indicating a reliable but very weak tendency (considering r^2) for high preoperative fear patients to remain high on fear following surgery.

The absence of substantial correlations between the pre- and postoperative measures could be attributed to any one or the combination of a large number of factors including the possible unreliability and invalidity of any of the measures or the intervention of uncontrolled variables such as differential quality of medical and nursing care and individual differences in stress-coping ability of the patients. The working assumption in studies of this type is that, other things being equal, differences in the amount and quality of care and coping ability will be equally distributed across the variables in such a way as to allow a correlation to appear. To the extent that such an assumption is inaccurate, real relationships may be masked. Considering the size of the samples in the present study, there were no obvious reasons for doubting the assumption. However, future research concerning the possible relationship between preoperative emotional distress in the form of anticipatory fear and anxiety and postoperative recovery would do well to assess and control for situational variables such as specific type of surgery, type and quality of medical and nursing care, both pre- and postoperatively, and patient's coping ability. It may well be, for example, that within the high anticipatory fear group, individual differences in coping ability reduce the possibility for a linear correlation between degree of preoperative fear and some measure of postoperative recovery because high-fear effective copers tend not to have unusual postoperative psychological and physical difficulties, whereas low-fear ineffective copers may have such difficulties. Janis seems to have assumed that the level of anticipatory fear itself was a reflection of a patient's coping behavior; that is, both high and low fear patients adjust poorly postoperatively compared to moderate fear patients.

A final problem when the assessment of the patient's emotional state is based on self-reports is the possibility of error due to response sets. For example, some respondents may feel it is socially undesirable to admit publicly any strong emotion, especially fear or anxiety. Hence, they may report they are less frightened than they really are. There has been a great deal of research on this problem and some investigators believe that most of the individual differences on chronic anxiety scales can be attributed to differences in willingness to admit socially undesirable traits (40). Although it has not been determined to what extent a social desirability response set influences more situationally-specific fear ratings, some of the patients who fall on the low end of the fear continuum may be "false lows." That is, they

Table 6. Intercorrelations for postoperative recovery measures in female sample (decimal points omitted)*

	1	*2*	*3*	*4*	*5*	*6*	*7*	*8*	*9*	*10*	*11*	*12*	*13*	*14*	*15*	*16*	*17*	*18*	*19*
1. Fear-anxiety I																			
2. Fear-anxiety II	38**																		
3. Positive affect I	−73	−30																	
4. Positive affect II	−31	−82	41																
5. Recovery inventory I	−31																		
6. Recovery inventory II		−71			38														
7. Pain amount I	49	30	−62	−32	−47	−32													
8. Pain intensity I	31	44	−38	−38		−38	58												
9. Pain amount II		53	−32	−59		−60	36	50											
10. Pain intensity II		54	−34	−54	−27	−57	49	55	84										
11. Nurse physical rating		37		32	34	38													
12. Nurse emotional rating				26	38	32	−32	−28	−32	−35	80								
13. Nurse family physical rating					33					33		30							
14. Family emotional rating	−31				42		−50		−36	−42			68						
15. No. days in hospital		47		−38		−52													
16. No. analgesics		39				−44	42	26	42	50		−30							
17. No. h.s. sedations				−27		−26					−36	−30							
18. No. elevated temps.															53				
19. No. complaints	43	46	−50	−49		−46	50	47	57	53	−46	−55	−26	−39		49			

*Only correlations significant at .05 level or better are listed
**N = 67-70; $r > .25$, $p < .05$; $r > .33$, $p < .01$

Table 7. Intercorrelations for postoperative recovery measures in male sample. (decimal points omitted)*

	1	2	5	4	5	6	7	8	9	10	11	12	13	14	15	16	17	18	19
1. Fear-anxiety I																			
2. Fear-anxiety II	64**																		
3. Positive affect I	−41																		
4. Positive affect II	−40	−59	50																
5. Recovery inventory I			43	30															
6. Recovery inventory II		−41		49	59														
7. Pain amount I	31		−41		−38														
8. Pain intensity I			−33	−32	−29		81												
9. Pain amount II	31	34	−34	−39	−42	−44	54	44											
10. Pain intensity II	29		−32	−45	−36	−46	34	34	74										
11. Nurse physical			34	29	29	47			−38	−31									
12. Nurse emotional			42	45		36	−34		−51	−43	74								
13. Family physical			29	29	31	45	−31		−39	−41	52	53							
14. Family emotional					31	36			−36	−46	42	39	74						
15. No. days in hospital						−29					−27		−36						
16. No. analgesics								25	36	41	−43	−36			29				
17. No. h.s. sedations																39			
18. No. elevated temp.											−38	−25							
19. No. complaints														32			−28		

*Only correlations significant at .05 level are listed
**N = 67-70; $r > .25$, $p < .05$; $r > .33$, $p < .01$

indicate they are lower in fear and anxiety than they really are. Further, when threat is great, some individuals will deny they are very frightened or anxious with varying degrees of awareness. Denial of anxiety has traditionally been viewed as one kind of "defense mechanism," particularly when the person is unaware of the process. Consequently, some of the low self-ratings may be from deniers and again represent "false lows." To the extent that self-ratings allow for false negatives they are, of course, invalid measures of fear or anxiety. These possible sources of error in the preoperative fear measure might have contributed to the low and zero-order correlations with postoperative recovery indicators and measures. The problem of accurately assessing the patient's fear levels requires much further work.

Relationships among postoperative measures. All the inventory and rating scores, including individual scales and items, and quantitative recovery indicators were intercorrelated for both samples separately. Tables 6 and 7 give only the intercorrelations for the total ratings and major indicators for the female and male samples respectively. Only correlations significant at the .05 level or better are listed.

One general question here is the extent to which the different recovery measures go together. Are there a few measures which correlate high enough with most of the other measures so that they could be used separately as main indicators of a patient's overall postoperative condition? Or are the measures sufficiently independent to contribute additional information about the patient's condition and therefore necessitate their inclusion as part of an operational definition of patient welfare? Further statistical analysis in the form of multivariate analysis will be necessary to answer these questions properly. This was not performed at this point because some of the individual measures may require further methodological work. Nevertheless, consideration of the correlation matrices will serve to illustrate some of the problems involved in selecting and developing patient recovery measures.

The first 14 variables listed in the tables are ratings; the last five are indicators. As can be seen, most of the ratings are intercorrelated from low to moderately high compared to the indicators where there are fewer intercorrelations, especially in the male sample (Table 7). With the exception of number of analgesics and number of complaints in the female sample, the indicators are comparatively independent of each other and of the ratings. One interpretation is that these generally different types of recovery measures reflect quite different aspects of patients' convalescences.

The Recovery Room Rating of the smoothness of emergence from anesthesia did not correlate with any of the other recovery variables. Whether a patient regains consciousness in an uneventful manner or does not, in terms of the amount and type of activity displayed, was not related to other aspects of his postoperative recovery.

The intercorrelations among the patients' self-ratings of Fear-Anxiety, Positive Affect, Physical Recovery, and amount and intensity of pain are all in the expected direction although lower, or absent, in some cases than might be expected. For example the correlation of .38 between the day I and II F-A ratings for the female patients might be interpreted as an indication of low test-retest reliability. However, it is highly likely that there are differential experiences within a 24-hour period that influence patients' emotional states so that they change their relative positions on the scales from one day to the next. Similarly, the correlations between the day I and day II Recovery Inventory ratings of .38 for the females and .59 for the males indicate that patients' relative positions on this recovery measure can vary considerably from one day to the next. It is doubtful that this is a sign of low reliability since the ratings on the subscales of the Inventory are quite consistent. Rather it may be an indication that although nearly all patients show improvement on the Inventory from day I to day II (as shown by the large and significant increase in the mean scores), they improve at different rates, with some patients showing decreases. Again, this suggests that a more useful recovery score might be a deviation from the daily mean score plotted over several postoperative days, which would provide an index of the daily relative position and the rate of improvement over time.

The intercorrelations for the amount versus the intensity of pain ratings are high enough (.74 to .84) with the exception of day I in the female sample (.58) to suggest that a single pain rating would suffice. Otherwise the intercorrelations for the self-ratings are, by and large, low enough to suggest these self-ratings reflect different facets of postoperative recovery as judged by the patients themselves. On the other hand, if the self-ratings were not correlated at all, the reliability and validity of the scales would be suspect.

The ratings of the patient's general physical and emotional progress by the staff nurses and family members correlate significantly with each other and with some of the patient's self-ratings. However, most of these correlations are of low or very low magnitude. As noted earlier, most of the family members expressed little confidence in their ratings.

Turning to the recovery indicators listed in Tables 6 and 7, it can be seen that number of analgesics in both samples, and number of complaints in the female sample were the only variables in this group that had several significant and moderately high correlations with the recovery ratings. Understandably, number of analgesics taken was significantly but not highly correlated with patients' pain ratings in most cases. That the total number of complaints was significantly correlated with most of the other recovery variables in the female sample but not in the male sample is of special interest. Female patients who complained a great deal tended to have higher Fear-Anxiety ratings, lower PA ratings, lower Recovery Inventory scores on day II, higher pain ratings, lower nurse and family member ratings of physical and emotional progress, and received more analgesics. Hence, number of complaints would seem to be a good single indicator of the general postoperative recovery of *female* patients because it is reliably associated with most of the other aspects of their convalescences. It was an almost completely independent measure for male patients. Although it is tempting to speculate about possible sex difference based on this finding, further research will be necessary to verify the trend.

There were no significant or substantial intercorrelations for the following recovery indicators: number of sedatives, number of anti-emetics, number of days until the catheter was removed, number of times catheterized, number of times out of bed on days I and II, incidence of nausea and vomiting, wound complications, and respiratory complications with those indicators listed in Tables 6 and 7.

The total amount of time patients spent in the operating room correlated with only a few recovery measures; in the female sample, .49 with number of elevated temperatures, −.40 with day II Recovery Inventory scores, .72 with number of days until the catheter was removed, and .40 with number of days in the hospital. In the male sample, time in the operating room did not correlate substantially with any of the postoperative measures. Similarly, the total time spent in the recovery room did not correlate significantly with any of the postoperative measures except with number of days until the catheter was removed, in the male sample (.51). Time in the operating room was not correlated with time in the recovery room in either sample. Insofar as the length of time spent in the operating room is a rough index of the duration of anesthesia and amount of surgical trauma, these situational variables were not strongly associated with most aspects of the patient's recovery status. Finally, the patient's age, number of previous surgeries, and number of days hospitalized before surgery did not correlate with any of the recovery measures.

SUMMARY

The purpose of this investigation was to examine problems in the assessment of surgery patients' preoperative recovery. Seventy-six female patients who underwent major gynecologic surgery and 70 male patients who underwent major abdominal surgery were given a variety of instruments designed to assess their preoperative fear and anxiety and postoperative recovery and adjustment. The results provided information regarding the incidence and variation of undesirable pre- and postoperative emotional and physical conditions, the relationship among different types of measures of preoperative affect and postoperative recovery, and the relationship between level of preoperative fear and anxiety and postoperative recovery. The major findings and conclusions were: 1) at least 15 per cent of the males and 30 per cent of the females reported a high degree of fear and anxiety the night before surgery; 2) female patients reported more fear and anxiety than male patients; 3) postoperative self-ratings of emotional state, pain, and various aspects of physical condition are promising criterion measures of postoperative recovery in terms of being sensitive to individual differences and changing in the expected direction from day to day following surgery; 4) some commonly used indicators of postoperative condition have such low incidences of occurrence under usual conditions that they would not be efficient criterion measures; 5) most of the different measures and indicators of recovery are intercorrelated but not sufficiently so to justify assessing postoperative welfare with only one or two criterion measures; and 6) there was no substantial relationship between patients' preoperative level of fear and anxiety and any aspect of their postoperative recovery. Methodological problems in connection with the assessment of patients' emotional and physical reactions to surgery are discussed and suggestions for future research are made.

REFERENCES

1. Janis, I. L. *Psychological Stress; Psychoanalytic and Behavioral Studies.* New York, John Wiley and Sons, 1958.
2. Sheffer, M. B., and Greifenstein, F. E. Emotional responses of patients to surgery and anesthesia. *Anesthesiology* 21:502-507, Sept.-Oct. 1960.
3. Abram, H. S., and Gill, B. F. Predictions of postoperative psychiatric complications. *New Eng J Med* 265:1123-1128, Dec. 7, 1961.
4. Dumas, Rhetaugh G., and Leonard, R. C. Effect of nursing on the incidence of postoperative vomiting; a clinical experiment. *Nurs Res* 12:12-15, Winter 1963.
5. Bursten, Ben, and Russ, J. J. Preoperative psychological state and corticosteriod levels of surgical patients. *Psychosom Med* 27:309-316, July-Aug. 1965.
6. Depee, Jane K. *Effective Therapeutic Communication in Nursing.* (Clinical Sessions, 1964 No. 8) New York, American Nurses' Association, 1964, pp. 17-26.
7. Carnevali, Doris L. Preoperative anxiety. *Amer J Nurs* 66:1536-1538, July 1966.
8. Giller, D. W. Some psychological correlates of recovery from surgery. *Texas Rep Biol Med* 20:366-376, Fall 1962.
9. Palmer, Irene S. Development of a measuring device; measuring patients' perception toward impending surgery. *Nurs Res* 14:100-105, Summer 1965.
10. Lynch, J. D., and others. Anxiety and anxiety reduction in surgical patients. *AORN* 6:58-60, July 1967.
11. Tsushima, W. T. Responses of Irish and Italian patients of two social classes under preoperative stress. *J Personality Soc Psychol* 8:43-48, Jan. 1968.
12. Spielberger, C. D. Theory and research on anxiety. In *Anxiety and Behavior*, ed. by C. D. Spielberger. New York, Academic Press, 1966, pp. 2-20.
13. Cattell, R. B., and Scheier, I. H. *Meaning and Measurement of Neuroticism and Anxiety.* New York, Ronald Press, 1961.
14. Taylor, J. A. Personality scale of manifest anxiety. *J Abnorm Soc Psychol* 48:285-290, Apr. 1953.
15. Zuckerman, M. The development of an affect adjective check list for the measurement of anxiety, *J Consult Psychol* 24:457-462, Oct. 1960.
16. Hodges, W. F., and Spielberger, C. E. The effects of threat shock on heart rate for subjects who differ in manifest anxiety and fear of shock. *Psychophysiology* 2:287-294, Apr. 1966.
17. Hodges, W. F. Effects of ego threat and threat of pain on state anxiety. *J Personality Soc Psychol* 8:364-372, Apr. 1968.
18. Henderson, Virginia. Overview of nursing research. *Nurs Res* 6:61-71, Oct. 1957.
19. Abdellah, F. G. Criterion measures in nursing. *Nurs Res* 10:21-26, Winter 1961.
20. Iowa University, nurse utilization project staff. *An Investigation of the Relation between Nursing Activity and Patient Welfare.* Principal coinvestigators, Myrtle K. Aydelotte and Marie E. Tener. Iowa City, Iowa, State University of Iowa, 1960.
21. DeLuca, Virginia M. *Some Observations on the Use of a Deliberative Nursing Process and the Incidence of Urinary Retention Following Surgery.* New Haven, Conn., Yale University School of Nursing, 1962. (M.S. thesis microfilm) (Abstracted in *Nursing Research* 13:275(139), Summer 1964.
22. Simon, R. J. Systematic ratings of patient welfare. *Nurs Outlook* 9:432, July 1961.
23. Egbert, L. D., and others. Reduction of postoperative pain by encouragement and instruction of patients. *New Eng J Med* 270:825-827, Apr. 16, 1964.
24. Johnson, J. E. Influence of purposeful nurse-patient interaction on the patient's postoperative course. In *Exploring Progress in Medical-Surgical Nursing Practice* A series of papers presented at the 1965 regional clinical conferences sponsored by the American Nurses' Association in Washington, D.C. and Chicago, Ill., 1965. New York, American Nurses' Association, 1966, No. 2, pp. 16-22.
25. Healy, K. M. Does preoperative instruction make a difference? *Amer J Nurs* 68:62-67, Jan. 1968.
26. Meehl, P. E., and Rosen, A. Antecedent probabil-

ity and the efficiency of psychometric signs, patterns, or cutting scores. *Psychol Bull* 52:194-216, May 1955.
27. Dumas and Leonard, *op. cit.*
28. Egbert and others, *op. cit.*
29. Janis, *op. cit.*
30. Bittle, S. P. *The Relationship between Preoperative Psychological Distress and Postoperative Recovery.* Salt Lake City, Utah, University of Utah College of Nursing, 1969. (Unpublished master's thesis)
31. Hutton, A. P. *Nursing Assessment of Emotional Distress and Postoperative Recovery in Heart Surgery Patients.* Salt Lake City, Utah, University of Utah College of Nursing, 1969. (Unpublished master's thesis)
32. Healy, *op. cit.*
33. Endler, N. S. and others. An S-R inventory of anxiousness. *Psychol Monogr* 76: (17 Whole No. 536) 1962.
34. Gelfand, S. Relationship of experimental pain tolerance to pain threshold. *Canad J Psychol* 18: 36-42, Mar. 1964.
35. Gelfand, D. M., and others. Some personality factors associated with placebo responsivity. *Psychol Rep* 17:555-562, Oct. 1965.
36. Coppolino, C. A. Incidence of postanesthetic delirium in a community hospital; a statistical study. *Milit Med* 128:238-241, Mar. 1963.
37. Smessaert, A., and others. Observations in the immediate postanaesthesia period. Part 2. Mode of recovery. *Brit J Anaesth* 32:181-185, Apr 1960.
38. *Ibid.*
39. Janis, *op. cit.*
40. Hodges, W. F. Effects of ego threat and threat of pain on state anxiety. *J Personality Soc Psychol* 8:364-372, Apr. 1968.

35

Case histories and shorter communications

An application of behavior modification technique to a problem of chronic pain

Wilbert E. Fordyce, Roy S. Fowler, and Barbara DeLateur

INTRODUCTION

The case study reported here treats as operants aspects of what we term "pain behavior". It describes applications of operant methods (Ayllon and Michael, 1959; Haughton, 1962) to modifying environmental contingencies to pain behavior and illustrates preliminary results.

Responses by others to overt pain behavior accompanying the subjective experience of pain may serve to reinforce or to extinguish aspects of that behavior. When the pain behavior occurs with some consistency over a protracted period of time, as in chronic pain problems, the environment may come to be shaped in such a way as to reinforce the pain behavior and thereby sustain it. In a hospital, overt expressions or demonstrations of discomfort are frequently followed by attention from professional personnel, just as at home family members may respond with attention and ministering behavior. If one can modify such environmental responses, pain behavior itself may be modified.

The case study reported was carried out in a comprehensive medical rehabilitation department of a teaching hospital.

Mrs. Y is a 37-yr-old, married, white female, high school graduate with one child, a teenage son. Her husband is a bright, upward mobile, school administrator. Since 1948, approximately 1 yr after her marriage, she has had virtually constant low-back pain and has been decreasingly able to carry out her normal homemaking activities.

At the time of admission to the hospital, she complained of a continuous aching pain in the low back which increased with any activity. She reported her maximum continuous period of activity without an interval of reclining rest was approximately 20 min. When one of these episodes of pain occurred, typically she ceased all activity, reclined on her bed or couch, took pain medication, and cried until the pain subsided. These episodes elicited much solicitous and ministering behavior from husband and son.

Medically, during the 18-yr history of back pain, the patient had undergone four surgical procedures. The first of these (1951) was removal of a herniated disc, which removed the symptoms of root irritation, but did not completely remove the localized back pain. The final operation (1962), a lumbosacral spine fusion, left her with a stable spine. A careful evaluation revealed no neurologic deficit. No signs of nerve root irritation were elicited.

It was decided that Mrs. Y's pain behavior would be treated as an operant. A treatment schedule was designed to modify her pain behavior and increase her general level of activity. The major reinforcers under our control were medication, attention, and rest.

When admitted, the patient was taking 4

Reprinted with permission from Fordyce, W. E., Fowler, R. S., and DeLateur, B.: An application of behavior modification technique to a problem of chronic pain. Behavior Research and Therapy **6:**105-107.

From the Department of Physical Medicine and Rehabilitation, University of Washington, School of Medicine, Seattle, Washington.

or 5 habit-forming analgesic tablets per day when she experienced pain. Such a regime has the effect of reinforcing pain behavior, with chemotherapeutic relief and attention from prestige figures. Her medicine regime was shifted from a pain to a time contingency program; i.e. medication was given at specified time intervals. Medication was never given when she complained of pain unless the complaint coincided with elapse of the time interval.

A color and taste masking vehicle was added to her medication. After the patient was solidly established in an activity regime, the narcotic content was decreased and by 40 days after admission was deleted altogether, without knowledge of the patient or nurses. Then the doses were decreased to every 4 hr, and 1 week later the dose in the middle of the night was omitted.

All treatment staff (physicians, nurses and other ward personnel, occupational therapist, physical therapist, and rehabilitation counselor) were instructed to be as neutral and socially unresponsive as possible to complaints by Mrs. Y of pain and discomfort (Ayllon and Michael, 1959). When the patient was observed participating in any kind of activity, other than lying in bed, the staff was instructed to make a positive effort to be friendly and socially responsive. They were instructed to be lavish in their praise of daily increases in her activity level. Thus, pain behavior received a minimum of social reinforcement while activity was maximally reinforced.

An occupational therapy program was designed which emphasized rest as the reinforcer. Mrs. Y was given the task of constructing a close-weave luncheon cloth on a standard 36-in floor loom. The task demanded considerable movement of her arms and legs and was accomplished sitting, a position she had described as one of her most painful. At the outset she was instructed "to work as long as you can." Several days of observation established her base line as approximately 25 threads within her 20 min activity tolerance. She was then instructed that each day she was to add ten more threads before she could leave occupational therapy to return to the ward to rest. At the end of 13 days she had completed a sizable tablecloth and was working continuously for more than 1 hr. She was then started on a new task which involved the construction of a small Turkish knot rug. At this point her rate of activity was so rapid and so efficient that she was able to complete this and several other occupational therapy projects before a stable base line of activity could be established. By the 30th day after admission she was working voluntarily for the full period of available occupational therapy time which was slightly under 2 hr.

A program was developed to increase her walking. A minimal physical therapy program of body baker and mild massage to the lower back area was begun. Concomitantly, on the ward she was assigned a daily walking schedule of 200-ft laps around the ward in the morning and again in the afternoon. Her initial trials demonstrated a base line of approximately 10 laps before she would complain of intolerable fatigue and/or pain. She was instructed to report to the nurses at the outset and completion of each series of laps. This provided a check on the reliability of her lap elapsed time recordings. It also alerted the ward staff to apply appropriate social reinforcement to this activity (Meichenbaum, 1966). The immediate reinforcers for the walking task were rest upon completion, social attention and praise from ward personnel both during and following her striding around the ward, and her own record, which she could observe herself and show to others. She was started at sets of 10 laps in the morning and 10 in the afternoon. Approximately every 10 days she was instructed to increase the number of laps in each set by five. At the end of seven weeks she was walking 25 laps or 5000 ft both morning and afternoon in very nearly the same time it had taken her to do 10 laps at the outset. She reached a walking speed approximately twice that of normal (Bard and Ralston, 1959).

Mrs. Y was given a small notebook to keep near her at all times in which she recorded unscheduled activities and their duration, in minutes. The staff referred to it often and made positive references to her daily increases in extra-schedule activities. The total number of minutes spent in activity each day, both scheduled and unscheduled were tabulated daily.

An approximate baseline of Mrs. Y's prehospitalization activities was provided by her husband who submitted a list which he felt was representative of her typical activities. It indicated a nonreclining activity schedule averaging approximately 2 hr per day. The balance of her day was spent reading, watching TV or sleeping.

Mrs. Y was seen daily for 10-15 min to construct graphs from her own records showing her daily progress. These sessions served to provide social reinforcement for her progress, as well as quality control checks on each component of the program.

At the outset of treatment, it was specified that her case would not be accepted unless her husband made himself available no less than 1 hr per week. He was seen by the same psychologist who was seeing the patient. The general outlines of the program were described to him. His cooperation was readily obtained. He was instructed on specific ways of being non-responsive to pain behavior and the importance of making reinforcing responses to her activity behavior.

He was asked to keep records of the amount of time she was engaged in active pursuits, rather than reclining and resting, when she was home on weekend passes. These records provided checks against Mrs. Y's records and served as reminders to him to be selectively responsive to activity and inactivity or pain behavior. They also served as a source of reinforcers to him in that he could observe tangible evidence of changes in her behavior as the treatment program went along. The length and frequency of passes granted to the patient to go home were increased on succeeding weeks. Concomitantly, sessions with the husband were used to explore specific activities which could be added during the times Mrs. Y was on pass. These included homemaking, cooking, washing, ironing, grooming, visiting with friends and relatives, and dining out.

Despite these various measures designed to provide generalization of her increasing levels of activity, when Mrs. Y moved to outpatient status there was, at first, a sharp drop in her activity and a sharp increase in her overt complaints of pain, as well as in the accompanying reclining behavior. She soon returned to her pattern of steady increase in activity. Figure 1 shows the record of her activity since admission.

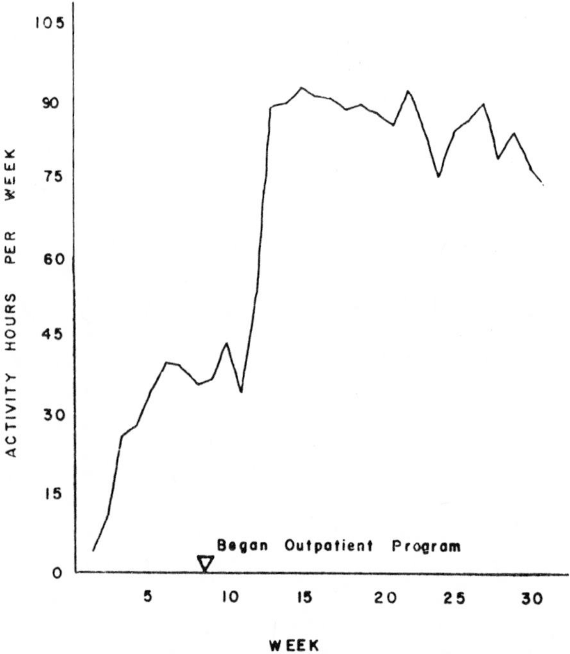

Fig. 1. Hours of non-reclining activity per week.

At the time of this report the program had consisted of eight weeks of inpatient care and 23 weeks of decreasingly frequent outpatient visits. She was being seen once a month for a brief recheck. The family had acquired a second car and she was taking driving lessons so as to be independently mobile in the community.

DISCUSSION

Results with this case suggest that the modification of some environmental contingencies influenced pain behavior. The methods described consider questions relating to whether the pain is "real" as irrelevant. The question dealt with is whether modification of environmental responses to pain behavior can produce measureable changes in that behavior and in other behavior identified as limited by virtue of the presence of a chronic pain problem.

The results suggest judicious use of three potential reinforcers (medication, rest and social attention), commonly available in medical settings, can produce significant effects on behavior relating to chronic pain.

There has been a marked increase in her activity level and virtual disappearance of complaints of pain in a period of eight weeks of comprehensive care following 18 yr of decreasing activity, during the past 5 yr of which she was in a state of virtually total immobilization. Fairly effective control has been gained over environmental responses to her behavior. How long these new patterns will continue remains to be seen.

ACKNOWLEDGEMENTS

This study was supported in part by VRA Research and Training Grant RT-3.

REFERENCES

Ayllon T. and Michael J. (1959) The psychiatric nurse as a behavioral engineer. *J. exp. Analysis Behav.* **2,** 323-334.

Bard G. and Ralston H. J. (1959) Measurement of energy expenditure during ambulation, with special reference to evaluation of assistive devices. *Arch. phys. Med. Rehabil.* **40,** 415-420.

Haughton E. (1962) Shaping participation in occupational therapy. Paper given at the Third International Congress World Federation of Occupational Therapists. November, 1962, Boston, Massachusetts, mimeo.

Meichenbaum D. H. (1966) Sequential strategies in two cases of hysteria. *Behav. Res. & Therapy* **4,** 89-94.

36

Pain and cancer

John M. Woodforde and Jennifer R. Fielding

Pain, destruction or loss of body parts, and death are the expected associates of cancer. In practice these pessimistic forbodings are not necessarily realised. In particular the incidence of severe, intractable pain is low contrary to the expectations of both the patients and their doctors. The pervasive sense of inevitability undoubtedly leads to the prescribing by doctors of addiction producing narcotics and it has been our observation that this hopelessness and helplessness may contribute to the complaint of pain by the patients.

The diagnosis of the cause of pain usually is seen as manifestly clear in patients with demonstrated tissue damage due to the neoplastic disease and the usually difficult question of whether there are "psychogenic" components to the pain is easily pushed aside. Yet it is clear that patients with neoplastic disease, like any other disease, often have complaints which have major emotional determinants. Furthermore, while all doctors agree that it is natural to have an emotional reaction following the diagnosis of neoplastic disease and its treatment, there are some who would prefer to agree with the patients who state or imply that the emotional effects are necessarily secondary to the pain, rather than involved in its causation. The tendency in clinical practice is to accept the "psychogenic-organic" dichotomy too easily.

Previous papers [1, 2] have described the evaluation and management of patients with intractable pain referred for consultation at a Pain Clinic. We, like many others [3-6] have sought more information about the patient's complaint of pain. This present paper reports some investigations into the pain of patients with cancer.

METHOD

The Cornell Index was introduced to this clinic in an attempt to provide, in a simple fashion, some more information about the emotional state of the patient. Weider *et al.* [7, 8] have described this test and its uses as an adjunct to the interview and as an instrument which "would statistically differentiate persons with serious personal and psychosomatic disturbances from the rest of the population".

As a practical point it was hoped that, by having more information about the patient's personality, it would be possible to predict those patients who would respond best to the recommended treatment. Querido [9] has shown that assessment of personality and social factors allowed prediction of the results of treatment in a general hospital. The first hypothesis in the present study was that patients referred to the Pain Clinic for treatment of intractable pain have more personality disturbance than those who have not been referred. The second hypothesis in this investigation is that patients with the greatest personality disturbance respond less well to pain relieving procedures.

Form N2 of the Cornell Index was used. This is a very simple pencil and paper test. It has 101 questions on two sides of a page. The patient has to answer "yes" or "no" to these questions which are phrased in informal English and can be understood by all those people who can read simple English. It can be completed usually within 15 min.

Each patient attending the Pain Clinic

Reprinted with permission from Woodforde, J. M., and Fielding, J. R.: Pain and cancer, Journal of Psychosomatic Research **14**:365-370. Copyright 1970, Pergamon Press.

From St. Vincent's Hospital, Sydney, N.S.W. Australia 2010.

was invited to complete the questionnaire in the waiting room of the Outpatient Department. He was then interviewed by the members of the clinic. The recommended treatment usually was performed by a member of the Pain Clinic and varied from nerve block, cordotomy, antidepressants, and/or alteration of analgesics. The results were assessed at a subsequent visit to the clinic or by contact with the referring doctor.

The result of treatment was assessed on a three point scale as (1) "complete" or "satisfactory" relief; (2) "slight" or "fair" or "some" relief; and (3) "unchanged" or "worse". It was occasionally difficult to make distinctions as the pain often varied from time to time and as to the informant. In the final analysis the distinction was between two categories only, "improved" or "unimproved".

The largest source of referral to the Pain Clinic was the Radiotherapy and Tumour Clinic of this hospital. And, although these patients formed a very small percentage of the population of the Radiotherapy and Tumour Clinic, it was decided to seek a sample of unreferred patients against which to compare the scores on the Index.

The sample of "unreferred" patients sought in the Radiotherapy and Tumour Clinic was matched with those referred to the Pain Clinic. This was done for age, diagnostic categories, and with the stipulation that they have active disease. It is of interest that there was a greater resistance to completing the questionnaire at the Radiotherapy and Tumour Clinic than at the Pain Clinic.

RESULTS

During the period of one year of investigation 80 patients attended the Pain Clinic. Of these 80 patients, 54 were undergoing, or had undergone, treatment in the Radiotherapy and Tumour Clinic of this hospital. It is this latter group which is the subject for investigation regarding response to procedures for pain relief. It is a percentage similar to that previously reported [1].

Of this group of 54 Pain Clinic patients two patients refused or were too ill to complete the Index. A further five patients could not be assessed regarding their response to treatment. The reasons for this were that they either refused to accept the recommendation regarding management, that they died before treatment or later assessment, or were otherwise lost to follow-up. This left 47 patients who had both completed the Index and were available for assessment of their response to treatment.

There was twice as many men (35) as women (17) in our group of Pain Clinic patients referred from the Tumour Clinic. This fact is largely related to the sex incidence of the particular site of the neoplasms. The average age was 55. 6 yr with a wide distribution from 25 to 80 yr but 86 per cent of patients fell within the range 40-79 (Table 1).

The diagnosis was malignant disease of some type. In the largest group the primary site (Table 2) was the head and neck on 19 occasions—lip, tongue, floor of the mouth, salivary glands, pharynx, palate, oesophagus and larynx, and in the skin of the head. On a further 12 occasions the primary lesion was in the genitourinary system—kidney, prostate, bladder, testes and cord, ovary, uterus. The next largest group (6) was those with primary lesions in

Table 1. Age distribution of the patients

Age	*Pain clinic (%)*		*Unreferred (%)*	
80-89	2	4	1	2
70-79	6	12	11	20
60-69	18	34	12	22
50-59	13	25	13	24
40-49	8	15	10	18
30-39	3	6	4	7
20-29	2	4	4	7
	$n = 52$		$n = 55$	

Table 2. Site distribution of the primary malignancy

Organs involved	*Pain clinic*	*Unreferred*
Head and neck	19	13
Lung	5	7
Breast	3	18
Bowel	6	1
Genitourinary	12	11
Other	7	5

the rectum and colon. Lesions in the bronchi occurred on five occasions. There was a smaller number of primary lesions in the breast (3) limbs (3 sarcomas).

The site of pain was the head and neck on 19 occasions, the chest 11 times, the shoulder and upper limbs 9 times, the abdomen 4 times and the pelvis and lower limbs on 12 occasions. There was no pattern of lateralisation of the site of pain. The pain was located on the left side by 20 patients, the right by 18 patients and a further 16 patients did not indicate whether the pain was localised to one particular side.

The total scores on the Index of the patients seen in the Pain Clinic were compared with their response to treatment. The scores were fairly symmetrically distributed about the median of 18 and ranged from a score of 1 to a score of 48 (Table 3).

Different methods of "cut-off levels" of score are used with this test. An Index score of 13 or more is reported [8] to include the majority of those with severe personality disturbance and a number of ostensibly healthy persons. A smaller percentage of serious personality disturbances but few ostensibly healthy persons are included when a cut-off level of 23 is used. In this investigation an intermediate "cut-off level" of 18 was chosen for statistical purposes. There was no significant correlation between the score on the Cornell Index and the response to treatment ($\chi^2 = 0.15$; $p = 0.70$).

Table 3. Distribution of Cornell Medical Index scores and the response to treatment of pain

	Response to treatment of pain		
Index score	*Good*	*Slight*	*None*
23+	9	1	6
18-22	5	2	0
13-17	6	3	0
0-12	5	5	5
	25	11	11

The second sample of patients given the Index were those who were under treatment in the Radiotherapy and Tumour Clinic but who had not been referred to the Pain Clinic i.e., the "unreferred" sample. There were 55 patients in this sample. The average age was 55.6 yr with 84 per cent lying between the age of 40 and 79. There were 25 men and 30 women. The sex distribution was more equal than in the group of patients referred to the Pain Clinic.

Comparison of the mean scores on the Index between the two samples of patients indicates some differences (Table 4). The Pain Clinic sample has a mean total score of 18.81 which is significantly greater than the 12.66 of the unreferred patients, i.e., in the direction of more personality disturbance.

Furthermore, it can be seen in the analysis of the scores that there are significant differences in the symptom complexes between the Pain Clinic sample and the "unreferred" sample. The patients referred to the Pain Clinic scored higher in the areas of Depression, Psychosomatic symptoms, Gastrointestinal symptoms, Hypochon-

Table 4. Comparison of Cornell Medical Index scores

	Pain clinic	*Unreferred*	*T*	*p*
Total score	18.81	12.66	2.764	<0.01
Fear and inadequacy	3.17	3.05	0.2276	>0.1
Depression	1.64	0.64	3.392	<0.01
Nervousness and anxiety	1.80	1.47	1.166	>0.05
Neurocirculatory	1.27	1.38	0.4919	>0.1
Startle reactions	1.19	1.4	0.664	>0.1
Psychosomatic symptoms	2.62	1.55	2.381	<0.02 >0.01
Hypochondriasis and asthenia	2.21	1.47	2.335	<0.05 >0.02
Gastrointestinal	3.19	1.47	3.946	<0.001
Sensitivity and suspiciousness	0.38	0.65	1.586	>0.1
Psychopathy	1.32	1.33	0.031	>0.1

Table 5. Comparison between sexes of Cornell Medical Index scores

	Pain clinic			*Unreferred*		
	Males	*Females*	*t*	*Males*	*Females*	*t*
Total score	19.66	17.06	0.8019	13.6	11.87	0.5091
Depression	1.77	1.35	0.7936	0.64	0.73	0.3243
Other psychosomatic symptoms	2.91	2.00	1.751	1.4	1.6	0.3922
Hypochondriasis and asthenia	2.2	2.23	0.061	1.44	1.50	0.013
Gastrointestinal	3.31	2.94	0.4944	1.52	1.43	0.016

driasis and Asthenia. The occurrence of depression among patients with pain referred to this clinic has been commented upon previously [1, 2].

It is possible that there would be differences in the Index scores between the men and women in each group both in the total scores and in the areas of the different symptom complexes. However it can be seen (Table 5) that in neither the Pain Clinic sample or the "unreferred" sample is there any significant difference in the mean scores between the sexes. The differences between the groups were not attributable to sex difference between the two groups.

DISCUSSION

The use of the Cornell Medical Index (C.M.I.) has confirmed our clinical impression that the group of "referred" cancer patients with intractable pain has more personality disturbance (higher mean total scores) than the "unreferred" group of cancer patients. The personality disturbance which distinguished the group of "referred" patients was in the areas of depression, psychosomatic symptoms, gastrointestinal symptoms, hypochondriasis and asthenia.

However there was no correlation between scores on the C.M.I. and the response to treatment within the group of referred patients. Therefore the use of the test as a screening tool at the Pain Clinic would be of little use with cancer patients similar to those in this group.

We had considered that personality features would be one factor significantly related to the complaint of pain, as would be the fear of helplessness of the patient and damage to the body image. It is worthwhile to look at each of these considerations and some of the relationships between them.

A wide range of emotional reactions can occur to cancer [10] or be associated with the complaint of pain [11, 12] but the occurrence of depression in our "referred" group was not unexpected. Yet the relationship of the depression to the intractable pain in the patients is not simply explained. The pain could be part of the depressive syndrome or it could be secondary to the pain resulting from the progression of the cancer. Of course, the latter too has its significance emotionally as well as due to local pressure on peripheral nerves.

The widespread occurrence of moderately severe depression presenting with physical symptoms, such as pain, is recognised frequently by psychiatrists but less often by other doctors [13]. Bradley [14] has drawn attention to the depression of patients presenting with persistent localised pain and this association has been observed in our experience at the Pain Clinic in the treatment of patients with postherpetic neuralgia [2]. The latter have some characteristics in common with cancer patients: the pain is persistent to the point of making both doctor and patient feel helpless, and there is a marked disturbance of body image. The pain is generally relieved by the use of antidepressant medication.

Cancer differs from most other conditions by the nature of its being a progressive disease. This progression depends on many factors including emotional factors and hormonal changes. West [10] has drawn attention to psychological defences which are utilised in cancer patients and how these may affect host resistance and result in success or failure of therapy for the disease. It is an important observation in this regard that many of the cancer patients with intractable pain referred to the Pain Clinic have subsequently died within a few months. It seems likely that the pain, depression and the progress of the disease are all indicative of the patient's helplessness to cope with the disease, the damage of his body and the threat of life on both the biochemical and the emotional level.

Childlike helplessness was a factor in the relationship between pain and depression recently discussed by Joffe and Sandler [15] who suggested that the depressive reaction is a "response to a state of pain, a response that reflects helplessness, capitulation, and resignation in the face of pain". They introduced the notion of a painful discrepancy in the self representation, in effect, a loss of self-image causing psychic pain which may result in depression or may be displaced to the idea of bodily pain. In those cases where there is pain and depression they regarded these as mixed clinical states in which no stable defensive solution has been reached.

Another aspect of the complaint of pain is its communication function. The pattern of communication between the doctor and the patient with cancer has been reviewed by Abrams [16]. She points to the changes in the communications from phase to phase of the disease. Many of the patients in the present study were in the phase of advancing disease (metastasis, etc.) when it is obvious to both the doctor and the patient that treatment has been unsuccessful in halting the disease. Abrams reminds us of the change from the optimism of the earlier treatment phase which gives way in this next phase to anxiety, euphemism and evasion, and dependency on the doctor with fears of abandonment. Abrams reports that patients rarely talk about the diagnosis at this stage but they wish to talk about questions related to bodily symptoms, diet, activity, etc. The complaint of pain can be an assurance of getting help in a euphemistic fashion without acknowledging the disease itself.

It is evident that the recognition and appropriate treatment of the depression and the implied requests for help will afford a great deal of relief to cancer patients who complain of pain.

SUMMARY

The Cornell Medical Index was used to provide more information regarding the personality disturbance of cancer patients referred to a Pain Clinic. There was no significant correlation between the scores of the Cornell Medical Index and the response to procedures for pain relief of a sample of 54 patients with persistent pain referred from the Radiotherapy and Tumour Clinics. There were significant differences between the scores of this referred sample and a sample of 55 patients at the Radiotherapy and Tumour Clinics who had not been referred. These differences indicate that the sample of patients referred to the Pain Clinic had more personality disturbance and that there were significant differences in the areas of Depression, Gastrointestinal symptoms, Hypochondriasis and Asthenia, and Psychosomatic symptoms. The relationship between the complaint of pain and the emotional state of the patient as a reaction to cancer has been discussed.

REFERENCES

1. McEwan B. W., de Wilde F. W., Dwyer B., Woodforde J. M., Bleasel K. and Connolley T. J. The pain clinic: a clinic for the management of intractable pain. *Med. J. Aust.* **1,** 676 (1965).
2. Woodforde J. M., Dwyer B., McEwan B. W., de Wilde F. W., Bleasel K., Connolley T. J. and Ho C. Y. Treatment of post-herpetic neuralgia. *Med. J. Aust.* **2,** 869 (1965).
3. Kolb L. C. *The Painful Phantom, Psychology, Physiology and Treatment.* Charles C Thomas, Springfield, Illinois (1954).
4. Szasz T. S. *Pain and Pleasure. A Study of Bodily Feelings.* Tavistock, London (1957).
5. Engel G. L. Psychogenic pain and the pain prone patient. *Am. J. Med.* **26,** 899 (1959).
6. Merskey H. and Spear F. G. The concept of pain. *J. Psychosom. Res.* **2,** 59 (1967).
7. Weider A., Brodman K., Mittelmann B., Wechsler D. and Wolff H. G. The Cornell Index. *Psychosom. Med.* **8,** 411 (1946).
8. Weider A., Wolff H. G., Brodman K., Mittelmann B. and Wechsler D. Cornell Index Manual. *Aust. Council of Educational Research.* Melbourne (1948).
9. Querido A. Forecast and Follow-up. An investigation into the clinical, social, and mental factors determining the results of hospital treatment. *Br. J. Prev. Soc. Med.* **13,** 33 (1959).
10. West P. M. Psychologic factors and host resistance to cancer, In *Year Book of Cancer* (Edited by Clark R. I. and Cumley R. W.), p. 542. (1956-1957).
11. Walters A. Psychogenic regional pain alias hysterical pain. *Brain* **84,** 1 (1961).
12. Merskey H. The characteristics of persistent pain

in psychological illness. *J. Psychosom. Res.* **9,** 291 (1965).

13. Watts C. A. H. The mild endogenous depression. *Br. Med. J.* **1,** 4 (1957).
14. Bradley J. J. Severe localised pain associated with the depressive syndrome. *Br. J. Psychiat.* **109,** 741 (1963).
15. Joffe W. G. and Sandler J. On the concept of pain with special reference to depression and psychogenic pain. *J. Psychosom. Res.* **2,** 69 (1967).
16. Abrams R. D. The patient with cancer—his changing pattern of communication. *New Engl. J. Med.* **274,** 317 (1966).

37

Pain and its management in malignant disease
Elucidation of staff-patient transactions

I. Pilowsky, MD, ChB, MANZCP, DPM, and M. R. Bond, MD

The need to study pain is "real" situations and the importance of taking into consideration its psychological aspects have been stressed by a number of authors.[1-4] A difficulty facing workers in this field is the multiplicity of variables involved and the lack of reliable methods for their measurement. This investigation was conducted in order to discover whether the use of a principal component analysis of data relating to the behavior of patients suffering from malignant disease, and the staff caring for them, would yield information regarding interactions between these two groups in relation to the management of pain. The settings chosen were the male and female radiotherapy wards of a general hospital. The measurements of patient and staff behavior were designed for acceptability and ease of use so that the subjects involved would be able to provide complete responses without any disruption of their activities.

Reprinted with permission of the American Psychosomatic Society from Psychosomatic Medicine **31**:400-404. Copyright 1969.

From the Department of Psychiatry, University of Sydney, Sydney, Australia (I. Pilowsky); and the Department of Psychiatry, University of Sheffield, Sheffield, England (M. R. Bond).

We wish to thank Dr. D. J. Evans, Director of the Computing Laboratory of the University of Sheffield, and Mrs. Anne Fairburn for the considerable help they have given us in the analysis of the data; as well as Professor E. Stengel and Dr. C. P. Seager for their advice and encouragement. We are grateful to the consultants of the Sheffield National Center for Radiotherapy for allowing us to investigate their patients, and to the nursing staff for their unfailing cooperation.

MATERIAL AND METHODS
Subjects

A total of 54 patients were studied, of whom 18 were excluded because of death or hospital discharge before the 5-day period of investigation was completed. Of the remaining 36, there were 21 females and 15 males, with ages ranging from 31 to 76, and 23 to 75 years, respectively. The conditions for which they were being treated are listed in Table 1.

Subjective assessment of pain

A graphic method was used by the patient for recording pain experienced at a series of fixed times during each of the 5 days. This procedure is a modification by Pilowsky and Kaufman[5] of the method devised by Clarke and Spear[6] for the subjective assessment of well-being.

The patient was required to make a pencil mark on a 10-cm line which contained the words "I have no pain at all" at the left end, and "my pain is as bad as it could possibly be" at the right end. The distance from the left end of the line to the point at which the patient's mark intersected it was measured in millimeters, and this figure was designated as a "pain score."

Patients were required to assess their pain in this way every 2 hr from 8 AM to 8 PM over a 5-day period, giving seven scores daily from each individual. From this data, each patient's mean pain score for the 5-day period was obtained.

Drugs were given according to the usual ward practice, and entirely at the discretion of the nursing and medical staff without reference to the investigators.

Table 1. Nature and sex distribution of lesions

Tumor type	*Females*	*Males*
Carcinoma – cervix	9	0
Carcinoma – bladder	0	5
Carcinoma – larynx	0	3
Carcinoma – tongue	2	2
Carcinoma – breast	2	0
Multiple myeloma	2	1
Hodgkin's disease	1	2
Lymphosarcoma	1	0
Carcinoma – lung	1	0
Carcinoma – maxillary antrum	1	1
Carcinoma – uterus	1	0
Spiral secondary deposits	0	1
Carcinoma – rectum	1	0

Cornell Medical Index (CMI)

This inventory was used in an attempt to gain some indication of the patient's physical and psychological symptom pattern. Originally intended as an adjunct to medical interviewing,[7] the CMI consists of an inventory of 195 questions to which the patient responds "yes" or "no." The questions are grouped by systems labeled A to R, with Sections A to L dealing with physical symptoms, and M to R being mainly concerned with psychiatric symptoms. A total score of 0 to 15 was considered "normal," a score of 16 to 30 "intermediate," and scores over 30 as "high."[8] Patients were categorized accordingly. In addition, Section J of the CMI was scored separately as an index of the patient's concept of himself as an "ill person" with some indication of his attitude toward his illness. The following questions were asked:

1. Are you frequently ill?
2. Are you frequently confined to bed by illness?
3. Are you always in poor health?
4. Are you considered a sickly person?
5. Do you come from a sickly family?
6. Do severe pains and aches make it impossible for you to do your work?
7. Do you wear yourself out worrying about your health?
8. Are you always ill and unhappy?
9. Are you constantly made miserable by poor health?

Communication of pain and staff response

The nursing staff was asked to fill in a "pain chart" on which they recorded the occasions and times that each patient was given medication for the relief of pain. The nature of the drug given was recorded and, in addition, whether it was given in response to a request by the patient or on the initiative of the staff. All requests for pain relief by patients were recorded, whether or not they were acceded to by the administration of analgesics.

From these charts, a number of scores were obtained for each patient relating to requests and drugs given. They were:

(1) total number of patient requests not acceded to, total number of patient requests acceded to, total number of treatments given on staff initiative; and (2) The number of occasions on which aspirin or Paracetamol were given, the number of occasions on which dihydrocodeine or codeine phosphate were given, and the number of occasions on which morphine or Pethidine were given.

Principal component analysis

The statistical procedures were carried out on the mercury electronic digital computer in the Computing Laboratory of the University of Sheffield. The 16 variables were intercorrelated, and the resultant matrix of product-moment correlations was then subjected to a principal-component analysis.[9] The factors which emerged were rotated by the Varimax method[10] in order to maximize loadings and facilitate interpretation.

RESULTS

Of the factors which emerged from this analysis, only the first three (accounting for 66% of the total variance) were amenable to interpretation (Table 2).

Each factor seemed to delineate a pattern of staff-patient transactions relating to the issues of pain experience, the communication of discomfort, and the staff response.

Factor 1

This factor had high positive loading on the CMI Section J score, the mean weekly subjective pain assessment, and the number of patient's requests for pain relief

Table 2. Rotated factor loadings

Variable	*Factor 1*	*Factor 2*	*Factor 3*
Sex (+ female)	−0.164	+0.548	+0.066
Age	−0.160	+0.123	+0.464
Attitude to ill health	+0.329	+0.189	−0.092
Lesion of head & neck	+0.158	−0.126	+0.271
Lesion of pelvis	−0.238	+0.047	+0.242
Other lesions	−0.242	+0.068	−0.517
CMI 0-15	−0.067	−0.260	−0.013
CMI 16-30	−0.092	−0.125	−0.089
CMI 31+	+0.154	+0.368	+0.101
Average pain score	+0.414	−0.053	−0.043
No. patient requests (no drug)	+0.394	−0.056	+0.031
No. patient requests (drug)	+0.374	+0.066	+0.086
No. times drugs given on staff initiative	+0.249	+0.207	−0.331
Aspirin	+0.260	+0.080	+0.083
Dihydrocodeine	+0.241	−0.091	+0.196
Morphine	+0.080	+0.203	−0.334

(with or without staff response). This factor, therefore, indicated a transaction in which patients who regarded themselves as "ill," and were concerned about this, assessed themselves as having considerable pain and frequently asked for relief. The loadings suggested that the nurses tended to respond variably to these requests. The staff response showed that, in terms of the relevant variables, they acted on their own initiative at times, but morphine and Pethidine were withheld in favor of the less powerful analgesics.

Factor 2

This factor indicated a sex-related transaction. There was a high positive loading for being female, having a high CMI score, and receiving drugs on staff initiative. Powerful analgesics such as morphine and Pethidine were more likely to be given.

Factor 3

Factor 3 appeared to be an age-related factor, indicating a tendency for older patients not to be given powerful analgesics and not to be treated by the nursing staff on their own initative.

DISCUSSION

As might be expected, a variety of treatment transactions have emerged from this study, once again supporting previous observations that the relationship between the experience of pain and its treatment is an exceedingly complex one. The types of staff-patient interaction which have emerged from this study inevitably must depend on the variables which have been included in the analysis, and there can be no doubt that the picture which has emerged constitutes an oversimplification of the actual situation. Nonetheless, it does suggest a method by which ward interactions may be studied, and possibly provide pointers relating to desirable and undesirable staff-patient relationships.

The findings of this study indicate that the tendency to complain of pain is very much related to the patient's assessment of his sick-role status rather than to his degree of neuroticism. Furthermore, there is a relationship between this and a tendency for the nursing staff to administer less effective analgesics. Clearly there is a difference in the way the patient's discomforts were evaluated by the patient himself, and by the nursing staff. Thus the patient's tendency to assess his pain as considerable, and to frequently request relief, may be as much related to his unquestioned organic pathology as to his feeling that the staff does not respond to his needs. The tendency for the staff to give minor analgesics may indicate a need to respond to requests in a "conventional" help-giving manner, coupled with a belief that the requests for pain relief do not indicate a need for powerful analgesics. In this supposition they may well be wrong of course, but there is the implication that the staff response is insufficient if it consists of tablet giving alone, without psychological support based on an understanding of the patient's subjective state.

The second factor suggests that in the female ward, the staff was more prepared to provide powerful analgesics without waiting for the patient to make a request. Although the CMI loading suggests that these patients are more "neurotic,"[8] it would seem that they do not feel the need to communicate pain to the same extent as those involved in the first transaction. This may be due in part to their less marked tendency to regard themselves as ill, as indicated by the lower loading on the CMI Section K score. At the same time, it is obvious that a readiness to provide powerful analgesia may result in less pain experience and pain communication, both for psychological and pharmacological reasons.

The third treatment transaction seems to be related to a different dimension of relationships. It seems likely that the desire to deny the nursing staff the initiative of giving analgesics, and the withholding of powerful agents, indicates a wish to avoid the possibly dangerous side-effects with the use of such drugs in older patients. It is interesting to note that this was not associated with high subjective pain assessments or requests for relief, and this may indicate that the staff attitude to the use of analgesics was not seen as a rejection, and furthermore, that the staff was relating satisfactorily to the older patients at the purely interpersonal level.

This study has been based on the conviction expressed by many authors that the experience of pain cannot be studied independently of the individual's view of its significance to his own illness, the setting in which it occurs, and the reactions of those to whom appeals for help are directed. The statistical method employed was intended to dissect out patient-staff transactions in a meaningful fashion. The results obtained suggest that this approach may prove a fruitful one, and that a considerable degree of self-awareness and psychological sophistication may be required of a staff working with the category of patients taking part in this study.

SUMMARY

In order to delineate staff-patient interactions in relation to the management of pain in patients with malignant disease, a principal component analysis has been carried out on variables presumed to be relevant. From this, three "transactions" have emerged: (1) a tendency for increased subjective assessment of pain with requests for analgesics from patients who regard themselves as ill people, were met with staff ambivalence and the withholding of powerful analgesics; (2) a correlation between high CMI scores, female sex, and the staff's tendency to provide powerful analgesics on their own initiative; and (3) an association between greater patient age and a reluctance to give powerful analgesics.

The significance of these findings is discussed.

REFERENCES

1. Beecher, H. K. *The Assessment of Pain in Man and Animals. UFAW Symposium.* Livingstone, Edinburgh, 1961.
2. Stengel, E. Pain and the psychiatrist. *Brit J Psychiat 111*:795, 1965.
3. Szasz, T. S. *Pain and Pleasure.* Tavistock Publications, London, 1957.
4. Rangell, L. Psychiatric aspects of pain. *Psychosom Med 15*:22, 1953.
5. Pilowsky, I., and Kaufman, A. An experimental study of atypical phantom pain. *Brit J Psychiat 111*:1185, 1965.
6. Clark, P. R. F., and Spear, F. G. Reliability and sensitivity in the self-assessment of well being. *Bull Brit Psychol Soc 17*:55, 18A, 1964.
7. Brodman, K., Erdmann, A. J., Large, I., Wolff, H. G., and Broadbent, T. H. The Cornell Medical Index—An adjunct to medical interview. *JAMA 140*:530, 1949.
8. Ryle, A., and Hamilton, M. Neurosis in fifty married couples. *J Ment Sci 108*:265, 1962.
9. Cooley, W. W., and Lohnes, P. R. *Multiveriate Procedures for the Behavioural Sciences.* Wiley, New York, 1962.
10. Kaiser, H. F. The varimax criterion for analytic rotation in factor analyses. *Psychometrika 23*:187, 1958.

38

Effects of a counterirritant on perceived pain and hand movement in patients with arthritis

James R. White, Ph.D.

Pathological restriction of range of motion in joints of patients with arthritis is usually referred to as partial ankylosis. Ankylosis may result from erosion of articular cartilage, fibrosis in the joint capsule, fibrous adhesion between joint surfaces, or fibrosis and contracture of muscles and tendons in and surrounding the joint. Any of these conditions may cause a sensation of pain in the joint and a resulting spasm in the surrounding muscles. Using electromyography, Wasserman and associates found abnormal levels of electrical activity in the muscles surrounding the joints of patients with arthritis.[1] Similarly, a coworker and I tested thirty patients suffering from arthritic involvement and found higher levels of electrical activity in the muscles surrounding the arthritic joints than in those surrounding the nonarthritic joints.[2] The patients reported that the application of a counterirritant produced a decrease in pain ($p < .001$), and a significant decrease in muscle spasm (demonstrated by reduced electrical activity) was observed after treatment ($p = .001$). In a later study, we found that shoulder joint range of motion significantly increased following application of the counterirritant.

Wasserman has shown that abnormal electromyographic readings occur more frequently in distal muscles than in proximal and more frequently in those muscles adjacent to arthritic joints than in those adjacent to uninvolved joints. The relatively higher levels of electrical activity found in the muscles adjacent to involved joints are probably the result of contraction of the muscles occurring in response to the unconscious effort of the patient to immobilize the painful joint. The contracting muscles produce metabolites which may irritate nerve endings causing pain. The pain brings about additional muscle spasm, which produces metabolites; thus, a vicious cycle is formed.

A reasonable hypothesis is that the application of a counterirritant over the muscles surrounding the affected joint should break the cycle in the following way: it should decrease subjective pain by increasing blood supply (the increase being elicited through the axon reflex), thus removing metabolites trapped in the tissue. The removal of metabolites should decrease muscle spasm and, as a result, increase the range of motion and digital dexterity which was limited by the muscle spasms related to the original pain.

INSTRUMENTATION

Audiometer

The purpose of the audiometer was to enable the patients to match decibel level at a given frequency with perceived pain. The device consisted of earphones and a signaling box (capable of producing sounds ranging from zero to 80 decibels and 500

From the Department of Physical Education, University of California, San Diego, Box 109, LaJolla, Calif. 92037.

to 6,000 Hz). The reliability of the instrument was established by the correlation of repeated trials ($r = .96$). The data represent the .01 level of confidence. The instrument is described in greater detail elsewhere.[4]

Flexometer

A flexometer was used to measure joint motion. The instrument, designed by Leighton, consists of a circular scale (360 degrees) with a weighted dial and a weighted pointer needle.[5] The instrument was strapped to the specific hand which was to be tested. The dial and pointer were set at zero degrees. The patient extended his wrist, and the pointer indicated the exact number of degrees through which the hand had moved. The mechanics of the instrument are based on the fact that gravity pulls the weighted end of the needle downward during the execution of the range-of-motion movement. Leighton reported reliabilities of r = .90 to r = .98 in the use of the flexometer. Similar results were found in test-retest correlations of the instrument in the author's laboratory.

Digital dexterity quantifier

A digital dexterity quantifier was used to measure finger dexterity. The instrument, designed in the author's laboratory, consists of a set of three keys mounted on a wooden panel. Each time a finger depresses one of the keys, the depression is mechanically recorded. In this study, the sum of the finger depressions taken for thirty seconds constituted the task. The patient worked the fingers of one hand for thirty seconds, rested for thirty seconds, then worked the fingers of the opposite hand for thirty seconds, and rested for thirty seconds for a total of five trials with each hand. A criterion score of the five trials was used, and a greater score indicated a greater degree of digital dexterity. The reliability of the instrument was established by the correlation of repeated trials (r = .93). The data represent the .01 level of confidence.[6]

METHOD

Patients

Selection of patients was made by a specialist in arthritis at the Riverside Medical Clinic and County Hospital in Riverside, California. Thirty patients, ten men and twenty women ranging in age from thirty-seven to eighty-one years with a mean age of fifty-nine, were tested. Sixteen patients were classified as having rheumatoid arthritis and fourteen were classified as having osteoarthritis. (Classification of patients for the study was based on standards prescribed by the American Rheumatism Association.)

Testing procedure

A questionnaire was administered to verify the existence of perceived pain and to gather pertinent information to be used in the analysis of data.

The patient was asked to sit in a comfortable chair. A mobile table containing the audiometer (frequency at 3,000 Hz) was wheeled to the side of the patient. Selection of the specific hand to be tested first was made by rotation on the Latin square design. The patient was seated in such a position that the numbers on the audiometer scale were concealed from his view. The experimenter then increased the intensity level (loudness) until the patient indicated that the sound intensity matched the level of perceived pain he was experiencing in the hand being tested. The procedure was repeated for the other hand. The decibel levels selected for both hands were recorded. To correlate the reliability of the test-retest, the entire audiometric procedure was repeated.

The patient was then asked to sit at a desk with his back erect. To ensure alignment during hand movement, the patient's arm was aligned with a horizontal mark drawn on the desk top. The flexometer was strapped to the hand just above the transverse metacarpal ligament. The patient's hand was gently placed against the table top with the palm flat, elbow in contact with the table top. The patient was then asked to slowly extend the hand at the wrist and continue the movement until he was unable to continue because of the resultant pain. (This point was called the limit of joint motion.) The degrees registered at the limit were recorded, and the subject was told to relax. The same procedure was repeated with the opposite hand.

For the test of finger dexterity, the patient was instructed to place the ring finger, index finger, and thumb on the keys of the dexterity quantifier, the fingers being comfortably stretched and the heel of the hand resting on a pad adjacent to the keys. Next, the patient was instructed to begin finger movements similar to those used in typing. The ring finger or the thumb was moved first, followed by the other fingers in sequence. The patient was given three five-second trials for each hand to acquaint him with the instrument. Following this introductory period, he was instructed to depress the keys in sequence as rapidly as possible. The task was performed for thirty seconds, a thirty-second rest was given, and the task was then performed for thirty seconds by the fingers of the opposite hand. Each subject performed the task five times. A criterion score was used for the five trials.

Each patient was assigned a box containing two coded tubes of cream. One tube contained the active counterirritant,* and the other contained the placebo (a cream base similar to that used in Ben-Gay in which the active ingredients were replaced by isopropyl myristate and water). The code numbers on each tube differed for each patient. The master code was not given to the experimenters until testing was completed. The research design was double blind. Approximately one centimeter of the contents of the coded tubes was applied to the wrist, hand, and fingers, accompanied by a thirty-second massage. Selection of the hand to first receive the contents of a tube was made by rotation on the Latin square design. The coded tube to be used on each hand was selected randomly.

Approximately five minutes after application of the cream, audiometer testing was repeated to gather postapplication readings. Approximately ten minutes after application of the cream, range-of-motion testing was repeated, and approximately fifteen minutes after application of the cream, dexterity testing was repeated to gather postapplication data.

*Ben-Gay greaseless/stainless (10% menthol and 15% methyl salicylate).

RESULTS

After the testing was completed, the samples were decoded and the data were grouped according to pretreatment and posttreatment readings on hands receiving placebo and active medication. Analysis of the data yielded the following results.

Audiometer

The mean audiometer readings taken before medication was applied indicated that similar pain levels were being experienced in both hands. Application of the placebo produced a nonsignificant decrease in perceived pain in that hand (Tab. 1).

Range of motion

No significant difference in limit of joint motion was found to exist in the preapplication flexometer readings between hands designated to receive placebo and counterirritant. Following the application of the placebo, the limit of joint motion significantly increased, and following the application of the counterirritant, the limit also significantly increased. Application of the counterirritant, however, produced a significantly greater increase in range of motion than did application of the placebo (Tab. 2).

Table 1. Audiometer—perceived pain matched to sound level measured in decibels before and following application of the counterirritant and placebo

	Decibels	*t*	*p*
Counterirritant			
Preapplication	35.53	3.438	.002
Postapplication	31.83		
Placebo			
Preapplication	33.23	1.863	.073
Postapplication	31.03		

Table 2. Flexometer—range of motion measured in degrees before and following application of the counterirritant and placebo

	ROM	*t*	*p*
Counterirritant			
Preapplication	39.73	4.92	<.001
Postapplication	46.93		
Placebo			
Preapplication	39.17	3.278	.003
Postapplication	41.23		

Table 3. Dexterity—dexterity measured by the sum of finger depressions executed in thirty seconds following the application of the counterirritant and placebo

	Number of depressions	*t*	*p*
Counterirritant			
Preapplication	73.7	6.067	<.001
Postapplication	88.23		
Placebo			
Preapplication	74.87	3.152	.004
Postapplication	78.93		

Digital dexterity

The preapplication digital dexterity scores for the hand designated to receive the placebo and the hand designated to receive the counterirritant indicated no significant differences between the hands. Following the application of both the placebo and counterirritant, the criterion score for dexterity increased significantly; however, application of the counterirritant produced a significantly greater increase in finger dexterity than did application of the placebo (Tab. 3).

QUESTIONNAIRE

Answers to the questionnaire showed that all the patients experienced varying degrees of pain and stiffness on the testing day. Twenty-seven of the thirty patients reported that, in past experiences, warmth or massage had aided in relieving pain and had improved the range of motion of the involved joint.

In this study, twenty-nine of the subjects reported temperature effects, i.e., a feeling of warmth or coolness in the hand receiving the active medication. Of these, twenty reported warmth and nine reported coolness. Of the thirty subjects, twenty-two reported temperature effects in the hand receiving the placebo, fifteen reporting warmth and seven reporting coolness.

Twenty-five patients reported that the active medication was effective in decreasing pain; twenty-four reported that the placebo did not alter the pain.

Twenty-eight patients reported that the medication reduced stiffness and increased the possibility of hand and finger movements; twenty-five reported that the placebo did not change the possibility of movement.

DISCUSSION

In this study, it was hypothesized that the counterirritant would reduce muscle spasm around arthritic joints and that the reduction of spasm would allow greater range of movement of the joints and greater digital dexterity.

The application of counterirritants does not actually increase tissue temperature,[7] but causes a sensation of heat, as well as a "flair" or flushed appearance of the skin, which results from active tissue hyperemia elicited through the axon reflex.[8-12] This hyperemia is helpful in terminating the ischemia which, in part, causes muscle pain.[13]

Treatment for soreness in muscles adjacent to arthritic joints usually involves changing body temperature. DonTigny and Sheldon have explained that heat reduces spasm by causing a decrease in frequency of gamma motor impulses with a "general rise in body temperature."[14]

According to Ochs, the hyperemia brought about by the axon reflex is only partially responsible for decreased gamma activity, as only a portion of the total impulses are used in the axon reflex.[11] The remaining impulses from the active hyperemia, resulting from the counterirritant action, may be perceived as heat acting through other possible areas in the central nervous system, such as the anterior hypothalamus, and subsequently bringing about the decreased gamma activity that has otherwise been demonstrated as a result of increasing body temperature.[15,16]

CONCLUSION

On the basis of the findings of this study, one can conclude that:

1. The audiometric technique used in this study was a reliable measure of subjective pain.
2. The application of the placebo did not decrease perceived pain.
3. The application of a counterirritant containing 10 percent menthol and 15 percent methyl salicylate decreased perceived pain.

4. The application of the placebo significantly increased the range of motion of the wrist joint.
5. The application of the counterirritant containing 10 percent menthol and 15 percent methyl salicylate significantly increased the range of motion of the wrist joint.
6. Comparison of the increase in range of motion in the wrist joints receiving applications of the placebo with the increase in those receiving applications of the counterirritant indicates that application of the counterirritant resulted in a significantly greater increase in range of motion than did application of the placebo.
7. The application of the placebo significantly increased digital dexterity.
8. The application of the counterirritant containing 10 percent menthol and 15 percent methyl salicylate significantly increased digital dexterity.
9. Comparison of the increase in digital dexterity after application of the placebo with the increase after application of the counterirritant indicates that application of the counterirritant resulted in significantly greater increase in digital dexterity than did application of the placebo.

REFERENCES

1. Wasserman RR: Electromyographic, electrodiagnostic, and motor nerve conduction observations in patients with rheumatoid arthritis. Arch Phys Med Rehabil 9:90-95, 1968
2. White JR, Sage JN: Effects of a counterirritant on muscular distress in patients with arthritis. Phys Ther 51:36-42, 1971
3. White JR, Sage JN: Effects of a counterirritant on shoulder joint range of movement in patients with arthritis. (in press)
4. Peck R: A precise technique for the measurement of pain. Headache 6:189-194, 1967
5. Leighton JR: An instrument and technic for the measurement of range of joint motion. Arch Phys Med Rehabil 36:571-578, 1955
6. White JR: The reliability between test versus retest of trials of rapid movement and digital dexterity. Unpublished data, San Diego, University of California, November 1972
7. White JR: Effects of rubefacients on local and general skin temperature. Unpublished data, Riverside, University of California, January 1969
8. Green JH: Introduction to Human Physiology. London, England, Oxford University Press, 1963
9. Guyton AC: Textbook of Medical Physiology 3rd ed. Philadelphia, W. B. Saunders Company, 1968.
10. McDowell RJS: Handbook of Physiology 43rd ed. Philadelphia, J. B. Lippincott Company, 1964
11. Ochs S: Elements of Neurophysiology. New York, John Wiley and Sons, Inc., 1967
12. Ruch TC, Fulton JF: Medical Physiology and Biophysics 18th ed. Philadelphia, W. B. Saunders Company, 1960
13. Karpovich PV: Physiology of Muscular Activity 6th ed. Philadelphia, W. B. Saunders Company, 1965
14. DonTigny RL, Sheldon KW: Simultaneous use of heat and cold in treatment of muscle spasm. Arch Phys Med Rehabil 43:235-237, 1962
15. Mathews PBC: Hypertonus and gamma motorneurones. Cerebral Palsy Bull 7:2-3, 1959
16. Euler Von C, Soderberg U: The relation between gamma motor activity and the electroencephalogram. Experientia 12:278, 1956

39

Pain and mood patterns in patients with rheumatoid arthritis

A prospective study

H. Moldofsky, MD, and W. J. Chester, PhD

For many years rheumatoid arthritis has been the subject of intensive investigations by various medical disciplines. Genetic, bacteriologic, virologic, endocrine, biochemical and immunologic specific hypotheses have been pursued more or less diligently. There is general consensus that the biologic components of the illness are influenced by broader psychosocial and possibly environmental factors. Yet while the quest for etiologically significant biologic factors has continued, the roles of the less palpable psychologic and social issues have stimulated much less careful enquiry.

Psychosomatic studies to date have been principally retrospective, searching for possible psychologic and/or social etiologic factors. However, a recent comprehensive critique on this particular subject (1) has emphasized that the majority of studies have not met minimal scientific criteria. The search for so-called stress situations, characteristic personality defects, or conflict difficulties left investigators open to the criticism that they were subject to retrospective bias or had unfavorable controls.

What is needed is an ongoing study which would make it possible to elucidate the precise nature of the association between psychic and somatic parameters. Studying the physical and psychologic state of the patient over an extended time period would allow the patient to serve as his own control. But this particular approach has not been used extensively because of methodologic difficulties within the areas of rheumatology and psychiatry. In both spheres, there has been difficulty finding instruments sufficiently sensitive and reliable to detect diurnal physiologic and psychologic change.

This paper reports a study in which a longitudinal psychophysiologic model was used. Mood states, which emerged empirically, were correlated with articular pain, quantified as a dimension of rheumatoid inflammatory activity.

METHOD

The study was carried out on 16 randomly selected patients with rheumatoid arthritis during their stay on a rheumatic disease unit of a general hospital. All patients fulfilled the American Rheumatism Association criteria for definite or classic rheumatoid arthritis (2). All were either experiencing an initial attack or an acute exacerbation of their disease.

Each patient was evaluated initially for his medical, rheumatologic and psychiat-

Reprinted with permission of the American Psychosomatic Society from Psychosomatic Medicine 32:309-318. Copyright 1970.
From the Rheumatic Diseases Unit, Wellesley Hospital, Toronto (H. Moldofsky), and the Department of Psychiatry, University of Toronto, Canada (W. J. Chester).
Supported by Grant 118 from the Ontario Mental Health Foundation.
The authors are much indebted to Mrs. Mary Reid, RN and Mrs. Carol Wilson, RN for their clinical assistance; and to Dr. M. A. Ogryzlo, Director of the Wellesley Rheumatic Diseases Unit, for his support and encouragement.

ric-social condition. Subsequently an assessment of mood and pain was made twice daily, morning and evening, by a registered nurse research assistant. A record was also kept of daily conversational themes, preoccupations, and the personally experienced stressful events of each patient. Mood state was assessed by an adjective check list rating technic of various emotional states. The list of adjectives was derived from a similar method employed by Nowlis and Nowlis (3) and included items relevant to concepts of helplessness and hopelessness (4). Each of the 27 adjectives was quantified along a six point gradient ranging from *not at all* to *extremely* evident. Simultaneously, pain indices were determined by both objective and subjective assessments. For quantifying pain in a reasonably objective manner, a dolorimeter was employed. This instrument, a modified strain gauge, gives rise to measures of pressure inducing joint tenderness when applied to the peripheral joints of the upper limb, 36 in all. This technic has been shown, in a recent rheumatologic study, to be a reasonably valid and reliable measure of joint inflammation (5). A subjective functional pain rating scale was employed also to determine, in each locomotor region, the degree of joint function that would produce pain.

A third technic for quantifying joint inflammation was used. Coincident diurnal heat loss was measured with a calorimetric device from the 36 peripheral joints to which the dolorimeter was applied. (Our findings relevant to heat loss and pain will be reported elsewhere.)

Each patient was studied throughout his hospital confinement and re-entered the study if readmitted at any time during the 2-year period of the research project. Two patients who had entered the study were subsequently withdrawn because they did not fit the diagnostic criteria established.

When the hospital stay terminated, the accumulated raw data were analyzed mathematically: standardized specific mood constellations derived from factor

Table 1. Personal and disease data of patients with a synchronous pain-mood pattern

Patient	*Sex*	*Age (years)*	*Marital status*	*Social class (6)*	*Duration of illness (years)*	*Functional class (7)*	*Radiologic stage (7)*
SR	F	48	Married	II	½	II	I
OW	F	56	Married	II	10	II	I
BQ	F	44	Married	IV	15	II	III
AK	F	62	Widow	IV	5	II	II
MF	F	67	Widow	IV	19	II	III
HS	M	32	Married	V	7	II	II
MC	M	42	Married	IV	6	II	II
RH	F	69	Widow	II	½	II	II

Table 2. Mood-pain correlation in patients with synchronous pattern

Patient	*Length of study (days)*	*Characteristic mood range*	*Mood-pain correlation ($p < 0.05$)*
SR	25	Anxiety, hopelessness – calm, confidence	+0.587
OW	22	Overt hostility – passivity	+0.478
BQ	21	Overt hostility	+0.490
AK			
1st study	25	Anxiety – calm	+0.800
2nd study	57	Anxiety, hostility – calm	+0.664
MF	31	Anxiety – calm	+0.530
HS	19	Anxiety, hopelessness – confidence	+0.670
MC	29	Anxiety, helplessness – energy	+0.365
RH	32	Apathy – energy	+0.505

analysis were correlated with the quantified dimensions of subjective joint pain experience and the dolorimeter tenderness scores.

FINDINGS

A total of 21 separate studies were carried out on 16 patients over the 2 years. Of the 16 patients, 2 were examined during an additional hospital admission; and 1 was studied on three further admissions. The average length of each study was approximately 36 days. The median correlation of dolorimeter and functional pain index in all 16 patients was 0.6. To achieve greater objectivity, the relationship between diurnal dolorimeter joint tenderness scores and mood constellations was studied. Two

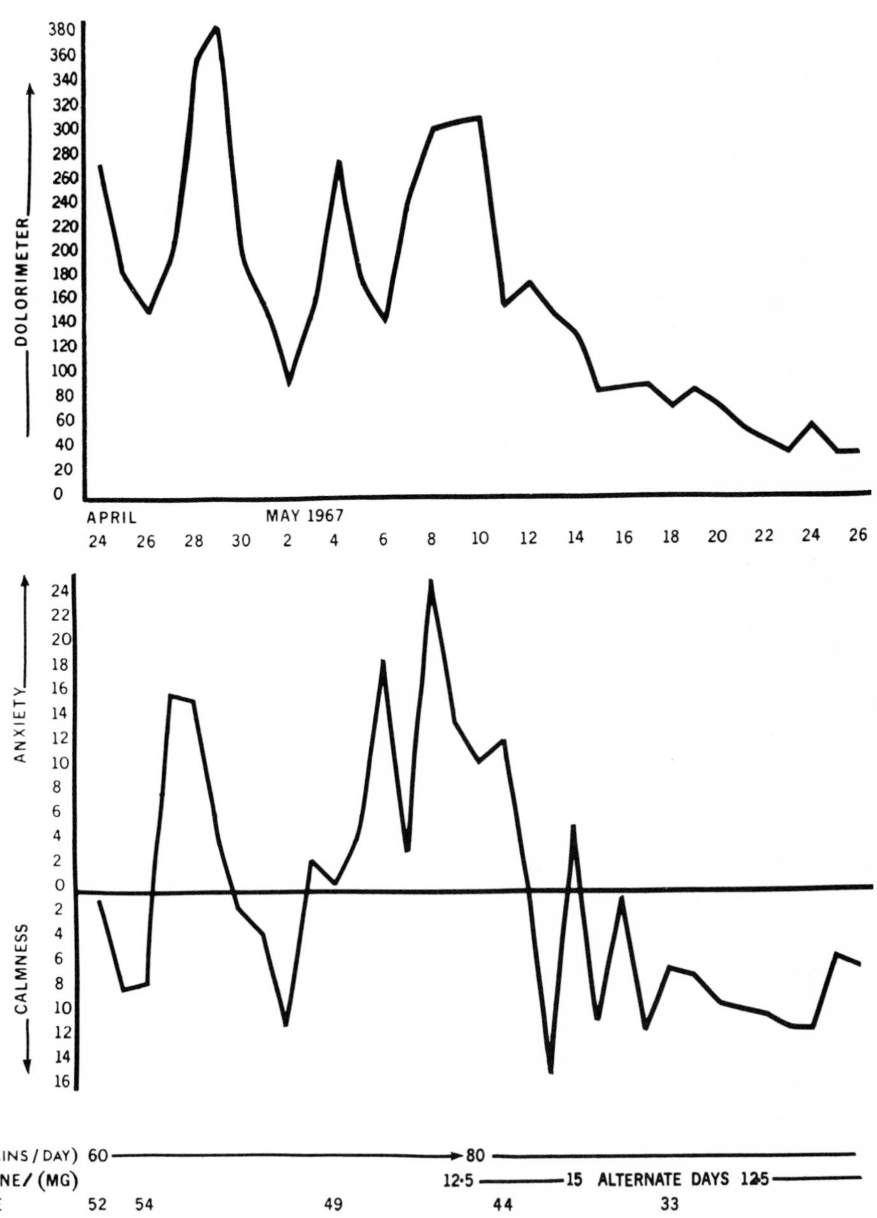

Fig. 1. Mood-pain pattern of Patient AK (first study) illustrating synchronous pattern.

characteristic pain-mood patterns emerged from this investigation.

Synchronous state

Eight patients were discovered to have a pattern of pain-mood association termed a *synchronous state*. In this group, the altered mood either preceded by 1 day or was simultaneously associated with changing dolorimeter pain readings. The characteristics of this group are given in Tables 1 and 2. There were 6 females and 2 males, with a mean age of 52 years and a mean duration of illness of 8 years. All were of uniform disability (according to functional Class II of Steinbrocker et al (6)—ie, "adequate for normal activities despite handicap of discomfort or limited motion at one or more joints"). The radiologic assessments, in accordance with designated criteria (7), revealed a wide range of joint destruction: On skeletal survey, 2 patients showed doubtful rheumatoid articular changes (Stage I); 4, minimal (Stage II); and 2, moderate (Stage III). The most characteristic mood in this group, as derived from the factor analysis, ranged along a bipolar continuum from degrees of manifest hostility or anxiety to degrees of calmness.

Patient AK, in Study 1, (Fig 1), dramatically illustrates such a synchronous configuration.

Paradoxical state

Eight other patients manifested a second pattern which the authors termed a *paradoxical* or asynchronous state. In this group, an inverse relationship existed between the intensity of mood disturbance and the quantified pain experience. The characteristics of this group of patients are given in Tables 3 and 4. The 5 women and 3 men, with a mean age of 51 years, were nearly all similarly disabled (1 patient in functional Class I, and 7 patients in Class II). Their mean duration of illness was 6 years, and their joint disease, as categorized by radiologic rating, were: 3 doubtful (Stage I), 3 minimal (Stage II), and 2 moderate (Stage III). The significant mood constellation ranged along a continuum from degrees of hopelessness to degrees of confidence. Patient DW (Fig 2) is illustrative of the paradoxical pattern.

The same individually characteristic pattern tended to reappear on each subsequent study of the 3 patients (AK, WS, JM) who required readmission to the hospital unit. Patient JM, in study 3, temporarily reverted to a synchronous pattern. This was associated with prospects of improved financial status and elevated self-esteem in his family. Immediately prior to his fourth hospital admission, his disability pension was withdrawn and his pain-mood pattern returned to its previous configuration.

In both patient groups, the correlation of all selected values of mood with dolorimeter values was significant at the 0.5 level or less.

Unfortunately, the ideal of maintaining constancy of medication could not be met. All patients received aspirin-type drugs and nearly all received hypnotics routinely at night. In the synchronous group, gold salts were given to 3 patients, antimalarial drugs to 1, corticosteroids to 5, and day sedatives to 1. In the paradoxical group, gold salts were given to 5 patients, antimalarials to 2, corticosteroids to 5, and day sedatives to 3. The physicians felt obliged to change medication dosage or to introduce different drugs—eg, corticosteroids, gold salts, or sedatives—in order to alleviate the patient's distress. However, the drugs employed did not seem to influence these particular pain-mood patterns directly.

When synchronous and paradoxical patterns were compared with personal and disease indices, no relationship was found to age, sex, social class, duration of illness, functional class or radiologic stage. Moreover, there was no relationship between pain-mood pattern and the particular rheumatologist supervising the patient's care.

DISCUSSION

The association between mood and pain as an indication of disease activity in rheumatoid arthritis has been demonstrated. A review of studies of pain perception or reaction and emotion (8) has suggested that anxiety is the main factor in lowering thresholds. Specifically, flares of joint pain, in rheumatoid arthritis, have been attributed to restrictive expression of hostile impulses and anxiety with its associated increase in muscle tension (9, 10).

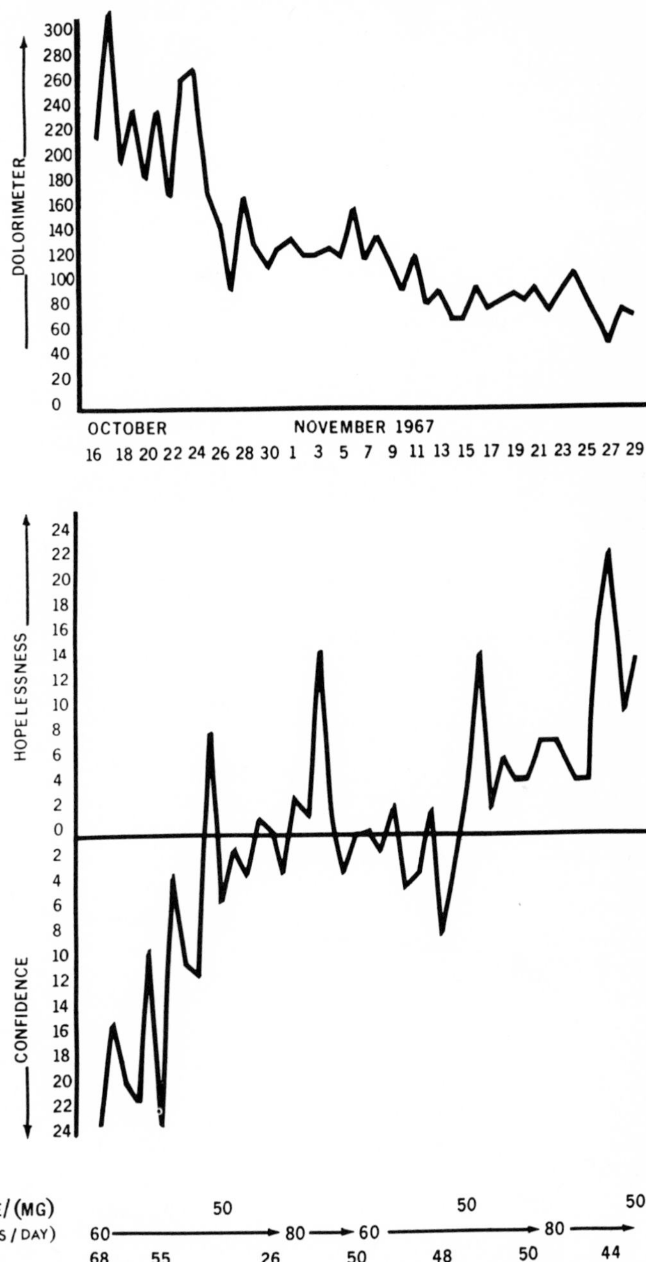

Fig. 2. Mood-pain pattern of Patient DW illustrating paradoxical pattern.

Table 3. Personal and disease data of patients with a paradoxical pain-mood pattern

Patient	*Sex*	*Age (years)*	*Marital status*	*Social class (6)*	*Duration of illness (years)*	*Functional class (7)*	*Radiologic stage (7)*
IA	F	60	Widow	IV	7	II	I
MB	F	32	Married	III	7	II	II
DW	F	52	Married	III	2	II	III
LT	M	64	Married	III	5	II	I
WS	M	54	Married	IV	7	II	III
JM	M	46	Married	V	4	II	II
ES	F	55	Married	I	5	II	II
DP	F	42	Married	II	6	I	I

Table 4. Mood-pain correlation in patients with paradoxical pattern

Patient	*Length of study (days)*	*Characteristic mood range*	*Mood-pain correlation ($p < 0.05$)*
IA	29	Helplessness, hopelessness – energetic confidence	−0.728
MB	51	Hopeless hostility – passivity	−0.303
DW	44	Hopelessness – calm, confidence	−0.766
LT	27	Helplessness, hopelessness – confidence	−0.741
WS			
1st study	41	Hopeless anxiety – calm, confidence	−0.453
2nd study	111	Anxiety, hopelessness – calm, confidence	−0.469
JM			
1st study	46	Helpless hostility – passivity	−0.700
2nd study	31	Hopelessness – confidence	−0.467
3rd study	33	Hopeless anxiety – calm, confidence	+0.715
4th study	11	Hostile hopelessness – calm	−0.749
ES	36	Hopelessness – confidence	−0.736
DP	25	Hopelessness – confidence	−0.407

Contrary to this view that painful experience is heightened in the presence of disturbed feelings, this ongoing study of day-to-day changes in mood and pain indicates that the relationship between intensity of pain and emotional reactivity is much more complex. A simple distinctive affective constellation was not found constantly in our factor analytic studies (Tables 2 and 4). For example, moods answering to adjectives descriptive of and including helplessness were found to be associated with moods descriptive of hopelessness. These moods were further associated in a mixed mood cluster which included adjectives descriptive of anxiety, energy and anger.

Furthermore, although there was confirmation of the significance of the direct association of pain with anxiety or hostility, as noted in our synchronous group, a surprising number of our patients displayed an inverse or asynchronous relationship. It was because this association of intensity of joint tenderness and mood disturbance was contrary to the hitherto accepted views that the configuration was termed a paradoxical state. Of particular significance in this state was the common finding of a hopelessness affective constellation. In this group, when an amelioration in the pain intensity of their disease took place, they displayed a mounting sense of despair concerning their immediate situation and pessimism about their future; when their joint pain increased, they would appear paradoxically calm and optimistic. These findings suggested that, even though the joint pain had subsided, the patients of the paradoxical group were not free of ill health.

FOLLOW-UP

Assuming that the patterns of pain-mood relationship were constant for a particular patient, the group exhibiting the paradoxical pattern would have an unfavorable outcome, whereas the group with a synchronous pattern would have a more favorable outcome. A second study was carried out to test this hypothesis.

Outcome, or course of illness, was defined to encompass clinical manifestations of rheumatoid activity—eg, pain, stiffness, swelling and limitation of movement—as well as the ability to cope with the disease, with key interpersonal and environmental issues. Some of these include need for rest, amount of physical activity or exercise, emotional state and outlook, and need for medical attention and drugs, and state of social and family relationships as revealed in work, recreation, living accommodation and finances. All the factors making up the general concept of outcome were graded and tabulated by our research assistant at approximately 6 months and 1 year after discharge from the hospital unit. A simultaneous independent rheumatologic-medical evaluation was carried out and the assessments were compared. Generally speaking, the two evaluations agreed as to whether the individual was functioning well, fairly, or poorly. (In 2 instances the patients' assessments of their conditions were contrary to medical evaluations: 1 in the synchronous group, Patient OW, who felt that her disease was worsening and her functioning deteriorating, displayed negligible rheumatologic findings and in fact was leading a reasonably active and independent life; the other, Patient IA in the paradoxical group, said that her disease activity and functional ability had remained unchanged or improved even though she had required two further hospitalizations within the year following the initial study. At the time of the last follow-up assessment she was once more a patient in the hospital.)

To this date, at least a 1-2 year follow-up has been carried out, and the outcome hypothesis has been reasonably confirmed: 7 of the 8 patients in the synchronous group are managing reasonably well. The patient who required readmission to the unit for a recurrent flare in her disease readily responded to medical management (1 year later this patient suddenly died of a myocardial infarction). Overall, the synchronous group appears to have coped with their disease more easily, required less medical attention, received more conservative treatment measures, and, in spite of physical limitations, have been able to carry on reasonably well with their work, family relationships and social involvements than the paradoxical pattern group.

Of the 8 in the paradoxical group, 6 have managed poorly. They have required further lengthy hospitalizations, and most have encountered major medical difficulties: Patient LT died of a pneumonitis after a cerebral vascular accident and coincident flare in rheumatoid disease; Patient MB experienced a temporary cardiac arrest associated with coronary angiography for unremittent nonspecific chest pain; Patient JM underwent metacarpalphalangeal synovectomy, then urinary tract problems requiring a ureterolithotomy for removal of a stone, and after that, required additional surgical intervention for a fistula; he also received a trial of immunosuppressant drug treatment. Most apparent was the rigidity of the mood state of this group. They experienced great difficulty in altering their pessimistic outlook and seemingly purposeless existence. Family, friends, associates and physicians were distrusted or were perceived as lacking sufficient interest and understanding. They deprecated the attempts of those who tried to provide encouragement or significance in their lives. This in turn frequently led to misunderstandings, interpersonal discord, brooding resentment with fear of loss of support, which led to further distrust and social withdrawal. With the giving up of their vocational and social pursuits, they came to depend increasingly upon magical solutions to their illness. They demanded and received additional medical and surgical attention. It was as if they succeeded in producing guilt in their physician because he seemed impotent to relieve their chronic distress. Less conservative measures—eg, narcotics and sedatives—were tried in an effort to placate them. These patients only appeared calm and confident while quietly suffering severe pain during their successive hospitalizations for more intensive and possibly hazardous treatments such as immunosuppressant drug trials or surgical intervention. Since they cooperated with whatever unpleasant investigation or treatment was rendered, they were the so-called "good patients." A measure of self-worth and recognition appeared to have been attained at the expense of being perceived as sick and helpless. Whenever there was relief from discomfort, they became frightened and despaired of being able to function satisfactorily. Notably, after leaving the protective environment of the hospital they would disregard advice to function within their prescribed limitations and push themselves beyond their physical capabilities. Once more they fell victim to recurrence of their painful distress; discouragement ensued, and their sense of futility was reinforced.

It is possible that these pain-mood patterns are changeable, for 2 of the paradoxical group, at follow-up, seem to be coping fairly well. Patient MB has been able to alter her life style by escaping from her unhappy domestic situation and has obtained gratification from her work as a saleswoman. She volunteered that if she gave up this work she would certainly become functionally incapacitated. Patient ES, who was initially pessimistic about her future prospects, seemed to manage well for several months, comforted by her faith in a second trial of gold salt injections; but soon after the medication was discontinued, because of a recurrence of its toxic side effects, her functional capacity deteriorated.

The prognosis (based on the short 1-2 year follow-up) for those patients characterized by a synchronous pain-mood posture would appear to be more favorable than for those of a paradoxical one. These observations, if confirmed, may help to clarify why some rheumatoid patients profit from relatively brief conservative treatment measures whereas others are poorly even with long-term and sometimes heroic therapeutic technics. Moreover, consideration of these groupings might be of importance in the assessment of pharmacologic, physiotherapeutic or surgical approaches to treatment.

CONCLUSIONS

An association appears to exist between emotional issues and articular pain as an index of rheumatoid arthritis inflammatory activity. The pain-mood constellation may be of a synchronous or paradoxical nature, and these patterns may have prognostic significance.

REFERENCES

1. Scotch N, Geiger HJ: The epidemiology of rheumatoid arthritis: a review with special attention to social factors. J Chron Dis 15:1037-1067, 1962
2. Primer on the Rheumatic Diseases. Sixth edition. New York, The Arthritis Foundation, 1963, p 63-64
3. Nowlis V, Nowlis HH: The description and analysis of mood. Ann NY Acad Sci 65:345-355, 1956-1957
4. Schmale AH: A genetic view of affects with special reference to the genesis of helplessness and hopelessness. Psychoanal Stud Child 19:287-310, 1964
5. McCarty DJ, Gatter A: A dolorimeter for quantification of articular tenderness. Arthritis Rheum 8:551-559, 1965
6. Steinbrocker O, Traeger CH, Batterman RC: Therapeutic criteria in rheumatoid arthritis. JAMA 140:659-662, 1949
7. Lansbury J: Methods for evaluating rheumatoid arthritis, Arthritis and Allied Conditions, Textbook of Rheumatology. Seventh edition. Edited by JL Hollander. Philadelphia, Lea. 1966, p 269-291
8. Merskey H, Spear FG: Pain, Psychological and Psychiatric Aspects. London, Bailliere, Tindall & Cassell, 1967, p 150
9. Cobb S: Contained hostility in rheumatoid arthritis. Arthritis Rheum 2:419-425, 1959
10. Moos RH: Personality factors associated with rheumatoid arthritis: a review. J Chron Dis 17:41-55, 1964
11. Hollingshead AB, Redlich FC: Social Class and Mental Illness. New York, Wiley, 1958

40

Meprobamate therapy for the myofascial pain-dysfunction (MPD) syndrome

A double-blind evaluation

Charles S. Greene, DDS, and Daniel M. Laskin, DDS, MS

The myofascial pain-dysfunction (MPD) syndrome which involves the masticatory apparatus is a clinical phenomenon that has been observed, described, and analyzed by many investigators. Patients experiencing the symptoms of pain, tenderness, clicking, and limitation of function which characterize this syndrome[1] have been subjected to a wide variety of therapeutic measures. Among these are a number of pharmacological agents that have been administered either orally, or by injection into the temporomandibular joint (TMJ) or the masticatory muscles.

Joint injections have been advocated by many clinicians who regard the TMJ itself as the locus of the pain and dysfunction. For example, drugs such as hydrocortisone have been used by some in an attempt to reduce the inflammation which they believe exists within the joint space,[2,3] whereas others have recommended the use of hyaluronidase to "restore normal fluid balance" within that area.[4-6] Even sclerosing solutions have been injected into the TMJ to produce a fibrosis of the joint capsule and ligaments, thereby preventing excessive movement (hypermobility) of the mandible.[7,8]

On the other hand, many recent investigators have concluded that masticatory muscle spasm or hypertonicity, rather than intra-articular trauma or inflammation, is responsible for the majority of TMJ symptoms.[1,9,10] This idea has led to the prescription of various muscle relaxant drugs,[6,11,12] as well as the injection of local anesthetic solutions into so-called trigger zones within the masticatory muscles, not only to block the pain temporarily, but presumably to "break the pain-spasm-pain cycle."[6,10,13] In addition, the injection of corticosteroid and local anesthetic combinations into the muscles has been recommended by some clinicians,[14,15] because they claim that these combinations are more effective than the anesthetic alone in obtaining a sustained improvement.

A third school of thought, although still regarding the muscles as the locus of dysfunction, has hypothesized that the psychological effects of stress and tension are significant in the etiology of MPD problems.[16-18] On this basis, some clinicians have used psychotropic drugs such as tranquilizers, sedatives, and hypnotics in an attempt to reduce this psychic tension and thereby diminish the muscular spasm.[6,13,19]

Thus, it is apparent that the selection of appropriate drug therapy for MPD patients usually has been based on the clinician's interpretation of the symptoms, and related to his particular ideas regarding the etiology of the problem. The effectiveness of most of the agents mentioned has never

From the Journal of the American Dental Association **82**:587-590.

From the Temporomandibular Joint Research Center, University of Illinois College of Dentistry, Chicago (C. S. Greene); and the Department of Oral and Maxillofacial Surgery and the TMJ Research Center, University of Illinois College of Dentistry, Chicago (D. M. Laskin).

This investigation was supported by USPHS research grant PHS-2899-01 from the National Institute of Dental Research, Bethesda, Md.

been established by any type of objective clinical investigation, although both Schwartz[20] and Franks[11] have reported double-blind evaluations of specific muscle relaxant drugs. Nevertheless, claims of high empirical success rates have generated widespread interest among clinicians in the use of various drugs, including some that subsequently were shown to be ineffective or, in some instances, actually harmful.[19-22]

Since previous research conducted at the University of Illinois TMJ Research Center has shown that MPD problems are generally associated with masticatory muscle fatigue, spasm, and tenderness,[1,23] and are often related to psychophysiologic etiologic factors,[18,23] it was decided to investigate the therapeutic effectiveness of a drug that, theoretically, could deal with both of these elements simultaneously. Meprobamate* was selected on the basis of its combined tranquilizing and muscle relaxant properties,[24,25] and also because of favorable experimental reports with its use in the treatment of other musculoskeletal disorders.[26,27]

*Supplied by Wyeth Laboratories, Philadelphia.

METHOD

Ninety patients with the MPD syndrome were selected randomly from the patient population of the TMJ Research Center. The diagnosis was made according to the criteria described in previous papers.[1,19] Patients with positive radiographic findings or other evidence of organic TMJ pathologic conditions were not included in this series.

Each patient was given a numbered bottle with a five-day supply of capsules that contained either 400 mg meprobamate or placebo, to be taken four times a day. At the end of the fifth day, the patients returned for a clinical evaluation of their response to these capsules. They were then given a second bottle, and again the response was evaluated after the fifth day. The drugs were distributed randomly, with the type unknown to the investigators, so that some patients received either meprobamate of placebo twice, whereas others received one bottle of each in any sequence.

To assess the patients' responses as objectively as possible, a special treatment evaluation form was developed (illustra-

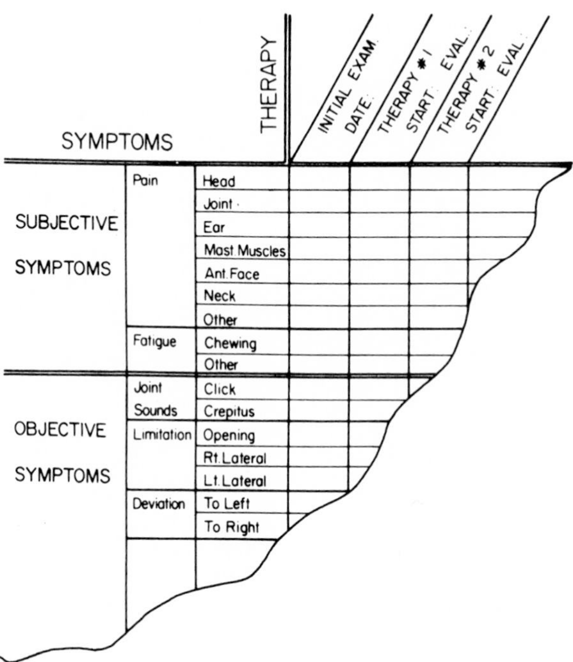
SYMPTOMS
THERAPY
INITIAL EXAM DATE:
THERAPY #1 START: EVAL.:
THERAPY #2 START: EVAL.:
SUBJECTIVE SYMPTOMS
Pain: Head, Joint, Ear, Mast Muscles, Ant. Face, Neck, Other
Fatigue: Chewing, Other
OBJECTIVE SYMPTOMS
Joint Sounds: Click, Crepitus
Limitation: Opening, Rt. Lateral, Lt. Lateral
Deviation: To Left, To Right

Treatment evaluation form. This form can be used for sequential evaluation of any therapy that is used for MPD patients.

tion). At the initial examination and history-taking appointment, this form was filled in with code symbols to describe the intensity of each subjective and objective symptom. The changes in these symptoms were then determined by examination at the end of each five-day period of therapy. The patients also were asked to comment generally on whether the medication seemed to make their symptoms better or worse, or if they remained unchanged.

RESULTS

The responses of the patients to the drugs that they received are shown in Tables 1 and 2. Side effects were also reported with each drug; these are shown in Table 3. Fifty-eight percent of the patients reported some improvement or remission of their symptoms after taking meprobamate, and 31% after taking the placebo drug (Table 1). This compares closely with the 60% and 37%, respectively, who, on clinical examination showed improvement of one or more symptoms with the same drugs (Table 2). Regardless of whether meprobamate or placebo was taken, it was the subjective symptoms that improved most frequently, whereas the more objective symptoms seemed to be less affected by either of the drugs.

A number of interesting contradictions were revealed during assessment of the patients' responses. More than a third of the 37 patients who took the same drug twice reported different results after each five-day period of therapy. Moreover, of the 38 patients who received one bottle of each drug, 13 did not respond to either drug, 15 reported a "normal" reaction, (that is, they improved with meprobamate but not with placebo), but 10 patients reported the opposite response to these two drugs.

To determine whether possible lingering effects of the first drug altered the response to the second one, we conducted a separate analysis on only first-drug responses (Table 4). These results closely paralleled the overall findings, with 66% responding positively to meprobamate and 30% to the placebo. Apparently, there was little or no distortion of patients' responses due to lingering effects.

Table 1. Effectiveness of drugs as reported by the patients

	Meprobamate %	*Placebo* %
Improved	58	31
Worse	5	7
No change	37	62

Table 2. Effectiveness of drugs based on clinical examination

	Meprobamate %	*Placebo* %
Pain		
Eliminated	20	6
Improved	36	31
Worse	13	8
No change	31	55
Click		
Eliminated	8	2
Improved	24	11
Worse	4	14
No change	64	73
Limitation		
Eliminated	None	None
Improved	12	5
Worse	4	4
No change	84	91
Tenderness		
Eliminated	13	7
Improved	40	23
Worse	6	14
No change	41	56
General effectiveness (Improvement of 1 or more symptoms)	60	37

Table 3. Number of drug side effects reported by patients

	Meprobamate	*Placebos*
Sleepiness	32	14
Dizziness	7	5
Nausea	4	6
Headache	1	3
Diarrhea	2	5

Table 4. Analysis of first-drug effectiveness

	No. patients	*No. improved*	*% improved*
Meprobamate taken first	36	24	66
Placebo taken first	54	16	30

DISCUSSION

In a primarily functional disorder such as the MPD syndrome, the clinical diagnosis necessarily is based on a combination of subjective complaints, objective findings, and the absence of pathologic changes. Once the diagnosis has been made, however, the clinician is still confronted with the problem of selecting appropriate therapy. Since the MPD patient population is not homogeneous with respect to symptoms, etiologic factors, or psychological variables,[1] the selection of therapy for any one person is far from being an automatic procedure. It follows that the assessment of any particular therapy applied to such a heterogeneous group will, in turn, be complicated by the same factors.

Overall, the results obtained in this study indicate that meprobamate can be effective for relieving symptoms in a significant number of MPD patients (Tables 1, 2). Unfortunately, it is not easy to make any direct comparisons with the results of other drug studies, even when they have been carried out with a double-blind protocol, since there are some variations in diagnostic criteria as well as a lack of uniform standards for judging symptomatic improvement. Nevertheless, the data seem to indicate that meprobamate, which is primarily a sedative and only secondarily a muscle relaxant, is more effective than the primary muscle relaxants which were evaluated by Schwartz[20] and Franks.[11] This finding tends to confirm the empirical observations of Shore,[6] Schwartz,[21] Henny[19] and others with respect to meprobamate, diazepam, and similar drugs.

However, the incidence of positive responses to placebo (Tables 1, 2), as well as the remarkable number of inconsistent and contradictory responses to both the placebo and the drug, illustrate just how complex the assessment of therapeutic effectiveness can be, not only for meprobamate, but for any treatment that is applied to MPD patients. The high success rates reported with nearly all treatments for the MPD syndrome become more understandable if it is recognized that placebo effects are inherent in all forms of therapy; if one is aware of the potential for exaggerated responses in MPD patients;[28] and if it is realized that significant psychological factors that affect both etiology and response to therapy are operating within this patient population.[18]

Ultimately, the success or failure of any treatment for the MPD syndrome depends to some extent on the psychodynamics of the individual patient. Even those patients with a traumatically or mechanically induced dysfunction must subjectively interpret and communicate their perception of the problem, and their response to therapy will be influenced by that perception as well as other intrinsic factors. Previous studies by Lupton[29] have shown that variations in the responses of MPD patients to different types of therapy are related to certain personality characteristics. Those he identified as "stress-reactors" seemed to respond well to definitive physical treatments combined with a cognitive teaching program, whereas those he designated as "psychoneurotics" responded rather equivocally to physical treatment, but often reacted favorably to an interpersonal type of psychological counseling. Lupton and Johnson[30] have shown a relationship between these same personality characteristics and the degree of tolerance for experimentally induced pain stimuli. In another clinical study, Greene and Laskin[28] have reported that the responses of MPD patients to a placebo varied greatly according to the presence or absence of these "stress-reactor" or "psychoneurotic" tendencies. In addition to these intrinsic factors, the effectiveness of any pharmacologic or mechanical treatment will be augmented or diminished by a number of extrinsic factors, not the least of which is the personality of the therapist himself.[16]

In a future paper, the significance of these relationships between personality factors and responses to therapy will be explored in greater detail. At this point, however, it is apparent that the clinical diagnosis of MPD syndrome must be refined psychologically for each individual patient and the patient must be subclassified according to more specific diagnostic criteria, so that truly appropriate therapy can be selected on a more rational basis. Until this type of diagnostic refinement becomes readily accomplishable, it seems reasonable to recommend the use of conservative and reversible modalities for the treatment of unclassified MPD patients, as long as these therapies are selected on a sound pharmacologic and physiologic basis. Certainly, the use of drugs such as meprobamate can be defended on this basis, since they generally can reduce or eliminate the psychic tension and the muscular spasm which are, in most instances, the major elements of the MPD syndrome.

REFERENCES

1. Greene, C. S., and others. The TMJ pain-dysfunction syndrome: heterogeneity of the patient population. JADA 79:1168 Nov 1969.
2. Henny, F. A. Intra-articular injection of cortisone into the temporomandibular joint. J Oral Surg 12: 314 Oct 1954.
3. Horton, C. P. Treatment of arthritic temporomandibular joints by intra-articular injection of hydrocortisone. Oral Surg 6:826 July 1953.
4. Kochan, E. Treatment of temporomandibular joint disturbances with hyaluronidase. Oral Surg 9:513 May 1956.
5. Nathan, A. S. The use of hyaluronidase in temporomandibular disturbances. Oral Surg 7:368 April 1954.
6. Shore, N. A. Occlusal equilibration and temporomandibular joint dysfunction. Philadelphia, J. B. Lippincott Co., 1959.
7. Schultz, L. W. A curative treatment for subluxation of the temporomandibular joint or any joint. JADA 24:1947 Dec 1937.
8. Schultz, L. W. Twenty years experience in treating hypermobility of the temporomandibular joint. Amer J Surg 92:925 Dec 1956.
9. Schwartz, L. Pain associated with the temporomandibular joint. JADA 51:394 Oct 1955.
10. Travell, J. Temporomandibular joint pain referred from muscles of the head and neck. J Prosth Dent 10:745 July-Aug 1960.
11. Franks, A. S. Mandibular muscle spasm: a double-blind study of a muscle relaxant drug. Brit J Clin Prac 19:281 May 1965.
12. Marlette, R. H. Adjunct treatment of TMJ pain with Equagesic. Milit Med 129:69 Jan 1964.
13. Kutscher, A. H., and others. Pharmacologic methods. In Schwartz, L., and Chayes, C. Facial pain and mandibular dysfunction. Philadelphia, W. B. Saunders Co., 1968.
14. Marbach, J. Personal communication, New York, 1969.
15. Finder, J., and Post, M. Local injection therapy for rheumatic diseases. JAMA 172:2021 April 30, 1960.
16. Moulton, R. E. Emotional factors in non-organic temporomandibular joint pain. Dent Clin N Amer Nov 1966, p 609.
17. Kydd, W. L. Psychosomatic aspects of temporomandibular joint dysfunction. JADA 59:31 July 1959.
18. Lupton, D. E. Psychological aspects of temporomandibular joint dysfunction. JADA 79:131 July 1969.
19. Henny, F. Surgical treatment of the painful temporomandibular joint. JADA 79:171 July 1969.
20. Schwartz, L., and others. Carisoprodol in the management of temporomandibular joint pain and dysfunction: a preliminary investigation. Ann NY Acad Sci 86:245 March 1960.
21. Schwartz, L. Disorders of the temporomandibular joint. Philadelphia, W. B. Saunders Co., 1959.
22. Poswillo, D. An experimental investigation of the effects of intra-articular hydrocortisone and high condylectomy on the mandibular condyle. Oral Surg 30:161 Aug 1970.
23. Laskin, D. M. Etiology of the pain-dysfunction syndrome. JADA 79:147 July 1969.
24. Berger, F. M. Meprobamate—its pharmacologic properties and clinical uses. Internat Rec 169:184 April 1956.
25. Borrus, M. D. Study of the effects of Miltown on psychiatric states. JAMA 157:1596 April 30, 1955.
26. Gillette, H. E. Relaxant effects of meprobamate in disabilities resulting from musculoskeletal and central nervous system disorders. Internat Rec 169:453 July 1956.
27. Cazort, R. J. Role of relaxants in treatment of traumatic musculoskeletal disorders: a double-blind study of three agents. Curr Ther Res 6:454 July 1964.
28. Greene, C. S., and Laskin, D. M. Correlation of placebo responses and psychological characteristics in myofascial pain-dysfunction (MPD) patients. IADR program and abstracts, No. 282, 1970.
29. Lupton, D. E. Differential patient response to instruction, counseling and dental treatment. PhD dissertation, University of Chicago, 1967.
30. Lupton, D. E., and Johnson, D. L. Personality characteristics of TMJ pain-dysfunction patients related to pain tolerance. J Psychother Psychosom. In press.

41

Pain in psychiatric patients

F. G. Spear

Although pain is most commonly regarded as a symptom of physical disorder it also occurs commonly in psychiatric patients [1-3]. Such pain often occurs in the absence of local tissue damage and even where there is such damage the treatment of the underlying psychiatric illness is often of great importance in the relief of the symptom. Certain ideas about the nature of pain of this type seem common, for instance, that it is described in a florid, bizarre and histrionic manner, but this belief finds no support in the literature [1, 2]. Unfortunately most published reports are concerned with isolated aspects of the problem such as headache [4, 5] chest pain [4-7] and muscular pain [8, 9]. In general it seems that the pain is often localized, is usually described in simple terms, may be more common on the left side [8]. Walters [10] in a general study confirms these impressions and finds that pain is most common in the head and neck, next in chest and upper arms, then low back and lower limbs. The present paper summarizes some investigations of these aspects of pain in psychiatric patients.

METHODS

If we accept Szasz's [11] view that the division of pain into 'organic' and 'psychogenic' is logically unsound and fundamentally misleading the problem of definition can be greatly simplified. Pain can then be operationally defined as present when the patient describes his symptom using the word 'pain', or agrees that he regards his symptom as 'a pain'.

Two investigations using questionnaires were made to examine the general statistical characteristics of pain in a psychiatric population. In the out-patient survey information about age, sex, diagnosis, and presence or absence of pain, was recorded at the initial examination of 200 consecutive new patients, while in the second part, report forms were completed weekly by the nurses and by the patients themselves for all patients in the clinic, either as in-patients or day patients, for a six-month period. In conjunction with these reports details of age, sex, diagnosis, marital status, number of siblings, ordinal position in family, history of operation, number of admissions as in-patients or day patients, duration of illness, approximate intelligence and social class (Hall Jones Scale [12]) were obtained from the case notes. Patients were categorized as suffering from anxiety states, including those where hysterical symptoms were prominent, depression of all types and 'other'. To examine the relationship between pain and other features of the illness all records in which less than four successive observations were made were discarded. The symptoms and features studied were regarded as present to an important extent if they were reported on more than 25 per cent of the opportunities available.

132 patients, 41 male, 91 female, mean age 43.3 yr, standard deviation 11.4 yr, who complained of pain as defined above were then examined. Physical and psychiatric examination was supplemented by asking the patients to describe and to draw their pain or pains on a chart. As it is pos-

Reprinted with permission from Spear, F. G.: Pain in psychiatric patients, Journal of Psychosomatic Research, **11:**187-193. Copyright 1967, Pergamon Press.
From Middlewood Hospital, Sheffeld 6.

Table 1. Relationship of report of pain to major psychiatric diagnosis in out-patients

Diagnosis	*Anxiety*	*Hysteria*	*Depression*	*Other*	*Total*
Pain	19	21	48	18	106
No pain	19	7	37	31	94
Total	38	28	85	49	200

$\chi^2 = 11.27$ d.f. = 3 $P < 0.02$.

Table 2. Relationship of report of pain to age on first attendance as an out-patient

Age	25	26-35	36-45	45+	Total
Pain	6	30	30	40	106
No pain	21	20	18	35	94
Total	27	50	48	75	200

$\chi^2 = 12.99$ d.f. = 3 $P < 0.01$.

sible that bizarre reports of neurotic pains are elicited by pressing the patient to describe sensations for which he has no vocabulary this description was elicited in a specific and limited way. After the complaint of the pain was made and the site or sites obtained the patient was asked "what is the pain like?" Where the response was non-qualitative, for example, a reiteration of the site, or a description of the intensity, the question was repeated but regardless of the nature of the second response the question was pressed no further. Verbatim records of all responses were made. Details of the time relationships, precipitating and relieving factors and of the relationship of the pains to other features of the illness were obtained.

The patients were followed up for periods ranging from one month to two years and six months, and were then classified as worse, unchanged, improved and recovered. A note was made as to whether the patient was still attending, had been discharged or had discharged himself. Some statistical tests were carried out on the results of this part of the investigation using the chi-squared test. Where appropriate and helpful in clarifying the findings the over-all chi-squared was partitioned [13].

RESULTS

The positive results of the questionnaire studies are presented in detail in Tables 1-10 where the statistics used and significance levels attained are given.

Briefly, pain occurs in 45-50 per cent of psychiatric patients and may have a lower incidence in summer than in winter. Pain, once established, tends to persist, and any change is in the direction of resolution of symptoms. The incidence is highest in patients with anxiety states, and of the 15 in-patients who were diagnosed as schizophrenics, only three reported pain. Pain is associated with a history of surgical operations, other somatic symptoms and overt anxiety. Membership of social class 5 in the Hall Jones Scale was associated with pain in the case of male patients only. In the out-patient group pain was less common in younger patients (Table 2) but this difference was not demonstrable in the hospital patients ($t = 0.18$ d.f. = 114 N.S.).

No association was established between pain and hostility, sex, marital status, duration of illness, clinical assessment of intelligence, number of admissions, number of siblings, ordinal position amongst siblings, overt depression, overt tension, nor overt agitation. Further, in female patients, there was no association between pain and social class nor between pain and dysmenorrhoea.

From the clinical investigations it is found that the 132 patients described a total of 222 pains, the number ranging from 1-5 for each patient. Three patients complained of pain 'all over' without further qualifications or localization. Of those who described localized pains several extended their description to include pain 'all over' when questioned (Table 11). Pain had been a symptom in these patients for periods ranging from its occurrence during the course of the present illness to 25 yr. The mean duration of all pains was 4.27 yr.

As pains related to psychiatric illness have been reported to be commonly left sided [8] criteria of laterality were set up

Table 3. Weekly incidence of pain expressed as a percentage of the hospital population

Week	1	2	3	4	5	6	7	8	9	10	11	12
Incidence (%)	65.9	58.6	45.5	56.7	51.1	53.3	47.8	51.1	63.0	51.1	40.4	51.3
Week	**13**	**14**	**15**	**16**	**17**	**18**	**19**	**20**	**21**	**22**	**23**	**24**
Incidence (%)	39.5	47.6	41.5	42.1	34.2	36.4	36.1	32.5	36.4	49.0	44.0	32.2

(Mean weeks 1-12 = 51.32% Weeks 13-24 = 39.29% $t = 4.19$ d.f. = 22 $P < 0.001$.)

Table 4. Relationship of pain to major diagnostic categories in hospital patients

	Depression	*Anxiety/ hysteria*	*Other*	*Total*
Pain	32	17	10	59
No pain	33	4	20	57
Total	65	21	30	116

$\chi^2 = 11.02$ d.f. = 2 $P < 0.01$.

Table 5. Relationship of pain to history of operation

	No history of operation	*History of one or more operations*	*Total*
Pain	32	27	59
No pain	44	13	57
Total	76	40	116

$\chi^2 = 5.78$ d.f. = 1 $P < 0.02$.

Table 6. Relationship of pain to social class in male patients

Class	*1-4*	*5*	*6*	*7*	*Total*
Pain	1	13	4	4	22
No pain	4	3	11	6	24
Total	5	16	15	10	46

$\chi^2 = 11.643$ d.f. = 3 $P < 0.01$.

Table 7. Relationship of pain to other somatic symptoms

	Other somatic symptoms present	*Other somatic symptoms absent*	*Total*
Pain	32	27	59
No pain	18	39	57
Total	50	66	116

$\chi^2 = 5.18$ d.f. = 1 $P < 0.05$.

Table 8. Relationship of pain to overt anxiety

	Anxiety	*No anxiety*	*Total*
Pain	54	5	59
No pain	41	16	57
Total	95	21	116

$\chi^2 = 6.24$ d.f. = 1 $P < 0.02$.

Table 9. Incidence of pain on 1st and 4th weeks of admission

	Number of patients
Pain on 1st and 4th weeks of admission	28
Pain on 1st week, no pain on 4th week of admission	13
No pain on 1st week, pain on 4th week of admission	3
No pain on 1st nor 4th week of admission	50

Binomial test for significance of change $N = 16$ $x = 3$ $P = 0.022$.

to examine this possibility. Lateral pains present no problem, asymmetric central, or central and lateral pains were localized to the side of the asymmetry while symmetrically bilateral pains and pains 'all over' were regarded as central. Sixty-five pains could be regarded as left sided, 27 as right sided. If the assumption be made that where pain is lateralized the probability of its occurrence on the left or right is equal the chi-squared test can be applied, giving $\chi^2 = 15.69$ d.f. $= 1$ $P < 0.001$. Pain associated with psychiatric illness tends to be located axially in the head, neck and trunk (Table 12). Radiation of the pain is not very common, occurring in only 29 of the 219 localized pains described.

162 (48.7%) of the 331 descriptions of the pain given by the patients were considered to be simple. The relative incidence of these types of description is the same in different parts of the body.

Patients describe two types of precipitating factor, first those factors which initiate individual episodes of pain, and second those which seem to start a pain response which continues whether or not the precipitating factor remains active. Mental work and emotional strain are the most common precipitating factors, initiating individual episodes of 20 pains and triggering a continued pain response on 13 occasions. Exertion was the next most common precipitant but applied only to individual episodes of pain. Its score here exceeded that of mental factors as it was implicated in relation to 21 pains. However, of the 132 patients, 69 (52.3%) could not relate a precipitating factor to any of their pains, whilst of the 222 pains reported 127 (57.2%) had no ascertainable precipitating factor.

Individual episodes of pain were usually continuous (117 pains) implying continuity from day to day, but not demanding that the patient be awake all night, or intermittent (69 pains) with episodes of pain last-

Table 10. Incidence of pain on discharge and 4 weeks before discharge

	Number of patients
Pain 4 weeks before discharge and on discharge	30
Pain 4 weeks before discharge, but not on discharge	10
No pain 4 weeks before discharge, but pain on discharge	1
No pain 4 weeks before discharge, nor on discharge	54

Binomial test for significance of change $N = 11$ $x = 1$ $P = 0.012$.

Table 11. Distribution of number of pains per patient

Number of pains complained of by the patient	*Number of patients*	*Number of patients extending pain to 'all over'*	*Total pains*
1	72	9	72
2	42	2	84
3	11	3	33
4	5	0	20
5	2	2	10
'All over' only	3		3

Table 12. Distribution of pain according to laterality (excluding pains 'all over')

	Head and face	*Back and neck*	*Abdomen*	*Chest*	*Limbs*	*Total*
Lateralized to left	21	13	11	13	7	65
Not lateralized	49	26	25	14	13	127
Lateralized to right	8	6	7	1	5	27
Total	78	45	43	28	25	219

Table 13. Relationship of pains to other features of illness

	Site						Total
	Head and face	*Back*	*Abdomen*	*Chest*	*Limbs*	*'All over'*	
Direct	36	18	18	16	10	1	99
Inverse	7	1	2	0	2	0	12
Invariant	25	19	19	10	9	2	84
Unrelated	10	7	4	2	4	0	27
Total	78	45	43	28	25	3	222

ing more than 1 hr, but less than one day. Transient episodes lasting 1 hr or less (21 pains) and prolonged episodes (15 pains) where the pain is present for two or more successive days but where there are intervals of at least 1 day between such episodes, were much less common.

Ninety-five (71.9%) patients were unable to relate the pain to any other regularly occurring events, and of the total 222 pains 179 (80.6%) had no discernible time relationship of this type.

Fifty patients (37.9%) failed to find relief for any of their pains; of these 19 had transient, and 13 intermittent pains. The standard mild analgesics, aspirin codeine, paracetamol were the most successful, alleviating 35 pains. Abdominal pains were most commonly (6 reports) relieved by antacids, but in general the most successful treatment after analgesics was the use of antidepressant drugs, which gave some relief to 23 pains. Rest (18 reports), rubbing and manipulation (12 reports), heat (11 reports), antacids (11 reports in all), sedatives and tranquilisers (10 reports in all) fairly commonly gave relief. A variety of other 'treatments' including electroencephalography, vomiting and admission to hospital were also described as giving relief.

The variation of pain with other features of the illness may be complete or partial but can be classified as direct, inverse, invariant and unrelated (Table 13). These types of variation define four groups of patients, two large and two small, according to the type of their dominant pain.

There are marked differences between the two larger groups. Some of these differences are amenable to statistical examination and for this purpose the smaller groups have been combined as the numbers would otherwise be too small for satisfactory conclusions to be drawn.

The first group contains 56 patients, 20 male, 36 female, age range 20-66, mean age 42.86, standard deviation 11.4, whose pain varied directly with other symptoms. Thirty-eight patients suffered from a predominantly depressive illness, 13 from anxiety/hysteria and five from various other conditions.

The dominant clinical feature of this group, apart from its selection criterion is the preponderance of depression. All forms of depressive illness are represented, but no attempt has been made to subdivide the diagnostic category further as such attempts could only decrease the reliability of the divisions made.

The second large group contained 60 patients, 19 male, 41 female, age range 20-66, mean age 44.00, standard deviation 11.5, whose pains were invariant with respect to other symptoms. Depression is less common in this group, occurring in 18 patients. The remaining patients fall into a variety of diagnostic categories, but most of them (29 patients) can be classified as anxiety/hysteria.

Pains which alternate with other symptoms occurred in a small group containing nine patients, seven female, two male, mean age 46.33, range 31-56. In three of them a depressive illness responded to treatment, to be replaced by pain, four of them showed alternation of the pain with other symptoms, one patient became depressed when a pain thought to be 'psychogenic' was found to be due to a hiatus hernia, and cured by operation, while the last patient showed a sequence of hysterical paralysis, endogenous type of depression, a headache and recovery.

Incidental pains occurred in seven patients, all female, mean age 37.43, range 25-57. Three were diagnosed as depressed, one as depressed with hysterical features,

Table 14. Relationship of pain groups to diagnosis

	Direct relationship	*Invariant*	*Other*	*Total*
Depression	38	18	8	64
Other	18	42	8	68
Total	56	60	16	132

$\chi^2 = 16.49$ d.f. = 2 $P < 0.001$.

Table 15. Relationship on pain group to response to treatment

	Direct relationship	*Invariant*	*Other*	*Total*
Well	16	4	5	25
Improved	19	14	3	36
Unchanged and worse	21	42	16	71

$\chi^2 = 16.33$ d.f. = 4 $P < 0.01$.

one as an anxiety state, one as an hysterical psychopath and one undiagnosed.

The two largest groups show considerable differences clinically, particularly in diagnostic distribution and apparent difficulty and complexity of the problems presented. There is no significant difference in age, sex, time since onset or duration of treatment from date first seen until discharge or the end of the follow-up period. When diagnoses were categorized simply as Depression and Other there was a significant difference between the groups ($\chi^2 = 16.49$ d.f. = 2 $P < 0.001$) due to the difference between the larger groups ($\chi^2 = 15.15$ d.f. = 1 $P < 0.001$) (Table 14). There was also a difference in response to treatment. Response was assessed on discharge, or at the end of the investigation as, no change or worse, improved and well. The 3×3 table (Table 15) between response and groups showed significant differences ($\chi^2 = 16.33$ d.f. = 4 $P < 0.01$) due to the better response in patients whose pain varied directly with their other symptoms. A comparison of the number of patients discharged, self-discharged and still attending, showed no significant difference between the groups.

DISCUSSION

It is clear that pain is a common symptom in psychiatric patients, particularly those with anxiety states. If Stoetzel's [14] figures be accepted the high incidence in depression is only the same as that to be found in a normal population, although it may be a depressive symptom to complain to others. Schizophrenic patients do not seem to complain much of pain, but the number in this series is small and should be substantiated from another population. The period of study was from January to July, and the weekly incidence suggests the possibility of a seasonal variation. Obviously this cannot be regarded as established on the basis of this investigation and figures should be obtained for at least two years.

It is widely believed that hostility, with or without associated guilt, is an important factor in the genesis of pain in psychiatric patients. If this belief is to be substantiated in its general form it should be possible to demonstrate a relationship between overt or covert hostility, or behaviour suggesting hostile or aggressive attitudes, or depression and guilt, with pain. No such relationship could be demonstrated in this investigation.

The association of pain with other somatic symptoms, with a history of operation, and possibly its association with anxiety tend to support Szasz's view [11] that pain is a consequence of a threat to the integrity of the body viewed as an object of the ego.

The results suggest that the pains which psychiatric patients report show certain general characteristics. They tend to be located centrally in the head and trunk, to be continuous from day to day and to be unrelated to temporal factors such as time of day, meals, awaking etc. The most notable feature is their behaviour in time; they tend to be continuous for long periods, but do not greatly interfere with sleep and do not vary throughout the day. In contrast the pains of organic illness are commonly related to various events, e.g. meals, and are episodic.

It would be unreasonable to regard one feature of a symptom as diagnostic, but it is suggested that enquiry about the temporal characteristics of a pain is a useful screening procedure both in the patient complaining primarily of pain and in the patient suffering from neurosis who develops a pain during his illness. Physical disorder is of importance at some stage in many of these patients. In this series organic factors were considered to be important in 31 pains (13.9%). A further 102 pains (45.9%) were considered to be related to bodily disturbance, particularly muscle tension. However, in all of these patients the mental state was of equal or greater importance. Successful treatment of the psychiatric illness resulted in many cases in resolution of the pain.

SUMMARY AND CONCLUSIONS

The incidence of pain and its relationship to other symptoms and social characteristics has been studied in patients attending the psychiatric department of a general hospital and university.

45-50 per cent of patients complained of pain, the incidence being lower in summer than winter.

Pain occurs most commonly in patients suffering from anxiety states and was associated significantly with a history of surgical operation, other non-painful somatic symptoms, overt anxiety, and, in men, membership of social class 5 on the Hall Jones Scale. Pain in these patients shows the following clinical characteristics: It tends to be continuous throughout the day and from day to day or to occur for periods of several hours but with no fixed temporal pattern. Patients are unable to describe well-defined precipitating factors for their pains. Similarly many patients are unable to define factors exacerbating the pain and such factors vary considerably from patient to patient. The pain is capricious in its response to treatment. Mild analgesics and anti-depressant drugs are the most effective. Pain is most commonly localized in the head or trunk, arising in the midline or bilaterally, but when lateralized it is most frequent on the left. Most people have only one or two pains although spread 'all over' may occur.

Pain descriptions vary widely from the simple to the highly complex or bizarre. The pain may vary directly or inversely with other features of the patient's illness, may persist regardless of changes in the mental state or may appear to be coincidental. Most patients have pain which persists regardless of changes in the other symptoms or which varies directly with those symptoms.

Pain which varies directly with the other symptoms is significantly associated with depression and with good short-term prognosis. Pain which persists regardless of the illness is significantly associated with anxiety states and hysteria and with a poor short-term prognosis.

ACKNOWLEDGEMENTS

This paper is based on part of a thesis accepted for the Degree of M.D. at Bristol University. The work was carried out in the Department of Psychiatry, Sheffield University, United Sheffield Hospitals. I should like to thank Professor E. Stengel and Dr. W. L. Tonge for permission to study patients under their care and for much valuable advice.

REFERENCES

1. Spear F. G. A study of pain as a symptom of psychiatric illness, M.D. Thesis, Bristol University (1964).
2. Merskey H. and Spear F. G. *Psychological and Psychiatric Aspects of Pain,* Balliere. Tindall & Cassell (1967).
3. Klee G. D., Ozilis S., Greenberg G. L. and Gallant L. J. Pain and other somatic complaints in a psychiatric clinic. *Md St. Med. J.* **8,** 188 (1959).
4. Douglas-Wilson I. Somatic manifestations of neurosis. *Br. Med. J.* **i,** 413 (1964).
5. Gittleson N. L. Psychiatric headache: A clinical study. *J. Ment. Sci.* **107,** 403 (1961).
6. Da Costa J. M. On irritable heart: A clinical study of a form of functional cardiac disorder and its consequences. *Am. J. Med. Sci.* **61,** 17 (1871).
7. Masters A. M., Jaffe H. L. and Pordy L. Cardiac and noncardiac chest pain: A statistical study of 'diagnostic' criterion. *Ann. Intern. Med.* **41,** 315 (1954).
8. Halliday J. L. Psychological factors in rheumatism. *Br. Med. J.* **i,** 213; 264 (1937).
9. Paulett J. D. Low back pain. *Lancet* **ii,** 272 (1947).
10. Walters A. Psychogenic regional pain alias hysterical pain. *Brain* **84,** 1 (1961).
11. Szasz T. S. *Pain and Pleasure,* Basic Books, New York (1957).
12. Hall J. and Jones D. C. The social gradings of occupations. *Br. J. Sociol.* **1,** 31 (1950).
13. Maxwell A. E. *Analysing Qualitative Data,* Methuen, London (1961).
14. Stoetzel J. Psychologie sociale appliqué – 3. Les malades dans la Société. *Bull. Psychol., Paris* **12,** 618 (1959).

Annotated bibliography

M. Weisenberg and N. A. Stilwell

This bibliography was compiled to provide the reader with an entré to the experimental and clinical literature scattered throughout the many journals. The emphasis has been placed on journal articles published mainly in the years 1965 to 1972. It is by no means exhaustive of the journal literature.

GENERAL AND THEORETICAL CONCEPTS OF PAIN

Beecher, H. K. 1962. Pain, placebos and physicians, The Practitioner **189:**141-155.
A thorough review of different kinds of pain and the drugs used to relieve pain. The role of the physician and the ethical considerations involved in administering placebos are discussed. 47 references.

Blaylock, J. 1968. The psychological and cultural influences on the reaction to pain: a review of the literature, Nursing Forum **7:**262-274.
A general discussion of the psychological components of pain and the role of culture in pain perception. 44 references.

Brena, S. 1970. The pain-prone patient, Northwest Medicine **69:**573-575.
A brief review of several theories on the pain-prone patient as well as a discussion of two different response patterns exhibited by such individuals. 6 references.

Cabanac, M. 1971. Physiological role of pleasure, Science **173:**1103-1107.
The thesis that any stimulus will be interpreted as pleasant or unpleasant depending on its usefulness as determined by internal signals. Experimental evidence is presented. 17 references.

Casey, K. L. 1973. Pain: a current view of neural mechanisms, American Scientist **61:**194-200.
A review of recent physiological and psychological literature. Evidence is cited to support several hypotheses updating earlier work on the gate control theory of pain. 46 references.

Dallenbach, K. M. 1939. Pain: history and present status, American Journal of Psychology **52:**331-347.
A review of the major philosophical, psychological, and physiological theories of pain from Aristotle's time to 1939. 67 references.

Edwards, W. 1950. Recent research on pain perception, Psychological Bulletin **47:**449-474.
An outline of four related problems: the definition of pain, the psychophysics of pain, the peripheral nervous mechanisms involved in pain perception, and the role of the central nervous system in certain abnormalities of pain perception. Conclusions are drawn. 101 references.

Fisher, A. J. 1970. A psychobiologic reconsideration of pain, Headache **9:**74-86.
A discussion of organic and psychogenic pain as viewed from different clinical perspectives. 8 references.

Hanken, A. F. 1966. Pain and systems analysis, Nursing Research **15:**139-143.
The development of a theoretical "patient model" as a first step toward predicting pain control. Author stresses the need for techniques to accurately quantify the intensity of pain. 13 references.

Keele, K. D. 1972. Pain, how it varies from person to person, Nursing Times **68:**890-892.
A discussion of sensitivity to pain, its measurement, its different forms, and its relationship to organic disease. No references.

Leffert, R. D. 1970. Neurophysiology of pain, Bulletin of the Hospital for Joint Diseases **31:**199-204.
A discussion of basic neurophysiological theories

and the different kinds of pain. Special attention is focused on causalgia. No references.

Melzack, R. 1968. Pain perception, Research Publication Association for Research in Nervous and Mental Diseases **48:**272-285.
A discussion of the gate control theory of pain. Audioanalgesia and cognitive control of pain are considered in light of this theory. 52 references.

Melzack, R., and Wall, P. D. 1965. Pain mechanisms: a new theory, Science **150:**971-979.
The original presentation and explanation of the gate control theory and a review of previous theories of pain perception. 77 references.

Mersky, H. 1970. On the development of pain, Headache **10:**116-123.
A review of evidence supporting the idea of pain as a learned experience depending on an interaction of the organism and its environment. 36 references.

Mersky, H. 1971. Pain, Nursing Times **67:**988-989.
A brief discussion of the nature of pain and psychological factors affecting its perception. Examples are given from hospital and outpatient situations. No references.

Mersky, H., and Spear, F. G. 1967. The concept of pain, Journal of Psychosomatic Research **11:** 59-67.
The definition of pain. Authors argue against separating pain into sensation and reactive components; they feel it should be considered as a whole entity and studied as such. 38 references.

Murray, J. B. 1969. The puzzle of pain, Perceptual and Motor Skills **28:**887-899.
A review of literature on pain as a complex experience involving sensory, cognitive, and affective components. Greatest attention is directed toward physiological research on the sensory aspect. 36 references.

Plainfield, S., and Adler, N. 1962. The meaning of pain, Dental Clinics of North America 659-669.
An examination of many aspects of the pain experience. Topics included are functions of pain, pain used to establish cultural and sexual identity, pain as a means of communication. Authors stress need to evaluate each person's pain individually. 4 references.

Prior, J. C. 1967. Some aspects of the clinical communication of pain, Journal of the American Women's Medical Association **22:**725-731.
A discussion of the various means of expressing pain and variations of these means among cultures. Author stresses the need for the physician to empathize with the patient. 34 references.

The problem of pain relief. 1970. British Journal of Anaesthesia **42:**1.
An editorial on the need to acknowledge pain relief as a major goal of medicine. Author feels that practitioners must cease judging patient by whether or not they verbally complain of pain. No references.

The psychology of pain. 1970. Nursing Times. **66:** 1577-1578.
An extract of a lecture by Dr. W. A. Lishman on studies of postoperative pain and the influence of pain on personality. An explanation of how environmental variables affect an individual's perception of pain is given. No references.

Thomson, A. H. 1965. The anatomy, physiology and psychology of pain, Journal of Occupational Medicine **7:**526-534.
A review of the three major components (anatomy, physiology, and psychology) of pain perception. Objectives of treatment and modes of action of pain-relieving drugs are also discussed. 22 references.

MEASUREMENT OF PAIN

Adair, E. R., and others. 1968. Thermally induced pain, the Dol scale, and the psychophysical power law, American Journal of Psychology **81:**147-164.
A series of experiments showing that pain produced by thermal irradiation of the skin follows the psychophysical power law proposed by S. S. Stevens. 18 references.

Auerbach, A. J. 1967. A pain-tolerance determination technique for evaluating analgesic drug efficacy, Canadian Journal of Psychology **21:**490-495.
A technique for measuring pain tolerance based on suprathreshold contact maintenance. Tolerance was greater under the effect of codeine than under a placebo. 12 references.

Beaugie, A., Askill, S., and Payne, J. P. 1972. Measurements of pain threshold, a preliminary report, British Journal of Anesthesiology **44:**901.
A description of a radiant heat apparatus for testing pain threshold based on length of exposure to the stimulus. 1 reference.

Beecher, H. K. 1956-1957. The measurement of pain, prototype for the quantitative study of subjective responses, Pharmacological Reviews **8-9:**60-209.
A major comprehensive literature review and discussion of all aspects of pain reaction and measurement. 687 references.

Beecher, H. K. 1966. Pain: one mystery solved, Science **151:**840-841.
A description of tourniquet pain as the appropriate laboratory analogue of pathological pain. 4 references.

Bloomfield, S. S., and Hurwitz, H. N. 1970. Tourniquet and episiotomy pain as test models for aspirin-like analgesics, Journal of Clinical Pharmacology **10:**361-369.
A study comparing the response to aspirin with the response to a placebo in patients with episiotomy pain who later were subjected to tourniquet pain. Authors conclude that tourniquet pain is unreliable for evaluating aspirin analgesia. 26 references.

Brown, R. L., Spern, R., Schmitt, K., and Solomon, A. 1966. Stimulus parameter considerations and individual differences in cutaneous sensitivity to electropulse stimulation, Perceptual Motor Skills **23:** 1215-1222.
Two experiments to define optimal parameter values for an electropulse stimulus and the extent of subject differences. 12 references.

Dillon, D. J. 1968. Stimulus intensity, site of stimulation, and individual reactivity as determinants of the energy threshold for pricking pain, Journal of Experimental Psychology **77:**559-566.
A study in which threshold energies were obtained at 3 stimulus intensities in 2 experimental sessions from 3 locations on the nonpreferred arm of 33 subjects. A latency measure was used, and differences were observed on each of 3 variables. 10 references.

Dinnerstein, A. J., Blitz, B., and Lowenthal, M. 1965. Effects of aspirin on detection and tolerance of electric shock, Journal of Applied Physiology **20:**1052-1055.

An experimental study in which it was found that aspirin increased sensitivity to shock-induced pain in a large minority of subjects. 8 references.

Forgione, A. G., and Barber, T. X. 1971. A strain gauge pain stimulator, Psychophysiology **8:**102-106. A description of a pain stimulator with a bonded strain gauge that eliminates methodological faults of previous applications of this method. 8 references.

Gelfand, S. 1964. The relationship of experimental pain tolerance to pain threshold, Canadian Journal of Psychology **18:**36-42.
An experimental study that yielded low correlations between pain threshold and pain tolerance. The type of instructions and the measure of tolerance used could have a significant effect on tolerance. 8 references.

Green, R. T. 1962. The absolute threshold of electric shock, British Journal of Psychology **53:**107-115.
An experimental study using variations in stimuli, size of electrode, and use of electrode jelly. Power seems to be the relevant variable in threshold sensitivity. 8 references.

Haslam, D. R. 1968. Some anomalies in the study of experimental pain, Quarterly Journal of Experimental Psychology **20:**208-211.
An investigation of anomalies connected with the assessment of pain threshold by the limiting method. An anchoring effect seems to account for the low pain threshold values found when a small stimulus interval is used. 8 references.

Haslam, D. R., and Thomas, E. A. C. 1967. An optimum interval in the assessment of pain threshold, Quarterly Journal of Experimental Psychology **19:** 54-58.
A continuation of authors' investigation of pain threshold measured by the limiting method. The results indicate that pain threshold is uniform over the population. 4 references.

Kast, E. C. 1968. Clinical measurement of pain, Medical Clinics of North America **52:**23-32.
Several methods of measuring clinical pain. Although the pain sensation itself cannot be measured, a comparative stimulus leading to the pain can serve as an analogue of the pain. 16 references.

Melzack, R., and Torgerson, W. S. 1971. On the language of pain, Anesthesiology **34:**50-59.
The development of valid and reliable terminology for describing the various types of pain. Words to describe pain are divided into subcategories and scaled. 20 references.

Merskey, H., and Spear, F. G. 1964. The reliability of the pressure algometer, British Journal of Social and Clinical Psychology **3:**130-136.
A study in which the pressure algometer method is shown to have a moderate degree of consistency and reliability when used independently by two observers. 22 references.

Peck, R. E. 1966. The application of thymometry to the measurement of anxiety, International Journal of Neuropsychiatry **2:**337-341.
Experimental evidence for thymometry, a technique measuring feelings and tension states by comparing the intensity of an unknown stimulus with a known stimulus. 10 references.

Riehl, J. P. 1965. The effect of a naturally occurring pain on the galvanic skin response and heart rate: a clinical study, American Nurses Association, Regional Clinical Conferences **3:**16-23.
A study of women during labor. The results confirm the hypothesis that the galvanic skin response and heart rate increase with increases in labor pain stimulus. 17 references.

Rogers, J. G. 1971. Blink test to establish threshold for reaction to pain, Postgraduate Medicine, **49:** 108-111.
Three case studies showing that a blink test is a satisfactory indicator of pain tolerance. 9 references.

Sharpley, R. P., and Holliday, A. R. 1966. The use of ultrasound as a method for assessing changes in sensitivity to pain, Proceedings of the Western Pharmacological Society **9:**54-56.
A conclusion after several studies, that ultrasound has no particular advantages over other techniques for evaluating anagesics. It may, however, be more dangerous. 7 references.

Sigel, H. 1951. Cutaneous sensory threshold stimulation with high frequency square-wave current, The Journal of Investigative Dermatology **18:**441-445.
An experimental study of the cutaneous sensory threshold, using high frequency square-wave current and five electrodes of different dimensions. 7 references.

Smith, G. M., Parry, W. L., Denton, J. E., and Beecher, H. K. 1970. Effect of morphine on pain produced in man by electric shock delivered through an annular disc cellulose sponge electrode. In: Proceedings, 78th Annual Convention, American Psychological Association, Washington, D.C., pp. 819-820.
A successful test of the Tursky-Watson procedure of using the pain of electric shock in humans to differentiate morphine and a placebo. 2 references.

Sullivan, R. 1968. Effect of different frequencies of vibration on pain-threshold detection, Experimental Neurology **20:**135-142.
An experimental study in which threshold detection of radiant heat pain was found to be altered as a function of the frequency of an applied vibratory stimulus. 12 references.

Troup, J. D. G. 1970. Some problems of measurement in clinical trials of physiotherapy, with particular reference to the assessment of pain, Physiotherapy **56:**491-496.
A discussion of measurement problems as a result of subjective interpretations, and the relationship to the gate control of pain. 31 references.

Tursky, B., and Watson, P. D. 1964. Controlled physical and subjective intensities of electric shock, Psychophysiology **1:**151-162.
A series of investigations to determine which physical parameters must be controlled to deliver constant electrical stimulation. 9 references.

Voevodsky, J. and others. 1967. The measurement of suprathreshold pain, American Journal of Psychology **80:**124-128.
A study in which suprathreshold pain was measured by subjects who subjectively reported increasing pain during hand-and-arm immersion in ice water. Consistent patterns were observed. No references.

Wolff, B. B. 1964. The relationship of experimental pain tolerance to pain threshold: a critique of Gelfand's paper, Canadian Journal of Psychology **18:** 249-253.

A discussion and critique of Gelfand's paper on differences between pain tolerance and pain threshold. 6 references.

Wolff, B. B., and Jarvik, M. E. 1963. Variations in cutaneous and deep somatic pain sensitivity, Canadian Journal of Psychology **17:**37-44.
A study in which deep somatic pain and cutaneous pain were experimentally induced in 20 human subjects by 3 techniques. From the results it was hypothesized that for different stimuli the highest correlations should occur when similar pain sensations, especially from the same body structure or tissue, are induced. However, there are differences between deep somatic and cutaneous pain. 8 references.

Wolff, B. B., and Jarvik, M. E. 1964. Relationship between superficial and deep somatic thresholds of pain with a note on handedness, The American Journal of Psychology **77:**589-599.
An experimental study in which authors found that different thresholds of pain elicited by different stimuli impinging on different body loci will be related if the resultant subjective pain is similar in quality. No references.

Woodforde, J. M., and Merskey, H. 1972. Some relationships between subjective measures of pain, Journal of Psychosomatic Research **16:**173-178.
An experimental study comparing pain reactions of psychiatric patients who had organic diseases with psychiatric patients who had pain but no related organic disease. No significant differences between groups were observed on measures of pain. 14 references.

SOCIAL AND PSYCHOLOGICAL CORRELATES OF PAIN PERCEPTION

Blitz, B., Dinnerstein, A. J., and Lowenthal, M. 1968. Performance in the pain apperception test and tolerance for experimental pain: a lack of relationship, Journal of Clinical Psychology **24:**73.
A study in which results from the pain apperception test were correlated with pain tolerance using electrical stimulation. No relationship between responses to the test and tolerance for actual pain was observed. 4 references.

Bronzo, A., Jr., and Powers, G. 1967. Relationship of anxiety with pain threshold, The Journal of Psychology **66:**181-183.
An experimental study (in which N = 1) carried out to show that anxiety lowers the pain threshold. 10 references.

Chapman, W. P. 1944. Measurements of pain sensitivity in normal control subjects and in psychoneurotic patients. Psychosomatic Medicine **6:**252-257.
A study in which no differences in pain perception were observed but differences in reaction to pain were observed. Psychoneurotics were less willing to tolerate pain.

Collins, G. L. 1965. Pain sensitivity and ratings of childhood experience, Perceptual and Motor Skills **21:**349-350.
A study showing a positive relationship of pain threshold and tolerance measures to childhood protection and a negative relationship to childhood independence scores on a childhood history questionnaire. 5 references.

Collins, G. L., and Stone, L. A. 1966. Family structure and pain reactivity, Journal of Clinical Psychology **22:**33.
A study of the relationship of birth order and family size to a pain complaint scale and three measures of experimental pain. No significant relationships were found. 3 references.

Davidson, P. O., and Bobey, M. J. 1970. Repressor-sensitizer differences on repeated exposure to pain, Perceptual and Motor Skills **31:**711-714.
A study of 72 female subjects who were categorized as repressors or sensitizers and then given heat and pressure algometer tests of pain tolerance. The groups differed in responses over time but not in overall pain tolerance. 17 references.

Friedman, R. 1972. Some characteristics of children with "psychogenic" pain: observations on prognosis and management, Clinical Pediatrics **7:**331-333.
A survey of 74 children with psychogenic pain. No differences from average children were found in intelligence, family size, or ordinal position. According to follow-up data, most children improved with or without treatment 1 to 3 years later. 6 references.

Gelfand, D. M., Gelfand, S., and Rardin, M. W. 1965. Some personality factors associated with placebo responsivity, Psychological Reports **17:**555-562.
An experimental study indicating that personality factors in placebo responsivity were related to pain tolerance but not to pain threshold. 22 references.

Gonda, T. A. 1962. The relation between complaints of persistent pain and family size, Journal of Neurology, Neurosurgery and Psychiatry **25:**277-281.
A study of outpatients, revealing that patients who persistently complain of pain to their doctors tend to come from larger families than patients who do not complain. 11 references.

Haslam, D. R. 1967. Individual differences in pain threshold and level of arousal, British Journal of Psychology **58:**139-142.
An assessment of pain thresholds for introverts and extraverts. Results showed introverts to have lower thresholds. The issue of perception of pain and level of arousal is also considered and related to introversion versus extraversion. 19 references.

Haslam, D. R. 1970. Lateral dominance in the perception of size and of pain, Quarterly Journal of Experimental Psychology **22:**503-507.
A study of size and pain perceptions in right-handed and left-handed subjects. For right-handed subjects a significant relationship was found between estimation of size and pain tolerance. 8 references.

Levine, F. M., Tursky, B., and Nichols, D. C. 1966. Tolerance for pain, extraversion, and neuroticism: failure to replicate results, Perceptual and Motor Skills **23:**847-850.
An experimental study that fails to confirm previous evidence showing a positive correlation between pain tolerance and extraversion. 10 references.

Martin, J. E., and Inglis, J. 1965. Pain tolerance and narcotic addiction, British Journal of Social and Clinical Psychology **4:**224-229.
An experimental study comparing former addicts and nonaddicts on pain tolerance. Former addicts exhibited lower tolerances on the cold pressor test. No relationship was found between pain tolerance and extraversion. 18 references.

Murray, F. S, and Safferstone, J. F. 1970. Pain threshold and tolerance of right and left hands, Journal of

Comparative and Physiological Psychology **71:**83-86.
A study measuring the pain of cold water stimulation in 41 women. Pain threshold and tolerance were greater for the right hand regardless of the hand preference of the subjects. 10 references.

Nichols, D. C., and Tursky, B. 1967. Body image, anxiety, and tolerance for experimental pain, Psychosomatic Medicine **29:**103-110.
A study of pain tolerance in relationship to body image and anxiety. A positive correlation was found between pain tolerance and definiteness of body boundaries, and a negative relationship was found between anxiety and pain tolerance. 19 references.

CULTURAL INFLUENCES ON PAIN PERCEPTION

Buss, A. H., and Portnoy, N. M. 1967. Pain tolerance and group identification, Journal of Personality and Social Psycology **6:**106-108.
A study in which groups were scaled for strength of identification. High, medium, and low groups were selected for a pain tolerance experiment. Subjects were given false norms for their group. The greater the subjects' identification, the greater the increase in tolerance levels. 1 reference.

Chapman, W. P., and Jones, C. M. 1944. Variations in cutaneous and visceral pain sensitivity in normal subjects, Journal of Clinical Investigation **23:**81-91.
A study in which 200 subjects of various races and ages were tested for cutaneous pain sensitivity. Significant differences were found for both variables. 12 references.

Mallam, R. A. 1966. Cultural influences on the patient's reaction to anxiety and pain, Ghana Nurse **3:**4-6.
A discussion of the ways in which cultural influences affect the behavior of the medical patient. Author argues that cultural influences must be taken into account when treating a patient. 4 references.

Sternbach, R. A., and Tursky, B. 1965. Ethnic differences among housewives in psychophysical and skin potential responses to electric shock, Psychophysiology **1:**241-246.
A study of Yankee, Irish, Jewish, and Italian housewives, supporting the hypothesis that subcultural differences in attitudes toward pain are reflected in psychophysiological correlates. 11 references.

Tsushima, W. T. 1968. Responses of Irish and Italian patients of two social classes under preoperative stress, Journal of Personality and Social Psychology **8:**43-48.
A study in which the hypothesis that Italian patients report more overt signs of emotional tension and hostility than do Irish patients was supported. It was also hypothesized that lower-class patients report more overt signs of tension and hostility than middle-class patients, but no class differences were observed. 19 references.

Zborowski, M. 1952. Cultural components in responses to pain, Journal of Social Issues **4:**16-30.
An exploration of the role of cultural patterns in attitudes toward and reactions to pain caused by disease and injury. No references.

Zola, I. K. 1966. Culture and symptoms—an analysis of patients' presenting complaints, American Sociological Review **31:**615-630.
The suggestion that a socially conditioned selective process may be operating to determine what problems cause patients to seek medical treatment. Two such processes are delineated. A comparison of Italian and Irish patients and the way they react to pain is presented. 107 references.

EXPERIMENTAL STUDIES OF PAIN

Pharmacological studies

Arieff, A. J., and Wetzel, N. 1967. Tegretol in the treatment of neuralgias, Diseases of the Nervous System **28:**820-823.
A study in which Tegretol produced a remission in 15 of 19 patients with classical trigeminal neuralgia; it was ineffective for the other neuralgias. 17 references.

Berguist, J. R. 1972. The relief of postpartum pain with Fiorinal, Therapy and Research **14:**264-269.
A study in which effective relief of postpartum pain was obtained with Fiorinal in 83% of patients 12 to 48 hours after delivery. 4 references.

Brena, S. 1969. Current status of regional analgesia for diagnosis and therapy, Clinical Anaesthesia **2:**167-191.
A discussion of basic concepts of pain and nerve block therapy, and the present status of regional analgesia in the management of common chronic pain problems. 76 references.

Cantor, J. K. 1972. Phenytoin treatment of thalamic pain. British Medical Journal **4:**490.
Two case studies where phenytoin was effective in relieving chronic thalmic pain. 8 references.

Carter, B. L. 1967. Comparison of individual pain reactions to injections of distilled water and normal saline. American Nurses Association, Regional Clinical Conferences 219-225.
A review of literature and a study comparing subjective reactions to injections of saline solution or distilled water. Subjects found saline to be less painful. Implications for placebo administration are considered. 16 references.

Cherkin, A., and Harroun P. 1971. Anesthesia and memory processes, Anesthesiology **34:**469-474.
A discussion of the causes of recall of events during surgery and the need for avoiding conversation during surgery on patients under light anesthesia. 121 references.

Economou, G., Monson, R., and Ward-McQuaid, J. N. 1971. Oral pentazocine and phenazocine: a comparison in postoperative pain, British Journal of Anaesthesia **43:**484-495.
A study of 284 patients with postoperative pain. Two types of orally administered pentazocine given in single doses were compared for analgesia and side effects. Both types were found to be effective. 13 references.

Espir, M. L. E., and Millac, P. 1970. Treatment of paroxysmal disorders in multiple sclerosis with carbamazepine (Tegretol), Journal of Neurology and Psychiatry **33:**528-531.
A study comparing the effects of Tegretol with those of a placebo on patients with paroxysmal disorders. The majority of patients experienced some relief. 9 references.

Finch, J. S., and DeKornfeld, T. J. 1971. Clonixin: a clinical evaluation of a new oral analgesic, Journal of Clinical Pharmacology and New Drugs **11:**371-377.

A study comparing the effectiveness of clonixin with standard analgesics in two controlled clinical evaluations. No references.

Forrest, W. H., and othres. 1969. Analgesix and other effects of the *d*- and *l*-isomers of pentazocine. Clinical Pharmacology and Therapeutics **4:**468-476.
Two randomized, double-blind assays involving 478 patients. *D*- and *l*-isomers of pentazocine were compared with morphine for analgesia and other effects. 5 references.

Giddon, D. B., Quadland, M., Rackwall, P. C., Springer, J., and Tursky, B. 1968. Development of a method for comparing topical anesthetics in different application and dosage forms, Journal of Oral Theraputics and Pharmacology **4:**270-274.
Techniques for comparison of topical anesthetics in different application and dosage forms. 8 references.

Hamilton, R. C., and others. 1967. Alterations in response to somatic pain associated with anaesthesia. XVIII. Studies with some opiate antagonists, British Journal of Anaesthesia **39:**490-502.
A study using tibial pressure algesimetry to determine the effects of several types of drugs on pain response. 44 references.

Houde, R. W., Wallenstein, S. L., and Rogers, A. 1960. Clinical pharmacology of analgesics. I. A method of assaying analgesic effect, Clinical Pharmacology and Therapeutics **1:**163-174.
A study comparing the effects of aspirin, morphine, and a combination of other analgesic drugs on patients in a clinical setting. 10 references.

Isaacs, W. A., Effiong, C. E., and Ayani, O. 1972. Steroid treatment in the prevention of painful epidodes in sickle-cell disease, Lancet **1:**570-571.
A comparison of testosterone and progesterone with a saline solution in a cross-over trial. Results showed a significant reduction in the frequency of painful episodes in 80% of steroid-treated patients. 25 references.

Jick, H., and others. 1971. A new method for assessing the clinical effects of oral analgesic drugs, Clinical Pharmacology and Theraputics **12:**456-463.
A comparison of aspirin, a placebo, and two salts of propoxyphene in a randomized double-blind trial. No difference was found between the two salts. 8 references.

Kerslake, D. 1973. Is your pain really necessary? British Medical Journal **2:**614-615.
A brief letter on the successful treatment of dysmenorrhea with cyclandelate. No references.

Kolliker, K. 1972. Pentazoxine, pethidine and placebo for postoperative pain, Acta Anaesthesiologica Scandinavica **16:**11-16.
An evaluation of subjective and objective methods of assessment of analgesia. Pentazoxine proved to be a more effective analgesic with fewer side effects than pethidine. 11 references.

Kolodny, A. L. 1966. A clinical determination of pain relief in office patients: a controlled comparative study, Psychosomatics **7:**11-13.
A study of the analgesic potency of hydromorphone in 102 office patients suffering from pain of varied causes. It was found to be significantly more effective than a placebo in this double-blind design. 8 references.

Lasagna, L., and Werner, G. 1966. Conjoint clinic on pain and analgesia, Journal of Chronic Diseases **19:** 695-709.
A review of several studies on pain mechanisms and reactions, as well as a discussion of various analgesics and their effects. 26 references.

Martinetti, L., and others. 1970. Clinical evaluation of an oral analgesic Z.424, in patients with chronic pain, Journal of Clinical Pharmacology **10:**390-399.
Two double-blind crossover studies comparing the analgesic activity and tolerability of a new compound, Z.424, for chronic pain with those of codeine and a placebo. The effects were found to be comparable to those of codeine. 13 references.

Marx, G. F., and others, 1971. Pain and awareness during surgical anesthesia, New York State Journal of Medicine **67:**2623-2624.
A case report of a 68-year-old woman who complained of pain during surgery and suggestions for avoiding such situations. No references.

McIntyre, J. W. R. 1966. Awareness during general anaesthesia: preliminary observations, Canadian Anaesthetist's Society Journal **13:**495-499.
A study of patients' awareness while under general anesthesia. Patients under nitrous oxide oxygen anaesthesia failed to recall a story told to them during surgery. Paired words applied to patients under methoxyflurane fentanyl droperidol anaesthesia were associated with signs of arousal in four of them. 25 references.

Merskey, H., and Hester, R. A. 1972. The treatment of chronic pain with psychotropic drugs, Postgraduate Medical Journal **48:**594-598.
A description of the treatment of 30 patients. It is suggested that the drugs used act partly by virtue of an effect on the multisynaptic neuronal systems whose activities are related to the experience of pain. 25 references.

Morrison, J. D. 1970. Alterations in response to somatic pain associated with anaesthesia. XIX. Studies with the drugs used in neurolepthanesthesia, British Journal of Anaesthesia **42:**838-848.
An investigation of the effects of several intravenously administered drugs on sensitivity to tibial pressure-induced somatic pain in a controlled, double-blind trial. 13 references.

Prostaglandins, pain and fever. 1972. Nature **240:**377-378.
A discussion of recent research on the mechanism of action of aspirin on pain and fever as related to the production of prostaglandins.

Sadove, M. S. 1971. A look at narcotic and nonnarcotic analgesics, Postgraduate Medicine **49:**102-105.
A consideration of the advantages and disadvantages of several narcotic and nonnarcotic drugs. Author contends that several widely used drugs are not as effective as some that are rarely used. No references.

Shira, R. B. 1967. A rational approach to drug therapy in modern dentistry, Bulletin Contra Costa Dental Society **12:**7-14.
A listing of different types of drugs and specific uses for them in dentistry. No references.

Shresta, B. L. 1971. Intrathecal cold saline for relief of intractable pain, Canadian Medical Association Journal **105:**345.
A letter confirming the effectiveness of intrathecal saline for relief of pain. No references.

Siegler, P. E., Fabiani, J. A., and Nodine, J. H. 1967. Double-blind comparison of intramuscular pheny-

ramidol and placebo in acute musculoskeletal pain syndromes, Current Therapeutic Research **9**:6-9.
A comparison of the effects of phenyramidol and a placebo, both by intramuscular injection, on 2 groups of 35 patients who suffered acute muscle pain. The drug produced a prompt response and is recommended. 2 references.

Vandam, L. D. 1972. Analgetic drugs—the mild analgetics, New England Journal of Medicine **286**:20-33.
A discussion of several analgetics and their effectiveness. Adverse effects and dosage levels are considered. No references.

Vuopala, U., Vesterinen, E., and Kaipainen, W. J. 1971. The analgetic action of dimethyl sulfoxide (DMSO) ointment in arthrosis—a double blind study, Acta Rheumatologica Scandanavica **17**:57-60.
A double-blind study of the analgetic action of 50% DMSO ointment and placebo ointment in patients with arthrosis. Relief was obtained with both ointments in 76% of the cases. 6 references.

Walike, B. C., and Meyer, B. 1966. Relation between placebo reactivity and selected personality factors, Nursing Research **15**:119-123.
A study of 29 patients to investigate the hypothesis that definite personality characteristics differentiate placebo reactors from nonreactors. The hypothesis was supported. 15 references.

Wolff, B. B., Kantor, T. G., Jarvik, M. E., and Laska, E. 1966. Response of experimental pain to analgesic drugs. I. Morphine, aspirin and placebo, Clinical Pharmacology and Theraputics **7**:224-238.
An evaluation of the effectiveness of morphine, aspirin, and a placebo in two experimental pain situations, ice water and electrical stimulation. Morphine significantly increased pain tolerance. 41 references.

Wolff, B. B., Kantor, T. G., Jarvik, M. E., and Laska, E. 1966. Response of experimental pain to analgesic drugs. II. Codeine and placebo, Clinical Pharmacology and Theraputics **7**:323-331.
An evaluation of the effects of codeine in several situations that produced experimental pain. Permissive and nonpermissive instructions were used in a randomized block design. Codeine increased pain tolerance but not threshold. 5 references.

Wolff, B. B., Kantor, T. G., Jarvik, M. E., and Laska, E. 1969. Response of experimental pain to analgesic drugs. III. Codeine, aspirin, secobarbital, and placebo. Clinical Pharmacology and Theraputics **10**:217-228.
A study of the effectiveness of several drugs in alleviating experimentally induced pain. The study considered cross-over and single-dose designs as well as pain threshold and pain tolerance as measures of drug effectiveness. 19 references.

World Health Organization. 1972. Opiates and their alternates for pain and cough relief. 1972. World Health Organization Technical Report Series **495**: 1-19.
A comparison of opiates and synthetic drugs and their effectiveness in controlling pain and cough. Several conclusions are drawn, and more research is recommended. 9 references.

Physiological studies

Akil, H., and Mayer, D. J. 1972. Antagonisms of stimulation-produced analgesia by p-CPA, a serotonin synthesis inhibitor, Brain Research **44**:692-697.
A study indicating the possibility that analgesic effects of morphine and brain stimulation have a similar neurochemical as well as anatomical basis. 30 references.

Anderson, D. J., Hannam, A. G., and Matthews, B. 1970. Sensory mechanisms in mammalian teeth and their supporting structures, Physiological Reviews **50**:171-195.
An extensive review of experiments, histological investigations, and electrophysiological investigations of the intradental and periodontal sensory mechanisms. 163 references.

Appenzeller, O., and Kornfeld, M. 1972. Indifference to pain, Archives of Neurology **27**:322-329.
A report of clinical features, laboratory investigations, and tests of autonomic function in two sisters with indifference to pain. 26 references.

Berkley, K. J., and Smith, O. A., Jr. 1970. Behavioral indices for neural systems involved in pain and fear responses of monkeys, Experimental Neurology **26**:527-542.
A study of monkeys trained to choose between an escape and an avoidance response by pressing one of two levers after electrodes were implanted in several areas in the brain. 34 references.

Cook, A. W., and Browder, E. J. 1964. Function of the posterior column, Transactions of the American Neurological Association **89**:193-194.
A consideration (in light of clinical evidence) of the theory of localization, adequacy of ablation experiments in elucidating neurological function, and capacity for compensation in the central nervous system. No references.

Denny-Brown, D. 1965. The release of deep pain by nerve injury, Brain Research **88**:725-738.
A discussion of two categories of persistent pain following injury to peripheral nerves: classical causalgia and posttrauma tic neuralgia. 52 references.

DeVries, H. A. 1966. Quantitative electromyographic investigation of the spasm theory of muscle pain, American Journal of Physical Medicine **45**:119-134.
An evaluation, using electromyography, of experimentally induced and accidentally induced muscle pain. A "spasm" theory that seems to explain all the experimental observations is elucidated. 23 references.

Dudley, D. L., and others. 1965. Psychophysiological studies of experimentally induced action oriented behavior, Journal of Psychosomatic Research **9**: 209-221.
A study of 26 subjects before, during, and after stimulation with a steel headband to determine physiological changes associated with the stimulus. 16 references.

Evans, R. J. 1972. Acid-base changes in patients with intractable pain and malignancy, Canadian Journal of Surgery **15**:37-42.
A study of metabolic alkalosis in proportion to the subjective severity of pain in 91 patients. Implications of the relationship between acid-base balance and pain are considered. 15 references.

Farley, F. H. 1967. The effect of auditory stimulation on blood pressure changes associated with pain, Psychonomic Science **7**:343-344.
A study of the effects of auditory stimulation on systolic blood pressure increases elicited by the cold

pressor procedure. Blood pressure increases were found to be significantly depressed in comparison with a no-stimulation control condition. 7 references.

Fibiger, H. C., Mertz, P. H. and Campbell, B. A. 1972. The effect of para-chlorophenylalanine on aversion threshold reactivity to foot shock, Physiology and Behavior **8:**259-263.
A study of the effect of para-chlorophenylalanine (p-CPA) on measures of sensitivity and reactivity to foot shock in the rat. Data indicate that p-CPA does not alter sensitivity to foot shock but induces changes in the reactivity to intense aversive stimulation. 22 references.

Garcia, F., McGowan, B. K., Ervin, F. R., and Koelling, R. A. 1968. Cues: their relative effectiveness as a function of the reinforcer, Science **160:**794.
A study in which either size or flavor of food pellets was conditionally paired with either malaise induced by x-ray or pain induced by shock in four groups of rats. Authors conclude that effective associate learning depends on central neural convergence of the paired afferent input. 7 references.

Guilbaud, G., Besson, J. M., Oliveras, J. L., and Liebeskind, J. C. 1973. Suppression by L.S.D. of the inhibitory effect exerted by dorsal raphe stimulation on certain spinal cord interneurons in the cat, Brain Research **61:**417-422.
A report of results indicating spinal inhibitory effects of electrical stimulation in the vicinity of the serotonin-containing cell bodies of the dorsal raphe nucleus. 19 references.

Jarabak, J. P. 1969. Neurological interpretation of oral pain, The Journal of the Oregon Dental Association **38:**11-20.
A classification of various kinds of pain into four groups and a consideration of them in the context of the categorization. 11 references.

Kesner, R. P. 1971. ECS as punishing stimulus: dependency on retrograde amnesia, duration of anterograde amnesia, and intensity of pain, Journal of Comparative and Physiological Psychology **74:**398-406.
A report of five experimental studies on the development of fear in rats in response to ECS treatment. Results agree with previous findings regarding mechanisms that account for the development of fear. 12 references.

Kimura, C. 1966. Visceral Sensation—clinical manifestation and experimental bases, Acta Neuroveg (Wien) **28:**405-436.
A review of experimentation and a conclusion that internal organs can evoke pain and some other sensations. 60 references.

Lichstein, L., and Sacketh, G. P. 1971. Reactions by differentially raised rhesus monkeys to noxious stimulations, Developmental Psychobiology **4:**339-352.
Two studies in which adult monkeys in social and sensory isolation showed anomalous reactions to noxious stimuli compared with socially raised controls. 12 references.

Liebeskind, J. C., Guilbaud, G., Besson, J. M., and Oliveras, J. L. 1973. Analgesia from electrical stimulation of the periaqueductal gray matter in the cat: behavioral observations and inhibitory effects on spinal cord interneurons, Brain Research **50:**441-446.
A study showing that stimulation in the vicinity of the dorsal raphe nucleus evokes in the cat, just as in the rat, a powerful analgesia. 26 references.

Liebeskind, J. C., Mayer, D. J., and Akil, H. 1974. Central mechanisms of pain inhibition, Advances in Neurology **4:**261-268.
A summary of research on the use of focal electrical stimulation of the brain as analgesia. Theoretical considerations and implications of the research are presented. 37 references.

Liebman, J. M., Mayer, D. J., and Liebeskind, J. C. 1973. Self-stimuation loci in the midbrain central gray matter of the rat, Behavioral Biology **9:**299-306.
A study in which rats with implanted electrodes in or near the mesencephalic gray matter were tested for self-stimulation behavior in an operant situation. Results indicated that important functional distinction exists between various portions of the central gray matter. 35 references.

Mayer, D. J., Wolfle, T. L., Akil, H., Carder, B., and Liebeskind, J. C. 1971. Analgesia from electrical stimulation in the brain stem of the rat, Science **174:** 1351-1354.
A study in which stimulation at several mesencephalic and diencephalic sites abolished responsiveness to intense pain in rats while leaving responsiveness to other sensory modes relatively unaffected. 14 references.

Meadows, J. C. 1970. Observations on muscle pain in man, with particular reference to pain during needle electromyography, Journal of Neurology, Neurosurgery and Psychiatry **33:**519-523.
A discussion of the presence of "pain spots" that are encountered as the needle pierces muscle tissue. This and other findings are considered in relation to experimental work on pressure-pain receptors in animals. 12 references.

Melzack, R. 1970. Phantom limbs, Psychology Today **4:**63-69.
A discussion of phantom limb pain and how it affects amputees physiologically. A model is proposed to acount for phantom limb phenomena. No references.

Melzack, R. 1971. Phantom limb pain: implications for treatment of pathologic pain, Anesthesiology **35:** 409-419.
A consideration of the properties of phantom limb pain, causal mechanisms, and a theoretical model building on gate control concepts. 49 references.

Mitchell, C. L., and Kaelber, W. W. 1967. Unilateral vs bilateral medial thalamic lesions and reactivity to noxious stimuli, Archives of Neurology **17:**653-660.
A study in which lesions of the medial thalamus were produced in cats trained to escape electrical stimuli delivered to two different sites. The cats were put in the escape apparatus repeatedly and killed after 1 month. It was found that much more destruction of tissue was necessary to abolish the escape response to paw stimulation than to tooth pulp stimulation. 11 references.

Mosso, J. A., and Kruger, L. 1972. Spinal trigeminal neurons excited by noxious and thermal stimuli, Brain Research **38:**206-210.
A discussion of physiological characteristics of pain perception in trigeminal neurons. 6 references.

Parker, C. E., Liederman, V., Edwards, A. E., and

Tuttle, S. G. 1963. Pressure changes in the esophagus to fear, pain and intense aural stimulation, Journal of Comparative and Physiological Psychology **56:**1074-1077.
A study of the effects of experimentally induced fear, pain, and loud noise on pressure transducers throughout the esophageal body and an electrode above the cardiac sphincter. 9 references.

Price, D. D. 1972. Characteristics of second pain and flexion reflexes indicative of prolonged central summation, Experimental Neurology **37:**371-387.
An investigation of the subjective responses and physiological factors involved in the second pain phenomenon. 30 references.

Sachs, E., Jr. 1968. The role of the nervus intermedius in facial neuralgia—report of four cases with observations on the pathways for taste, lacrimation, and pain in the face, Journal of Neurosurgery **28:**54-60.
A report of four cases of intractable face and head pain relieved by section of the nervus intermedius. Inferences are drawn regarding the seventh and eighth cranial nerves and nervus intermedius. 18 references.

Shealy, C. N. 1966. The physiological substrate of pain, Headache **6:**101-108.
A description and investigations of a central nervous system pathway that is uniquely related to painful stimuli. 10 references.

Spiegel, E. A., and Wycis, H. T. 1968. Multiplicity of subcortical localization of various functions, Journal of Nervous and Mental Diseases **147:**45-48.
A study showing that multiple subcortical representations seem to exist for various functions, including pain. It has important implications for the takeover of functions following injury. 23 references.

Vierck, C. J., Hamilton, D. M., and Thornby, J. I. 1971. Pain reactivity of monkeys after lesions to the dorsal and lateral columns of the spinal cord, Experimental Brain Research **13:**140-158.
A study in which the force, latency, and threshold of escape responses were measured as a function of stimulation intensity before and after lesion of the spinal cord. 85 references.

Webber, T. D. 1972. Travell myofascial trigger points and the osteopathic lesion, Journal of the American Osteophatic Association **71:**543-544.
A discussion of pain patterns and the association between trigger points and reference areas. Treatments of such pain problems are also considered. No references.

Wirth, F. P., Jr., and Van Buren, J. M. 1971. Referral of pain from dural stimulation in man, Journal of Neurosurgery **34:**630-642.
A study in which electrical stimulation of the dura was carried out in 25 patients. Chronically implanted electrodes were used to determine areas of referred pain. 36 references.

Wyke, B. 1970. The neurological basis of thoracic spinal pain, Rheumatology and Physical Medicine **10:** 356-367.
A description of the distribution of pain receptor nerve endings in the tissues of the vertebral column in light of recent neurological research and in relationship to diagnostic classification of types of spinal pain. 55 references.

Psychological studies

Blitz, B., and Dinnerstein, A. J. 1968. Effects of different types of instructions on pain parameters, Journal of Abnormal Psychology **73:**276-280.
A study in which varying instructions were shown to have significant effects on subjects' pain tolerance levels. Findings demonstrate analgesic potential of verbal instructions. 6 references.

Blitz, B., Dinnerstein, A. J., and Lowenthal, M. 1966. Relationship between pain tolerance and kinesthetic size judgment, Perceptual and Motor Skills **22:**463-469.
An experiment showing that pain tolerance and kinesthetic size judgment (KSJ) are related. Subjects were tested in tasks, and subjects lower in pain tolerance made larger errors in KSJ than subjects higher in pain tolerance. 15 references.

Bobey, M. J., and Davidson, P. O. 1970. Psychological factors affecting pain tolerance, Journal of Psychosomatic Research **14:**371-376.
A study investigating the effects of three instructional tapes and a control tape on coping with pain. Instruction in relaxation proved to be most effective. 28 references.

Bowers, K. S. 1968. Pain, anxiety and perceived control, Journal of Consulting and Clinical Psychology **32:**596-602.
A study indicating that subjects who believe they have control over electric shock experience less anxiety and perceive shocks as less painful than subjects in a no-control condition. 17 references.

Bowers, K. S. 1971. The effects of UCS temporal uncertainty on heart rate and pain, Psychophysiology **8:**382-389.
A study in which subjects underwent shock trials under two conditions: in one they knew when the shock would be delivered, and in the other they were uncertain. Lower heart rates were observed in the uncertain condition. 12 references.

Chessick, R. C., Massan, M., and Shattan, S. 1966. A comparison of the effect of infused catecholamines and certain affect states, American Journal of Psychiatry **123:**156-165.
A study of the physiological effects of two drugs and a placebo in contrived situations of anxiety, pain, and anger. Results offer no clear pattern in correlation. 11 references.

Clark, W. C. 1969. Sensory-decision theory analysis of the placebo effect on the criterion for pain and thermal sensitivity, Journal of Abnormal Psychology **74:**363-371.
A study in which a placebo described as a powerful analgesic was administered to 22 subjects. The results indicated no change in pain sensitivity but a change in willingness to call the stimulation painful. 36 references.

Clark, W. C., and Mehl, L. 1971. Thermal pain: a sensory decision theory analysis of the effect of age and sex on *d'*, various response criteria, on *d'* 50% pain threshold, Journal of Abnormal Psychology **78:**202-212.
A study indicating that with thermal pain stimulation older subjects were less likely to label the stimulation painful. Older women also showed a drop in pain sensitivity. 27 references.

Craig, K. D., and Weiss, S. M. 1971. Vicarious influ-

ences on pain-threshold determinations, Journal of Personality and Social Psychology **19:**53-59.
An experimental study showing the social influence of a model on increasing pain tolerance to incremental elective shock. 22 references.

Feather, B. W., Chapman, C. R., and Fisher, S. B. 1972. The effect of a placebo on the perception of painful radiant heat stimuli, Psychosomatic Medicine **34:**290-294.
A laboratory study in which a placebo failed to affect sensitivity to thermal stimulation but significant decreases in willingness to report pain were observed. 9 references.

Greene, R. J., and Reyher, J. 1972. Pain tolerance in hypnotic analgesia and imagination states, Journal of Abnormal Psychology **79:**29-38.
A study investigating the use of hypnosis and pleasant imagery for increasing pain tolerances. Hypnotic analgesia conditions produced the highest tolerance increases. 46 references.

Haslam, D. R. 1966. Repetition effect in the determination of pain threshold, Journal of General Psychology **75:**297-303.
A study investigating "repetition effect." Findings support a psychological rather than physiological explanation for the phenomenon. 6 references.

Haslam, D. R. 1972. Field dependence in relation to pain threshold, British Journal of Psychology **63:**85-87.
An experiment in which a significant positive correlation was found between the amount by which a subject's pain threshold was lowered and the extent of his field dependence. 8 references.

Higgins, J. D., Tursky, B., and Schwartz, G. E. 1971. Shock-elicited pain and its reduction by oncurrent tactile stimulation, Science **172:**866-867.
A study in which human affective reactions to nociceptive electrical stimulation were attenuated by application of a tactile stimulus to the shocked site. Results support the Melzack-Wall gate control theory. 14 references.

Hill, H. E., Kornetsky, C. H., Flanary, H. G., and Wikler, A. 1952. Studies on anxiety associated with anticipation of pain. I. Effects of morphine, Archives of Neurology and Psychiatry **67:**612-619.
A study of the effects of morphine on the reaction time of former addicts. It was concluded that morphine reduces the disruptive effects on performance that are associated with anxiety produced by anticipation of pain. 10 references.

Jarvik, M. E., and Wolff, B. B. 1962. Differences between deep pain responses to hypertonic and hypotonic saline solutions. Journal of Applied Physiology **17:**841-843.
A study in which different concentrations of hypertonic and hypotonic saline solutions produced three significant differences in deep pain responses. 8 references.

Jones, A., Bentler, P. M., and Petry, G. 1966. The reduction of uncertainty concerning future pain, Journal of Abnormal Psychology **71:**87-94.
A study finding that providing information regarding timing and intensity of shocks was a strong positive reinforcement for most subjects. 6 references.

Kanfer, F. H., and Goldfoot, D. A. 1966. Self-control and tolerance of noxious stimulation, Psychological Reports **18:**79-85.
A study investigating the effects of several behaviors as potential self-controlling devices in the tolerance of a noxious stimulus. 7 references.

Lazarus, R. S., Opton, E. M., Nomikos, M. S., and Rankin, N. O. 1965. The principle of short-circuiting of threat: further evidence, Journal of Personality **33:**622-635.
An experimental study designed to illustrate reactions to a threatening film under three conditions intended to elicit (1) denial, (2) intellectualization, and (3) control. 11 references.

LeBlanc, J., and Potvin, P. 1966. Studies on habituation to cold pain, Canadian Journal of Physiology and Pharmacology **44:**287-293.
Studies indicating that adaption of one hand does not transfer to the other hand and that no adaption occurs if subjects are distracted from discomfort. Findings suggest the role of the central nervous system in adaption to cold pain and tend to minimize the importance of local peripheral changes. 6 references.

Lepanto, R., Moroney, W., and Zenhausern, R. 1965. The contribution of anxiety to the laboratory investigation of pain, Psychonomic Science **3:**475-476.
An attempt to introduce anxiety into the laboratory situation to study its effect on absolute pain thresholds in light of Beecher's belief that laboratory pain, since it usually involved no anxiety, was not comparable to clinical pain. No references.

Lerner, M. J., and Mathews G. 1967. Reactions to suffering of others under conditions of indirect responsibility, Journal of Personality and Social Psychology **5:**319-325.
A study in which subjects were led to believe that their partners in a learning task would receive strong shocks and that they were in a more desirable situation. The dependent measure was the subjects' rating of the partners. Significant differences in ratings were observed depending on the degree to which subjects felt responsible for partners' suffering. 6 references.

Levin, R. H., and McGuire, F. L. 1966. Electrical anesthesia. VI. Anesthesia and Analgesia **45:**222-225.
A study in which application of continuous subconvulsive electric current to the head as a means for inducing surgical analgesia provided an opportunity for measuring effects on intellectual functioning (memory and subjective verbal reports). No adverse effects were observed, and some degree of analgesia was obtained. 19 references.

Lewin, I. 1966. The effect of reward on the experience of pain, Dissertation Abstracts **27:**2122-2123.
An experiment that varied the amount of monetary reward for subjects undergoing shock. Results support the adaption level theory.

Lovallo, W. 1971. The cold pressor effect and models of homeostasis: a review and integration, unpublished manuscript, University of Oklahoma Health Center.
A review of literature on the cold pressor test and integration of known results in light of two models of homeostasis. 60 references.

Lovallo, W. Parsons, O. A., and Holloway, F. A. 1972. Autonomic arousal in normal, alcoholic, and brain-damaged subjects as measured by the plethysmograph response to cold pressor stimulation, un-

published manuscript, University of Oklahoma Health Center.
A study of the role of central factors in controlling autonomic arousal. Brain-damaged, alcoholic, and control subjects were tested for responsivity to the cold pressor test. 18 references.

Newton, A. V., and Mumford, J. M. 1972. Lateral dominance, pain perception, and pain tolerance, Journal of Dental Research **51:**940-942.
A study in which the suggestion that lateral dominance influences pain perception and pain tolerance was not substantiated when electric stimulation was applied to human teeth. 10 references.

Nisbett, R. E., and Schachter, S. 1966. Cognitive manipulation of pain, Journal of Experimental Social Psychology **2:**227-236.
A study in which subjects who were told that they had been given a drug that would cause arousal when, in fact, the drug was a placebo tolerated more shocks and tended to attribute arousal to the drug instead of the shock. 6 references.

Sadler, T. G., Mefferd, R. B., Wieland, B. A., Benton, R. G., and McDaniel, C. D. 1969. Physiological effects of combinations of painful and cognitive stimuli, Psychophysiology **5:**370-375.
A study that varied the order of presentation of a cognitive task and a cold pressor. Sympathetic activity was the dependent measure. Results indicate that competition between the task and cold pressor occurs at a level below that of cognition. 5 references.

Sadler, T. G., Wieland, B. A. Mefferd, R. B., Jr., Benton, R. G., and McDaniel, C. D. 1967. Modification in autonomically mediated physiological responses to cold pressor by cognitive activity: an extension, Psychophysiology **4:**229-230.
A study of the sympathetic nervous system response decrement when a cognitive task was imposed during a painful stimulus. The decrement was reproduced with 15 subjects under conditions involving minimal motor activity, supporting the conclusion that cognitive activity is the major determinant of the decrement. 1 reference.

Satran, R., and Goldstein, M. N. 1973. Pain perception: modification of threshold of intolerance and cortical potentials by cutaneous stimulation, Science **180:**1201-1202.
A study finding that cutaneous electrical stimulation temporarily raises the threshold of intolerance for pain elicited by electric shock. 5 references.

Smith, R., Keele, K. D., and Keele, C. A. 1967. Pain: its experimental investigation, Proceedings of the Royal Society of Medicine **60:**415-422.
Experimental findings and discussions of theoretical considerations for pain measurement by pressure and chemical means and their use in practice. 32 references.

Sternbach, R. 1964. The effects of instructional sets on autonomic responsivity, Psychophysiology **1:**67-72.
A study designed to determine whether instructional sets would influence the pattern of autonomic response. Instructions produced expected physiological responses in the majority of subjects. No references.

Strassberg, D. S., and Klinger, B. G. 1972. The effect on pain tolerance of social pressure within the laboratory setting, Journal of Social Psychology **88:**123-130.
A study examining the effects of group pressure, instruction, and the subject's sex on pain tolerance. Results indicate that these variables interact in a complex manner. 12 references.

Sweeney, D. R. 1966. Pain reactivity and kinesthetic aftereffect, Perceptual and Motor Skills **22:**763-769.
Results of a study substantiating a previously reported relationship between reaction to suprathreshold pain and kinesthetic aftereffect. 13 references.

Ulrich, R. 1967. Unconditioned and conditioned agression and its relation to pain, Activitas Nervosa Superior (Praha) **9:**80-92.
A consideration of various experiments in which pain and aggressive responses were studied in animals. Author generalizes to humans and discusses implications for research on human behavior. 48 references.

Walster, E., and Aronson, E. 1966. Choosing to suffer as a consequence of expecting to suffer: an unexpected finding, Journal of Experimental Social Psychology **2:**400-406.
A study in which subjects were allowed to shock themselves in private before being placed in one of three situations of which they were aware beforehand. It was found that subjects who knew they would be in an unpleasant situation gave themselves more shock than others. 2 references.

Wolff, B. B., and Harland, A. A. 1967. Effect of suggestion upon experimental pain: a validation study, Journal of Abnormal Psychology **72:**402-407.
An experimental study to investigate Gelfand's hypothesis that pain threshold and pain tolerance have different loadings of physiological and psychological components. The basic hypothesis was supported. 8 references.

Wolff, B. B., Krasnegor, N. A., and Farr, R. S. 1965. Effect of suggestion upon experimental pain response parameters, Perceptual and Motor Skills **21:**675-683.
An experimental study supporting Gelfand's hypothesis. Authors also found that the nondominant hand was more sensitive to pain. 13 references.

EFFECTS OF HYPNOSIS AND ACUPUNCTURE ON PAIN

Acupuncture

Bowsher, D., Mumford, J., Lipton S., and Miles, J. 1973. Treatment of intractable pain by acupuncture, Lancet **2:**57-60.
A series of 18 well-documented case reports of intractable pain that was resistant to orthodox procedures. The patients were treated by acupuncture and were relieved for varying periods. 16 references.

Chaves, J. F., and Barber, T. X. 1973. Acupuncture analgesia, Human Behavior **2:**19-24.
A skeptical analysis of the efficacy of acupuncture as an analgesic. Many of the same arguments that apply to hypnosis are used for acupuncture. 48 references.

Dimond, E. G. 1971. Acupuncture anesthesia—western medicine and Chinese traditional medicine, Journal of the American Medical Association **218:**1558-1563.

Case reports of surgery done in China with the patients under acupuncture analgesia. 3 references.

Hudson, N. C. 1972. Yesterday and today: dentistry in China, Journal of the American Dental Association **84:**985-993.
The history of dentistry in China and current practices, including acupuncture. 5 references.

Leung, S. J. 1973. Acupuncture treatment for pain syndrome. I. Treatment for sciatica, American Journal of Chinese Medicine **1:**317-326.
The use of acupuncture on 90 patients suffering from sciatica. It was found to be most effective in those cases caused by a herniated disc of the lumbar vertebrae.

Li, Choh-luh 1973. Neurological bases of pain and its possible relationship to acupuncture analgesia, American Journal of Chinese Medicine **1:**61-72.
A discussion of the theory and physiology of pain and its possible relationship to the mechanism of action of acupuncture. 83 references.

Mann, F. 1972. Acupuncture analgesia in dentistry, Lancet **1:**898-899.
Case studies of four dental patients treated under acupuncture analgesia. Results were good but not as complete as results with local anesthetics. No references.

Melzack, R. 1973. Stimulus/response—how acupuncture works, Psychology Today **7:**28-37.
A general description of acupuncture. Its potential in the United States is discussed, and it is compared with hypnosis. No references.

Van Nghi, N., Fisch, G., and Kao, J. 1973. An introduction to classical acupuncture, American Journal of Chinese Medicine **1:**75-83.
The classical concepts of acupuncture. A discussion of the organs of the body and the meridians is included. No references.

Clinical reports of hypnosis

Bartlett, E. F. 1971. Hypnoanesthesia for bilateral oophorectomy—a case report, The American Journal of Clinical Hypnosis **14:**122-130.
A detailed account of one case study. Hypnoanesthesia was used for surgery on a patient with terminal cancer. No references.

Crasilneck, H. B., Stirwan, J. A., Wilson, B. J., McCranie, E. J., and Fogelman, M. J. 1955. Use of hypnosis in the management of patients with burns, Journal of the American Medical Association **158:**103-106.
An account of hypnotic and posthypnotic suggestion successfully used as an anesthetic and analgesic for eight burn patients. Further implications are discussed. 8 references.

Dudley, D. L., Holmes, T. H., Martin, C. J., and Ripley, H. S.: 1966. Hypnotically induced facsimile of pain, Archives of General Psychiatry **15:**198-204.
An experimental study comparing reactions to noxious stimulation of the head and its hypnotically induced facsimile. No references.

Gilbert, A. S. 1967. Hypnotherapy and problems of pain, Proceedings of the Annual Clinical Spinal Cord Injury Conference **16:**105-107.
Techniques for inducing hypnosis and the use of posthypnotic suggestions for injured patients. No references.

Golan, H. P. 1971. Control of fear reaction in dental patients by hypnosis: three case reports, The American Journal of Clinical Hypnosis **13:**279-284.
Three case reports illustrating the use of hypnosis for overcoming fear in the dental situation. 4 references.

Hightower, P. R. 1966. The control of pain, American Journal of Clinical Hypnosis **9:**67-70.
Six case studies illustrating the use of hypnosis for controlling pain. No references.

Kaplan, E. A. 1960. Hypnosis and pain, Archives of General Psychiatry **2:**567-568.
A review of the use of hypnosis as an analgesia in light of an experiment in which pain is perceived despite hypnotic "anesthesia." Author suggests that hypnosis is ineffective and should not be used by physicians. 3 references.

Lauer, J. W. 1968. Hypnosis in the relief of pain, Medical Clinics of North America **52:**217-224.
A general discussion of hypnosis, including a historical perspective, emotional reactions to pain, and the hazards of hypnosis. 34 references.

Sacerdote, P. 1965-1966. The uses of hypnosis in cancer patients, Annals of the New York Academy of Sciences **125:**1011-1019.
A discussion of the uses of hypnosis and possible methods of evaluation. Obstacles and limitations are considered. 11 references.

Sacerdote, P. 1970. Theory and practice of pain control in malignancy and other protracted or recurring painful illnesses, International Journal of Clinical and Experimental Hypnosis **18:**160-180.
Methods for hypnotic alteration of pain. Case presentations illustrate multiple psychological and physiological approaches to pain control through the use of hypnosis. 28 references.

Zane, M. D. 1966. The hypnotic situation and changes in ulcer pain, International Journal of Clinical and Experimental Hypnosis **14:**292-304.
A detailed account of the treatment by hypnosis of a patient with a duodenal ulcer. 19 references.

Experimental studies of hypnosis

Barber, T. X. 1959. Toward a theory of pain: relief of chronic pain by prefrontal leucotomy, opiates, placebos, and hypnosis, Psychological Bulletin **56:**430-460.
A discussion of the neurological correlates of the pain response and how this response or some components of it can be mitigated or eliminated by prefrontal leucotomy, opiates, placebos, and hypnosis. 174 references.

Barber, T. X. 1963. The effects of "hypnosis" on pain, Psychosomatic Medicine **25:**303-333.
A critical evaluation of experimental and clinical studies concerned with the effects of hypnotically induced analgesia. Author suggests that the hypnotic trance state is an extraneous variable in ameliorating pain experience in situations described as hypnosis. 152 references.

Barber, T. X., and Hahn, K. W., Jr. 1962. Physiological and subjective responses to pain-producing stimulation and hypnotically suggested and waking-imagined "analgesia," Journal of Abnormal and Social Psychology **65:**411-418.
An experimental study to determine if hypnotically suggested analgesia is more effective than "waking-imagined analgesia" in attentuating subjective and

physiological responses to a stimulus eliciting pain over a longer duration than stimuli used in previous studies. 33 references.

Black, S. 1968. Effects of emotion and pain on adreno-cortical function investigated by hypnosis, British Medical Journal **1:**477-481.
An investigation by hypnosis of the effects of emotion and pain on plasma cortisol levels in eight deep-trance hypnotic subjects. 16 references.

Chaves, J. F. 1968. Hypnosis reconceptualized: an overview of Barber's theoretical and empirical work, Psychological Reports **22:**587-608.
A summary and clarification of Barber's theory of hypnosis, which differs from the traditional "special state of consciousness" paradigm. Criticisms of Barber's work are discussed and evaluated. 64 references.

Dudley, D. L., and others. 1966. Hypnotically induced facsimile of pain, Archives of General Psychiatry **15:**198-204.
A report of hypnotic suggestion used in a group of ten male subjects to reproduce an actual stimulus with its emotional and physiological components. 9 references.

Evans, M. B., and Paul, G. L. 1970. Effects of hypnotically suggested analgesia on physiological and subjective responses to cold stress, Journal of Consulting and Clinical Psychology **35:**362-371.
An experimental study in which suggestion rather than hypnotic induction produced reductions in the self-report of distress. The degree of reduction was related to hypnotic susceptibility. 37 references.

Greene, R. J., and Reyher, J. 1972. Pain tolerance in hypnotic analgesic and imagination states, Journal of Abnormal Psychology **1:**29-38.
An experimental investigation of the effects of hypnotically suggested analgesia and pleasant imagery. Results indicate the effectiveness of analgesia and a mixed result for imagery. 45 references.

Hilgard, E. R. 1967. A quantitative study of pain and its reduction through hypnotic suggestion, Proceedings of the National Academy of Science of the United States of America **57:**1581-1586.
An experimental study that supports the hypothesis that hypnosis can reduce laboratory pain as well as clinical pain. 8 references.

Hilgard, E. R. 1969. Pain as a puzzle for psychology and physiology, American Psychologist **24:**103-113.
A consideration of pain reduction techniques through hypnosis and of the effects of pain on blood pressure. 41 references.

Hilgard, E. R. 1971. Pain: its reduction and production under hypnosis, Proceedings of the American Philosophical Society **115:**470-476.
A summary of several of the author's experiments on pain. Emphasis is on the study of hypnosis; a rigorous scientific design is used. 2 references.

Hilgard, E. R., Cooper, L. M., Lenox, J., Morgan, A. H., and Voesodsky, J. 1967. The use of pain-state reports in the study of hypnotic analgesia to the pain of ice water, The Journal of Nervous and Mental Disease **144:**506-513.
An experimental study in which subjects of high and low hypnotic susceptibility were subjected to ice water stress. Several conclusions regarding hypnotic analgesia are drawn from the reseearch. 20 references.

Kehoe, J. 1971. Pain and gastric acid secretion, Journal of Psychosomatic Research **15:**47-53.
A study of the effect of spontaneous experiences of pain on gastric secretion in 9 subjects. Hypnosis was used to evoke depressive responses. 9 references.

Lenox, J. R. 1970. Effect of hypnotic analgesia on verbal report and cardiovascular responses to ischemic pain, Journal of Abnormal Psychology **75:**199-206.
An experimental study in which it was shown that hypnotic analgesia effectively reduced reported pain of ischemia along with heart rate and systolic blood pressure. 13 references.

London, R., and McDevitt, R. A. 1970. Effects of hypnotic susceptibility and training on responses to stress, Journal of Abnormal Psychology **76:**336-348.
An experimental study in which 32 subjects with a high susceptibility to hypnosis and 32 subjects with a low susceptibility were exposed to shock and cold stress treatments. Significant differences were observed after half the subjects in each group were trained in autohypnosis. 38 references.

McGlashan, T. H., Evans, F. J., and Orne, M. T. 1969. The nature of hypnotic analgesia and placebo response to experimental pain, Psychosomatic Medicine **31:**227-246.
A theoretical review and experimental study of the effects of hypnotically induced analgesia and placebo response to an analgesic drug. Both subjects with high susceptibilities to hypnosis and those with low ones were used. 38 references.

Sachs, L. B. 1970. Comparison of hypnotic analgesia and hypnotic relaxation during stimulation by a continuous pain source, Journal of Abnormal Psychology **76:**206-210.
A comparison of the reactions of five subjects to ice water immersion under hypnotic-relaxed and hypnotic-analgesic states. Physiological measures concurred with subjective reports of pain. 8 references.

Spanos, N. P., and Chaves, J. F. 1970. Hypnosis research: a methodological critique of experiments generated by two alternative paradigms, American Journal of Clinical Hypnosis **13:**108-127.
A theoretical comparison of the hypnotic state or trance paradigm with the alternative that rejects this view. Three criteria for evaluating experiments in this area are presented. 78 references.

SURGICAL INTERVENTION TO RELIEVE PAIN

Adams, J. E. 1961. The future of stereotaxic surgery, Journal of the American Medical Association **198:**180-184.
A discussion of movement disorders, pain control, and convulsive states in relation to stereotaxic surgery. 19 references.

Albe-Fessard, D., Dondey, M., Nicolaidis, S., and LeBeau, J. 1970. Remarks concerning the effect of diencephalic lesions on pain and sensitivity with special reference to lemniscally mediated control of noxious afferences, Confinia Neurologica **32:**174-184.
An account of discriminative sensory loss observed in ten patients who underwent posterior subthalamotomy. Authors hypothesize the cause of the losses. 20 references.

Burton, C. 1972. Neurosurgical treatment of intractable pain, Pennsylvania Medicine **75:**53-55.
A review of surgical techniques used in the past to alleviate pain and a description of newer techniques: percutaneous cordotomy, dorsal column stimulation, and telethermocoagulation. 9 references.

Cooper, I. S. 1965. Clinical and physiologic implications of thalamic surgery for disorders of sensory communication. I. Thalamic surgery for intractable pain, Journal of the Neurological Sciences **2:**493-519.
A comprehensive review of studies of thalamic surgery to relieve pain plus a discussion of the implications of this type of procedure. 35 references.

Faillace, L. A., Allen, R. P., McQueen, J. D., and Northrup, B. 1971. Cognitive deficits from bilateral cingulotomy for intractable pain in man, Diseases of the Nervous System **18:**171-175.
Results of psychological tests performed preoperatively and postoperatively on nine patients who underwent bilateral stereotaxic cingulotomy for relief of intractable pain. Small behavioral changes were noted. 9 references.

Fairman, D. 1967. Unilateral thalamic tractotomy for the relief of bilateral pain in malignant tumors, Confinia Neurologica **29:**146-152.
An account of satisfactory pain relief obtained for 80% of patients who had a unilateral thalamic tractotomy. It lasted between 2 and 12 months, the length of patient survival. 6 references.

Fedio, P., and Ayub, K. 1970. Bilateral cingulum lesions and stimulation in man with lateralized impairment in short-term verbal memory. Experimental Neurology **29:**84-91.
Result of examinations of patients undergoing bilateral cingulumotomy for relief of pain. Severe impairment in recall for verbal memoranda accompanied left, but not right, cingulum stimulation. 27 references.

Foltz, E. L., and White, L. E. 1968. The role of rostral cingulumotomy in pain relief. International Journal of Neurology **6:**353-373.
A discussion of the technique and effects of rostral cingulumotomy for alleviating symptoms of 35 patients with psychogenic or organic pain accompanied by strong emotional factors. 32 references.

Fox, J. L. 1971. Recent advances in neurological surgery, Medical Annals of the District of Columbia **40:**88-91.
A general discussion of recent advances in the field with regard to relief of pain, control of intracranial pressure, diagnostic advances, and operative care. 15 references.

Gildenberg, P. L. 1972. Stereotaxic lower cervical cordotomy for the treatment of intractable pain, Confinia Neurologica **34:**275-278.
A technique for introducing a needle electrode into the spinal cord to interrupt pain pathways of the spinothalamic tract. No references.

Gol, A. 1967. Relief of pain by electrical stimulation of the septal area, Journal of the Neurological Sciences **5:**115-120.
An investigation of the effect of deep cerebral stimulation in six cases of severe pain caused by terminal carcinomatosis. Author found a low probability of achieving success with this method. 11 references.

Gol, A., and Faibish, G. M. 1967. Effects of human hippocampal ablation, Journal of Neurosurgery **26:**390-398.
Seven case studies where hippocampectomy was performed to alleviate intractable pain. Pain relief was satisfactory temporarily, but intellectual and affective functions were disturbed. 9 references.

Hosobuchi, Y., Adams, J. E., and Weinstein, P. R. 1972. Preliminary percutaneous dorsal column stimulation prior to permanent implantation, Journal of Neurosurgery **37:**242-245.
An account of percutaneous dorsal column stimulation performed prior to implantation of a dorsal column stimulator. It provided useful information to both doctor and patient by forecasting tolerance to vibratory sensation and efficacy of the device in relieving pain. 12 references.

Kandel, E., and Chebotaryova, N. M. 1972. Conray ventriculography in stereotaxic surgery experience with 320 operations, Confinia Neurologica **34:**34-40.
The use of Conray in ventriculography. It seems to provide clearer visibility than injection of air and produces fewer side effects. 16 references.

Leskell, L., Meyerson, B. A., and Forster, D. M. C. 1972. Radiosurgical thalamotomy for intractable pain, Confinia Neurologica **34:**264.
The technique of treating chronic pain by a bloodless surgical intervention in the centrum medianum and parafasciculus complex. No references.

Moffie, D. 1971. Late results of bulbar trigeminal tractotomy—some remarks on recovery of sensibility, Journal of Neurology, Neurosurgery and Psychiatry **34:**270-274.
A study of 8 patients in whom bulbar trigeminal tractotomy had been performed 13 to 15 years previously. Four had no complaints about pain and the other 4 had only minor complaints. 21 references.

Morgan, M., and Robson, J. G. 1972. A step towards the more rational treatment of chronic pain by nerve block, British Journal of Anaesthesia **44:**893-894.
The rationale for a case in which nerve block distal to the site of the lesion produced relief of pain. 3 references.

Nashold, B. S., Jr., and Wilson, W. P. 1966. Central pain: observation in man with chronic implanted electrodes in the midbrain tegmentum. Confinia Neurologica **27:**30-44.
A single case study of a woman treated for facial pain following subarachnoid hemorrhage. 17 references.

Onofrio, B. M., and Campa, K. 1972. Evaluation of rhizotomy review of 12 years experience, Journal of Neurosurgery **36:**751-755.
An evaluation of 286 Mayo Clinic patients who had dorsal rhizotomies for pain. Overall long-term success rates were low. 10 references.

Richardson, D. E. 1967. Thalamotomy for intractable pain, Confinia Neurologica **29:**139-145.
A discussion of 45 operations (on 38 patients) that were carried out utilizing stereotaxic methods to destroy portions of the posterior thalamus to control intractable pain. Temporary results were good; long-lasting results were more difficult to achieve. 14 references.

Sheldon, C. H., Pudenz, R. H., and Bullara, L. 1972. Development and clinical capabilities of a new im-

plantable biostimulator, American Journal of Surgery **124:**212-217.
An explanation and discussion of the use of implantable electronic units with particular reference to electronic control of pain secondary to malignant disease. 9 references.

Spangfort, E. V. 1972. The lumbar disc herniation, a computer aided analysis, Acta Orthopaedica Scandinavica **142:**1-95.
A comprehensive consideration of past research, characteristics of patients, radiological and surgical techniques, and results of surgery. 191 references.

Sugita, K., Mutsuga, N., Takaoka, Y., and Doi, T. 1972. Results of stereotaxic thalamotomy for pain, Confinia Neurologica **34:**265-274.
A study of nine patients in whom stereotaxic thalamotomy was effective in relieving pain. 9 references.

Sweet, W. H., and Wepsic, J. G. 1970. Relation of fiber size in trigeminal posterior root to conduction of impulses for pain and touch; production of analgesia without anesthesia in the effective treatment of trigeminal neuralgia, Transactions of the American Neurological Association **95:**134-139.
A study indicating that no A-alpha or beta group fibers exist for noxious stimuli in the human trigeminal posterior root. When many of these are destroyed, the quality of the residual touch sensation is only modestly impaired. No references.

Tsubokawa, T. 1967. The correlation of pain relief, neurological sign, EEG and anatomical lesion sites in pain patients treated by stereotaxic thalamotomy, Folia Psychiatrica et Neurologica Japonica **21:**41-50.
A description of clinical syndromes on the basis of anatomical correlations in nine patients who had stereotaxic thalomotomies for the relief of intractable pain. 14 references.

Udvarhelyi, G. B., and Aronson, N. I. 1969. Pain and motor disorders, Progress in Neurology and Psychiatry **24:**332-368.
A comprehensive review of research and literature dealing with various types of pain and motor disorders and the effectiveness of treatments. 147 references.

CLINICAL STUDIES OF PAIN

Abdominal and gastrointestinal pain

Abatso, G. W. 1972. Should the asymptomatic patient have surgery? Illinois Medical Journal **142:**131-133.
A review of 1,530 appendectomies. Ten percent of those patients admitted with symptoms and 54% of those without symptoms had normal appendices. 11 references.

Bockus, H. L. 1968. Abdominal pain—mechanisms and philosophic concepts, Lahey Clinic Foundation Bulletin **17:**77-88.
The clinical, theoretical, and philosophical implications of the pain experience with special reference to abdominal pain. 2 references.

Davies, R. J. 1972. Dysphagia, abdominal pain and sarcoid granulomata, British Medical Journal **3:**564-565.
A case study of a patient with severe abdominal sarcoid granulomata that were found in both the esophagus and the abdominal lymph nodes. 8 references.

Dilawari, J. B., Blendis, L. M., and Edwards, D. A. W. 1973. The epigastric pain in duodenal ulcer, Gut **14:**422.
A study in which perfusion of the lower esophagus with acid reproduced the central epigastric pain in only a minority of patients with duodenal ulcer. 2 references.

Dugan, R. E. 1972. Familial rectal pain, Lancet **1:**854.
The rectal pain syndrome and its genetic pattern. No references.

Earlam, R. J. 1972. Further experience with epigastric pain reproduction test in duodenal ulceration, British Medical Journal **2:**683-685.
Experimental evidence that epigastric pain of duodenal ulceration arises from the lower esophagus. 4 references.

Hislop, I. G. 1971. Psychological significance of the irritable colon syndrome, Gut **12:**452-457.
A study of 67 patients with the irritable colon syndrome. The symptom complex is considered to be a concomitant of an affective disorder. Possible psychological origins are discussed. Eighty percent of 56 patients treated with antidepressant therapy reported improvement. 30 references.

Howell, T. H. 1972. Abdominal-wall pain of bony origin: two clinical entities in geriatric patients, Journal of the American Geriatric Society **20:**312-313.
Two clinical entities of pain in the anterior abdominal wall. Author warns against mistaking the pain for a symptom of acute or chronic intraabdominal disease. 3 references.

Jurko, M. F., and Andy, O. J. 1966. Gastrointestinal pain and electroencephalographic abnormality in adults, International Journal of Neuropsychiatry, **2:**212-215.
A study in which EEG's were performed on 31 male veterans with a history of gastrointestinal pain. The incidence of EEG abnormality was over twice that found in the normal adult population. It is suggested that cerebral pathophysiology is operative in the gastrointestinal symptoms of certain types of subjects. 13 references.

Kajtor, F., and Kaszas, T. 1966. Epileptiform EEG changes in the syndrome of periodic abdominal pain, Acta Medica Academiae Scientiarum Hungaricae Tomus **22:**309-324.
A study of EEG recordings made in the waking state and during hexobarbital anesthesia of 38 children with abdominal pain. In 31% of the cases the findings suggested the possibility of an epileptogenic brain lesion. 27 references.

Mann, T. P., and Cree, J. E. 1972. Familial rectal pain, Lancet **1:**1016-1017.
A description of a syndrome that appears to be hereditary. Authors believe, however, that it is not etiologically related to proctalgia fugax.

Mazier, W. P. 1971. The treatment and care of anal fistulas: a study of 1,000 patients, Diseases of the Colon and Rectum **14:**134-144.
A discussion of symptoms, diagnosis, and treatments in reference to 1,000 patients treated for anal fistulas at the Ferguson Clinic. 9 references.

Papatheophilou, R., Jeavons, P. M., and Disney, M. E. 1972. Recurrent abdominal pain: a clinical and electroenciphalographic study, Developmental Medicine and Child Neurology **14:**31-44.
Results of a study of 50 patients with recurrent abdominal pain. EEG studies indicate that the syn-

drome appears to be an epileptic phenomenon in only a small proportion of cases. 34 references.

Pilling, L. F., Swenson, W. M., Hill, J. R. 1967. The psychologic aspects of proctalgia fugax, Canadian Medical Association Journal **97**:387-394.
A psychiatric study of 48 patients with proctalgia fugax to determine whether psychological factors were important in causing the disorder. Literature on the topic is reviewed. 31 references.

Rang, E. H., Fairbairn, A. S., and Acheson, E. D. 1970. An inquiry into the incidence and prognosis of undiagnosed abdominal pain treated in hospital, British Journal of Preventive Social Medicine **24**:47-51.
An investigation into the incidence and prognosis of unexplained abdominal pain causing admission to a hospital. In females, there was a high incidence in the younger age groups, with a steady decline thereafter; but in males, the trend was reversed. 6 references.

Ritchie, J. A., Ardan, G. M., and Truelove, S. C. 1972. Observations on experimentally induced colonic pain **13**:841.
A study of patients with diverticular disease or irritable colon syndrome. They were liable to develop pain at much lower levels of inflation of a balloon in the pelvic colon than were normal subjects. No references.

Siegler, J. 1972. Isotope renography in the diagnosis of recurrent abdominal pain of children, Acta Paediatrica Academiae Scientiarun Hungaricae **13**:57-62.
A study of isotope renography for the diagnosis of recurrent abdominal pain in 45 children. The procedure was of diagnostic use both in cases of suspected nephrological disease and in cases where routing examination failed to reveal the cause of complaints. 6 references.

Stone, R. L., and Barbero, G. J. 1970. Recurrent abdominal pain in childhood, Pediatrics **45**:732-738.
A study and follow-up through hospitalization of 102 children with recurrent abdominal pain. The syndrome is described as the irritable bowel syndrome in childhood. 10 references.

Thiele, G. H. 1972. Anorectal pain, American Family Physician **6**:54-62.
A description of several types of anorectal pain symptoms. Diagnosis and treatment are presented. No references.

Arthritis, rheumatism, bone and joint dysfunction

Currey, H. L. F. 1970. Osteoarthrosis of the hip joint and sexual activity, Annals of the Rheumatic Diseases **29**:488-493.
An analysis of a questionnaire sent to 235 patients, aged 60 years or less, who had undergone surgery for osteoarthritis of the hip. Results indicate that two thirds of the patients had sexual difficulties caused by arthritis. 2 references.

Frost, H. M. 1972. Managing the skeletal pain and disability of osteoporosis, Orthopedic Clinics of North America **3**:561-570.
A discussion of the causes and treatment of osteoporosis. Author concludes that in almost all cases the pain of osteoporosis is self-limiting. 13 references.

Hart, F. D., and Huskisson, E. C. 1972. Pain patterns in the rheumatic disorders. British Medical Journal **4**:213-216.
A discussion of several rheumatic disorders and suggestions for physical, psychological, and pharmacological therapy. 17 references.

Hart, F. D., Taylor, R. T., and Huskisson, E. C. 1970. Pain at night, Lancet **1**:881-884.
A discussion of pain and stiffness at night caused by chronic rheumatoid disorders. Measures for alleviating such pain are considered. 31 references.

Hazleman, B. L. 1972. The painful stiff shoulder, Rheumatology and Physical Medicine **11**:413-421.
An assessment of three types of treatment for the painful stiff shoulder. Little difference among treatments was observed. 23 references.

Huskisson, E. C., and Hart, F. D. 1972. Pain threshold and arthritis, British Medical Journal **4**:193-195.
A study of pain threshold in 50 patients with ankylosing spondylitis and in 50 normal patients. There was no evidence that pain threshold affected the cause or outcome of rheumatoid arthritis in any way. 16 references.

McCarroll, H. R., Priest, W. S., Compere, E. L., Beattie, E. J., and Bucy, P. C. 1964. Neck, shoulder and arm pain, Postgraduate Medicine **36**:385-399.
A discussion of the relationship between arm pain and coronary disorders, and other causes of neck, shoulder, and arm pain. No references.

Macnab, I. 1969. Pain and disability in degenerative disc disease, Texas Medicine **65**:56-63.
A consideration of the relationship between the amount of pain perceived and the anatomical disc degeneration. Surgical and pharmacological treatments are discussed. 3 references.

Opio, E., and Barnes, P. M. 1972. Intravenous urea in treatment of bone-pain crises of sickle-cell disease: a double-blind trial, Lancet **2**:160-162.
In a double-blind trial of 23 episodes of bone pain in 19 patients with sickle-cell disease, a 16% solution of intravenous urea in 10% invert sugar was not found to be successful. 9 references.

Reynolds, G. G., Pavot, A. P., and Kenrick, M. M. 1968. Electromyographic evaluation of patients with posttramatic cervical pain, Archives of Physical Medicine **49**:170-172.
An evaluation of 17 patients with pain in the neck region following an automobile accident. Authors hypothesize that injury to nerve roots is the cause of pain. 5 references.

Robinson, H., Kirk, R.. F., Frye, R. F., and Robertson, J. T. 1972. A psychological study of patients with rheumatoid arthritis and other painful diseases, Journal of Psychosomatic Research **16**:53-56.
A correlational study supporting the hypothesis that rheumatoid arthritis is a condition in which the personality dynamics of the patient are a factor in the onset and progression of the disease. 5 references.

Sheldon, P. J. H. 1972. Retrospective survey of 102 cases of shoulder pain, Rheumatology and Physical Medicine **11**:422-427.
A retrospective study of 102 patients with shoulder pain. Sex, obesity, diabetes, and carcinoma are important factors. 3 references.

White, J. R., and Sage, J. N. 1971. Effects of counterirritant on muscular distress in patients with arthritis, Physical Therapy **51**:36-42.
A study in which 30 patients with osteoarthritis or rheumatoid arthritis were tested electromyographically and subjectively regarding pain in joints and surrounding muscles after either a topical anal-

gesic or placebo was applied. The placebo was found to be ineffective in reducing muscle action potential. 17 references.

Behavioral and nursing intervention

Baer, E., Davitz, L. J., and Lieb, R. 1970. Inferences of physical pain and psychological distress. I. In relation to verbal and nonverbal patient communication, Nursing Research **19:**388-392.
A study assessing the inferences of physical pain and psychological distress in relation to verbal and nonverbal patient communication. No references.

Billars, K. S. 1970. You have pain? I think this will help, American Journal of Nursing **70:**2143-2145.
A study evaluating the effectiveness of the suggestion of pain relief in reducing patients' pain. 10 references.

Cashatt, B. 1972. Pain: a patient's view, American Journal of Nursing **72:**281.
An account of a nurse's own pain experience from the patient's side. No references.

Copple, D. 1972. What can a nurse do to relieve pain without resort to drugs? Nursing Times **68:**584.
Specific suggestions for relieving patient anxiety, improving general physical comfort, and relieving specific pains. 1 reference.

Fordyce, W. E. 1970. Operant conditioning as a treatment method in management of selected chronic pain problems, Northwest Medicine **69:**580-581.
A brief overview of the application of operant conditioning methods to certain problems of chronic clinical pain. 6 references.

Fordyce, W. E., Fowler, R. S., Lehmann, J. F., and DeLateur, B. J. 1968. Some implications of learning in problems of chronic pain, Journal of Chronic Diseases **21:**179-190.
A behavior modification approach to chronic pain and its comparison with a medical model. The behavioral model is applied to situations of chronic pain. 8 references.

Hackett, T. P. 1971. Pain and prejudice—why do we doubt that the patient is in pain? Medical Times **99:** 130-141.
Several prejudices and various medical attitudes toward patients in pain, including narcotic addiction and the use of placebos. No references.

Lenburg, C. B., Burnside, H., and Davitz, L. J. 1970. Inferences of physical pain and psychological distress. III. In relation to length of time in the nursing education program, Nursing Research **19:**399-401.
A study evaluating levels of educational experience in nursing as related to inferences of physical pain and psychological distress of hospitalized patients. 9 references.

Lenburg, C. B., Glass, H. P., and Davitz, L. J. 1970. Inferences of physical pain and psychological distress. II. In relation to the stage of the patient's illness and occupation of the perceiver, Nursing Research **19:**392-398.
A study on how four different occupational groups view pain and psychological distress in patients. No references.

McCaffery, M., and Moss, F. 1967. Nursing intervention for bodily pain, American Journal of Nursing **67:**1224-1227.
A discussion of three factors that nurses can use to help alleviate the patient's pain. 16 references.

Swerdlow, M. 1972. The pain clinic, British Journal of Clinical Practice **26:**403-407.
A discussion of a pain clinic and how it operates. 6 references.

Vernon, D. T., Schulman, J. L., and Foley, J. M. 1966. Changes in children's behavior after hospitalization, American Journal of the Diseases of Children **111:** 581-593.
A study in which changes in behavior of 387 children after hospitalization were assessed through a questionnaire sent to the parents. Factor analysis revealed 6 distinct types of behavioral changes. 24 references.

Villegas, E. L. 1967. Placebo reaction—the effect of the nurse-patient communication process on patient attitude to pain, The Anphi Papers, The Academy of Nursing of the Philippines **2:**12-23.
A discussion of literature plus a study investigating the effects of the relationship between nurse and patient on the placebo phenomenon. 27 references.

Webb, C. 1966. Tactics to reduce a child's fear of pain, American Journal of Nursing **66:**2698-2701.
Practical suggestions for management of the child in pain. No references.

Cancer

Berry, C. L., and Keeling, J. W. 1970. Gastrointestinal lymphoma in childhood, Journal of Clinical Pathology **23:**459-463.
Thirteen case studies of lymphoma of the bowel in infancy and childhood. 11 references.

Bond, M. R., and Pearson, I. B. 1969. Psychological aspects of pain in women with advanced cancer of the cervix, Journal of Psychosomatic Research **13:** 13-19.
A clinical study comparing patients experiencing pain with patients free of pain. Personality factors, methods of communicating pain, and pain thresholds are considered. 18 references.

Cole, R. 1965. The problem of pain in persistent cancer, The Medical Journal of Australia **1:**682-686.
A discussion of persistent pain in cancer with regard to patient management at a pain clinic. Various treatments are evaluated, and suggestions for supportive therapy are offered. 22 references.

Dickey, R. P., and Minton, J. P. 1972. Levodopa relief of bone pain from breast cancer, New England Journal of Medicine **286:**843.
Two case studies in which L-dopa was used as an alternative to steroid therapy for hormone-sensitive breast cancer. 3 references.

Frankendal, B., and Kjellgren, O. 1971. Severe pain in gynecologic cancer, Cancer **27:**842-847.
A clinical study comparing the effectiveness of pentazocine morphine and a placebo in treating severe pain of gynecological cancer. 19 references.

Lewis, J. L. 1969. Palliative therapy of advanced ovarian cancer, Clinical Obstetrics and Gynecology **12:** 1038-1049.
A discussion of clinical mangement of patients whose ovarian cancer has recurred or persisted following initial therapy. 6 references.

Mathews, G. J., Zarro, V., and Osterholm, J. L. 1973. Cancer pain and its treatment, Seminars in Drug Treatment **3:**45-53.
A consideration of the stages of progressive cancer and appropriate use of analgesics at each stage.

Stress is placed on the need for sensitivity to the patient's feelings and state of mind. 28 references.

Montgomery, W., and Cousins, M. J. 1972. Aspects of the management of chronic pain illustrated by the ninth nerve block, British Hournal of Anaesthesiology **44:**383-385.
An account of a glossopharyngeal nerve block used to relieve severe pain of oropharyngeal carcinoma. Management of pain caused by malignancy is discussed. 3 references.

Moore, C. H. 1966. Management of pain in cancer with special reference to pain caused by pelvic malignancy, Texas Reports on Biology and Medicine **24:**34-45.
A consideration of physiological causes of pain and methods of alleviating painful complications of cancer. 44 references.

Robbie, D. S. 1969. General management of intractable pain in advanced carcinoma of rectum, Proceedings of the Royal Society of Medicine **62:**1225.
A short discussion of the physical and psychological techniques for managing the terminal patient. No references.

Skutsch, G. M. 1972. Prolactin and breast cancer, Lancet **2:**1258.
A letter discussing the causal role of prolactin and the suppressor role of progesterone in the pain of cancer. No references.

Turnbull, F. 1971. Pain and suffering in cancer, The Canadian Nurse **67:**28-30.
A discussion of pain caused by various types of cancer and techniques for the management of pain in nine specific syndromes. 4 references.

Dentistry

American Dental Association, Council on Dental Education, 1972. Guidelines for the teaching of pain and anxiety control in dentistry, Journal of Dental Education **36:**62-67.
An outline of objectives, course content, course length, faculty, and facilities for teaching pain control. No references.

Anderson, D. J. 1972. Human and animal studies on sensory mechanisms in teeth, International Dental Journal **22:**33-38.
A discussion of sensations arising in both the dentine and pulp and problems in recording and interpreting electrical activity of dental nerves in response to stimulation. 9 references.

Baldwin, D. C., Jr. 1966. An investigation of psychological and behavioral responses to dental extraction in children, Journal of Dental Research **45:**1637-1651.
A clinical experiment to study the psychological and behavioral responses of children to the stress of dental extraction. 12 references.

Banasik, M. P., and Lasken, D. M. 1972. Production of masticatory muscle spasm and secondary tooth movement: an experimental model for MPD syndrome, Journal of Oral Surgery **30:**491-498.
An experimental study to produce masticatory muscle contraction in animals. Two changes occurred: (1) muscular spasm and (2) tooth movement. Findings support the premise that chronic masticatory activity can lead to the development of MPD syndrome. 16 references.

Brännström, M., and Aström, A. 1972. The hydrodynamics of the dentine: its possible relationship to dentinal pain, International Dental Journal **22:**219-227.
A study supporting the hypothesis that a hydrodynamic factor is responsible for the transmission of pain stimuli from the dentine surface to the nerve endings in the pulpodentinal area or the pulp, or both. 18 references.

Budzynski, T., and Stoyva, J. 1973. An electromyographic feedback technique for teaching voluntary relaxation of the masseter muscle, Journal of Dental Research **52:**116-119.
A technique for muscle relaxation, using auditory or visual electromyographic feedback. Experimental results are included. 7 references.

Chambiras, P. G. 1970. Sedation in dentistry: some pharmacological aspects of pain control, Australian Dental Journal **45:**294-298.
The hypothesis that consciousness is the consequence of the interaction and integration of two distinct neural mechanisms: perception and conceptualization. Several drugs are discussed in relationship to their effects on these mechanisms. 25 references.

Chasens, A. I. 1972. Facial pain. I. Journal of Oral Medicine **27:**43-48.
A review and classification of many conditions that produce facial pain. Differentiation of pain of dental origin from pain of other sources is emphasized. 8 references.

Chasens, A. I. 1972. Facial pain. II. Facial pain with dysfunction, Journal of Oral Medicine **27:**59-63.
Diagnosis and management of facial pain associated with dysfunction. Classification and descriptions of various conditions are presented to aid in differentiating pain of dental origin from pain referred from other areas. 19 references.

Christensen, L. V. 1971. Facial pain and internal pressure of masseter muscle in experimental bruxism in man. Archives of Oral Biology **16:**1021-1031.
A study in which 9 subjects performed right-sided bruxism for 30 minutes to assess whether unaccustomed exercise could induce pain in the masseter muscle. This pain occurred in 8 subjects, and it is suggested that such pain is a result of excess interstitial fluid in the muscle tissue. 21 references.

Dachi, S. F., and Stein, L. F. 1968. Diagnosis and management of orofacial pain of emotional origin, Journal of Oral Surgery **26:**345-348.
A discussion on recognizing clinical characteristics of facial pain and the barriers to therapeutic management of such patients. No references.

DeLeon, E. L. 1968. Facial pain of non-odontogenic origin, Journal of Oral Medicine **23:**119-131.
An article stressing the need to evaluate all possibilities in each case of facial pain. The primary role of the dentist in seeing a patient with facial pain is to systematically rule out oral structures as possible causes. 55 references.

Donaldson, K. I. 1967. Pain: the chief complaint, Australian Dental Journal **12:**9-11.
A general discussion of the nature of pain and the management of the patient with pain as a major symptom. 16 references.

Dworkin, S. F. 1967. Anxiety and performance in the dental environment: an experimental investigation, Journal of the American Society of Psychosomatic Dentistry and Medicine **14:**88-103.
An experimental study testing the hypothesis that

behavior in the dental situation is a function of the patient's predisposition to anxiety arousal when certain oral manipulations are contemplated. 14 references.

Elfenbaum, A. 1972. Defiant denture pain in older patients, Dental Digest **78:**254-257.
A discussion of several possible causes of toothaches that are difficult to diagnose in older patients with dentures. No references.

Evaskus, D. S. and Laskin, D. M. 1972. A biochemical measure of stress in patients with myofacial pain-dysfunction syndrome, Journal of Dental Research **51:**1464-1466.
A study in which physiological measures indicated that patients with MPD syndrome are under greater emotional stress than control individuals. These findings support the psychophysiological theory of the etiology of this syndrome. 18 references.

Friedman, A., and Carton, C. A. 1960. Facial pain, Transactions of the American Academy of Ophthalmology and Otolaryngology **64:**713-719.
A discussion of three categories of facial pain: (1) typical neuralgias, (2) atypical neuralgias, and (3) facial pain secondary to other causes, Management and treatments are considered. 4 references.

Gelb, H., Calderone, J. P., Gross, S. M., and Kantor, M. E. 1967. The role of the dentist and the otolaryngologist in evaluating temporomandibular joint syndromes, Journal of Prosthetic Dentistry **18:**497-503.
A discussion of the etiology, diagnosis, and treatment of TMJ syndromes and a survey of patients with TMJ symptoms. 18 references.

Goldstein, N. P., Gibilisco, J. A., and Rushton, J. G. 1963. Trigeminal Neuropathy and Neuritis, Journal of the American Medical Association **184:**458-462.
A clinical study and discussion of the etiology and treatment of trigeminal neuropathy and neuritis. 4 references.

Gordon, F. 1968. The telephone call from the patient in pain, Dental Assistant **37:**15.
The information to be obtained in a short time over the telephone from a patient in pain. No references.

Grainger, J. K. 1972. Perception: its meaning, significance, and control in dental procedures. I. Introduction and neurophysiological aspects, Australian Dental Journal **17:**24-30.
A consideration of the factors affecting perception and a discussion of the use of analgesics and anesthetics to modify perception. 52 references.

Greene, C. S. 1973. A survey of current professional concepts and opinions about the myofacial pain-dysfunction (MPD) syndrome, Journal of the American Dental Association **86:**128-136.
Findings from an opinion survey of physicians and dentists on existence and etiology of MPD syndrome. The findings indicate great diversity of opinions and much use of inappropriate therapies in treatment. 44 references.

Greene, C. S., Lerman, M. D., Sutcher, H. D., and Laskin, D. M. 1969. The TMJ pain-dysfunction syndrome: heterogeneity of the patient population, Journal of the American Dental Association **79:** 1168-1172.
A discussion of the diagnosis of the TMJ syndrome. Author believes TMJ patients cannot be considered a homogeneous group and cannot be treated identically despite a similar clinical appearance. 25 references.

Hardie, J. B. 1970. Premedication, Society for the Advancement of Anaesthesia in Dentistry Digest **1:** 52-55.
A summary and short analysis of various methods of premedication and anesthesia. No references.

Jacoby, J. D. 1960. Statistical report on general practice hypnodontics: tape recorded conditioning, International Journal of Clinical and Experimental Hypnosis **8:**115-119.
General statistical findings with case study examples on the practice of hypnodontics in 308 patients. 5 references.

Johnson, R., and Baldwin, D. C., Jr. 1968. Relationship of maternal anxiety to the behavior of young children undergoing dental extraction, Journal of Dental Research **47:**801-805.
A study establishing a significant relationship between the behavior of 60 children undergoing dental extraction and the anxiety level of their mothers. 13 references.

Katcher, A. H., Brightman, V., Luborsky, L., and Shep, G. 1973. Prediction of the incidence of recurrent herpes labialis and systemic illness from psychological measurements, Journal of Dental Research **52:**49-58.
A study in which approximately a third of the variance in a year's incidence of recurrent herpes labialis was predicted from psychological and sociometric variables. 23 references.

Knapp, D. E. 1968. Therapeutic control of apprehension and pain in adult dental patients, Dental Clinics of North America **2:**229-242.
Approaches for controlling apprehension and pain to improve patient attitudes regarding the dentist and dental treatment. 2 references.

Kominek, J., and Rozkovcova, E. 1966. Psychology of children's dental treatment, International Dental Journal **16:**1-29.
A discussion of children's anxieties in the dental situation and procedures for effective management. No references.

Lantz, B. 1970. Effects of placebo administration on the postoperative course of oral surgery, Swedish Dental Journal **63:**621-626.
A study of the placebo effects on 189 patients who had impacted molars surgically removed. 17 references.

Laskin, D. M. 1969. Etiology of the pain-dysfunction syndrome, Journal of the American Dental Association **79:**148-153.
Five types of experimental evidence for a psychophysiological theory of the pain-dysfunction syndrome. 35 references.

Laskin, D. M., and Greene, C. S. 1972. Influence of the doctor-patient relationship on placebo therapy for patients with myofacial pain-dysfunction (MPD) syndrome, Journal of the American Dental Association **85:**892-894.
A clinical study using a placebo drug endorsed by the dentist for patients with MPD syndrome. Findings indicate the importance and potential of the doctor-patient relationship. 6 references.

Liebman, F. M. 1972. Pain and pressure in the human pulp, Oral Surgery **33:**122-128.
A discussion supporting the gate control theory of pain as it affects pain in the pulp of human teeth. 13 references.

Lipton, D. E. 1969. Psychosomatic aspects of TMJ

dysfunction, Journal of the American Dental Dental Association **79:**131-136.
A conclusion (after review of literature and current research) that a significant relationship exists between psychological factors and nonorganic TMJ dysfunction. 14 references.

McCall, C. M., Szmyd, L., and Ritter, R. M. 1960. Personality characteristics in patients with temporomandibular joint symptoms, Journal of the American Dental Association **62:**694-696.
A study in which patients with TMJ symptoms differed significantly on a standard personality inventory from patients without TMJ symptoms. 9 references.

Mackenzie, R. S. 1968. Psychodynamics of pain, Journal of Oral Medicine **23:**75-84.
A review of variables affecting psychological perception and reaction to pain. Included are the following variables: (1) cultural, (2) personal history, (3) personality, (4) emotional, and (5) cognitive. 55 references.

McKenzie, R. E., Szmyd, L., and Hartman, B. O. 1967. A study of selected personality factors in oral surgery patients, Journal of the American Dental Association **74:**763-765.
A clinical study of selected personality factors as related to criteria of stress or difficult postoperative recovery from oral surgery. Results indicated no significant association between test scores and the established criteria. 17 references.

Molin, C., and Seeman, K. 1970. Disproportionate dental anxiety: clinical and nosological considerations, Acta Odontologica Scandinavica **28:**198-212.
Definitions and discussion of conditions causing disproportionate dental anxiety. It was found that in most patients fear was in connection with a specific form of treatment and could be managed by a considerate practitioner. 17 references.

Moulton, R. E. 1966. Emotional factors in non-organic temporomandibular joint pain, The Dental Clinics of North America **2:**609-620.
A comprehensive article on pain and anxiety, symptomatology and characteristics of TMJ symdrome, and the psychological aspects of treatment. 13 references.

Mumford, J. M. 1965. Pain perception threshold and adaptation of normal human teeth, Archives of Oral Biology **10:**957-968.
An experimental study investigating methods of raising low pain perception thesholds in human teeth via a cathodal electrode. Characteristics of the sensation were also analyzed. 17 references.

Mumford, J. M., and Newton, A. V. 1971. Convergence in the trigeminal system following stimulation of human teeth, Archives of Oral Biology **16:**1089-1098.
A study in which single teeth and groups of teeth were stimulated by square wave electrical impulses. It was found that as the size of the stimulation area increased, there was a decrease in pain threshold. 8 references.

Perry, H. T. 1968. They symptomatology of temporomandibular joint disturbance, Journal of Prosthetic Dentistry **19:**288-298.
The etiology and symptoms of TMJ syndrome, including common elements among patients and treatment procedures. 17 references.

Pollack, S. 1966. Pain control by suggestion, Journal of Oral Medicine **21:**89-95.
An experimental study to test hypotheses that suggestion from the dentist is an important element in producing a calm reaction from the patient during injection of analgesia. 12 references.

Rood, J. P. 1972. Chest pain of dental origin: a case report, British Dental Journal **33:**110.
A short case report of a 20-year-old man who experienced chest pain as a result of an infected tooth. Appropriate endodontic treatment relieved the pain. No references.

Rushton, J. G., Gibilisco, J. A., and Goldstein, N. P. 1959. Atypical face pain, Journal of the American Medical Association **171:**1331-1361.
A clinical study of 100 patients with facial pain. Conservative treatment is advised for patients with TMJ syndrome. No references.

Scott, D., Jr. 1972. Arousal and suppression of pain in the tooth, International Dental Journal **22:**20-32.
A discussion of electrical impulses recorded from human teeth and the mechanisms that give rise to painful sensations, as well as the use of analgesics. 7 references.

Shane, S. M. 1967. Intravenous amnesia to: obliterate fear, anxiety and pain in ambulatory dental patients, TIC **26:**13-16.
A clinical study assessing the effects of amnesia induced by intravenous injection. Findings support the technique and encourage wider application. 6 references.

Shane, S. M., and Kessler, S. 1967. Electricity for sedation in dentistry, Journal of the American Dental Association **75:**1369-1375.
A clinical study of 12 patients who underwent electrosedation. Results were moderately successful. 12 references.

Shoben, E. J., and Borland, L. 1954. An empirical study of the etiology of dental fears, Journal of Clinical Psychology **10:**171-174.
A comparison of fearful and nonfearful patients and a conclusion that the significant element in the etiology of dental fears is the attitude of the patient's family. The specific dental situation was not relevant. 5 references.

Soni, N. N., Thatcher, J. W., Higa, L., and Tade, W. H. 1972. Dental findings in a case of indifference-to-pain syndrome, Journal of Dentistry for Children **39:**436-439.
A case study of a young child with the indifference-to-pain syndrome. Several complications are discussed; particular reference is given to tooth eruption and abnormalities of tooth structure. 6 references.

Weiss, J. 1972. Some psychological aspects of dental pain, New York State Dental Journal **38:**32-35.
A discussion of the practitioner's need to be aware of the psychological aspects of pain. Particular reference is given to the psychological factors impinging on the orthodontic patient. 21 references.

Whinery, J. G. 1968. Examination of patients with facial pain, Journal of Oral Surgery **26:**110-113.
Suggestions for accurate diagnosis, good communication, and successful treatment of patients with facial pain. 1 reference.

Winkler, H. P. 1966. Educating the patient about pain, Dental Survey **42:**53-55.
An emphais on primary prevention and treatment to

alleviate potentially painful conditions. No references.

Zarem, P. 1966. The psychology of pain, Bulletin of Michigan State Dental Hygienists's Association **12:** 16-18.
A brief discussion of the relationship between fear and pain. Author suggests techniques for reducing fear in the dental treatment situation. 6 references.

Headache

Anderson, S. 1971. Warm hands mean a cool, quiet head, Midway, Magazine of the Topeka Capital–Journal **1**-8.
A first-person account of experience for the technique of mentally directing the flow of blood into the hands to avert migraine pain. No references.

Budzynski, T., Stoyva, J., and Adler, C. 1970. Feedback-induced muscle relaxation: application to tension headache, Journal of Behavior Therapy and Experimental Psychiatry **1:**205-211.
An account of five tension headache patients who learned to produce low frontalis EMG levels and showed subsequent reductions in tension headache activity. 12 references.

Dengrove, E. 1968. Behavior therapy of headache, Journal of the American Society of Psychosomatic Dentistry and Medicine **15:**41-48.
A discussion of various behavior therapy techniques in the treatment of headaches of psychogenic origin. 6 references.

Hobbs, H. E. 1964. Headache, Transactions of the Ophthalmological Societies of the United Kingdom **74:**637-661.
A comprehensive discussion of various causes of head pain and possible treatments. 12 references.

Lederer, F. L., Tenta, L. T., and Tardy, M. E. 1971. Otorhinolaryngologic aspects of headache and head pains, Headache **11:**19-30.
A discussion of headaches associated with visual disorders. Migraine, brain tumors, and ocular headaches and considered. No references.

Sargent, J. D., Green, E. E., and Walters, E. D. 1973. Preliminary report on the use of autogenic feedback in training in the treatment of migraine and tension headaches, Psychosomatic Medicine **35:**129-135.
The use of autogenic feedback in teaching the handwarming tehcnique. Twenty-eight migraine patients participated in the study. 13 references.

Miscellaneous grouping

Dyck, P. J., Johnson, W. J., and others. 1971. Segmental demyelination secondary to axonal degeneration in uremic neuropathy, Mayo Clinic Proceedings **46:**400-431.
A study in which thresholds of touch-pressure, temperature discriminations, and pain sensations were determined in two patients with uremic neuropathy. Metabolic failure of the neuron is postulated to be the cause. 78 references.

Flinn, D. E. 1967. Functional chest pain, Clinical Aviation and Aerospace Medicine **38:**1167-1170.
A discussion of the importance of accurate diagnosis and treatment of chest pain in aviation medicine. Various causes are considered. 8 references.

Golden, G. S. 1971. Neurologic disease of an adolescent service, American Journal of Diseases of Children **121:**24-29.
A report that neurological diseases or neurological complications of medical diseases accounted for 17% of all admissions to an adolescent service over a 2½-year period. Classifications of these cases are presented, and the implications of neurological diseases are discussed. 11 references.

Haaxma, R., Korver, M. F., and Willemse, J. 1971. Congenital indifference to pain associated with a defect in calcium metabolism Acta Neurologica Scandinavica **47:**194-208.
Case histories of two siblings with congenitial indifference to pain and disturbances of calcium metabolism. 16 references.

Haddow, J. E., Shapiro, S. R., and Gale, D. G. 1970. Congenital sensory neuropathy in siblings, Pediatrics **45:**651-655.
A discussion of two siblings with congenital sensory neuropathy. Inheritance is considered along with the factor of low cerebrospinal fluid protein levels in both siblings. 11 references.

Ham, P. 1972. Personal experience of chest pain, Medical Journal of Australia **1:**547.
A discussion of the effectiveness of different drugs for angina and hiatal hernia and the interaction of the two syndromes by an individual with both. 2 references.

Hawksley, J. C. 1972. Growing pains, British Medical Journal **3:**642.
A letter taking issue with a previous article that defined growing pain intensity as "severe enough to interrupt normal activities." He feels the definition is unsatisfactory and suggests the inclusion of emotional factors when evaluating growing pains. 6 references.

Herzberg, B. N. 1971. Body composition and premenstrual tension, Journal of Psychosomatic Research **15:**251-257.
A study in which the prevalence of certain premenstrual symptoms was assessed in a group of 113 nuns. Severe depressive symptoms occurred less frequently in the nuns than in a group of single British women. 16 references.

Hyslop, R. S. 1972. Some thoughts on pelvic pain, Australian and New Zealand Journal of Obstetrics and Gynecology **12:**40-42.
A description of the pelvic congestion syndrome and suggestions for treatment. No references.

James, J. L., and Miles, D. W. 1966. Neuralgic amyotraphy: a clinical and electromyographic study, British Medical Journal **2:**1042-1043.
A clinical and electromyographic report of 38 patients with neurologic amyotrophy. The etiology is unknown, and the study reveals nothing unusual in the population examined. 15 references.

Kane, F. J., Downie, A. W., Marcotte, D. B., and Perez-Reyes, M. 1968. A case of congenital indifference to pain, Diseases of the Nervous System **29:** 409-412.
A psychiatric and neurological evaluation of one patient with congenital indifference to pain. The personality pattern deviated from other reported cases. 8 references.

Knoblock, V. 1971. Influence of parturient's personality on the pain during labor, Ceskoslovenska Gynekologie (English Abstract) **36:**153-155.
A psychological evaluation of 70 primigravidae during the tenth month of pregnancy and during labor. No relationship was observed between such

characteristics as neuroticism, extraversion, introversion, masculinity, and feminity and the women's report of pain intensity. No references.

Krzeminska, P. M. 1971. Diagnosis of coronary pain in the young, Przegland Lekarski (English Abstract) **27:**465-467.
An analysis of the symptoms in the course of coronary disease in 90 patients who had had cardiac infarction before age 45. No references.

Lowell, R. R. H., and Verghese, A. 1967. Personality traits associated with different chest pains after myocardial infarction, British Medical Journal **3:** 327-330.
A study in which 97 men who had had a myocardial infarction were classified according to their subsequent experience of chest pain. Personality traits were measured. Neuroticism was correlated with some types of chest pain. 28 references.

Mills, W. G. 1971. Pelvic pain, British Medical Journal **1:**385-387.
A discussion of pelvic pain as a symptom among women and a consideration of various specific causes. No references.

Oster, J. 1972. Growing pain, a symptom and its significance, Danish Medical Bulletin **19:**72-79.
A review of the literature on growing pains and a history of its hypothesized causes and correlates. 40 references.

Oster, J. 1972. Recurrent abdominal pain, headache and limb pains in children and adolescents, Pediatrics **50:**429-436.
An 8-year longitudinal study of the prevalence of recurrent abdominal pain, headache, and limb pains in a nonselected population of school children. All types of pain showed a declining frequency with approaching adulthood. 34 references.

Oster, J., and Nielsen, A. **1972.** Growing pains: a clinical investigation of a school population, Acta Paediatrica Scandinavica **61:**329-334.
A study of growing pains in 2178 children. The symptom complex appears to be a clinically well-defined one that may belong to a special emotional familial pattern. 10 references.

Payten, R. J. 1972. Facial pain as the first symptom in acoustis neuroma, Journal of Laryngology and Otology **86:**523-534.
Records of two patients with acoustic neuromas in which pressure on the sensory root of the trigeminal nerve resulted in development of facial pain before the onset of any otological symptoms. 15 references.

Smith, T. R. 1972. The thalamic pain syndrome, Minnesota Medicine **55:**257-261.
A consideration of the sensory and motor physiological aspects of the thalamic pain syndrome, as well as the treatment. 13 references.

Tremble, G. E. 1965. Referred pain in the ear, Archives of Otolaryngology. **81:**57-63.
A discussion of the etiology of ear pain and its classification according to intrinsic or extrinsic causation. 14 references.

Warren, S. E. 1972. The painful arm: evaluation and treatment of vascular causes, Angiology **23:**392: 400.
A discussion of the causes and treatments for arm pain. 15 references.

Preparation for surgery and postoperative pain

Abram, H. S., and Gill, B. F. 1961. Predictions of postoperative psychiatric complications, New England Journal of Medicine **265:**1123-1128.
Predictions of patients' postoperative psychological course from preoperative interview data. Parameters were marital adjustment, health, SES, and so on. 14 references.

Bellville, J. W., Forrest, Jr., W. H., Miller, E., and Brown, B. W., Jr. 1971. Influence of age on pain relief from analgesics—a study of postoperative patients, Journal of the American Medical Association **217:**1835-1841.
A study of 712 patients who received analgesics for postoperative pain, to determine possible correlations between pain relief and patient characteristics. Age proved to be the most stable indicator, suggesting that dosages should be determined by age rather than size. 16 references.

Bird, B. 1955. Psychological aspects of preoperative and postoperative care, American Journal of Nursing **55:**685-687.
An article stressing the need for nurses to accept the responsibility for keeping communication lines open between the medical staff and the patient. No references.

Boyar, J. I., and Gramlech, E. P. 1970. Unusual post-surgical pain, Surgical Clinics of North America **50:** 309-318.
A review of the literature and a discussion of intense postoperative pain as a syndrome to be treated medically and psychologically. 28 references.

Brown, W. A. 1968. Post amputation phantom limb pain, Diseases of the Nervous System **29:**301-306.
An investigation of 52 subjects with postamputation phantom limb pain, regarding circumstances of amputation, site of amputation, procedure of amputation, and description of phantom limb pain. There were many more upper-extremity amputations than lower-extremity amputations. 23 references.

Bruegel, M. A. 1971. Relationship of preoperative anxiety to perception of postoperative pain, Nursing Research **20:**26-31.
A study of anxiety, other psychological variables, and surgical variables as influences on patients' perceptions of postoperative pain. Only marital status, occupation, and surgical variables were found to have significant influences. 31 references.

Bursten, B., and Russ, J. J. 1965. Preoperative psychological state and corticosteroid levels of surgical patients, Psychosomatic Medicine **27:**309-316.
A study of correlations between the anxiety levels and plasma cortiocosteriod levels of ten patients undergoing surgery. A positive correlation was found between the two measures. No references.

Carnevali, D. L. 1966. Preoperative anxiety, American Journal of Nursing **66:**1536-1538.
An informal study of how accurately nurses perceive patients' fears. 3 references.

Corman, H. H., Hornick, E. J., Kritchman, M., and Terestman, N. 1958. Emotional reactions of surgical patients to hospitalization, anesthesia, and surgery, American Journal of Surgery **96:**646-653.
A series of case studies illustrating various psychological reactions to surgery. 10 references.

Cummings, G. S., and Girling, J. 1971. A clinical assessment of immediate postoperative fitting of pros-

thesis for amputee rehabilitation, Physical Therapy **51:**1007-1011.
A study in which 23 patients were fitted with immediate postoperative prostheses following lower-extremity amputations. This method was found to have several advantages over the conventional method. 6 references.

Dalrymple, D. G., Parbrook, G. D., and Steel, D. F. 1972. The effect of personality on postoperative pain and vital capacity impairment, British Journal of Anaesthesiology **44:**902.
A study of 50 women undergoing surgery, to assess the relationship between personality and postoperative factors. Several strong correlations were observed. 3 references.

Dalrymple, D. G., Parbrook, G. D., and Steel, D. F. 1973. Factors predisposing to postoperative pain and pulmonary complications, British Journal of Anaesthesia **45:**589-598.
A study of 50 women, in which significant relationships were found between preoperative neuroticism scores and postoperative vital capacity impairments and chest complications. 17 references.

Egbert, L. D., Battit, G. E., Turndorf, H., and Beecher, H. K. 1963. The value of the preoperative visit by an anesthetist, Journal of the American Medical Association **185:**553-555.
A comparison of the psychological effect of the preoperative visit by an anesthetist with the effect of pentabarbital for preanesthetic medication. The preoperative visit had a more calming effect on the patients. 4 references.

Egbert, L. D., Battit, G. E., Welch, C. E., and Bartlett, M. K. 1964. Reduction of postoperative pain by encouragement and instruction of patients, New England Journal of Medicine **270:**825-827.
A study in which 97 experimental patients were given encouragement and education both preoperatively and postoperatively. In comparison with a control sample, they required less postoperative analgesia and were discharged from the hospital earlier. 8 references.

Jeffries, M. 1970. Postoperative analgesia, The American Surgeon **36:**296-302.
A discussion and evaluation of various types of postoperative analgesics. Authors recommend better evaluation of circumstances rather than routine prescription of narcotics. 25 references.

Johnson, B. A., Johnson, J. E., and Dumas, R. G. 1970. Research in nursing practice: the problem of uncontrolled situational variables, Nursing Research **19:**337-342.
A clinical study investigating relationships of the type of surgery, duration of anesthesia, and race to postoperative recovery. Several significant correlations were revealed. 9 references.

Gildea, J. 1968. The relief of postoperative pain, Medical Clinics of North America **52:**81-90.
A discussion of postoperative pain and various methods, both past and present, used to control it. 35 references.

Hewitt, P. B. 1970. Subjective follow-up of patients from a surgical intensive therapy ward, British Medical Journal **4:**669-673.
A study in which 100 consecutive patients on an intensive therapy ward completed forms regarding impressions of their experience. Most patients were not unduly worried and were satisfied with the care they received. 17 references.

Loan, W. B., and Morrison, J. D. 1967. The incidence and severity of postoperative pain, British Journal of Anaesthesia **39:**695-698.
A reveiw of postoperative pain and relevant correlates. 31 references.

McBride, M. A. B. 1967. Nursing approach, pain and relief: an exploratory experiment, Nursing Research **16:**337-341.
A study, using an experimental design, of three nursing approaches to the relief of surgical pain. Results indicate that a psychosomatic view of pain is a most effective approach. 27 references.

Melzack, R. 1971. Phantom limb pain: implications for treatment of pathologic pain, Anesthesiology **35:**409-419.
A theoretical hypothesis, supported by clinical evidence, of the cause and physiology of phantom limb pain. 49 references.

Moss, F. T., and Meyer, B. 1966. The effects of nursing interaction upon pain relief in patients, Nursing Research **15:**303-306.
An article on the capability of nurses to provide care that effectively reduces or relieves a patient's pain without the use of analgesics. 17 references.

Paddock, R., Beer, G., Bellville, J. W., Ciliberti, B. J., Forrest, W. H., and Miller, E. V. 1969. Analgesic and side effects of pentazocine and morphine in a large population of postoperative patients, Clinical Pharmacology and Therapeutics **10:**355-365.
A comparison of the analgesic and side effects of pentazocine with those of morphine in 1,074 surgical patients. 12 references.

Pilowsky, I., and Kaufman, A. 1965. An experimental study of atypical phantom pain, British Journal of Psychiatry **111:**1185-1187.
One case study of phantom limb pain to illustrate psychological correlates. The TAT was used to determine what factors precipitated the pain. 7 references.

Quimby, C. W., Jr. 1968. Preoperative prophylaxis of postoperative pain, Medical Clinics of North America **52:**73-80.
A discussion of the psychological impact of surgery and various techniques used to support the patient both preoperatively and postoperatively. 22 references.

Wolfer, J. A., and Davis, C. E. 1970. Assessment of surgical patients' preoperative emotional condition and postoperative welfare Nursing Research **19:**402-414.
A preliminary study to test the effects of preoperative psychological preparation on the postoperative recovery of 76 female and 70 male patients. 40 references.

Psychiatry

Albronda, H. F. 1957. Psychologic aspects of pain, California Medicine **86:**296-298.
A consideration of clinical pain as a syndrome with both psychic and somatic elements. Guidelines for evaluating pain are suggested. 15 references.

Apley, J. 1971. Their question to us, Clinical Pediatrics **10:**135-137.
A compelling article advocating the union of pediatrics and child psychiatry. 7 references.

Bothe, A., and Galdston, R. 1972. The child's loss of consciousness: a psychiatric view of pediatric anesthesia, Pediatrics **50:**252-263.
A clinical study of 50 pediatric patients receiving general anesthesia, to assess how children experience and conceptualize induced unconsciousness. Techniques to minimize psychological stress were observed and analyzed. Theoretical implications are considered. 27 references.

Caston, J., Cooper, L., and Paley, H. W. 1970. Psychological comparison of patients with cardiac neurotic chest pain and angina pectoris, Psychosomatics **11:**543-550.
A clinical study in which patients with cardiac neurotic chest pain were compared with and found to be psychologically similar to patients with angina pectoris. Specific reference is made to hyperventilation. 37 references.

Cheek, D. B. 1965. Emotional factors in persistent pain states, American Journal of Clinical Hypnosis **8:**100-110.
A discussion of factors initiating, reinforcing, and continuing an exaggerated awareness for discomfort, and methods of treatment. 12 references.

Cheek, D. B. 1966. Therapy of persistent pain states. 1. Neck and shoulder pain of five years' duration, American Journal of Clinical Hypnosis **8:**281-286.
One detailed case study of chronic pain following an accident. Psychotherapy eventually relieved all symptoms. 4 references

Clark, D. S.: 1965. Psychosomatic implications of obsessive-compulsive disorders and their resemblance to certain types of central pain, Guy Hospital Report **114:**209-222.
Author's hypothesis and clinical cases to support it. A discussion of other theories is included. 17 references.

Devine, R., and Merskey, H. 1965. The description of pain in psychiatric and general medical patients, Journal of Psychosomatic Research **9:**311-316.
A clinical study comparing psychiatric patients who had persistent pain with medical outpatients.

Farnsworth, D. L. 1956. Pain and the individual, The New England Journal of Medicine **254:**559-562.
Some aspects of the interaction between pain and the individual. Author urges physicians to be sensitive to the suffering of patients as well as to specific inquiries or illnesses. 5 references.

Fisher, A. L. 1970. A psychobiologic reconsideration of pain, Headache **9:**74-86.
Clinical facts and observations that seem to have a vital bearing on the problem of functional pain and its probable psychological significance. 8 references.

Hill, O. W. 1968. Psychogenic vomiting, Gut **9:**348-352.
A comparison of a group of patients suffering from psychogenic vomiting with a group having psychogenic abdominal pain without vomiting. It was found that the first group tended to be involved in hostile familial relationships. Treatments are discussed. No references.

Hirschfeld, A. H., and Behan, R. C. 1966. The accident process, Journal of the American Medical Association **197:**85-89.
A clinical study of 200 workers who were disabled following an injury. The prodromal state during which the worker predicted and prepared for the accident and later used the disability to justify his depression or maladjustment is discussed.

Hopwood, M. 1965-1966. A case of severe psychogenic pain, Guy Hospital Reports **114-115:**325-327.
A case study of a man with long-standing pain in the leg. The pain was so severe that amputation was contemplated. He was eventually completely relieved by psychiatric treatment. No references.

Joffee, W. B., and Sandler, J. 1965. Note on pain, depression, and individuation, Psychoanalytic Study of the Child **20:**394-424.
A psychoanalytically oriented discussion of several authors' views on depression and individuation. 10 references.

Kane, E. M., Nutter, R. W., and Weckowicz, T. E. 1971. Response to cutaneous pain in mental hospital patients, Journal of Abnormal Psychology **77:**52-60.
A study in which process schizophrenics, reactive schizophrenics, nonschizophrenics, and normal subjects were tested for warmth threshold, pain threshold, and pain tolerance. Results indicate that chronic institutionalized psychiatric patients display weaker reactions to potentially harmful stimuli. 43 references.

Kolb, L. C. 1956. Pain as a biosocial phenomenon, Connecticut State Medical Journal **20:**116-123.
An explanation of the familial and cultural influences that determine individual reaction to pain and their application in facilitating the patient-physician relationship. Specific reference is made to phantom limb pain. No references.

Kollar, E. J. 1966. Psychology of the acutely sick and injured, International Psychiatry Clinics **3:**83-91.
A discussion of various aspects of the acutely ill patient, including the role of psychological regression, the role of denial, and the clinical management of pain. No references.

Kurland, H. D., and Hammer, M. 1968. Emotional evaluation of medical patients, Archives of General Psychiatry **19:**72-78.
A clinical study using the MMPI and CICMI to identify and quantify neurotic behavior in medical patients. The pros and cons of using computer-analyzed psychological tests in the medical field are discussed. 7 references.

Marshall W. 1970. The psychology of being hurt, Journal of the Louisiana State Medical Society **122:**180-184.
A brief introduction to the immunological approach to psychology and psychiatry. 5 references.

Merskey, H. 1965. The characteristics of persistent pain in psychological illness, Journal of Psychosomatic Research **9:**291-298.
Results of clinical examinations of patients in whom pain was a persistent, prominent complaint. These patients tended to be older and were responsive to psychiatric treatment. 27 references.

Merskey, H. 1965. Psychiatric patients with persistent pain, Journal of Psychomatic Research **9:**299-309.
A clinical study comparing psychiatric patients who had pain with those who did not have pain. Parameters were family size, birth order, SES, marital status, and so on. Results show that pain is more prevalent in a specific type of patient. 44 references.

Merskey, H. 1966. Pain and the psychiatrist, British Journal of Psychiatry. **112:**637-638.

A letter in which author defends his definition of pain. 10 references.

Merskey, H. 1972. Personality traits of psychiatric patients with pain, Journal of Psychosomatic Research **16:**163-166.
Scores on the Maudsley Personality Inventory for normal subjects and for psychiatric patients with or without pain. Findings contrast with earlier studies. 8 references.

Pilling, L. F., Brannick, T. L., and Swenson, W. M. 1967. Psychologic characteristics of psychiatric patients having pain as a presenting symptom, Canadian Medical Association Journal **97:**387;394.
A clinical study designed to identify psychological and social correlates in patients with psychogenic pain. Results concur with those of other studies, and author concludes that pain is often a cover for other symptoms of emotional conflicts. 11 references.

Raney, J. O. 1970. Pain, emotion and a rationale for therapy, Northwest Medicine **69:**659-661.
Five case studies dealing with chronic pain. Pain is discussed as a conversion symptom. 5 references.

Rangell, L. 1953. Psychiatric aspects of pain, Psychosomatic Medicine **15:**22-37.
An examination of the reciprocal interaction between symptomatic pain and emotional factors. Therapeutic approaches to symptomatic pain and emotional involvement are discussed. 27 references.

Riemer, M. D. 1967. Disability determinations of disorders based on emotional factors, Industrial Medicine and Surgery **36:**347-351.
An outline, discussion, and comparison of three categories of disabilities based on emotional disturbances: (1) inertia, (2) hypochondriasis, and (3) pain. 2 references.

Rose, A. R. 1970. Anxiety and pain, Medical Trial Technique Quarterly **17:**147-155.
A discussion of the multiple aspects of the pain experience. Emphasis is on the interaction between pain and anxiety. Several illustrative cases are reported. No references.

Schoenberg, B., and Senescu, R. 1966. Group psychotherapy for patients with chronic multiple somatic complaints, Journal of Chronic Diseases **19:**649-657.
A clinical study of women with chronic multiple somatic complaints. Group psychotherapy was provided for 18 months. The technique was evaluated and compared with other alternatives. 22 references.

Sgarlato, T. E., and Ginsburg, A. 1970. Psychic pain, a case report, Journal of the American Podiatry Association **60:**247-248.
A case study of a woman suffering from burning sensations in both feet. Her condition was eventually diagnosed as a psychoneurotic conversion reaction. No references.

Spear, F. G. 1967. Pain in psychiatric patients, Journal of Psychosomatic Research **11:**187-193.
A clinical study designed to investigate and summarize the work of several authors on complaints of localized pains in psychiatric patients. 14 references.

Szasz, T. S. 1955. The nature of pain, Archives of Neurology and Psychiatry **74:**174-181.
An examination of the nature of pain, based on clinical observations and on a consideration of philosophical, semantic, and psychiatric knowledge. 6 references.

Tinling, D. C., and Klein, R. F. 1966. Psychogenic pain and aggression: the syndrome of the solitary hunter, Psychosomatic Medicine **28:**738-748.
An analysis of a cluster of factors appearing in common among a sample of men with psychogenic pain. Pain is discussed in relationship to aggression, and some recommendations concerning treatment are offered. 5 references.

Waldman, R. D. 1968. Pain as fiction: a perspective on psychotherapy and responsibility, American Journal of Psychotherapy **22:**481-490.
A philosophical discussion of pain as a means and an end, in contrast to the medical model of pain based on physical events. The examples used are the hysteric and the malingerer. 9 references.

Weinberg, S. 1970. Suicidal intent in adolescence: a hypothesis about the role of physical illness, The Journal of Pediatrics **77:**579-586.
An exploration of the relationship between suicidal tendencies and illness. Thirteen case studies are reported, and a sex difference hypothesis is proposed. 6 references.

Wilson, W. P., and Nashold, B. S., Jr. 1967. Psychiatric considerations of certain neurological diseases treated neurosurgically, International Psychiatry Clinics **4:**189-204.
A discussion of the psychiatric implications of various categories of disease, including dyskinesias, pain itself, and epilepsy. A section on problems resulting from surgery is included. 22 references.

Wilson, W. P., and Nashold, B. S., Jr. 1970. Pain and emotion, Postgraduate Medicine **47:**183-187.
The thesis that an emotion of pain exists. Authors describe some of the more common emotional concomitants of pain. 21 references.